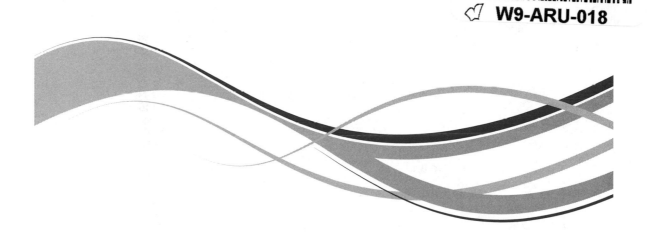

PHARMACY CERTIFIED
TECHNICIAN

Training Manual

EDITORS

Leah M. Godzina, B.A.
Dianne E. Miller, R.Ph.
Derek J. Quinn, Pharm.D.

TWELFTH EDITION

Michigan Pharmacists Association
408 Kalamazoo Plaza, Lansing, MI 48933
MichiganPharmacists.org

The Pharmacy Certified Technician Training Manual was developed by
Michigan Pharmacists Association.

The authors and publisher have made a conscientious effort to ensure that the drug information and
recommendations in this book are accurate and in accord with accepted standards at the time of
publication. However, pharmacology is a rapidly changing science, so readers are advised to check
package inserts provided by the manufacturer for the recommended dose, contraindications for administration, and added warnings and precautions. This recommendation is particularly important for
new, infrequently used or highly toxic drugs. The drugs referenced in this publication are included
strictly for teaching purposes and do not constitute an endorsement of the products.

CPhT™ is a federally registered trademark of the Pharmacy Technician Certification Board (PTCB®).
This book is in no way authorized by PTCB®.

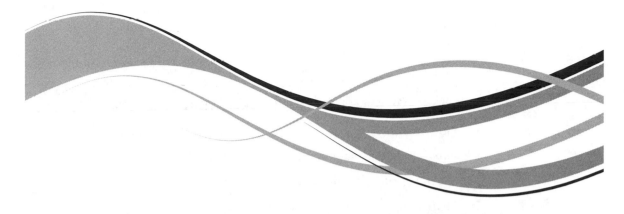

TABLE OF CONTENTS

About the Authors vi

Acknowledgements xiv

Associations and Organizations xvii

Introduction xxviii

PHARMACY PRACTICE

1 Introduction to Pharmacy Technician Practice 1

2 Pharmacy Terminology 15

PRACTICE AREAS

3 Community Pharmacy Practice 37

4 Third Party Insurance Issues 61

5 Pharmacy Compounding 83

6 Health-System Pharmacy Practice 97

7 Aseptic Technique and Sterile Product Preparation 111

8 Consultant and Long-term Care Pharmacy Practice 149

9 Medical Equipment 161

PRACTICE ESSENTIALS

10 Patient and Medication Safety... 175

11 Law and Ethics for Pharmacy Technicians............................. 197

12 Pharmacy Operations and Administration.............................. 221

13 Emergency Preparedness 243

14 Immunizations 259

15 Poisonings and Emergency Medicine....................................... 277

HUMAN SYSTEMS AND PHARMACY INTERVENTION

16 How Drugs Work 287

17 Drugs and Drug Names 299

18 Vitamins and Minerals 313

19 Herbal Supplements 333

20 Brain 349

21 Psychiatric Disorders 365

22 Central and Peripheral Nervous System 399

23 Cardiovascular System 425

24 Upper Respiratory System 449

25 Lower Respiratory System 465

26 Digestive System 487

27 Hepatic System 505

28 Reproductive System 525

29 Urinary System 553

30 Renal System 567

31 Endocrine System 583

32 Blood 605

33 Immune System 631

34 Musculoskeletal System 651

35 Skin 669

36 Cancer 689

Index 711

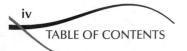

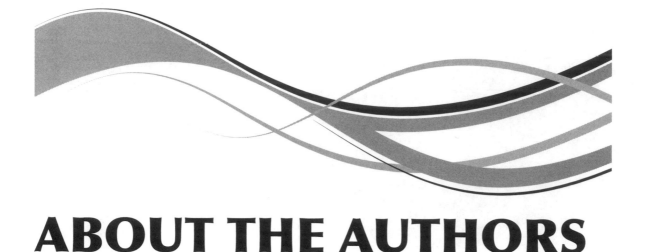

ABOUT THE AUTHORS

■ **Jessica M. Bessner, Pharm.D.,** received her Doctor of Pharmacy degree in 2006 from Ferris State University College of Pharmacy in Big Rapids, Mich. She is currently the director of pharmacy of Aspirus Keweenaw Hospital in Laurium, Mich. *(Author of Chapter 30: Renal System)*

■ **Andrew E. Britton, MBA, R.Ph.,** is a staff pharmacist for Professional Village Pharmacies, Inc. in Monroe, Mich. He received a Bachelor of Science degree from Wayne State University (WSU) in 2001, as well as a Master of Business Administration degree from Davenport University in 2004. Britton served on the Michigan Pharmacists Association Professional Affairs Committee for more than six years, and was the vice president of professional affairs for the WSU chapter of student pharmacists. He is also a former Board member for Wayne County Pharmacists Association. *(Author of Chapter 29: Urinary System)*

■ **Mary E. Burkhardt, M.S., R.Ph., FASHP,** is an independent medication safety consultant from Belleville, Mich. She is presently a contract consultant for the Institute for Safe Medication Practices and the Purdue Center for Medication Safety Advancement, as well as a contingent medication safety consultant for the Karmanos Cancer Center in Detroit, Mich. She is also adjunct faculty at Ferris State University. Burkhardt formerly worked as the director of medication safety at Medco Health Solutions, and as pharmacist program manager for the Department of Veterans Affairs National Center for Patient Safety. She graduated from Wayne State University (WSU) Eugene Applebaum College of Pharmacy and Health Sciences with a Bachelor of Science degree in pharmacy and a Master of Science degree in hospital pharmacy administration. A fellow of the American Society of Health-System Pharmacists (ASHP), she completed a generalized ASHP residency at the Detroit Medical Center. She was named Pharmacist of the Year twice (once from the Michigan Society of Health-System Pharmacists in 1994 and again in 2001 from the Michigan Pharmacists Association); and in 2004, she received the WSU Alumnus of the Year Award from the WSU Alumni Association. *(Author of Chapter 10: Patient and Medication Safety)*

■ **Hannah M. Bursiek, Pharm.D.,** is a pharmacy practice resident at St. John Hospital and Medical Center in Detroit. She graduated from Ohio Northern University Rabbe College of Pharmacy in 2010 with a Doctor of Pharmacy degree. *(Author of Chapter 22: Central and Peripheral Nervous System)*

- **Paul W. Bush, Pharm.D., MBA,** is the chief pharmacy officer for Duke University Hospital in Durham, N.C. and program director for Duke's health system pharmacy administration residency. He previously served as director of pharmacy services for the Medical University of South Carolina Medical Center, a position he held from 1999-2009. He also previously served as faculty at Wayne State University (1984-1999). Bush is a past treasurer of Michigan Pharmacists Association and member of the Michigan Society of Health-System Pharmacists Board of Directors. He is also a past chair of the American Society of Health-System Pharmacists Section of Pharmacy Practice Managers. *(Author of Chapter 12: Pharmacy Operations and Administration)*

- **Allen R. Doan, Pharm.D., ARRT,** received his Bachelor of Science degree in nuclear medicine technology and his Doctor of Pharmacy degree from Ferris State University (FSU) in Big Rapids, Mich. Doan is currently the pharmacy director at Hot Shots Nuclear Medicine in Lansing, Mich. He also holds an adjunct clinical faculty position with FSU. His research interests include radio-pharmaceutical preparation stability, quality control and aseptic compounding of radio-pharmaceuticals. He has extensive experience providing clinical training to pharmacists, nuclear medicine technologists, physicians and technical staff in commercial radiopharmacy, preparation of compounded sterile preparations in a hospital setting and compounding of immediate use radiopharmaceuticals in a hospital setting. *(Author of Chapter 7: Aseptic Technique and Sterile Product Preparation)*

- **Jodie L. Elder, Pharm.D., BCPS,** received her Doctor of Pharmacy degree in 2001 from Ferris State University (FSU) in Big Rapids, Mich. She completed a community pharmacy residency, co-sponsored by Meijer Pharmacy, FSU and Pfizer, in 2002. Elder is currently an assistant professor of pharmacy practice at FSU College of Pharmacy. *(Author of Chapter 35: Skin)*

- **Stephanie L. Freed, Pharm.D.,** is a pharmacy practice resident at Diplomat Specialty Pharmacy in Flint. She earned her Doctor of Pharmacy degree from Ferris State University (FSU) College of Pharmacy in 2011. In 2009, she was inducted into Rho Chi for academic excellence. Freed was also a recipient of the Doctor of Pharmacy Scholarship, which is a four-year scholarship given to select College of Pharmacy students. She is currently a Board member of the Genesee County Pharmacists Association, and has worked in the community pharmacy setting for more than eight years. *(Author of Chapter 24: Upper Respiratory System)*

- **Victoria A. Gates, Pharm.D.,** is a pharmacist at Sparrow Health System in Lansing, Mich. She graduated with a Doctor of Pharmacy degree from the Raabe College of Pharmacy of Ohio Northern University, along with the Honors College, in 2009. After graduation, she completed a PGY-1 at Sparrow Health System in 2010. During her residency, Gates was an adjunct faculty member at Ferris State University. *(Author of Chapter 22: Central and Peripheral Nervous System)*

- **Leah M. Godzina, B.A.,** is the director of communications at Michigan Pharmacists Association. She received a Bachelor of Arts degree in journalism from Michigan State University in 2007, with a concentration in publication design. In her role at MPA, Godzina manages all publications, including *Michigan Pharmacist* journal, the Michigan Society of Health-System Pharmacist (MSHP) newsletter (the *MSHP Monitor*) and *e-news weekly*. She also manages the Association Web site, MichiganPharmacists.org; social media; advertising sales; photography and videography; and other communication efforts. Prior to serving as director of communications, Godzina was the MPA Communications Assistant, and also worked at a media software company. *(Editor)*

■ **Andrea D. Goodrich, Pharm.D., BCPS**, works at Saint Mary's Hospital in Grand Rapids, Mich., where she is a clinical pharmacist in the area of orthopedics, a residency preceptor and an adjunct faculty member for Ferris State University (FSU). She graduated with her Bachelor of Science degree in pharmacy from FSU and completed her Doctor of Pharmacy degree at Midwestern University in Chicago. *(Author of Chapter 18: Vitamins and Minerals)*

■ **Jennifer K. Hagerman, Pharm.D., AE-C**, is the director of education for Diplomat Specialty Pharmacy. Previously, she was a faculty member at Ferris State University (FSU) College of Pharmacy for six years, first as an assistant professor, then becoming an associate professor in 2008. She has also been a course coordinator and lecturer at the University of Michigan-Flint for several years. Hagerman continues to serve as an adjunct professor at FSU. She received her Doctor of Pharmacy degree from FSU in 2003 and completed her pharmacy practice residency at Borgess Medical Center in 2004. Hagerman has also served as a member of the Michigan Pharmacists Association Executive Board. *(Author of Chapter 24: Upper Respiratory System)*

■ **Douglas L. Jennings, Pharm.D., BCPS (AQ Cardiology)**, is a clinical pharmacy specialist in the cardiovascular intensive care unit (ICU) at Henry Ford Hospital in Detroit, Mich. He provides daily pharmaceutical care to patients in the cardiac ICU, cardiothoracic ICU and advanced heart failure/ventricular assist device teams. He is also adjunct faculty in the Department of Pharmacy Practice at Wayne State University (WSU) Eugene Applebaum College of Pharmacy and Health Sciences. Jennings received his Doctor of Pharmacy degree from WSU in 2005. *(Author of Chapter 23: Cardiovascular System)*

■ **David W. Kaiser, Pharm.D.**, is the director of pharmacy for Forest View Hospital in Grand Rapids, Mich. He also serves as the program chair for pharmacy technology for Baker College of Muskegon, Mich., and is an adjunct professor in the physician assistant program at Grand Valley State University. Kaiser received his Bachelor of Science in pharmacy from Ferris State University and his Doctor of Pharmacy degree from the University of Florida. *(Author of Chapter 21: Psychiatric Disorders)*

■ **Pramodini B. Kale-Pradhan, Pharm.D.**, received her Bachelor of Science degree in pharmacy from the University of Wisconsin-Madison College of Pharmacy in 1981 and her Doctor of Pharmacy degree from the Philadelphia College of Pharmacy and Science in Philadelphia, Penn., in 1989. Kale-Pradhan completed an advanced residency in infectious diseases and surgery at the University of Illinois at Chicago (UIC) College of Pharmacy in 1990 and became a Fellow in Infectious Diseases and Surgery from that institution in 1991. Presently, she is an associate professor of pharmacy practice at Wayne State University (WSU) Eugene Applebaum College of Pharmacy and Health Sciences in Detroit, Mich. Her previous experience includes serving as a clinical pharmacist in the infectious diseases and dapsone clinics at UIC. Kale-Pradhan has delivered several presentations on topics related to the gastrointestinal system. She was the recipient of the 1998 and 2001 Hoffman LaRoche Hospital Preceptor of the Year Award and the 1992-1993 and 2000 Southeastern Michigan Society of Hospital Pharmacists Preceptor of the Year Award. Additionally, she received the WSU College of Pharmacy Excellence in Teaching Award in 2001. *(Author of Chapter 26: Digestive System)*

■ **Sister Phyllis Klonowski, Pharm.D.**, is a pharmacist at the Caro Center in Caro, Mich. She is also the founder and pharmacy director of Community Prescription Support Program, an organization that serves needy populations, such as the elderly, mental health patients and the working poor. In that capacity, she helps provide necessary medications, in addition to supporting efforts to obtain federal financial assistance for these patients. She is a graduate of Ferris State University College of Pharmacy with a Bachelor of Science degree in pharmacy. She received her Master of Science degree in clinical pharmacy from Purdue University. Prior to her current position, she was a clinical pharmacist consultant and worked in several positions in health-system pharmacy. *(Author of Chapter 20: Brain)*

■ **Renee R. Koski, Pharm.D., CACP**, received her Bachelor of Science degree in pharmacy in 1995 and her Doctor of Pharmacy degree in 1998 from Ferris State University (FSU) in Big Rapids, Mich. She then completed a general pharmacy practice residency at Bronson Methodist Hospital in Kalamazoo, Mich. Koski is currently professor of pharmacy practice with the FSU College of Pharmacy. She precepts fourth-year student pharmacists in ambulatory care and internal medicine at Marquette General Health System in Marquette, Mich. She also teaches pharmacotherapeutics and practice skills lab courses to third-year students. *(Author of Chapter 32: Blood)*

■ **Cherry Kwong, Pharm.D.**, received her Doctor of Pharmacy degree from Ferris State University. She is currently an infusion pharmacist at Metro Health Cancer Center in Wyoming, Mich. *(Author of Chapter 15: Poisonings and Emergency Medicine)*

■ **Claire T. Lee, Pharm.D.**, graduated in 2011 with a Doctor of Pharmacy degree from Wayne State University Eugene Applebaum College of Pharmacy and Health Sciences in Detroit, Mich. She was a member of the American Pharmacists Association student affairs policy standing committee, and has been an active leader in advocacy efforts among her peers, receiving national recognition for her involvement. She is currently practicing at Target Pharmacy. *(Author of Chapter 34: Musculoskeletal System)*

■ **Jean C. Lee, Pharm.D., BCPS, AAHIVE**, works as a clinical pharmacist in HIV medicine at Saint Mary's Health Care in Grand Rapids, Mich. She graduated with her Bachelor of Science degree in pharmacy in 1994 from Memorial University of Newfoundland and subsequently completed her residency program at The Hospital for Sick Children in Toronto. After completing her Doctor of Pharmacy degree at Ferris State University (FSU) in 2001, she began work in the area of HIV medicine in one of the largest HIV clinics in Michigan and works as a consultant to the HIV Continuum of Care Unit at the Michigan Department of Community Health. She is also an adjunct assistant clinical professor for the HIV Medicine Clerkship rotation with FSU. *(Author of Chapter 19: Herbal Supplements)*

■ **James M. Lile, Pharm.D.**, received his Bachelor of Science and Doctor of Pharmacy degrees from Purdue University and completed a clinical pharmacokinetic residency at Saint Joseph Hospital in Omaha, Neb. Lile is currently clinical pharmacy manager at St. Mary's of Michigan in Saginaw, Mich. He has been on the Board of Directors and served as president of the Michigan Society of Health-System Pharmacists. *(Author of Chapter 6: Health-System Pharmacy Practice)*

■ **Tracey L. Mersfelder, Pharm.D., BCPS**, received her Bachelor of Science and Doctor of Pharmacy degrees from the University of Cincinnati College of Pharmacy. She then attended the Medical University of South Carolina to complete general and specialized residencies. Currently, Mersfelder is an associate professor for Ferris State University, where she specializes in adult internal medicine. She is also a clinical preceptor for Borgess Medical Center. *(Author of Chapter 25: Lower Respiratory System)*

- **Dianne E. Miller, R.Ph.**, received her Bachelor of Science degrees in pharmacy and applied biology in 1987 from Ferris State University in Big Rapids, Mich. She has completed a variety of certificate courses and post-graduate training, including the University of Pittsburgh's Smoking Cessation Specialist Certification Program, the National Institute for Pharmacists Outcomes Osteoporosis Care Certificate Program, University of Tennessee's Asthma Patient Management Certification Program and American Pharmacists Association's Pharmacy-Based Immunization Delivery certificate course. Miller is the chief operations officer of Michigan Pharmacists Association and Pharmacy Services Inc. in Lansing, Mich. In addition, Miller served as the co-owner of an independent pharmacy in Grand Ledge, Mich. Prior to joining the staff at the Association, she was a staff pharmacist at Ingham Regional Medical Center in Lansing, Mich. *(Editor; Author of Chapter 12: Pharmacy Operations and Administration, and Chapter 28: Reproductive System)*

- **Jacqueline A. Morse, Pharm.D., BCPS**, received her Doctor of Pharmacy degree from Ferris State University (FSU) in 2006. She then completed a community pharmacy practice residency through Meijer, Pfizer and FSU, and joined the FSU College of Pharmacy as a faculty member in 2007. Morse holds a shared position between the College of Pharmacy and Meijer Pharmacy, where she coordinates an elective course, precepts student pharmacists and participates in the development and implementation of patient care services. Morse became a Board Certified Pharmacotherapy Specialist in 2008. She completed the American Pharmacists Association Pharmacy-Based Immunization Delivery certificate course in 2007 and became a faculty trainer for the course in 2009. *(Author of Chapter 14: Immunizations)*

- **Rita E. Naoum, Pharm.D.**, is a clinical pharmacist for Blue Cross Blue Shield of Michigan. She previously served in this role for the Genesys Regional Medical Center in Grand Blanc, Mich. Naoum earned her Doctor of Pharmacy degree from Ferris State University College of Pharmacy in 2006 as well as a Bachelor of Arts degree in biological sciences from Wayne State University in 2002. *(Author of Chapter 28: Reproductive System)*

- **Franz Neubrecht, Pharm.D.**, received a Bachelor of Science degree in pharmacy from the University of Michigan College of Pharmacy in Ann Arbor, Mich., a Master of Science degree in hospital pharmacy from Wayne State University in Detroit, Mich., and a Doctor of Pharmacy degree from Creighton University in Omaha, Neb. Neubrecht was formerly the director of pharmacy resources for Michigan Pharmacists Association in Lansing, Mich., before retiring in April 2006. Previous positions include owner of an independent community pharmacy, director of pharmacy at Port Huron Hospital in Port Huron, Mich.; staff pharmacist at Algonac Drug in Algonac, Mich.; and associate director at St. Clair Community Hospital, St. Clair, Mich. *(Author of Chapter 4: Third Party Insurance Issues)*

- **Tracey A. Okabe-Yamamura, Pharm.D.**, is clinical pharmacy specialist at Mercy San Juan Medical Center in Carmichael, Calif. The medical center is part of a multi-facility region of hospitals in the greater Sacramento area and includes services for neurology, cardiology, trauma, oncology and other acute care specialties. Her current responsibilities include coordination of facility clinical pharmacy services, clinical staff development, continuous quality improvement, preceptorship for student pharmacists and residents, and participation on the facility's Pain Support Team. Okabe-Yamamura is a graduate of the University of California, San Francisco, School of Pharmacy, and completed a clinical pharmacy residency at the University of California, Irvine. Her past positions include clinical coordinator at Pacific Hospital of Long Beach and clinical pharmacist for FHP, Inc. *(Author of Chapter 16: How Drugs Work)*

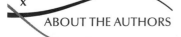

- **Kuldip R. Patel, Pharm.D.**, is associate chief pharmacy officer for central pharmacy services at Duke University Hospital in Durham, N.C. He has also served on the American Society of Health-System Pharmacists Section Advisory Group on Quality and Compliance. *(Author of Chapter 12: Pharmacy Operations and Administration)*

- **Cynthia Peitzsch, R.Ph.**, is the clinical coordinator for Pharmerica, in Warren, Mich. A long-time long-term care pharmacist, she has served as secretary, treasurer, president and chairman of the Consultant Pharmacists Society of Michigan. She received a Bachelor of Science degree in pharmacy from the Wayne State University Eugene Applebaum College of Pharmacy and Health Sciences in Detroit, Mich., in 1981. *(Author of Chapter 8: Consultant and Long-term Care Pharmacy Practice)*

- **D. Joshua Potter** is a compliance officer for PRS Pharmacy in Latrobe, Penn. Potter has been involved in retail pharmacy since the early 1990s. He has worked as a pharmacy technician and managed retail pharmacy stores. Potter has also been the primary developer for several programs for PRS, including its Health Insurance Portability and Accountability Act Compliance Program, Durable Medical Equipment, Prosthetics, Orthotics and Supplies Accreditation Prep Program (DAPP), and the Medicare Part D Fraud, Waste, and Abuse Prevention Program. Potter also serves as the privacy officer for a retail pharmacy. *(Author of Chapter 9: Medical Equipment)*

- **Gregg S. Potter, Ph.D., R.Ph.**, is an associate professor at Ferris State University College of Pharmacy, specializing in pharmacology. He served on the Michigan Pharmacists Association Professional Affairs Committee for six years, and he is a current member of the Pharmacy Response Network. *(Author of Chapter 28: Reproductive System, and Chapter 29: Urinary System)*

- **Gregory A. Pratt, R.Ph.**, is the emergency preparedness coordinator with Michigan Pharmacists Association (MPA) and is a pharmacist with Pharmacy Plus of Lansing, Mich., where he has practiced since 1988. As emergency preparedness coordinator, Pratt oversees recruitment, training and involvement of pharmacy professionals in emergency preparedness activities and planning. Pratt received his Bachelor of Science degree in pharmacy in 1984 from Ferris State University. Pratt is past chair of MPA's Public Relations and Membership Committees and has served as president of the Capital Area Pharmacists Association. He received the Distinguished Young Pharmacist Practitioner Award in 1984 and the Fred W. Arnold Public Relations Award In 1997. *(Author of Chapter 13: Emergency Preparedness)*

- **Derek J. Quinn, Pharm.D.**, is the pharmacy manager for Westlake Drug, Inc. in Kalamazoo, Mich. He received his Doctor of Pharmacy degree from Ferris State University in 2006 and has since received an immunization administration certificate and a diabetes medication therapy management certificate from the University of Findlay College of Pharmacy. Quinn is a preceptor for both student pharmacists and student pharmacy technicians. He has also served as an Executive Board member for Michigan Pharmacists Association. *(Editor; Author of Chapter 1: Introduction to Pharmacy Technician Practice, Chapter 3: Community Pharmacy Practice and Chapter 17: Drugs and Drug Names)*

- **Justin K. Rak, Pharm.D.**, received his Doctor of Pharmacy degree from the University of Toledo. After graduation, he completed a PGY-1 pharmacy practice residency and a PGY-2 critical care residency at the University Hospital in Cincinnati, Ohio. He is currently a clinical pharmacy specialist in critical care at Borgess Medical Center in Kalamazoo, Mich. *(Author of Chapter 15: Poisonings and Emergency Medicine)*

- **Joan M. Rider, Pharm.D., CDE, BC-ADM**, is a pharmacist for A-Line Staffing Solutions. For more than 17 years, she was a professor of pharmacy practice at Ferris State University College of Pharmacy, supervising fourth-year student pharmacists on experiential rotations in diabetes, internal medicine, ambulatory care and academics. Rider was also a clinical pharmacist for St. Mary's Hospital for 10 years. She has been actively involved in Michigan Pharmacists Association (MPA) for a number of years, serving as a past president of both the Association and the Michigan Society of Health-System Pharmacists (MSHP). Rider was also a member of the Michigan Pharmacy Foundation Board of Trustees, and several MPA and MSHP Committees. *(Author of Chapter 31: Endocrine System)*

- **Claire E. Saadeh, Pharm.D., BCOP**, is an associate professor at Ferris State University (FSU) College of Pharmacy and a Board Certified Oncology Pharmacist, specializing in the areas of oncology, pain management and palliative care. Saadeh received her Bachelor of Science degree in pharmacy in 1989 from Brighton University in England and a Doctor of Pharmacy degree in 1994 from Wayne State University. Following this, she pursued a specialty residency in oncology at the University of Florida, Shands Hospital. Saadeh has been with FSU since 2000, and her current clinical practice site is at Sparrow Health System in Lansing, Mich. *(Author of Chapter 36: Cancer)*

- **Linda J. Stuckey, Pharm.D., BCPS**, earned her Doctor of Pharmacy degree from University of Missouri-Kansas City and completed her pharmacy practice residency and critical care residency at the Hospital of the University of Pennsylvania in Philadelphia, Penn. Stuckey is currently practicing as a clinical transplant pharmacist at the University of Michigan Hospital and Health Centers and is a clinical adjunct instructor at the University of Michigan College of Pharmacy. Her practice area is a combination of inpatient and outpatient roles for the lung and liver transplant programs. *(Author of Chapter 27: Hepatic System)*

- **James B. Vander Linde, Pharm.D.**, received his Bachelor of Science degree in pharmacy from Ferris State University College of Pharmacy in Big Rapids, Mich., in 1979 and his Doctor of Pharmacy degree from Wayne State University Eugene Applebaum College of Pharmacy and Health Sciences in Detroit, Mich., in 1982. He completed an American Society of Health-System Pharmacist-accredited pharmacy practice residency at St. Lawrence Hospital in Lansing, Mich. Vander Linde is currently the pharmacy manager at Saint Joseph Mercy Livingston Hospital in Howell, Mich., which is part of the St. Joseph Mercy Health System. He has served on the Michigan Pharmacists Association Executive Board as chairman and president, as well as on the Michigan Pharmacy Foundation Board of Trustees. *(Author of Chapter 2: Pharmacy Terminology)*

- **Kali M. VanLangen, Pharm.D., BCPS**, received her Doctor of Pharmacy degree from Ferris State University in 2007. She then went on to complete a PGY-1 pharmacy practice residency at Saint Mary's Health Care in Grand Rapids, Mich., in 2008. Upon completion of her residency, VanLangen accepted a position with Ferris State University, where she is currently an assistant professor of pharmacy practice. She served as president of the Western Michigan Society of Health-System Pharmacists (WMSHP) in 2012 and as the WMSHP representative on the Michigan Society of Health-System Pharmacists Board of Directors. *(Author of Chapter 25: Lower Respiratory System)*

- **Dean A. Van Loo, Pharm.D., BCPS**, received his Doctor of Pharmacy degree in 1994 from the University of Michigan College of Pharmacy and completed a pharmacy practice residency at Bronson Methodist Hospital in Kalamazoo, Mich. Van Loo is currently an associate professor of pharmacy practice with Ferris State University College of Pharmacy in Kalamazoo, Mich. He also serves as a preceptor for student pharmacists in infectious disease, internal medicine and trauma care at Bronson Methodist Hospital. He previously served on the Michigan Pharmacists Association Executive Board. *(Author of Chapter 33: Immune System)*

ABOUT THE AUTHORS

- **Kari L. Vavra, Pharm.D.,** is an assistant professor of pharmacy practice at Ferris State University (FSU) College of Pharmacy. Her general medicine clinical practice site is at Spectrum Health-Butterworth Campus in Grand Rapids, Mich. Vavra received her Doctor of Pharmacy degree in 2009 from FSU College of Pharmacy. After obtaining her Pharm.D., she completed a pharmacy practice residency at Sparrow Health System in Lansing, Mich. *(Author of Chapter 22: Central and Peripheral Nervous System, and Chapter 36: Cancer)*

- **Kristin M. Verfaillie, Pharm.D.,** received her Doctor of Pharmacy degree from Wayne State University Eugene Applebaum College of Pharmacy and Health Sciences in 2011. She is a member of the Macomb County Pharmacists Association, and she also completed clinical rotations at St. John Hospital and Medical Center in Detroit, Mich. *(Author of Chapter 26: Digestive System)*

- **Jesse C. Vivian, R.Ph., J.D.,** received his Bachelor of Science in pharmacy and Juris Doctor degree from the University of Michigan College of Pharmacy and Wayne State University (WSU) Law School, respectively. He teaches pharmacy jurisprudence, pharmacy ethics and health care policy in the Department of Pharmacy Practice at WSU Eugene Applebaum College of Pharmacy and Health Sciences. He is also general counsel to the Michigan Pharmacists Association and is of counsel to the law firm of Cummings, McClorey and Acho, PC, in Livonia, Mich. He is a past president of the American Society for Pharmacy Law and served on the Committee that drafted the 1994 Code of Ethics for Pharmacists developed by the American Pharmaceutical Association. He is a frequent lecturer and author of several texts and articles dealing with pharmacy law and ethics. Further information is available at http://JesseVivian.org. *(Author of Chapter 11: Law and Ethics for Pharmacy Technicians)*

- **Kenny R. Walkup, Jr., R.Ph., FIACP**, received his Bachelor of Science degree in pharmacy from the Raabe College of Pharmacy at Ohio Northern University in Ada, Ohio. He is the president and owner of Specialty Medicine Compounding Pharmacy in South Lyon, Mich. He is a member of the Michigan Pharmacists Association and the National Community Pharmacists Association, as well as a member and Fellow of the International Academy of Compounding Pharmacists. In addition, Walkup, Jr. has been the executive director of the national pharmacy fraternity Phi Delta Chi; a task force member for state-wide regulation of compounding pharmacies; and a speaker at national compounding seminars. *(Author of Chapter 5: Pharmacy Compounding)*

- **John Watkins, MBA**, serves as the director of sales and as a sales account executive for PRS Pharmacy Services in Latrobe, Penn. Watkins represents the company at various seminars and tradeshows, as well as conducts webinars and audio seminars on topics such as durable medical equipment, prosthetics, orthotics and supplies (DMEPOS) accreditation and third party contracting for DMEPOS. Watkins also gives continuing education presentations on pharmacy compliance. *(Author of Chapter 9: Medical Equipment)*

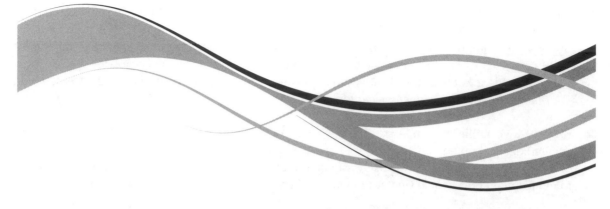

ACKNOWLEDGEMENTS

Michigan Pharmacists Association (MPA) would like to thank Jill Cobb and Stephanie Sisco for assistance in the editing process. In addition to the editors and authors, MPA also acknowledges the following individuals for their contributions to the Manual: Linda Branoff, CPhT; Tabitha Cross; Cathryn Poll, Pharm.D.; Michelle Richardson, CPhT; Cynthia Rowe; and La Vone Swanson.

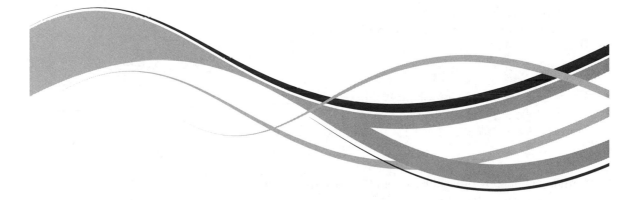

ASSOCIATIONS AND ORGANIZATIONS

Pharmacy Organizations

Accreditation Council for Pharmacy Education (ACPE)
20 N. Clark St., Suite 2500, Chicago, IL 60602
(312) 664-3575; Fax (312) 664-4652
www.acpe-accredit.org

American Association of Colleges of Pharmacy (AACP)
1727 King St., Alexandria, VA 22314
(703) 739-2330; Fax (703) 836-8982
www.aacp.org

American Hospital Association (AHA)
155 N. Wacker Drive, Chicago, Illinois 60606
(312) 422-3000
325 7th St. NW, Washington, D.C. 20004
(202) 638-1100
www.aha.org

American Pharmacists Association (APhA)
2215 Constitution Ave. NW, Washington, D.C. 20037
(202) 628-4410; Fax (202) 783-2351
www.pharmacist.com

American Society for Pharmacy Law (ASPL)
3085 Stevenson Drive, Suite 200, Springfield, IL 62703
(217) 529-6948
www.aspl.org

American Society of Consultant Pharmacists (ASCP)
1321 Duke St., Alexandria, VA 22314
(800) 355-2727 or (703) 739-1300; Fax (800) 220-1321 or (703) 739-1321
www.ascp.com

American Society of Health-System Pharmacists (ASHP)
7272 Wisconsin Ave., Bethesda, MD 20814
(301) 657-3000 or (866) 279-0681
www.ashp.org

Joint Commission on Accreditation of Health Care Organizations (JCAHO)
One Renaissance Blvd., Oakbrook Terrace, IL 60181
(630) 792-5000; Fax (630) 792-5005
www.jcaho.org

National Association of Boards of Pharmacy (NABP)
1600 Feehanville Drive, Mount Prospect, IL 60056
(847) 391-4406; Fax (847) 391-4502
www.nabp.net

National Association of Chain Drug Stores (NACDS)
413 North Lee St., Alexandria, VA 22314
(703) 549-3001
www.nacds.org

National Community Pharmacists Association (NCPA)
205 Daingerfield Road, Alexandria, VA 22314
(703) 683-8200; Fax (703) 683-3619
www.ncpanet.org

National Council for Prescription Drug Programs, Inc. (NCPDP)
9240 E. Raintree Drive, Scottsdale, AZ 85260
(480) 477-1000; Fax (480) 767-1042
www.ncpdp.org

National Council on Patient Information and Education (NCPIE)
200-A Monroe St., Suite 212, Rockville, MD 20850
(301) 340-3940; Fax (301) 340-3944
www.talkaboutrx.org

National Pharmaceutical Council (NPC)
1894 Preston White Drive, Reston, VA 20191
(703) 620-6390; Fax (703) 476-0904
www.npcnow.org

Pharmaceutical Research and Manufacturers of America (PhRMA)
950 F St., NW, Suite 200, Washington, D.C. 20004
(202) 835-3400; Fax (202) 835-3414
www.phrma.org

Pharmacy Technician Organizations

American Association of Pharmacy Technicians (AAPT)
P.O. Box 1447, Greensboro, NC 27402
(877) 368-4771 or (336) 333-9356; Fax (336) 333-9068
www.pharmacytechnician.com

National Pharmacy Technician Association (NPTA)
P.O. Box 683148, Houston, TX 77268
(888) 247-8700; Fax (888) 247-8706
www.pharmacytechnician.org

Pharmacy Technician Certification Board (PTCB)
2215 Constitution Ave. NW, Washington, D.C. 20037
(800) 363-8012; Fax (202) 429-7596
www.ptcb.org

Pharmacy Technician Educators Council (PTEC)
www.rxptec.org

Government Agencies

Drug Enforcement Administration, regional offices
www.justice.gov/dea
   Atlanta Division (404) 893-7000
   Boston Division (617) 557-2100
   Caribbean Division (787) 277-4700
   Chicago Division (312) 353-7875
   Dallas Division (214) 366-6900
   Denver Division (720) 895-4040
   Detroit Division (313) 234-4000
   El Paso Division (915) 832-6000
   Houston Division (713) 693-3000
   Los Angeles Division (213) 621-6700
   Miami Division (954) 660-4500
   New Jersey Division (973) 776-1100
   New Orleans Division (504) 840-1100
   New York Division (212) 337-3900
   Philadelphia Division (215) 861-3474
   Phoenix Division (602) 664-5600
   San Diego Division (858) 616-4100
   San Francisco Division (415) 436-7900
   Seattle Division (206) 553-5443
   St. Louis Division (314) 538-4600
   Washington, D.C. Division (202) 305-8500

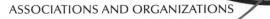

U.S. Food and Drug Administration
(888) INFO-FDA or (888) 463-6332, www.fda.gov

U.S. Food and Drug Administration MEDWATCH program
(800) 332-1088, www.fda.gov/Safety/MedWatch

State Boards of Pharmacy

Alabama (205) 981-2280, www.albop.com
Alaska (907) 465-2589, www.commerce.state.ak.us/occ/ppha.htm
Arizona (602) 771-2736, www.azpharmacy.gov
Arkansas (501) 682-0190, www.arkansas.gov/asbp
California (916) 574-7900, www.pharmacy.ca.gov
Colorado (303) 894-7800, www.dora.state.co.us/pharmacy
Connecticut (860) 713-6070, www.ct.gov/dcp
Delaware (302) 744-4500, www.dpr.delaware.gov
District of Columbia (202) 727-9856,
    http://hpla.doh.dc.gov/hpla/cwp/view,A,1195,Q,488414,hplaNav,%7C30661%7C,.asp
Florida (850) 245-4292, www.doh.state.fl.us/mqa/pharmacy
Georgia (478) 207-2440, www.sos.ga.gov
Hawaii (808) 586-2694, www.hawaii.gov/dcca/areas/pvl/boards/pharmacy
Idaho (208) 334-2356, www.idaho.gov/bop
Illinois (217) 782-8556, www.idfpr.com
Indiana (317) 234-2067, www.in.gov/pla/pharmacy.htm
Iowa (515) 281-5944, www.state.ia.us/ibpe
Kansas (785) 296-4056, www.kansas.gov/pharmacy
Kentucky (502) 564-7910, http://pharmacy.ky.gov
Louisiana (225) 925-6496, www.pharmacy.la.gov
Maine (207) 624-8603, www.maine.gov/professionallicensing
Maryland (410) 764-4755, www.dhmh.state.md.us/pharmacyboard
Massachusetts (617) 973-0950, www.mass.gov/reg/boards/ph
Michigan (517) 335-7212, www.michigan.gov/healthlicense
Minnesota (651) 201-2825, www.pharmacy.state.mn.us
Mississippi (601) 605-5388, www.mbp.state.ms.us
Missouri (573) 751-0091, www.pr.mo.gov/pharmacists.asp
Montana (406) 841-2371, http://mt.gov/dli/bsd/license/bsd_boards/pha_board/board_page.asp
Nebraska (402) 471-2118, www.hhs.state.ne.us
Nevada (775) 850-1440, http://bop.nv.gov
New Hampshire (603) 271-2350, www.nh.gov/pharmacy
New Jersey (973) 504-6450, www.state.nj.us/lps/ca/boards.htm
New Mexico (505) 222-9830, www.rld.state.nm.us/Pharmacy
New York (518) 474-3817, ext. 130, www.op.nysed.gov
North Carolina (919) 246-1050, www.ncbop.org
North Dakota (701) 328-9535, www.nodakpharmacy.com
Ohio (614) 466-4143, www.pharmacy.ohio.gov
Oklahoma (405) 521-3815, www.pharmacy.ok.gov
Oregon (971) 673-0001, www.pharmacy.state.or.us
Pennsylvania (717) 783-7156, www.dos.state.pa.us/pharm
Rhode Island (401) 222-2840, www.health.ri.gov/hsr/professions/pharmacy.php
South Carolina (803) 896-4700, www.llr.state.sc.us/pol/pharmacy

South Dakota (605) 362-2737, www.pharmacy.sd.gov
Tennessee (615) 741-2718, http://health.state.tn.us/Boards/Pharmacy
Texas (512) 305-8000, www.tsbp.state.tx.us
Utah (801) 530-6789, www.dopl.utah.gov
Vermont (802) 828-2373, www.vtprofessionals.org
Virginia (804) 367-4456, www.dhp.virginia.gov/pharmacy
Washington (360) 236-4700, www.doh.wa.gov/hsqa/Professions/Pharmacy
West Virginia (304) 558-0558, www.wvbop.com
Wisconsin (608) 266-2112, www.drl.state.wi.us
Wyoming (307) 634-9636, http://pharmacyboard.state.wy.us

State Pharmacy Associations

Alabama Pharmacy Association
1211 Carmichael Way, Montgomery, AL 36106
(334) 271-4222; Fax (334) 271-5423
www.aparx.org

Alaska Pharmacists Association
203 W. 15th Ave. #100, Anchorage, AK 99501
(907) 563-8880; Fax (907) 563-7880
www.alaskapharmacy.org

Arizona Pharmacy Alliance
1845 E. Southern Ave., Tempe, AZ 85282
(480) 838-3385; Fax (480) 838-3557
www.azpharmacy.org

Arkansas Pharmacists Association
417 South Victory St., Little Rock, AR 72201
(501) 372-5250; Fax (501) 372-0546
www.arrx.org

California Pharmacists Association
4030 Lennane Drive, Sacramento, CA 95834
(916) 779-1400, ext. 400; Fax (916) 779-1401
www.cpha.com

Colegio de Farmaceuticos de Puerto Rico
289 Cale Ing. Colon, Hato Rey, PR 00918
(787) 753-7157; Fax (787) 759-9793
www.colegiofarmaceuticos.com

Colorado Pharmacists Society
6825 E. Tennessee Ave., Suite 440, Denver, CO 80224
(303) 756-3069; Fax (303) 756-3649
www.copharm.org

Connecticut Pharmacists Association
35 Cold Spring Road, Suite 121, Rocky Hill, CT 06067
(860) 563-4619; Fax (860) 257-8241
www.ctpharmacists.org

Delaware Pharmacists Society
P.O. Box 454, Smyrna, DE 19977
(302) 659-3088; Fax (302) 659-3089
www.dpsrx.org

Florida Pharmacy Association
610 North Adams St., Tallahassee, FL 32301
(850) 222-2400; Fax (850) 561-6758
www.pharmview.com

Georgia Pharmacy Association
50 Lenox Pointe, NE, Atlanta, GA 30324
(404) 231-5074 or (404) 419-8119; Fax (404) 237-8435
www.gpha.org

Hawaii Pharmacists Association
P.O. Box 1510, Aiea, HI 96701
www.hipharm.org

Idaho State Pharmacy Association
P.O. Box 140117, Garden City, ID 83714
(208) 841-2843
www.idahopharmacists.com

Illinois Pharmacists Association
204 W. Cook St., Springfield, IL 62704
(217) 522-7300 or (217) 522-7349
www.ipha.org

Indiana Pharmacists Alliance
729 N. Pennsylvania St., Indianapolis, IN 46204
(317) 634-4968; Fax (317) 632-1219
www.indianapharmacists.org

Iowa Pharmacy Association
8515 Douglas Ave., Suite 16, Des Moines, IA 50322
(515) 270-0713; Fax (515) 270-2979
www.iarx.org

Kansas Pharmacists Association
1020 SW Fairlawn Road, Topeka, KS 66604
(785) 228-2327; Fax 785-228-9147
www.ksrx.org

Kentucky Pharmacists Association
1228 U.S. 127 South, Frankfort, KY 40601
(502) 227-2303; Fax (502) 227-2258
www.kphanet.org

Louisiana Pharmacists Association
450 Laurel St., Suite 1400, Baton Rouge, LA 70801
(225) 346-6883; Fax (225) 344-1132
www.louisianapharmacists.com

Maine Pharmacy Association
P.O. Box 174, Turner, ME 04282
(207) 225-5205
www.mparx.com

Maryland Pharmacists Association
1800 Washington Blvd., Suite 333, Baltimore, MD 21230
(410) 727-0746; Fax (410) 727-2253
www.marylandpharmacist.org

Massachusetts Pharmacists Association
500 West Cummings Park, Suite 3475, Woburn, MA 01801
(781) 933-1107; Fax (781) 933-1109
www.masspharmacists.org

Michigan Pharmacists Association
408 Kalamazoo Plaza, Lansing, MI 48933
(517) 484-1466; Fax (517) 484-4893
www.michiganpharmacists.org

Minnesota Pharmacists Association
1000 Westgate Drive, Suite 252, St. Paul, MN 55114
(651) 697-1771; Fax (651) 290-2266
www.mpha.org

Mississippi Pharmacists Association
341 Edgewood Terrace Drive, Jackson, MS 39206
(601) 981-0416; Fax (601) 981 0451
www.mspharm.org

Missouri Pharmacy Association
211 E. Capitol Ave., Jefferson City, MO 65101
(573) 636-7522; Fax (573) 636-7485
www.morx.com

Montana Pharmacy Association
P.O. Box 1569, Helena, MT 59624
(406) 442-5490; Fax (406) 442-8018
www.rxmt.org

Nebraska Pharmacists Association
6221 South 58th St., Suite A, Lincoln, NE 68516
(402) 420-1500; Fax (402) 420-1406
www.npharm.org

Nevada Pharmacy Association
7211 Falvo Ave., Las Vegas, NV 89131
(702) 683-1955

New Hampshire Pharmacists Association
26 S. Main St., PMB #188, Concord, NH 03301
(603) 229-0292
www.nhpharmacists.net

New Jersey Pharmacists Association
760 Alexander Road, Princeton, NJ 08543
(609) 275-4246
www.njpharma.org

New Mexico Pharmacists Association
2716 San Pedro NE, Suite C, Albuquerque, NM 87110
(800) 464-8729; Fax (505) 255-8476
www.nm-pharmacy.com

Pharmacists Society of the State of New York
210 Washington Ave., Albany, NY 12203
(518) 869-6595; Fax (518) 464-0618
www.pssny.org

North Carolina Association of Pharmacists
109 Church St., Chapel Hill, NC 27516
(919) 967-2237; Fax (919) 968-9430
www.ncpharmacists.org

North Dakota Pharmacists Association
1641 Capitol Way, Bismarck, ND 58501
(701) 258-4968 or (701) 258-4922; Fax (701) 258-9312
www.nodakpharmacy.net

Ohio Pharmacists Association
2674 Federated Blvd., Columbus, OH 43235
(614) 389-3236; Fax (614) 389-4582
www.ohiopharmacists.org

Oklahoma Pharmacists Association
Box 18731, Oklahoma City, OK 73154
(405) 557-5772; Fax (405) 528-1417
www.opha.com

Oregon State Pharmacy Association
147 SE 102nd Ave., Portland, OR 97216
(503) 582-9055; Fax (503) 253-9172
www.oregonpharmacy.org

Pennsylvania Pharmacists Association
508 North 3rd St., Harrisburg, PA 17101
(717) 234-6151; Fax (717) 236-1618
www.papharmacists.com

Rhode Island Pharmacists Association
1643 Warwick Ave., PMB 113, Warwick, RI 02889
(401) 737-2600; Fax (401) 739-0959
www.ripharmacists.org

South Carolina Pharmacy Association
1350 Browning Road, Columbia, SC 29210
(803) 354-9977; Fax (803) 354-9207
www.scrx.org

South Dakota Pharmacists Association
320 E. Capitol, P.O. Box 518, Pierre, SD 57501
(605) 224-2338; Fax (605) 224-1280
www.sdpha.org

Tennessee Pharmacists Association
500 Church St., Suite 650, Nashville, TN 37219
(615) 256-3023; Fax (615) 255-3528
www.tnpharm.org

Texas Pharmacy Association
12007 Research Blvd., Suite 201, Austin, TX 78759
(512) 615-9170; Fax (512) 836-0308
www.texaspharmacy.org

Utah Pharmacists Association
1125 S. Blackhawk Drive, Suite B, Mount Pleasant, UT 84647
(435) 462-5323; Fax (435) 462-5325
www.upha.com

Vermont Pharmacists Association
P.O. Box 90, Woodstock, VT 05091
(877) 483-2646; Fax (877) 483-2646
www.vtpharmacists.com

Virginia Pharmacists Association
2530 Professional Road, Richmond, VA 23235
(804) 285-4145; Fax (804) 285-4227
www.virginiapharmacists.org

Washington, D.C., Pharmaceutical Association
908 Caddington Ave., Silver Spring, MD 20901
(301) 593-3292; Fax (301) 593-7215

Washington State Pharmacy Association
411 Williams Ave. South, Renton, WA 98055
(425) 228-7171; Fax (425) 277-3897
www.wsparx.org

West Virginia Pharmacists Association
2016 1/2 Kanawha Blvd. East, Charleston, WV 25311
(304) 344-5302; Fax (304) 344-5316
www.wvpharmacy.org

Pharmacy Society of Wisconsin
701 Heartland Trail, Madison, WI 53717
(608) 827-9200; Fax (608) 827-9292
www.pswi.org

Wyoming Pharmacy Association
P.O. Box 228, Byron, WY 82412
(307) 272-3361; Fax (307) 548-6259
www.wpha.net

INTRODUCTION

Pharmacy technicians continue to be in high demand across the country in community pharmacies, health-systems, long-term care practices and other specialized health care settings. As the pharmacist's role in health care expands, educated and trained technicians become even more important in the medication delivery system, keeping patients safe and helping to improve their care.

Becoming a pharmacy technician is becoming part of the health care team. This important career choice will allow you the opportunity to, for example, interact with patients, assist and support pharmacists in clinical roles, prepare prescriptions, compound (create) specialized medications and assist in the compliance and administrative functions of a pharmacy or business, all dependent on your practice site.

That is why it is critical for those just entering the pharmacy technician field and those with years of experience in pharmacy to continue their education and earn national certification, the very reason this edition of the Pharmacy Certified Technician Training Manual was created.

The publication of the 12th edition marks 20 years in quality pharmacy technician education for Michigan Pharmacists Association (MPA), helping thousands of people prepare for and excel in their technician careers. This book is the compilation of pharmacy knowledge from experts across the United States. It addresses pharmacy technician practice, solidly prepares technicians for everyday functions of the job in major practice settings, and gives a well-rounded perspective on the body's systems, common disorders and drug treatment.

In addition to pharmacy education, MPA was a founder, along with the American Pharmacists Association, the American Society of Health-System Pharmacists and the Illinois Council of Health-System Pharmacists, in the creation of one consolidated, national certification program for pharmacy technicians: the Pharmacy Technician Certification Board (PTCB®).

In 2002, the National Association of Boards of Pharmacy (NABP®) joined the PTCB® founders to continue to advance the national certification program for pharmacy technicians. NABP® also works with the state Boards of Pharmacy to encourage acceptance of the PTCB® certification program as a recognized assessment tool.

What's New in This Edition

The 12th edition of the Pharmacy Certified Technician Training Manual includes freshly written and completely updated content, to help the pharmacy technician address the challenges of the pharmacy practice today, as well as current drug therapies.

To give pharmacy technicians a broad overview of the profession and the value technicians bring, the first section of the book, "Pharmacy Practice," addresses the three major practice settings for a technician and critical information about job function and responsibility in the community pharmacy, health-system and long-term care practice. Then, this section prepares technicians for essentials in pharmacy, including patient and medication safety, laws and regulations, operations, emergency preparedness and clinical opportunities.

Accompanying many chapters are real-life stories from pharmacy technicians around the nation and their perspective on pharmacy practice, bringing home the concepts discussed.

Then, in "Human Systems and Pharmacy Intervention," the Manual helps pharmacy technicians understand how drugs work, gives familiarity to the most common medications, and reviews each system of the body. As a bonus with this edition of the Manual, the accompanying CD-ROM includes a master spreadsheet table of all medications listed throughout the book, an incredible resource and tool for students and practicing pharmacy technicians.

All review questions are original to this edition, allowing those who own previous editions room for review and growth.

Finally, the previous edition included pharmacy calculations to create one reference book for pharmacy technicians. After careful collaboration with instructors, colleges, state associations and pharmacy technician students, it was overwhelmingly determined that the calculations portion of the training is more useful when provided separately in workbook form. As such, MPA produced a companion Pharmacy Certified Technician Calculations Workbook, as a necessary companion to this Manual (learn more under "Companion Calculations Workbook").

How to Use This Manual

Each chapter contains three basic elements: learning objectives, the main text with clinical information and practical applications, and practice problems.

The learning objectives will give the reader a broad overview of the core concepts in each chapter. These are the elements that need to be mastered, so be sure to review before diving into the chapter, in order to measure understanding.

The main text of the chapters will provide key terms and definitions, memorization drug charts and discussion of primary applications for pharmacy technicians.

At the end of each chapter, practice problems follow that reinforce key concepts and allow the learner to practically review.

To view the answers to the practice problems, purchase the accompanying CD-ROM—Pharmacy Certified Technician Training Manual Answers and Supplemental Materials. You may order at MichiganPharmacists.org/store or from your partnering state pharmacy association.

Companion Calculations Workbook

Pharmacists depend on pharmacy technicians to accurately perform pharmacy calculations to support the medication distribution process. The Pharmacy Certified Technician Calculations Workbook has been developed to provide pharmacy technicians a foundation for commonly used pharmacy calculation functions. Not only does it review basic mathematic principles, but it brings pharmacy formulas and equations into real-life situations that pharmacy technicians will encounter in practice.

The Calculations Workbook educates pharmacy technicians on essential pharmacy formulas and equations, as well as real-life situations to which these calculations are applied. Each chapter includes working examples that take the learner step-by-step through the process. Available with the Calculations Workbook is the accompanying CD-ROM—Pharmacy Certified Technician Calculations, which includes the answers to practice problems, along with the detailed work to solve.

You may order the Pharmacy Certified Technician Calculations Workbook and CD-ROM at MichiganPharmacists.org/store or from your partnering state pharmacy association.

After Completion of This Manual

After studying the entirety of this Manual, and mastering the Calculations Workbook, congratulate yourself! You have just completed a major milestone in the progress of your pharmacy technician education and career! It is now time to put your knowledge into action.

Technicians who have mastered the learning objectives and successfully completed the practice problems will want to become nationally certified to confirm and recognize their groundwork in the pharmacy field. The Pharmacy Technician Certification Board will help you complete this process, so you can proudly place the designation CPhT™ (certified pharmacy technician) behind your name. Visit www.ptcb.org for a practice exam, additional test preparation and management of your certification.

Next, begin using the information gleaned in the Manual and Calculations Workbook in your practice and career. Interface with your pharmacist and other experienced pharmacy technicians on what you learned, and hone your skills to further advance your education and your practice.

Finally, use this Manual as a reference and resource. It is not meant to be used for only a one-time college or training course, or as a independent study guide for certification, though it is certainly a great option for each! Along with the professional judgment of your pharmacist, this Manual can act as a handy, go-to reference for general practice questions and more in-depth guide for body system functioning.

Considering the quickly-changing field of pharmacy, pharmacy technicians must commit to on-going learning. Though every effort has been made to include the very latest in the pharmacy field, the most recent medication information and pharmacist guidance should be consulted in addition to the content of this publication.

Chapter 1

INTRODUCTION TO PHARMACY TECHNICIAN PRACTICE

By Derek J. Quinn, Pharm.D.

Learning Objectives

This chapter seeks to prepare a pharmacy technician to:

- be familiar with the skills, knowledge and training prerequisite to becoming a pharmacy technician.
- overview the practice of pharmacy, what a pharmacist does and how pharmacy technicians are essential to assisting pharmacists in the practice of pharmacy.
- compare and contrast the practice sites available to pharmacy technicians.
- compare and contrast certification, licensure and registration of health care professionals and para-professionals.
- evaluate the role of third parties (insurance companies) and regulatory agencies in the practice of pharmacy.

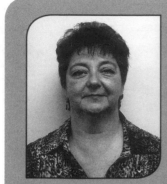

Introduction

Pharmacy technicians are essential to the practice of pharmacy. Most pharmacists could not accomplish the volume of patient care activities required of them without the assistance of pharmacy technicians. This means that there is much work to be done, and the profession of pharmacy needs qualified pharmacy technicians to fill an ever-expanding set of responsibilities that range from processing prescriptions for dispensing, to administering immunizations, to fitting patients for customizable medical equipment. Before starting to assist in this exciting world of patient care services, pharmacy technicians must come to the position with confidence in their training and knowledge. Pharmacy technicians need training in math, science and communications, as well as basic knowledge of available drugs, how drugs work, how the body works, the laws and rules that govern pharmacy, and where to find information on these topics. Some states have specific requirements that one must meet before becoming a pharmacy technician; these requirements may or may not include a required course of study at a college or training program. This manual serves to introduce a prospective pharmacy technician to all of these areas and can be used throughout a pharmacy technician's career as a reference.

What Does a Pharmacist Do?

To understand where pharmacy technicians fit into the health care team, a pharmacy technician must first understand where the pharmacist that they will assist fits into the health care team. Pharmacists are medication experts who are trained to evaluate drug therapies, assist patients with taking or using their drug therapies, and assist patients with medical devices related to managing their disease states. To be a pharmacist, one must have a Doctor of Pharmacy degree from an **accredited** university (or a Bachelor of Pharmacy degree if the pharmacist graduated before 1990) and be licensed to practice pharmacy in the state where he or she practices. Further, many pharmacists continue their training by completing residencies, fellowships and post-graduate certificates in specialty areas. Finally, to be a pharmacist, one must have a willingness to help patients and their community. Regardless of a pharmacist's practice setting and whether the pharmacist has direct contact with patients, pharmacists are there to help patients by working toward better therapy outcomes. Pharmacy technicians help ensure that caring for patients is the focus of the pharmacist they assist.

Practice Settings

The range of practice settings for a pharmacy technician is nearly endless. To get a better understanding of what skills and education are necessary to practice as a pharmacy technician, one must examine, at least, the more common settings for pharmacy practice.

Ambulatory Care Pharmacy

Ambulatory care is a general category for practice settings where patients walk into a pharmacy or clinic on either an as needed basis or with an appointment. Another way to look at ambulatory care pharmacy is that after coming to an ambulatory care pharmacy, the patient returns home to their own bed (outpatient); whereas, in an institutional practice setting, the patient is usually admitted to a hospital or other institution overnight (inpatient). This umbrella also generally covers working for a health insurance provider, health maintenance organization or as a consultant pharmacist.

Community pharmacy is one type of ambulatory care pharmacy and is the most recognizable practice setting for a pharmacy technician. Community pharmacies are the local pharmacies in every town throughout the world; this is where patients go to fill prescriptions, receive advice on the proper use of their drugs and often obtain medical devices and supplies. Pharmacy technicians practicing in this setting often spend much of their time interacting with patients by taking in prescriptions and refill requests for processing and assisting in the process of dispensing medications. Further, some pharmacies utilize pharmacy technicians in the process of **compounding**, administering immunizations and dispensing medical devices. Then, in addition to those clinical services, pharmacy technicians can be instrumental in the process of billing insurance companies, in inventory management procedures, in compliance with regulatory requirements and in human resource management. Finally, pharmacy technicians are often responsible for interacting with physician offices and insurance companies whenever prescriptions need clarification or when insurance companies require more detailed information before a claim can be paid.

Many community pharmacies do compounding to some degree, and a few pharmacies focus primarily on compounding (those that more heavily focus on compounding are often called compounding pharmacies, even if they also dispense noncompounded medications). Most drugs used today are manufactured by a drug company and then sold to the pharmacy (usually through a drug wholesaler); at the pharmacy, the finished product provided by the drug company is provided to the patient without being fundamentally changed. When a patient needs a product that is not commercially available, a pharmacist can use commercially-available raw ingredients to prepare a specific batch of medication for that patient. Pharmacists can utilize pharmacy technicians to help with this preparation work. Compounding includes everything from grinding tablets to be made into suspensions, mixing drugs into cream and ointment bases for topical use, molding suppositories, filling capsules, pressing tablets, preparing IV (intravenous) bags for home use and more.

Another type of ambulatory care pharmacy is the clinic setting. Many practices that once only employed physicians and nurses now employ a team of health care professionals and para-professionals, including pharmacists and pharmacy technicians. In this setting, the dispensing of medications is not a primary focus of caring for patients; instead, collaborating with physicians in the education of patients and assisting the rest of the health care team to prescribe medications more effectively are the primary focus. Pharmacy technicians in this setting, once trained, can assist in taking basic **vital signs**; help patients with medical devices such as **nebulizers** used for breathing treatments and blood glucose (sugar) monitors used to monitor patients with diabetes; and perform many clerical tasks required by their pharmacist. In this type of setting, pharmacists can also run monitoring centers for anticoagulation (blood-thinning) drugs and use pharmacy technicians throughout that process.

Health insurance providers and Health Management Organizations (HMOs) utilize pharmacy technicians for a variety of roles. Pharmacy technicians assist in both clinical and technical call centers to not only answer patient questions, but provider questions as well. Providers can be physicians, nurses, pharmacists, other pharmacy technicians or anyone who is part of the process of providing care or billing the insurance company. Pharmacy technicians are also utilized as **audit** specialists, especially if they have experience from practicing in another setting. Pharmacy technicians are utilized in cost-containment programs, delivery of clinical programs to patients and in provider education programs. Pharmacy technicians can also be involved in the process of assisting patients in receiving prior authorization to receive a therapy; some drugs require prior authorization from the insurance company before the drug is dispensed. The reasons that drugs require prior authorization are many and varied, but pharmacy technicians can be a vital part of making sure this process occurs smoothly.

Home infusion pharmacies are also considered ambulatory care pharmacies. Home infusion pharmacies prepare IV and injectable medications for use at home. Home IV medications are administered by patients and their families, after training, or by visiting nurses or other licensed caregivers. Pharmacy technicians are utilized throughout the process of receiving orders for home infusion medications, preparing the drugs for dispensing, billing insurance companies and delivering medication to patients in their homes.

Pharmacists are also beginning to offer their services of patient education without attaching dispensed medications to the process. Although the term consultant pharmacist covers many pharmacists in different settings, this is one growing area for consultant pharmacists. This process usually works by patients contacting the office of the consultant pharmacist to set up an appointment, where the pharmacist will review all of the medications (prescription, over-the-counter and herbal) that the patient is using, go over those medications with the patient and contact the patient's physician(s) when a patient's therapy may need adjusting. Pharmacy technicians can help at every step of this process, from scheduling appointments to contacting physician offices to provide them with the pharmacist's recommendations on changing therapy.

Institutional Care Pharmacy

There are two main types of institutions generally covered by the institutional care practice section: hospitals/health-systems and long-term care facilities. In a hospital, there are two main roles for pharmacists (and therefore two main roles for pharmacy technicians): processing prescription orders at the pharmacy and seeing patients on the floors (or wards) of the hospital. Pharmacy technicians are vital to fulfilling medication orders; responsibilities include filling a patient's daily medication box, preparing injectable and IV drugs for use, preparing **chemotherapy** for injection, maintaining required paperwork, transporting drugs to the floors or drug distribution rooms, and taking calls from the staff on the hospital floors regarding drugs being administered. Pharmacy technicians also support the pharmacist while he/she visits patients in their rooms. The pharmacist may be reviewing charts, checking lab values, ordering lab tests, talking with patients, calculating drug doses, reviewing possible adverse events from medication use and making recommendations for therapy changes to physicians; pharmacy technicians can assist in making sure that this process happens smoothly and efficiently.

The other main type of institutional practice is long-term care pharmacy. Long-term care includes nursing homes, skilled-nursing facilities or any other institution where the patient receives continuous care for extended periods of time. Much like pharmacists in the hospital, long-term care pharmacists (also called consultant pharmacists) spend time seeing patients in their rooms and talking with patients about their health and the therapies that they are using. Pharmacy technicians can be instrumental in preparing charts for pharmacists to review, collecting information from new patients about the medications they were using before coming into the facility and following up on recommendations made by the pharmacist for changes in therapy.

Other Pharmacy Practice Settings

There are many more ways in which pharmacists and pharmacy technicians assist patients. Although less common than the ambulatory care or institutional care environments, these settings can be a rewarding and often very necessary service niche in the delivery of health care services. Some other practice settings include:

- **Mail-Order, Central-Fill and Internet Pharmacies**
  These closed-door (not open to the public) pharmacies process prescriptions to either be delivered by mail or by a local community pharmacy. Mail-order pharmacies employ pharmacy technicians to assist in the high-volume of prescriptions that are being processed by these facilities, as well as by answering calls from patients. A central-fill pharmacy is one that does not generally interact directly with patients; instead, a central-fill pharmacy fills prescriptions and delivers them to a local community pharmacy, where they are dispensed to a patient by their local pharmacist. Finally, an Internet pharmacy is one where the patient orders prescriptions (and sometimes over-the-counter medications) online and then receives the drugs by mail or delivery. Internet pharmacies employ pharmacy technicians both on the filling and dispensing side of their operation and on the technical web-development and maintenance side of their operation.

- **Nuclear Pharmacy**
  A nuclear pharmacy prepares **radioactive contrast dyes** used in lab testing (such as **CT scans**) as well as other radioactive drugs used to treat cancers and other conditions. These closed-door facilities generally operate during the third shift to prepare the medications and dyes needed during the upcoming day. The safe use of these otherwise unstable materials is a vital part of current medical treatment.

- **Pharmaceutical Manufacturing**
  Pharmacy technicians employed by a drug company can serve in multiple capacities, ranging from clerical tasks, to answering patient and provider phone calls, to directly working on manufacturing products. Each drug company maintains a drug information center with information on the products that they manufacture, and pharmacy technicians can play a vital role in maintaining these centers and fielding questions from health care providers about those products.

- **Academia**
  As the number of pharmacy technician training programs increase, the need for qualified instructors also increases. A pharmacy technician with practice experience can be an invaluable asset to any training program.

- **Military**
  All branches of the military have a need for pharmacists and, therefore, pharmacy technicians to assist them. Due to most military property being federal land, rather than land of a state, pharmacy technicians are often granted rights and responsibilities that cannot exist outside of the military structure.

- **Professional Organizations**
  Pharmacy technicians are needed by the professional organizations for pharmacists and pharmacy technicians. Roles for pharmacy technicians with such organizations include lobbying the government, preparing educational materials for patients and providers,

organizing patient care events, coordinating continuing education events and producing pharmacy technician training manuals.

■ **Pharmacy Services Companies**
Pharmacies today use a wide variety of technology to be more efficient in preparing medications for dispensing so that more time can be spent on patient care. This presents an opportunity for pharmacy technicians to work with software providers, computer hardware providers, robotics manufacturers, retail management system providers, drug wholesalers, medical device suppliers, accreditation agencies and any other company that provides products and services to any of the other pharmacy practice settings.

Skills and Knowledge Required for Practicing as a Pharmacy Technician

Even with the wide range of practice sites available for pharmacy technicians, there are some skills that may not be common to all sites but that are generally recognized as required by a pharmacy technician practicing in ambulatory care or institutional care settings.

■ **Intake of Medication Orders**
Pharmacy technicians must be familiar with the procedures for the proper receipt of a prescription (medication order). This includes what is required to be on a medication order, how orders can be received by the pharmacy (e.g., can all prescriptions be received by fax?) and what steps are required to begin processing that medication order. Further, it requires knowing who is able to **prescribe** medications in the state where the pharmacy is located (e.g., can a physician's assistant prescribe narcotics or can an optometrist write prescriptions in your state?).

■ **Inventory Management**
Pharmacy technicians are expected to maintain and manage pharmacy inventories. This includes processing drugs as they are received by the pharmacy (according to the procedures of the pharmacy and the laws of the state where the pharmacy is located), stocking those medications properly, maintaining a rotation of inventory to ensure that the most recently received medications are used last, processing invoices for drugs received by the pharmacy and correcting errors in the inventory records. This also includes recognizing that many drugs require special storage; some drugs require a certain temperature (refrigeration or freezing), protection from light, protections from shaking or must be stored in a separate area of the pharmacy. Also, pharmacy technicians are usually tasked with preparing orders for drugs that the pharmacy needs.

■ **Preparing Medications for Dispensing**
Pharmacy technicians, in most modern pharmacies, do most of the typing, labeling, counting, mixing and pouring activities. In a community pharmacy, this looks mostly like retrieving stock bottles from the pharmacy inventory and counting out the correct number of tablets or capsules needed to fill a prescription. This may, however, include compounding activities as determined by the pharmacist being assisted. In the institutional setting, this looks more like filling medication boxes for each patient in the hospital and preparing IV bags to be dispensed to patients.

■ **Billing Prescription Claims to Insurance Companies**
Pharmacists are medication experts, and most pharmacists agree that pharmacy technicians are billing experts. Pharmacy technicians must be able to successfully process prescription claims and submit them to insurance companies. Each pharmacy software does this slightly different; however, it is expected that pharmacy technicians will be able to handle rejections and paid claims from insurance companies.

■ **Billing Durable Medical Equipment (DME) Claims to Insurance Companies**
Pharmacies are continuing to expand their roles to meet the needs of patients; for many pharmacies, this means dispensing DME, such as diabetic testing strips, oxygen and supplies, power wheelchairs, aerochambers and peak flow meters for asthma management. Pharmacists are relying more and more on pharmacy technicians to be able to bill Medicare Part B, Medicaid and some private insurances for DME, supplies and related services.

■ **Assessing Medication Orders for Completeness**
Pharmacy technicians are expected to review a medication order (prescription) and assess whether or not all of the essential information is present. If it is not, a pharmacy technician is expected to follow their pharmacy's procedure for obtaining the missing information. This could include contacting the prescriber, speaking with the patient or consulting with a pharmacist.

■ **Maintaining Pharmacy Records**
Most state Boards of Pharmacy have extensive requirements on maintaining prescriptions, invoices, medical charts and other records of the pharmacy. Further, state and federal laws govern the storage, use and disclosure of pharmacy records. Pharmacy technicians are expected to be familiar with the requirements for pharmacy records and assist their pharmacy in compliance with these requirements.

■ **Using Pharmacy/Lab Equipment**
Pharmacy technicians are expected to be able to use a tablet/capsule counting tray – the basic tool of modern community pharmacy. Also, a pharmacy technician must know how to use a mortar and pestle (to grind tablets), read a graduated cylinder (to measure liquid volume), properly use a syringe/needle and prevent a needle-stick, handle a balance (scale), read a thermometer and other basic lab functions. This also includes how to properly clean and maintain these instruments and devices.

■ **Understand the Basics of Drug Delivery Systems**
Pharmacy technicians are expected to understand that suspensions must be shaken before a portion is poured, that suppositories often must be refrigerated because they are designed to melt at body temperature, which is not significantly higher than room temperature, and that capsules should not be chewed. Further, understanding the process for medication use, like that most suppositories come wrapped in either foil or plastic and must be unwrapped before they are inserted, is essential.

■ **Perform Calculations Required in the Dispensing Process**
Pharmacy technicians are often called upon to calculate values not present on a medication order. This can include calculating the volume of suspension necessary to fill an order, how much of two creams to mix together to reach the desired strength, what the final volume of a mixture will be or how long a prescription will last a patient, as examples.

One of the most important skills for a pharmacy technician to possess is a command of the mathematics required in the practice of pharmacy.

- ■ **Demonstrate Understanding of How Drugs are Used**
  Pharmacy technicians are expected to know which drugs are used for blood pressure, which are used to lower cholesterol, which are for diabetes, which are for infections, etc. Although a pharmacy technician will increase their knowledge throughout their professional career, it is expected that a pharmacy technician will begin by knowing at least the top 200 or so medications and their use.

Certification, Licensure, Registration and Exclusion Listing

Each state is responsible for determining the requirements for pharmacy technicians to practice within that state. Some states have no requirements, and some have very restrictive requirements. Regardless, the goal of such regulations is to ensure patient safety. Beyond the requirements of a state, a pharmacy technician may elect to complete training that enhances their practice and allows them to assist the pharmacist they work with in a more comprehensive way.

Certification is one option for credentialing pharmacy technicians. The Pharmacy Technician Certification Board (PTCB) provides nationally-recognized certification for pharmacy technicians. To obtain PTCB certification, a pharmacy technician must sit for an exam administered by PTCB. Once certified, a pharmacy technician must maintain his/her certification by completing continuing education requirements and then must apply for recertification on the schedule determined by PTCB. Currently, a certification cycle is two years and a pharmacy technician must complete 20 hours of continuing education to remain certified with PTCB. A certified pharmacy technician may use the designation "CPhT" after his or her name as a title of accomplishment. Although each pharmacy differs in exactly how responsibilities are delegated to pharmacy technicians, many pharmacies reserve certain responsibilities only for pharmacy technicians who have been PTCB certified. For example, in some pharmacies, only certified pharmacy technicians may take medication orders over the phone from prescribers, may compound prescriptions or may order prescription drugs for the pharmacy. Further, compensation may differ between pharmacy technicians with and without certification; generally, PTCB-certified pharmacy technicians have greater access to company-provided benefits and higher compensation.

Not to be confused with PTCB certification, pharmacy technicians may also obtain specialization certificates at the direction of the pharmacist that they assist. Depending on the laws of the state where a pharmacy technician practices, they may be able to be certified to administer immunizations, be a certified phlebotomist (someone who draws blood from patients), be certified as a diabetes educator, be certified as a fitter for specialty medical devices such as diabetic shoes, just to name a few opportunities. This type of certification is generally available for PTCB-certified pharmacy technicians as part of continuing education requirements. The reason for obtaining such certifications is both for the advancement of the pharmacy technician and also so the pharmacy technician can better assist a pharmacist in his/her patient care activities.

Although some states require PTCB certification to practice as a pharmacy technician, some leave it up to the pharmacist as to whom she/he believes is qualified to assist them. Further, some states require that a prospective pharmacy technician obtain their PTCB certificate before applying for a license to practice. These states use the PTCB certificate as a licensing examination to show that at least minimum competency to practice as a pharmacy technician has been met before the state issues a license. When a state issues a license, the license-holder is subject to all of the Rules of the licensing Board or Department that governs that license. There is a higher level of responsibility that comes with holding a license because when a pharmacy technician acts outside the scope of their practice or acts unethically, the Board or Department may sanction or revoke their license. Holding this ability gives a state greater influence over who practices as a pharmacy technician and therefore assists in the state's goal of ensuring patient safety by protecting patients against those who, for good reason, should not be practicing. Some states take a slightly different approach in their pharmacy technician regulations.

These states hold that since pharmacy technicians practice under the direction of a pharmacist, who holds a license, those pharmacy technicians should not be issued licenses. Instead, some of these states established registries and require that anyone practicing as a pharmacy technician register with the state. This allows the state to track those who practice as pharmacy technicians, and it allows the state to separate individuals who are banned from practicing as a pharmacy technician due to inappropriate behaviors. This, like licensure, accomplishes a similar patient safety goal.

The United States government also maintains a list of individuals and businesses that are excluded from providing services to federal beneficiaries, such as those patients with Medicare or Medicaid. Again, the goal of these lists is to improve patient safety by preventing those with a history of inappropriate actions from continuing that behavior. If a company participates in federal programs, they are required to check the federal lists to ensure that they do not hire anyone on those lists, and then they are required to regularly check these lists to ensure that their employees do not appear on these lists while employed.

A pharmacy technician should investigate the requirements in his/her state before applying to work in a pharmacy. This may be done by contacting the state's Board of Pharmacy, Department of Community Health, Department of Health and Human Services or similar department within the state. Further, these requirements are continuing to evolve and standardization amongst the states is a goal; so, pharmacy technicians must be vigilant at keeping up on changes to the requirements of their state. There has also been a recent effort at the federal level to have minimum federal standards established that would likely include required PTCB certification for anyone wishing to practice as a pharmacy technician in the United States.

Third Party Regulation of Pharmacy Practice

Another influence on the practice of pharmacy is outside companies and agencies that a pharmacy interacts with or that have jurisdiction over the practice of pharmacy. These can be governmental agencies or private companies. Pharmacies must comply with many sets of rules and regulations that come from multiple sources. Some of the sources for regulations include (but are certainly not limited to): federal law, **Food and Drug Administration (FDA)** Rules, **Drug Enforcement Administration (DEA)** Rules, **Internal Revenue Service (IRS)** rules, **Centers for Medicare and Medicaid Services (CMS)** Rules, state law, Board of Pharmacy Rules, Department of Community Health (or similar state department) Rules, accreditation standards and insurance company contracts. Some of these rules limit the scope of practice for pharmacy technicians and some are so complex that having a pharmacy technician be the pharmacy's expert on the subject is the only way for compliance to be achievable.

It is essential that a pharmacy technician be familiar with the many sources for regulation in pharmacy so that pharmacists can reliably call on pharmacy technicians to assist in keeping the pharmacy compliant. Many companies now have a compliance officer who is responsible for keeping the company up-to-date on all of these regulations and ensuring that everyone is following them; a pharmacy technician is a perfect person to fill this role and should, if nothing else, be an involved part of this process for a pharmacy. This is part of why the PTCB currently requires that at least one hour of continuing education for each certified pharmacy technician be in law during each two-year recertification cycle.

Conclusion

This Manual seeks to prepare a prospective pharmacy technician to practice as a pharmacy technician. This book may be one helpful resource in preparing for the PTCB examination, it may be used as a textbook during a pharmacy technician training program or it may be a resource for a practicing pharmacy technician. The focus of this Manual is to give a prospective pharmacy technician insights and basic knowledge from the perspective of those pharmacists and pharmacy technicians currently in practice. By the end of this Manual, a prospective pharmacy technician will have been given exposure to a basic understanding of the human body, how drugs work in the human body, how pharmacy is practiced, how pharmacy is regulated and how pharmacy technicians are absolutely essential to making this exciting and growing field, pharmacy, meet the goal of helping patients safely and effectively use medications and medical devices to manage their overall health.

Chapter 1
REVIEW QUESTIONS

1. A licensed pharmacist who recently graduated from an accredited College of Pharmacy received which of the following degrees?
    a. Bachelor of Science in Pharmacy (B.S. Pharm.)
    b. Doctor of Philosophy in Pharmacy (Ph.D. Pharm.)
    c. Doctor of Pharmacy (Pharm.D.)
    d. Masters of Medicinal Practice (M.M.P.)

2. The primary role of pharmacy technicians is to allow a pharmacist to focus on:
    a. helping patients with their medication use.
    b. dispensing medications.
    c. office work, business operations and management functions.
    d. claim submission and billing processes.

3. The two primary practice settings for pharmacy technicians are:
    a. ambulatory care and nuclear medicine.
    b. institutional and mail-order pharmacy.
    c. pharmacy organizations and ambulatory care.
    d. institutional and ambulatory care.

4. Pharmacy technicians are not allowed to assist a pharmacist in compounding.
    a. True
    b. False

5. Which of the following is generally true of suppositories?
    a. Suppositories are generally taken orally
    b. Suppositories are generally designed to melt at body temperature
    c. Suppositories must always be compounded and are never commercially produced
    d. Suppositories must never be handled by pharmacy technicians because only a pharmacist may handle suppositories

6. Durable medical equipment can be billed to which of the following insurances?
   a. Medicare Part B
   b. Medicaid
   c. Some commercial insurance companies
   d. All of the above

7. A PTCB-certified pharmacy technician may use which designation?
   a. CPhT
   b. PhCT
   c. PTCB
   d. RphT

8. PTCB-certified pharmacy technicians must complete continuing education that includes at least one hour of which subject area in each two-year cycle to meet the requirements of PTCB?
   a. Pain management
   b. Compounding
   c. Law
   d. Billing and coding

9. Currently, a pharmacy technician must be licensed before beginning to practice as a pharmacy technician anywhere in the United States.
   a. True
   b. False

10. Which agency of the federal government does not have regulatory jurisdiction over some part of the practice of pharmacy?
    a. FDA
    b. FAA
    c. DEA
    d. CMS

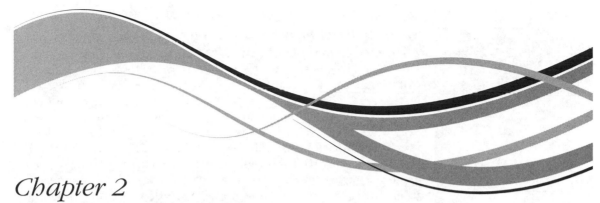

Chapter 2

PHARMACY TERMINOLOGY

By James B. Vander Linde, Pharm.D.

Learning Objectives

This chapter seeks to prepare a pharmacy technician to:
- define the listed medical and pharmacy terminology.
- explain the routes of medication administration.
- describe the types of pharmaceutical dosage forms.
- define the meaning of symbols and abbreviations used in pharmacy.

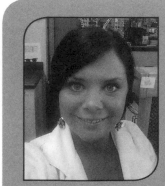

What are the primary resources you have used to study pharmacy terminology? How were they useful to you?

"Over the years, I have learned to use many tools and resources to improve my knowledge of pharmaceuticals. Most reference guides are readily available at your local bookstore, but it is important the guides are not outdated. I have referred to the Generic-Brand Comparison Handbook by UDL Laboratories frequently, and it's small enough to carry with you. Most importantly, I have worked closely with pharmacists who have many years experience.

Using trusted and reliable Web sites is also useful. I recommend using any resources you have to their full extent so you can help patients and yourself understand the importance of pharmacology and products that improve the quality of life."

Elizabeth Stewart, CPhT,
The Prescription Shop,
Traverse City, Mich.

How has your knowledge of pharmacy terminology developed over the years? Have you found that hands-on experience assisted you more than other learning methods?

"My knowledge of pharmacy terminology has vastly improved with my years of experience. Having hands-on practice has given me the opportunity to be exposed to new methods, terms, techniques and the ever-growing changes within the profession of pharmacy. Over the years, I have learned new terms, laws and techniques that I haven't been exposed to before. I feel it is very important and find pharmacy terminology to be easily understood having practical experience."

Introduction

Pharmacy technicians must have the ability to communicate and understand terminology that is used in various health care settings. To that end, this chapter contains definitions of terminology, discussion of medication administration routes and explanations of pharmaceutical dosage forms used in pharmacy practice. Also included are prefixes, suffixes, symbols and abbreviations commonly used in the practice of pharmacy, medicine and related health professions. Pharmacy technicians should be well-versed with this information, as it will be encountered on a regular, if not daily, basis. While the information in this chapter is by no means exhaustive, a mastery of these terms and concepts will provide a solid foundation. It is important to note that each area of pharmacy practice (e.g., community, health-system, long-term care, etc.) will have its own approved list of symbols, abbreviations and terminology, and its own list of banned symbols, abbreviations and terminology. Pharmacy technicians would do well to learn and utilize the symbols and abbreviations that are approved by their practice site. There is also a general shift in practice to avoid, when possible, abbreviations to lessen ambiguity and improve patient safety. This process to reduce the use of symbols and abbreviations will take time, and a pharmacy technician must have a mastery of the information presented in this chapter to best assist the pharmacist and care for patients.

Basic Principles of Pharmacy and Medical Terminology

To understand pharmacy and medical terminology, there are three important word parts that will help dissect and describe common words used in pharmacy practice. The three parts of words include:

- word roots.
- suffixes.
- prefixes.

The **word root** is the core of a word. Some medical terms may contain more than one word root; this potential combination of word roots leads to such large words as cardiopulmonary (referring to the heart and the lungs.) The **suffix** is a word part placed at the end of a word root to modify its meaning. Each medical term may contain a word root and may be modified, or clarified, by adding one or more suffix(es) to the end of the word. Therefore, -itis, meaning inflammation, is added to the word root cardio- or hepato- to create carditis (inflammation of the heart) and hepatitis (inflammation of the liver). A **prefix** is the word part placed at the beginning of a word root to modify its meaning. Medical terms may contain a word root plus one or more prefixes to modify, or clarify, the word. Examples of this include adding the prefix hyper- (excessive, more than normal) to the word root kinetic (motion) or the prefix hypo- (deficient, less than normal) to the word root tension (referring to blood pressure) to create the terms hyperkinetic and hypotension. Table 1 provides several forms of each word part and their definition for a comprehensive review.

Table 1
Medical Word Parts and Their Common English Equivalents

Medical Word Part	Common English Equivalent	Example
a-, an-	Absence of, lacking, no	Achlorhydria (a lack of hydrochloric acid)
-algia	Painful condition	Arthralgia (pain in the joints)
ant-, anti-	Inhibiting, opposing, relieving	Antihistamine (a drug that inhibits histamine)
ante-	Before, forward	Antecubital (before the elbow)
arter-, arteri-, arterio-	Artery	Arteriosclerosis (hardening of the arteries)
arthr-, arthro-	Joint	Arthroscopic (looking into a joint with a camera)
audi-, audio-	Hearing, sound	Audiologist (a hearing specialist)
brady-	Slow	Bradycardia (a slow heart beat)
cardi-, cardio-	Heart	Cardiac arrest (a stopping of the heart)
cervic-, cervico-	Neck	Cervical vertebrae (the spinal bones in the neck)
-cidal, -cide	Killing, killer	Bactericidal (a drug that kills bacteria)
col-, coli-, colo-	Colon	Colitis (inflammation of the colon)

Table 1 *cont.*
Medical Word Parts and Their Common English Equivalents

Medical Word Part	Common English Equivalent	Example
contra-	Against, in opposition	Contraindicated (against the listed indications)
cyst-, cysto-, cyst-	Bladder, sac	Cholecystitis (gall bladder inflammation)
derm-, dermat-, derma-, dermato-, dermo-, -derm	Skin	Dermatologist (a skin expert)
dys-	Abnormal, difficult, impaired	Dysrhythmia (an abnormal heart rhythm)
ect-, ecto-	Outside, external	Ectopic pregnancy (a pregnancy outside the uterus)
-ectomy	Surgical removal	Apendectomy (to remove the appendix by surgery)
-emia	Condition of the blood	Bacteremia (bacterial infection of the blood)
end-, endo-	Inside, within	Endocarditis (inflammation inside the heart)
enter-, entero-	Intestine	Gastroenteritis (inflammation of the stomach and intestines)
-itis	Inflammation	Myelitis (inflammation of the muscles)
macr-, macro-	Large, long	Macrocytic anemia (anemia involving larger than normal red blood cells)
micr-, micro-	Small, minute; one millionth part	Microvascular complications (effects on the small blood vessels)
my-, myo-	Muscle	Myocardial infarction (tissue death of the heart muscle)
nephr-, nephro-	Kidney	Nephrologist (a kidney specialist)
-oma	Tumor	Lymphoma (cancer of the lymph nodes)
ophthalm-, ophthalmo-	Eye	Exophthalmos (a condition where the eyes appear to be protruding from the head)
-osis	Any condition; abnormal or diseased condition	Psychosis (a disease of the mind)
oste-, osteo-	Bone	Osteoporosis (bone loss)

Medical Word Part	Common English Equivalent	Example
ot-, oto-	Ear	Otitis media (inflammation of the middle ear)
path-, patho-, -pathy	Disease	Pathophysiology (study of diseases affecting the body)
-penia	Deficiency	Osteopenia (diminished bone density)
peri-	Around, enclosing	Peri-menopausal (around the time of menopause)
phag-, phago-	Eating	Polyphagia (eating a lot)
phleb-, phlebo-	Vein	Phlebotomy (drawing blood from a vein)
pneum-, pneumo-	Air, gas; lung	Pneumonitis (inflammation of the lung)
proct-, procto-	Anus, rectum	Proctology (study of the anus and rectum)
psych-, psycho-	Mind, mental	Antipsychotics (drugs that treat diseases of the mind)
pulmo-	Lung	Pulmonary edema (fluid in the lungs)
rhine-, rhino-	Nose	Rhinorrhea (a runny nose)
-stomy, -ostomy	Surgical opening	Cholostomy (a hole in the colon)
sub-	Below, underlying; slightly, inadequately	Sublingual (under the tongue)
tachy-	Fast	Tachycardia (fast heart rate)
ther-, thermo-	Heat, temperature	Hypothermia (lower than normal body temperature)
tox-, toxi-, toxo-, toxic-, toxico-	Poisonous	Cytotoxic agent (a drug that kills cells)
uria-	Condition of urine or urination	Polyuria (urinating frequently)
vaso-	Blood vessels	Vasoconstriction (a closing of the blood vessels)

Medical Abbreviations

Most abbreviations used in medicine come from Latin, though some are from Greek, French, German and other languages. Many new abbreviations come from English, but the use of Latin is still alive and well in medical jargon. Technicians must be able to convert freely between the common abbreviations and the English interpretation of those abbreviations. Abbreviation misinterpretation can be a source for medication errors, as many common abbreviations are very close to others. Some patient safety organizations and accrediting groups have lists of banned abbreviations; an abbreviation is usually considered banned if it is commonly involved in medication errors or is more likely to cause medication errors because it looks or sounds like another abbreviation.

The following chart is a list of common abbreviations seen on prescriptions, the Latin that the abbreviation is based upon (when appropriate) and the English interpretation of the abbreviation that will be used when typing a prescription label for a patient. Abbreviations for common measurements (e.g., "mL") and elements on the periodic table (e.g., $FeSO_4$) appear elsewhere and are not included in this list. This list is not meant to be complete; rather, it is a place to begin.

⬥ CAUTION Some of the abbreviations in the following list have been reported to the Institute for Safe Medication Practices (ISMP) as being frequently misinterpreted and involved in harmful medication errors. They are provided here because, unfortunately, they are still often used, and pharmacy technicians must be diligent to make sure they correctly understand a prescription. Do not use these abbreviations at your pharmacy in communicating with other medical professionals. Be sure to check the ISMP's List of Error-Prone Abbreviations, Symbols and Dose Designations at www.ismp.org.

Table 2
Common Pharmacy Medical Abbreviations

Abbreviation	Full Latin Text	English Interpretation
✳ AC (a.c.)	**A**nte **C**ibum	Before a meal or meals
✳ ⬥CAUTION AD (a.d)	**A**uris **D**extra	Right ear
APAP		N-**A**cetyl-**P**-**A**mino**P**henol (the active component in acetaminophen)
AQ (a.q.)	**Aq**ua	Water
✳ ⬥CAUTION AS (a.s.)	**A**uris **S**inistra	Left ear
ASA		**A**cetyl**S**alicylic **A**cid (aspirin)
⬥CAUTION AU (a.u.)	**A**uris **U**traque	Both ears
BID	**B**is **I**n **D**ie	Twice daily
BIW		Twice weekly
BSA		**B**ody **S**urface **A**rea
c or c/	**C**um	With
cc	**C**um **C**ibo	With food
⬥CAUTION cc		**C**ubic **C**entimeter
CR		**C**ontrolled **R**elease
D5W		**D**extrose **5**% in **W**ater

Abbreviation	Full Latin Text	English Interpretation
D5NS		Dextrose 5% in Normal Saline
DAW (d.a.w.)		Dispense As Written
⬥ DC		DisCharge
⬥ d/c or DC		DisContinue
EC		Enteric-Coated
ER		Extended Release
FBS		Fasting Blood Sugar
gtt or gtts	Gutta (plural = Guttae)	Drop(s)
HCTZ		HydroChloroThiaZide
HS (h.s.)	Hora Somni	At bedtime
HTN		HyperTeNsion (high blood pressure)
IEN or EN		In Each Nostril
IM		IntraMuscular (into the muscle)
IR		Immediate Release
IV		IntraVenous (into the vein)
IVP		IntraVenous Push
IVPB		IntraVenous PiggyBack
mEq		milli-Equivalent
MVI		Multi-VItamin
noc or noct	Nocte	At night
NS		Normal Saline (0.9% NaCl)
1/2NS		Half (1/2) Normal Saline (0.45% NaCl)
⬥ OD (o.d.)	Oculus Dexter	Right eye
ODT		Orally Disintegrating Tablet
⬥ OS (o.s.)	Oculus Sinister	Left eye
⬥ OU (o.u.)	Oculus Utraque	Both eyes
Per	Per	Through
PC (p.c.)	Post Cibum (plural = Post Cibos)	After a meal or meals
PRN	Pro Re Nata	As needed
✱ PRN/Anx or P/Anx or prnax		As needed for anxiety
PRN/NV or PNV or P/NV		As needed for nausea and vomiting
PRN/P or P/P		As needed for pain

Table 2 cont.
Common Pharmacy Medical Abbreviations

Abbreviation	Full Latin Text	English Interpretation
PO (p.o.)	**P**er **O**s	By mouth
PR (p.r.)		Through the rectum
PV (p.v.)		Through the vagina
Q	**Q**uaque	Every
QAM	**Q**uaque (die) **A**nte **M**eridiem	Every day, in the morning
◆ QD (q.d.)	**Q**uaque **D**ie	(Once) Every day
QH (q.h.)	**Q**uaque **H**ora	Every hour
◆ QHS (q.h.s.)	**Q**uaque (die) **H**ora **S**omnis	Every day, at bedtime
QID (q.i.d.)	**Q**uater **I**n **D**ie	Four times each day
QOD (q.o.d.)		Every other day
QPM	**Q**uaque (die) **P**ost **M**eridiem	Every day, in the evening
Q4h		Every four hours
Q6h		Every six hours
Q4-6h		Every four to six hours
QS (q.s.)	**Q**uantum **S**ufficiat	**Q**uantity **S**ufficient
s or s/	**S**ine	Without
SA		**S**ustained **A**ction
◆ SC, SubQ, SQ		**S**ub**C**utaneous (below the skin)
Sig		Write on label / post this sign
SL		**S**ub**L**ingual (under the tongue)
SR		**S**ustained **R**elease
Stat	**Stat**im	Immediately
†		One
††		Two
†††		Three
TID	**T**er **I**n **D**ie	Three times daily
◆ TIW		Three times weekly
TPN		**T**otal **P**arenteral **N**utrition
◆ UD or UAD or UtD or UtDict	**U**t **D**ictum	As directed
XL		**EX**tended re**L**ease
XR		**EX**tended **R**elease

The presence of a symbol or abbreviation on one of these lists does not imply that these symbols and abbreviations are official, unambiguous or universally recognized. In fact, though commonly used, several of these abbreviations may be misinterpreted, or may be associated with only one particular practice setting. In some instances, it is valuable to interpret the abbreviation in the context it's used.

Examples:

PT, meaning the allied health specialty of **Physical Therapy**

PT, meaning **P**rothrombin **T**ime

Pt, meaning patient

Pt, meaning part

For more on pharmacy medical abbreviations and interpreting medication orders and prescriptions, see Chapter 5 of this Manual's accompanying Pharmacy Certified Technician Calculations Workbook.

Administration Route

The following are multiple methods of administering medications.

- **Buccal:** the administration of a drug by placing it between the cheek and gum, (the buccal pouch) where it will dissolve or disintegrate slowly
- **Hyperalimentation:** the administration of nutrients intravenously
- **Infusion:** the slow injection of a solution or emulsion into a vein or subcutaneous tissue
- **Inhalation:** the administration of a drug into the lungs or the respiratory tract by air /Nebulizer pathway
- **Intracardiac:** the administration of a drug by injection into the heart
- **Intradermal.** the administration of a drug by injection into the skin
- **Intranasal:** the administration of a drug into the nasal passage via the nares
- **Intraoseous:** the administration of a drug by injection into the bone
- **Intrathecal:** the administration of a drug by injection into the subarachnoid space surrounding the brain and spinal cord
- **Nasogastric:** the administration of a drug through a tube passed through the nose into the stomach
- **Ophthalmic:** the administration of a drug into the eye
- **Otic:** the administration of a drug into the ear
- **Parenteral #1:** the administration of a drug by routes other than orally; not intestinal
- **Parenteral #2:** the administration of a drug by injection; the most common injectable routes are intradermal, intramuscular, intravenous and subcutaneous
- **Rectal:** the administration of a drug into the rectum or lower intestine
- **Topical:** the administration of a drug applied to the skin on the skin only
- **Transdermal:** the administration of a drug across the skin barrier inside the body
- **Vaginal:** the administration of a drug into the vagina

Dosage Forms

The following terminology includes the dosage forms commercially and professionally prepared, along with their definitions or descriptions. Please note that where appropriate, abbreviations are presented in parentheses after the word.

- **Aerosols:** sprayable products employing propellants (liquefied gasses) and valve systems to deliver medication, used for topical application to the skin, inhalation into the lungs and local application in the nose and mouth; medicinal agent may be a liquid or a fine powder; when used for inhalation therapy, a standard amount of drug must be delivered with each activation of the system; metered-dose inhalers are used for this purpose
- **Ampule (Amp):** sterile glass or plastic container with a single dose of parenteral solution
- **Caplet:** tablet that is shaped like a capsule
- **Capsule (Cap):** solid dosage form with the drug enclosed in soluble shells of either hard or soft gelatin; can mask the unpleasant taste and odor of a drug by enclosing them in the almost tasteless shell; sizes range from the smallest (No. 5) to the largest (No. 000); hard gelatin capsules typically contain powders or granules; soft gelatin capsules typically contain liquids; capsules usually dissolve and release their contents in the stomach within 10-15 minutes; extended-release or time-release capsules are formulated to release the drug over a prolonged period of time (usually between eight and 24 hours)
- **Chewable:** tablet that is pleasant tasting and intended to be chewed or dissolved in the mouth and then swallowed
- **Colloidal suspensions:** see Gels
- **Creams:** viscous liquid or semi-solid emulsions of oil and water, generally applied topically to the skin, into the vagina or into the rectum
- **Effervescent:** tablet that contains a mixture of acid and sodium bicarbonate in addition to the active ingredient(s). (These tablets release carbon dioxide and dissolve rapidly when placed in water.)
- **Elixir (El, Elix):** clear, sweetened, liquid dosage form whose primary solvents are water and alcohol; it may contain flavoring substances; medicated elixirs contain active medicinal agents
- **Emulsions:** semi-liquid or solid preparations containing fats and oils suspended with the aid of an agent that promotes and stabilizes the formation of the preparation
- **Enemas:** rectal preparations used to evacuate the bowel (evacuation enemas), for a system's absorption of drugs (retention enema) or for local effect on the lower intestine
- **Enteric-coated (EC):** tablets that have a special coating to prevent dissolution in the stomach so they will dissolve in the intestine instead
- **Extended-release (ER):** tablets that are formulated to release the drug over a prolonged period of time; also referred to as controlled-release, sustained-action, sustained-release or timed-release tablets
- **Eye insert:** small, wafer-like pad designed for insertion under the eyelid where medication is released for an extended period of time
- **Gels:** semi-solid suspension of very small particles, usually in water; may be referred to as a colloidal suspension
- **Inhalers:** delivery devices that are used to administer aerosolized medications; three main types of inhalers are metered-dose aerosol, nebulizer and dry powder inhaler

- **Liniments:** mixtures of various substances in oil, alcohol solutions of soap or emulsions intended for external application; often used for their rubefacient, or heat-producing, effects
- **Lotions:** fluid emulsions or suspensions intended for external application to the body
- **Lozenges:** tablets held in the mouth for slow dissolution; the medication stays in contact with mouth and throat for an extended period of time; also known as troches
- **Matrix:** tablet that contains the active drug in a wax substance, formulated to provide a controlled release of the drug to minimize high concentrations in the gastrointestinal tract
- **Nebulizer:** inhaler device that converts a drug solution into a fine aerosol mist (usually using compressed air or oxygen); the aerosolized medication is then inhaled from a mouthpiece or mask
- **Ointments (Oint., Ung., Ugt.):** semi-solid preparations intended for external application to the skin or mucous membranes
- **Pellets (implanted tablets):** tablets intended for surgical implantation in the subcutaneous tissue. These highly-purified products release a drug over a long period of time.
- **Pledgets:** These are very small sponge-like or wafer-like materials that are impregnated with medication that is then released from the sponge to exert a pharmacologic effect; some ophthalmic medications may be administered in this manner
- **Powders (Pulv.):** fine solid materials intended for use internally or externally
- **Solutions:** liquid preparations containing one or more soluble chemical substances usually dissolved in water
- **Sprays:** liquid medications that are applied in a fine mist or aerosol most commonly for topical application to the skin, throat or nose; may be administered with the assistance of a propellant, a pump spray mechanism or via a squeeze bottle method
- **Sublingual (Subling.):** tablets that are placed under the tongue; sublingual tablets dissolve rapidly when the active ingredient is absorbed directly without passing through the gastrointestinal tract
- **Suppositories (Supp., Suppos.):** solid dosage forms that are usually manufactured in cylindrical, egg or pear shapes for insertion into the rectum, vagina or urethra
- **Suspensions (Susp.):** finely divided, undissolved drugs dispersed in a liquid; often supplied as powder intended for suspension in a suitable liquid vehicle prior to use; suspensions must be well shaken before use
- **Syrup (Syr.):** concentrated solutions of sugar (e.g., sucrose) in water or other aqueous liquid
- **Tablets:** solid dosage forms that vary greatly in shape, size, weight and other properties; most common dosage forms used in the United States, most are swallowed-whole with water and later disintegrate in the gastrointestinal tract; most tablets are made by compression in a large-scale facility; the granular medicinal substances are mixed with fillers, binders and other agents; this granular mixture is subjected to high pressure, utilizing dies and punches to form compressed tablets
- **Tinctures (Tr., Tinct.):** alcoholic or hydroalcoholic solutions prepared from an animal, vegetable or chemical substance; usually contain 10-20 percent (w/v) of the drug
- **Transdermal:** flat, topical systems (patches) intended to provide continuous, controlled release of a drug through a semi-permeable membrane; applied to intact skin
- **Vaginal:** tablets, suppositories, cream or ointments that deliver medication to the vagina; may be inserted with the fingers or a delivery device

Elemental Chemical Symbols and Molecular Formulae

Elemental chemical symbols, and the subsequent molecular formulae using those symbols, are universally recognized and should not be ambiguous. Table 3 contains some commonly used chemical symbols. Refer to any current chemistry text for additional formulae.

Table 3
Chemical Symbols

Chemical Symbol	Chemical
C	Carbon, elemental
Ca	Calcium
Cl	Chlorine
Cl-	Chloride
Cr	Chromium
Cu	Copper
Fe	Iron, elemental
H	Hydrogen
I	Iodine, elemental
K	Potassium, elemental
Mg	Magnesium
Mn	Manganese, elemental
Na	Sodium, elemental
O	Oxygen, elemental
O_2	Oxygen
P	Phosphorous, elemental
PO_4	Phosphate
S	Sulfur, elemental
SO_4	Sulfate
Zn	Zinc, elemental

Pharmacy Terms

Certain terminology is used in the practice of pharmacy when discussing pharmacy law, administrative rules, management and scope of pharmacy practice. See Table 4 for other pharmacy practice abbreviations.

- **Ambulatory pharmacy service:** health care provided by pharmacy professionals to the walk-in (ambulatory) patient
- **Auxiliary labels:** labels affixed to medication containers that provide additional information, reminders or warnings to the patient about medication use and are used to supplement direct patient counseling and the prescription label
- **Brand name:** name assigned to a drug by its manufacturer; often called the proprietary or trade name of a drug
- **Chemical name:** usually the full systematic name for the drug substance
- **Generic name:** convenient and concise name in the public domain used instead of the often unwieldy chemical name of a drug; also referred to as the nonproprietary name
- **Nonprescription:** medication that does not require a prescription; sometimes called over-the-counter (OTC)
- **Patient medication profile:** record of all medications and devices prescribed for an individual patient; may identify patient characteristics, including age, height, sex, diagnoses, previous adverse drug effects and allergies; may also include nonprescription and herbal medications; could also be called a chart, file, record or one of many other names
- **Prescription:** order for a patient's medication or device issued by an appropriately licensed health care professional with prescriptive authority in the state, or country, where the order is given
- **Sterilize:** to render objects, wounds, etc., free of microorganisms usually by destroying them with heat, chemicals or by other means
- **Synergistic response:** when the effect of two or more combined drugs is greater than the sum of their individual effects
- **Toxicity:** harmful or poisonous effect on the human body
- **Toxin:** poison produced by a living organism, often by a bacterium

Table 4
Pharmacy Practice Abbreviations

Abbreviation	Equivalent
aa	Of each
Aq dist	Distilled water
AWP	Average wholesale price
Cpd., cmpd	Compound
CQI	Continuous quality improvement
DEA	Drug Enforcement Administration
Disp.	Dispense
DNA	Deoxyribonucleic acid
DRG	Diagnosis-related group
DUE	Drug utilization evaluation; see also drug utilization review
DUR	Drug utilization review; see also drug utilization evaluation
HMO	Health maintenance organization
Hx	History, as in medical history
ICU	Intensive care unit
LR	Lactated ringers
m. ft.	Mix and make
MAC	Maximum allowable cost
MUE	Medication use evaluation
OBRA	Omnibus Budget Reconciliation Act
OP	Outpatient
OTC	Nonprescription; over-the-counter
PPO	Preferred provider organization
sol., soln.	Solution
Tx	Treatment
USP	United States Pharmacopeia
VO	Verbal order

Weights and Measures

The terminology found in pharmaceutical weights and measures for liquids and solids is based on the metric system (see Table 5 for common weight and measure abbreviations). There is limited reference to the apothecary system; the apothecary system is seldom used in current pharmacy practice.

Examples:

mg, milligram, meaning one one-thousandth of a gram

mL, milliliter, meaning one one-thousandth of a liter

For additional weight and measure abbreviations, see Table 5 below.

Table 5
*Weight and Measure Abbreviations**

Abbreviation	Weight / Measure
cc	Cubic centimeter
cm	Centimeter
g, gm.	Gram
Gr.	Grain
Gtt.	Drop
Kg	Kilogram
L	Liter
lb.	Pound
mcg	Microgram
mEq	Milliequivalent
mg	Milligram
mL	Milliliter
mm	Millimeter
mmol	Millimole
oz.	Ounce
Tbsp.	Tablespoon
Tsp.	Teaspoon
u.; un.	Unit

Although it is important to recognize these abbreviations, it may not always be good practice to use them, as they may be misinterpreted (see "Safety Concerns" section and Table 6.)

For more on pharmacy measurement systems and conversions, see Chapter 3 of this Manual's accompanying Pharmacy Certified Technician Calculations Workbook.

Safety Concerns with Abbreviations, Symbols and Acronyms

While using abbreviations, acronyms and symbols may be convenient, and appear to save time in the medication ordering process, this practice has the potential to lead to misinterpretation and can be the cause of medication errors. There are many instances documented in medical and pharmacy literature of serious medication errors resulting in patient harm and death due to misinterpretation of abbreviations, acronyms and symbols that were used in the medication ordering process. This is particularly true when two similar drugs share the same dose range and route of administration. As an example, "HCTZ 50 mg" could be interpreted as 50 mg of the diuretic hydrochlorothiazide or as 50 mg of the steroid hydrocortisone. It is always the safest practice to spell out clearly the full name of the medication being prescribed. Where possible, the diagnosis or condition being treated may be included in order to provide further clarification of the intended use of the medication. Whenever there is a question or doubt about what is meant by a particular abbreviation, symbol or acronym, the prescriber must be contacted for clarification in order to avoid a medication error.

Another source of documented medication errors that a pharmacy technician must be vigilant about is the use of the decimal point. Many medication errors occur when a decimal point is used in conjunction with a zero. It is easy to miss a written decimal point, resulting in an incorrect interpretation of a dose. When using the decimal point in relation to a zero, the rule is to always use a zero preceding a decimal point but never use a zero trailing a decimal point. As an example, 0.1 is correctly written to indicate one-tenth; however, 1.0 is incorrectly written to indicate one. The correct way to depict the value one is 1 without the decimal point and trailing zero.

The concern for the safety issues associated with the use of abbreviations is such that the Joint Commission on the Accreditation of Health Care Organizations has incorporated the requirement for the safe use of abbreviations into its National Patient Safety Standards. For health care organizations, there is now the expectation that each organization will standardize those abbreviations, symbols and acronyms that are used along with a list of abbreviations, symbols and acronyms that are not approved for use. Further, it is recommended that there be a process to identify abbreviations to be used and a means of communicating the information to all applicable staff and other individuals.

Table 6 represents several abbreviations and symbols that may be misinterpreted.

Table 6
Abbreviations and Symbols Commonly Misinterpreted

Abbreviation	Potential Problem	Preferred Term
U	Mistaken as zero, four or cc	Write the word "unit"
Q.D.	Mistaken for QOD (every other day) or QID (four times daily)	Write "daily" or "once daily"
Q.O.D.	Mistaken for QD (once daily) or QID (four times daily)	Write "every other day"
Trailing zero (X.0 mg), Lack of leading zero (.X mg)	Decimal point is missed	Never write a zero by itself after a decimal point (.X mg). Always use a zero before a decimal point (0.X mg).
$MgSO_4$	Mistaken as morphine sulfate	Write "magnesium sulfate"
MSO_4, MS	Mistaken for magnesium sulfate	Write "morphine sulfate"

Abbreviation	Potential Problem	Preferred Term
μg	Mistaken for mg (milligram), resulting in a one thousand-fold increase in dose	Write "mcg" or spell out "microgram"
H.S.	This can be mistaken for half-strength or at bedtime (writing q. H.S. can be mistaken for every hour.)	Write out "half-strength" or "at bedtime"
T.I.W.	Mistaken for three times per day or twice weekly	Write "3 times weekly" or "three times weekly"
S.C. or S.Q.	Mistaken as SL for sublingual, or "5 every"	Write "Sub-Q", subQ, or "subcutaneously"
D/C	Interpreted as discontinue whatever medications follow (typically discharge meds)	Write "discharge"
c.c.	Mistaken for U (units) when poorly written	Write "mL" for milliliters to express volumes of liquids
A.S., A.D., A.U. (for left ear, right ear or both ears)	Mistaken for each other (e.g., A.S. for O.S., A.D. for O.D., A.U. for O.U., etc.)	Write "left ear," "right ear" or "both ears"
O.S., O.D., O.U (for left eye, right eye or both eyes)		Write "left eye," "right eye" or "both eyes"
ss (for sliding scale)	Mistaken for 55 or half	Write out "sliding scale"
>	Easily confused	Write out "greater than"
<	Easily confused	Write out "less than"

Conclusion

Understanding commonly used terminology and abbreviations is essential to the practice of pharmacy. Pharmacy technicians in all practice settings will utilize this information on a daily basis when interpreting medication directions for computer entry, calculating appropriate amounts of additives for intravenous solutions, understanding a patient's therapy for a particular diagnosis and many other circumstances. Pharmacy technicians increase their ability to function more efficiently in the pharmacy and provide greater support to pharmacists when they enhance their knowledge of the items discussed in this chapter.

Bibliography

- Brooks, M.L., Exploring Medical Language, A Student-Directed Approach, 4th edition, Mosby, 1998.
- Chabner, Davi-Ellen, The Language of Medicine, 5th edition, 1996.
- Facts and Comparisons, J. B. Lippincott Company, St. Louis, MO, 1995.
- Masters, T., Masters, R., Terminology for Allied Health Professions with Medical Terminology, A Visual Guide, 1997.
- Michigan Pharmacists Association, Pharmacy Certified Technician Training Manual, Lansing, MI, 2010.
- Shargel, et al., Comprehensive Pharmacy Review, 3rd edition, 1997.
- Traupman, John C., The Bantam New College Latin & English Dictionary, New York, NY: Bantam Books, 1995.

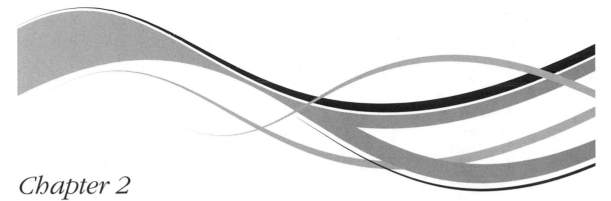

Chapter 2

REVIEW QUESTIONS

1. What does the abbreviation "a.c." mean?
    a. Before meals
    b. Left ear
    c. In the morning
    d. As directed

2. What does the abbreviation "IM" mean?
    a. In the morning
    b. Intramuscular
    c. Intravenous
    d. Right ear

3. What does the abbreviation "q.h." mean?
    a. Before noon
    b. Four times daily
    c. Daily, every day
    d. Every hour

4. What does the chemical symbol "K" represent?
    a. Calcium
    b. Potassium
    c. Iron
    d. Sulfate

5. What does the chemical symbol "$MgPO_4$" represent?
    a. Magnesium phosphate
    b. Manganese phosphate
    c. Magnesium sulfate
    d. Morphine sulfate

6. What is the most common dosage form in the United States?
   a. Tablet
   b. Capsule
   c. Lozenge
   d. Emulsion

7. Which route of medication administration involves dissolving a tablet under the tongue?
   a. Intraoseous
   b. Sublingual
   c. Intravenous
   d. Intrathecal

8. Which of the following is a semi-solid suspension of very small particles, usually in water?
   a. Suspension
   b. Solution
   c. Emulsion
   d. Gel

9. In pharmacy weights and measures, what does a "gtt" represent?
   a. Gram
   b. Tetrigram
   c. Drop
   d. Grain

10. Which of the following terms can be misinterpreted?
    a. Q.D.
    b. T.I.W.
    c. Q.O.D.
    d. All of the above

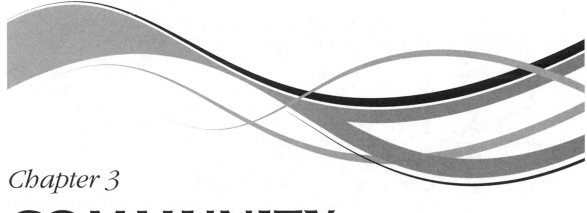

Chapter 3

COMMUNITY PHARMACY PRACTICE

By Derek J. Quinn, Pharm.D.

Learning Objectives

This chapter seeks to prepare a pharmacy technician to:
- distinguish between items that require a prescription and items that do not.
- distinguish between those who may prescribe medications and those who may not.
- recognize the anatomy of a prescription (including appropriate methods to handle missing or incorrect information).
- discuss the ways a prescription can be transmitted to a pharmacy and the special requirements for each type of transmission.
- examine the prescription dispensing process and how pharmacy technicians can be involved at each step of that process.
- discuss the common technologies used in community pharmacy practice and how pharmacy technicians commonly interact with these technologies.
- examine common billing errors, as well as common claim rejections, and what those rejections mean.
- recognize the anatomy of a prescription label.
- discuss the methods, verbal and written, for providing drug/medical information to patients, with a focus on those methods that can be delegated to a pharmacy technician.
- discuss the administrative roles that pharmacy technicians may be asked to fill in a community pharmacy.

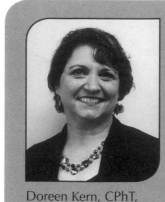

How do you believe the role of a pharmacy technician in a community setting differs from other environments?

"Community pharmacy, also known as retail ambulatory pharmacy, is as diversified as it is in varied names. It also includes independent, department/grocery store, franchise, chain and mail-order pharmacies. I believe the role of a pharmacy technician in a community setting differs from other environments in the importance of customer service. Any pharmacy (sometimes with one on each corner) can fill prescriptions and sell aspirin or bandages, but building relationships, greeting customers by name and becoming a part of the community is what is going to bring them back again and again."

Doreen Kern, CPhT,
The Prescription Shop,
Glen Arbor, Mich.

Why is the role of a technician vital to community pharmacy practice?

"Community pharmacy is always evolving, consistently finding ways to advance the role of the pharmacist, such as with medication therapy management (MTM), immunizations, compounding and medical clinics. Along with the usual responsibilities of filling prescriptions, inventory control, third party adjudication and reconciliation, telephone calls, patient questions and consultations, the role of a technician is vital to the community pharmacy practice to pick up many other duties traditionally done by a pharmacist, providing many opportunities for technicians to shine in leadership roles."

Introduction

Pharmacy technicians in the community pharmacy practice setting are often the first point of contact for patients interacting with the pharmacy. Pharmacy technicians enter prescription orders into electronic medical records, prepare prescription drugs for dispensing, ready durable medical equipment and supplies for dispensing, and often are the last point of contact at the pharmacy after a pharmacist has interacted with the patient. After observing a seasoned pharmacy technician for only a few moments, it is clear that extensive multitasking is a required part of practicing as a pharmacy technician, as they are answering the telephone, greeting patients, typing prescriptions, preparing medications for dispensing, interacting with prescribers and their office staff, and keeping it all in order. This chapter seeks to break down many of these tasks and highlight the essential knowledge that every pharmacy technician must have before walking into a community pharmacy.

Which Drugs and Devices Require a Prescription?

Some drugs require a prescription, and some do not; some medical devices and supplies require a prescription, and some do not. How is a pharmacy technician supposed to know what needs a prescription? Unfortunately, there is no automatic or easy way to look at a drug and know if it requires a prescription. There are, however, some general guidelines that will help a pharmacy technician distinguish between prescription and nonprescription items. In general, the drugs kept behind the pharmacy counter require a prescription and the drugs kept over-the-counter do not require a prescription.

Drugs are regulated at both the federal and state level. A state legislature, and sometimes a Board of Pharmacy, has the right to list a drug as requiring a prescription (or not). Further, the Food and

Drug Administration (FDA) and the U.S. Congress have the right to list a drug as requiring a prescription (or not). Since it is considered more restrictive to require a prescription than to not require one, if either the state or the federal government requires a prescription (even if the other does not), then the item requires a prescription. Generally, medications that are considered prescription drugs must include information from the manufacturer (called a package insert or prescribing information) that is regulated by the FDA. Further, drugs that require a prescription generally have the note "R$_x$ Only" on the package. Generally, drugs that are considered over-the-counter have a panel on the outside of the package labeled "Drug Facts" that is regulated by the FDA.

Some drugs require more regulation, and those drugs are called controlled substances. The Drug Enforcement Administration (DEA), the U.S. Congress, a state legislature and sometimes a Board of Pharmacy can designate a drug as being a controlled substance. These drugs are usually prescription drugs. They are placed in schedules; a schedule is a ranking based on either how addictive the drug can be or on how likely it is to be abused and misused. Schedule I controlled substances are "street drugs," like heroin, that the FDA has determined have no legitimate medicinal purpose. Schedule 2 controlled substances have a high potential for abuse, such as morphine and amphetamines. Schedules 3 and 4 contain pain relievers, anti-anxiety drugs and many other potential drugs of abuse that are not quite as likely to be as abused as Schedule 2 drugs. Schedule 5 drugs can be tricky; some require a prescription from a physician and some require a prescription from a pharmacist. Some states allow codeine-based cough syrups, generally listed in Schedule 5, to be dispensed based on a pharmacist's recommendation, but they must be kept behind the counter. Other Schedule 5 drugs require a physician's order.

Within over-the-counter drugs, there are a few oddities. The FDA has listed emergency oral contraception (sold under the brand name Plan B®, or the generic Next Choice®, etc.) as requiring a prescription for purchasers under the age of 17 but are over-the-counter for patients 17 and older. Some states have placed further restrictions on the sale of these products—either way, a pharmacist needs to be involved in the dispensing and sale of these products. There are also products that the FDA considers food (or dietary supplements) rather than drugs, even if these products exhibit effects on the body just like drugs do. These products are regulated under a different set of rules. There are also homeopathic products, which the FDA regulates in the same way that over-the-counter drugs are regulated.

Finally, there are medical devices. Some medical devices require a prescription according to the FDA; generally the more complex devices that are necessary to treat a disease require a prescription under the FDA's rules. States are also free to regulate medical devices; some states have laws requiring all medical devices to be dispensed only with a prescription and some allow the federal rules to determine the requirements within the state. Patients are generally encouraged to have a prescription written for any drug, device or supplement that is recommended to them by a physician. This helps the pharmacy to maintain an accurate record of the products used by the patient and may allow for the cost of the device, drug or supply to be covered by an insurance company (insurance companies generally do not cover items purchased without a prescription from a pharmacy).

Who May Write Prescriptions

Most people who are unfamiliar with the prescribing laws are shocked to find out just how many different professions can prescribe. Again, each state can regulate the practice of prescribing, but the following can commonly prescribe noncontrolled substances: medical doctors (MD), doctors of osteopathy (DO), physician's assistants (PA), nurse practitioners (NP, CNM, CNA, etc.), dentists/oral surgeons (DDS), podiatrists (DPM) and veterinarians (DVM). Generally, physician's assistants and nurse practitioners may not prescribe independently; instead, they are delegated the right to prescribe from the physician whom they are working under. Further, some states allow physicians to delegate limited prescribing authority to others. For instance, pharmacists may sometimes enter into collaborative practice agreements in order to prescribe. Some states also allow optometrists (OD) and psychologists (PhD Psych.) to prescribe after receiving appropriate training to do so. Regardless of the specialty, prescribers must stick to their scope of practice (e.g., podiatrists specialize in the hands and feet and therefore are not permitted in most cases to manage a patient's blood pressure with prescription drugs.) Controlled substances are generally more restricted by many states; commonly, states prevent some or all prescribing authority for controlled substances from being delegated.

The list of who generally cannot prescribe is also of some importance. Commonly, people expect that chiropractors (DC), physical therapists (DPT), respiratory therapists, certified diabetes educators and others have prescribing rights. Although exceptions may exist, generally these valuable health professionals are not granted prescribing rights because their specialty does not include the appropriate training necessary for prescriptive authority. A pharmacy technician is encouraged to always consult his or her pharmacist if a prescription looks unusual or appears to be written outside the scope of practice for the prescriber.

The Anatomy of a Prescription

It must once again be said that each state has different requirements for exactly what must be on a prescription; however, there are common elements that can be examined. Further, prescriptions for controlled substances have requirements that are generally stricter than prescriptions for noncontrolled substances. The following example is a typical prescription for a controlled substance (Norco® is a Schedule 3 controlled substance). Use the bold numbers in brackets **[1]** to identify the parts of this prescription; an explanation of each item, including some of the rules surrounding each item, are listed below the prescription example.

---

[1] Rex Exempli, M.D.
8822 Portage Road
Portage, IN 46368

608.892.4385 Phone
608.892.4386 Fax

[2] NPI 1124049176
[3] DEA FE8043159

[4] Rhonda Kingslight, P.A.
[2] NPI 8763019287
[3] DEA MK6561876

[4] Jeff Jamerson, N.P.
[2] NPI 6532856987

[4] JoAnne Langdon, C.N.M.
[2] NPI 1121134523
[3] DEA ML8888543

---

[5] Patient: _____ Heather Allen _____   D.O.B.: __ 10/18/1952 __
Address: __ 6909 West Q Avenue West LaFayette, IN 47907 __

[6] Date: __ 07 May 2013 __

[7] Norco® 10 mg/325 mg Tablets
[8] Sig †/†† PO Q4/6h P/P

[9] Dispense: __ 40 (forty) tablets __   **[10]** Refills: __ 5 (five) __

[11] DAW*: _____   **[12]** Signature: _____ *JoAnne Langdon* _____

*If manufacturer specification is medically necessary, then "DAW" must appear in the prescriber's own handwriting.

---

[1] Physician

This information is often pre-printed onto the prescription blank. This includes the degree of the physician (M.D., D.O., D.P.M., etc.) after his/her name. Also, the telephone number and practice address for the physician is listed. If many physicians have come together as part of a single practice, only the practice information may appear. In most states, it is not required to have the physician's name pre-printed onto the prescription.

[2] National Provider Identifier

The **National Provider Identifier (NPI)** is a number assigned to each health care provider and each health care facility. Physicians, pharmacists, nurse practitioners, dentists and many other professionals (including student pharmacists) may register for an NPI. Further, each pharmacy, hospital and clinic has its own NPI. This number is essential for completing the process of billing a prescription claim to an insurance company. In most situations, this number is not required by law to appear on a prescription, but all prescribers are encourage to list their NPI as it is required for the prescription to be properly billed.

[3] DEA Number

Any prescriber who is licensed to prescribe controlled substances and wishes to do so must register with the DEA to receive a registration number. Mid-level prescribers, such as physician's assistants or certified nurse mid-wives, may obtain their own DEA number but must show proof that a physician has delegated prescribing authority to them; however, a prescriber may elect not to register with the DEA if he/she does not wish to ever prescribe controlled substances. Notice that one of the mid-level prescribers on this prescription, Jeff Jamerson, has not reported a DEA registration number and has therefore not likely registered with the DEA to prescribe controlled substances. Many prescribers do not have their DEA number pre-printed on the prescription blanks that they use because it is only required, in most instances, to appear on prescriptions for controlled substances.

[4] Mid-Level Practitioners

Mid-level practitioners must work under a physician (generally an M.D. or D.O.) and have their prescribing authority delegated to them from that physician. Mid-level practitioners include physician's assistants, nurse practitioners, certified nurse midwives and many others.

[5] Patient

Although the patient's name is essential, the patient's address is only required by many states on prescriptions for controlled substances. Further, it is standard practice to include the patient's date of birth on a prescription to help ensure that the right patient chart is identified throughout the prescription filling process.

[6] Date Written

Prescriptions must be dated. This must be the date that the prescriber actually writes the prescription; prescribers may not pre-date or post-date prescriptions. This is important as prescriptions are only valid for a period of time after they are written.

[7] Drug, Strength and Dose Form

The name of the drug (either by brand name or by the generic name—in this case, Norco® is the brand name and hydrocodone/acetaminophen is the generic name) must be on the prescription. Further, the strength of the drug to be dispensed must appear; it is strongly encouraged that even if only one strength exists that it be included on the prescription. Finally, the dose form is only required when multiple dose-forms exist; however, prescribers are encouraged to list the dose form on each prescription.

[8] Sig

On a prescription, the term "sig" refers to the directions. Sig is an abbreviation from Latin and loosely means "write on the label." What follows is usually written in a short-hand that includes mostly Latin abbreviations (though many abbreviations from English are becoming common). On this particular prescription, the sig would expand to appear on the label as: "Take one or two tablets, by mouth, every four to six hours as needed for pain."

[9] Quantity to Dispense

This instructs the pharmacy on how many tablets to dispense. For controlled substance prescriptions, this must be written in both numbers (40) and words (forty). For other dose forms, such as nasal sprays, this quantity may either be the number of nasal spray bottles (e.g., one, two or three) or may be the metric quantity (e.g., 16 mL) to dispense.

[10] Refills

This indicates the number of refills allowed to the patient. Prescriptions for controlled substances are generally allowed only five refills (except for Schedule 2 drugs, which may not have any refills), while prescriptions for noncontrolled substances are generally not restricted as to the number of refills allowed. When allowed, a prescriber may indicate "prn" or "*pro re nata*" for refills, which is Latin for "as needed" and allows the patient as many refills as they desire until the prescription expires (a limit may be imposed by insurance coverage or as determined to be appropriate by a pharmacist). If refills are not indicated on the prescription, then it is assumed that no refills have been indicated.

[11] DAW

DAW stands for "Dispense As Written," which means that the prescriber is mandating which manufacturer's product must be used to fill the prescription. Generally, this is only used to indicate that the original brand may be used; however, a prescriber may specify a manufacturer on the prescription and then write DAW to indicate that this manufacturer's product is medically necessary for the patient. States vary on the requirements for putting a "DAW" on a prescription; some states require that the initials DAW appear in the prescriber's own handwriting, some require only that a box on the prescription be checked, and some have two separate signature lines on the prescription and the prescriber signs above the statement "brand medically necessary" or "substitution permitted" based on his/her choice.

[12] Signature

The prescriber must sign the prescription for it to be valid. If the prescription is transmitted to the pharmacy electronically, then the signature must be an electronic signature. If the prescription arrives by hand or by fax, the signature must be a hand-written signature applied to the piece of paper. Prescriptions telephoned into the pharmacy do not have to include a signature but must include the name of the prescriber and the prescription must indicate that it was telephoned in.

Transmitting a Prescription to a Pharmacy

A prescriber may transmit a prescription to the pharmacy in one of four ways. The prescription may be physically brought to the pharmacy (written), telephoned to the pharmacy, electronically transmitted to the pharmacy or transmitted by fax to the pharmacy. Prescriptions, especially for controlled substances, may have different restrictions in each state for how they may be transmitted. DEA regulations were revised in 2010 to allow controlled substances to be electronically transmitted to a pharmacy after a specific set of security measures is adopted by both the prescriber and pharmacy;

transmission of a prescription for a controlled substance to a pharmacy, even if all of the federal requirements are met, must be legal in the state where the pharmacy resides. Many insurance companies now require that the method of transmission for the prescription be indicated on all submitted claims.

Prescriptions that are hand written and brought to the pharmacy may either be completely hand-written or may be typed and then manually signed by the prescriber. In most states, a prescriber may have someone else prepare the prescription for them to review and sign, so the handwriting on the prescription may differ from the signature. Generally, all schedules of controlled substances (and noncontrolled substances) may be prescribed on a hand-written prescription. Some states, and some insurance companies, require that hand-written prescriptions be written on tamper-resistant or tamper-evident paper. In some cases, what qualifies as tamper-resistant is strictly specified by the state; however, in some cases, the requirements for tamper resistance simply specify the types of resistance that must be present but not how to achieve that resistance. For instance, Medicaid may require that the prescription prevents duplication on a photocopy machine. This may be achieved by a watermark that only appears when photocopied or it may be achieved by having a multicolored background that will not reproduce properly on a photocopier.

Prescriptions that are telephoned into the pharmacy must, generally, include the names of the people at each end of the telephone conversation and be immediately written down. Although states differ on who may call in and who may receive telephoned prescriptions, generally all prescriptions for noncontrolled substances and prescriptions for controlled substances in Schedules 3–5 may be transmitted to the pharmacy by telephone. It is prudent for a modern pharmacy to have telephones with caller ID to assist in preventing fraudulent prescriptions from being transmitted to the pharmacy. Prescriptions being telephoned to the pharmacy must come directly from the prescriber or the prescriber's office; patients may not telephone their own prescriptions into the pharmacy even if they have a written order in their possession. Some states restrict receiving prescriptions over the telephone to only licensed pharmacists; however, many states allow a pharmacist to delegate this responsibility to a pharmacy technician if the pharmacist assesses that the pharmacy technician is properly trained to do so. Many pharmacists require that pharmacy technicians obtain PTCB certification before taking oral orders over the telephone from a prescriber. Anyone taking prescriptions over the phone must be familiar with commonly available medications, common dosages for those medications, common directions for use, approved and banned abbreviations used (or not used) on prescriptions and requirements for what must appear on a prescription received by telephone.

Electronically-transmitted prescriptions are becoming more common as adoption of the necessary software by both pharmacies and prescribers is becoming more widespread. Prescriptions that are transmitted electronically to pharmacies must be electronically signed; what constitutes a valid electronic signature is defined by each sate and therefore will differ from state to state. Further, what constitutes an electronically-transmitted prescription differs in each jurisdiction; some states consider a prescription that is generated by a computer in the prescriber's office and received by the pharmacy's fax machine to be an electronic prescription. Some states only allow prescriptions transmitted from a computer to a computer to be considered valid electronic prescriptions. In either case, there is no paper record of the prescription ever generated in the prescriber's office—the prescription is generated on a computer and the record is stored on a computer. As previously mentioned, the DEA began allowing controlled substances in all Schedules (2–5) to be transmitted electronically as long as such transmission is allowed in the state where the pharmacy is located and if both the prescriber's software and the pharmacy's software meet certain security and functionality standards. In some cases, prescribing software allows a prescription for a controlled substance to be sent electronically to a pharmacy when either the prescriber or the pharmacy is not yet meeting the DEA standards; these prescriptions may not be accepted by the pharmacy without calling the prescriber to authenticate the prescription (or, for prescriptions for controlled substances in Schedule 2, the prescriber must transmit a handwritten prescription to replace the electronic prescription transmitted incorrectly).

Finally, prescribers may transmit a prescription via fax machine. A faxed prescription is one that is generated in the prescriber's office (either by hand or typed), manually signed in the prescriber's office and then placed on a fax machine for transmission to the pharmacy. In this case, the original paper prescription is retained by the prescriber for his/her records. Faxed prescriptions may not be electronically signed (even if they are typed). Although each state differs on its requirements, generally prescriptions for noncontrolled substances and prescriptions for controlled substances in Schedules 3–5 may be transmitted by fax. Pharmacy technicians must properly identify prescriptions that arrive via fax as being faxed prescriptions or as being electronic prescriptions that arrive by fax.

The Prescription Dispensing Process

Upon receiving a prescription, the first step (generally performed by a pharmacy technician) is to review the prescription to ensure that all required information is present. If the patient is bringing in the prescription, information about the patient should be verified for completeness and correctness (i.e., proper spelling of the patient's name, the patient's date of birth is on the prescription and correct, and who prescribed the medication). If any information is missing or incomplete, the pharmacy technician who finds the prescription to be incomplete should alert his or her pharmacist for instructions or follow the pharmacy's standard procedures for obtaining the missing information. Many times, the prescriber can be reached by telephone to clarify his or her intentions; in most cases involving Schedule 2 controlled substances, the prescription must be returned to the prescriber for manual correction. Any information changed or added to a prescription must be accompanied by identifying who authorized the change or addition, as well as the date and time that the change was authorized. Pharmacy technician involvement in this process is at the discretion of the pharmacist on duty.

The next step is for a pharmacy technician (or pharmacist) to enter the information on the prescription into the patient's electronic medical record (EMR), often called a chart or profile, at the pharmacy. This will involve finding the correct EMR using the patient's name and any other identifier provided on the prescription (such as a date of birth, address or phone number). Further, it will involve entering the product ordered by the prescriber and then, based on the state laws on substitution and the direction of the pharmacist on duty, select the actual product to be dispensed. In many cases, a prescription will be written for a brand name of a drug but a less expensive product of equal quality (a generic) will be dispensed. This part of the process will also, likely, include generating and transmitting a claim to an insurance company, or pharmacy benefit manager, for that prescription. Finally, after receiving a paid claim by the patient's insurance company, if one is being billed, a label is generated that will be used in the next step of the process to label the vial or product being dispensed to the patient.

Next, a pharmacy technician (or pharmacist) reads the label and the prescription to verify that the label was prepared correctly. Then, the person preparing the prescription selects the correct product from the pharmacy's inventory and separates the ordered quantity from the pharmacy inventory for dispensing to the patient. For tablets and capsules, this means using a counting tray and spatula to count out the required number of tablets or capsules from the stock bottle. For pre-packaged dose forms, such as inhalers or nasal sprays, this involves selecting the correct number of inhalers or nasal sprays from the pharmacy inventory. Certain drugs must include a MedGuide or a patient handout with each fill; this information must be retrieved (or printed) and included with the product being dispensed. Further, most pharmacies provide a handout (called a monograph) to each patient receiving a new drug for the first time; some pharmacies provide a monograph at each refill, some provide the monograph at least once each year and some provide it only at the first fill of that drug for the patient. Each pharmacy determines its own policy on providing monographs. The FDA mandates that a Medication Guide (or MedGuide) be provided to a patient at both the time of first fill and at each refill thereafter (without exception unless the prescriber exempts the patient from the MedGuide requirement by writing so on the prescription). Some drugs have a patient handout included in their labeling that is neither a MedGuide nor a monograph, and it is generally under the pharmacist's discretion as to when these are provided to a patient.

The last step before presenting a prescription to a pharmacist for verification is that the drug, if it is a tablet or capsule, is put into a vial, the vial is labeled and the vial, the prescription, any paperwork prepared for the patient and usually the stock bottle that the tablets or capsules came from are presented to a pharmacist. Exactly how this is presented varies based on the pharmacy's policies. Some pharmacies use a system of baskets or bins to hold everything for one patient, some want all of this piled in a specific way on the counter. Regardless of the system, it is important to be consistent so as to prevent errors; by making this part of the process standardized, a pattern can be established that will help prevent errors. At this point, a pharmacist must verify that the work done by her or his pharmacy technician(s) has been done correctly and that the prescription is appropriate (the dose is correct, the drug is appropriate for the patient and that the prescription is complete and properly written). This verification step includes ensuring that the label was prepared properly, that the correct product was selected from the pharmacy inventory and that the correct amount of product is being dispensed to the patient. After being checked (verified) by a pharmacist, the finished product and all of the information prepared for the patient are bagged and placed in a will-call system awaiting the patient to come in to pick up the medication. The process of bagging prescriptions may be done by a pharmacist but also may be delegated to a pharmacy technician at the pharmacist's discretion. Medication must NEVER leave the pharmacy (and generally must not be bagged) without a pharmacist reviewing the appropriateness of the therapy and the preparation work done by his or her pharmacy technician(s). Finally, prescriptions that were bagged and placed in the will-call system are picked up by patients and a pharmacist provides verbal information to the patient (or the patient's caregiver) on the proper use of the medication; this process is usually referred to as counseling. Counseling requires the training that a pharmacist undergoes and may NEVER be delegated to a pharmacy technician.

Other than verification and counseling, unless a state's laws are more restrictive, a pharmacist may delegate all other steps in processing a prescription to pharmacy technicians. Generally, states require that a pharmacist prepare a written manual of what has been delegated to a pharmacy technician, and this manual includes very detailed policies and procedures for pharmacy technicians to follow. In most cases, pharmacy technicians who work with a particular pharmacy software become the billing and filling experts with that software and serve as a resource for the pharmacists that they assist. Further, inventory management is often delegated to pharmacy technicians. Although everything that occurs in the pharmacy is the responsibility of the licensed pharmacist, it is the responsibility of every pharmacy technician to know exactly what tasks have been delegated to them, how to do those tasks and when to involve a pharmacist.

Common Technologies Used in Pharmacy Practice

The practice of pharmacy has changed a lot in the last 100 years. It wasn't that long ago that very few drugs were made by pharmaceutical companies in pressed tablets or filled capsules. A pharmacist would order raw ingredients and then combine ingredients at the time of a prescription being received into a finished product. At that time, an accurate balance (scale) and a mortar and pestle were the essential tools of the trade. Now, balances, mortars and pestles are still a part of the process, but counting robots, interactive voice-response telephone systems, digital scales, inventory management systems and electronic medical records are standard in many pharmacies. Further, because new technology continues to transform the practice, the following overview may change significantly in the next few years.

Hardware

■ **Computers**

Without first recognizing the role of computers in modern pharmacy practice, the other technologies, all of which stem from the main computers, cannot be fully appreciated. Pharmacy technicians are generally the chief person in the pharmacy responsible for interacting with the pharmacy computers.

■ **Interactive Voice-Response Systems**

Interactive voice-response (IVR) systems connect the pharmacy's telephone to the pharmacy's computers. An IVR can do as much as handling every call that comes into the pharmacy to as little as being an after-hours answering machine. The IVR handles incoming telephone calls and helps route calls to the appropriate recipient. Some even allow patients to type in refill requests over the phone that are then received by the pharmacy computers and presented to a pharmacy technician for processing. Pharmacy technicians can have responsibilities such as retrieving voice mail, retrieving refill requests and recording messages that play through the IVR for patients on hold or who are preparing to leave a message.

■ **Counting Robots**

Many companies offer counting robots for pharmacies to use instead of counting out each prescription by hand. Generally, robots handle a finite number of drugs, usually the drugs dispensed most frequently by the pharmacy, and do the counting work. Generally, these robots interact with the pharmacy computers to receive which prescriptions are to be filled by the robot. Before pharmacy technicians decide to fear robots replacing qualified personnel, a pharmacy technician must remember that most modern robots begin with a pharmacy technician entering a prescription order into a computer that is then sent to the robot for counting. This allows for the pharmacy technician to have more time to assist the pharmacist with his/her duties and spend less time at the counting tray.

■ **Counting Assistants**

These can be scales that weigh tablets to decide how many have been counted out, optical scanners that record how many tablets/capsules pass by the scanner or visual counting devices that actually count the number of tablets that appear in an image (just to name a few types of devices). These tools assist pharmacists and pharmacy technicians to be more efficient at counting prescription orders.

■ **Digital Scales**

Although many pharmacies continue to use analog balances (called torsion balances), some have chosen to invest in a digital scale for use in compounding. Digital scales are easier to setup and calibrate than torsion balances, but are often more expensive.

■ **Barcode Scanners**

In some capacity, most pharmacies now employ barcode scanners. Nearly all stock bottles that a pharmacy will order from a wholesaler will have a bar-code matching the **National Drug Code (NDC)** of the drug, which is a unique, three-segment number identified and reported for these products. The NDC will be explained further on page 53. Many pharmacy software products suggest or require that the stock package be scanned during the filling process to complete the fill. Further, some pharmacy software will print a barcode corresponding to a particular refill onto each label printed in the dispensing process. Some require a pharmacist to scan the barcode on the prescription vial and the stock bottle as a final check that the right drug is being dispensed.

■ **Signature Capture Pads**
Prescriptions generally cannot leave the pharmacy without being signed for by the person picking up the prescription. This is not only good record-keeping practice, but is also required by most insurance companies. Traditionally, a paper log was signed by patients picking up prescriptions; however, these logs are difficult to store, create issues protecting patient privacy and can make it a lengthy process to retrieve a specific record during an audit. Thus, digital signature capture devices are used by many pharmacies to digitally store signatures and attach those signatures directly to the prescription record for easy retrieval in an audit.

■ **Scanners**
Although paper records are often required to be kept by state law or for insurance companies, pharmacies may elect to scan prescriptions received on paper into their pharmacy software (if the software allows). This allows for easy retrieval of originals and often makes it more convenient for a pharmacist to verify on refills that the prescription was originally filled correctly.

Software

■ **Prescription Processing Software/Electronic Medical Records**
Nearly all (if not all) pharmacies employ an **electronic medical record (EMR)** system that allows each prescription presented to the pharmacy to be turned into a digital record, used to generate a typed label placed on the dispensing vial and be billed to any insurance company the patient may have. The EMR may also allow a pharmacist to enter clinical notes (also called chart notes or progress notes) on his or her interactions with patients.

■ **Inventory Management Software**
Although this may be an integrated feature of the EMR software, it may also be separate. Many pharmacies utilize a "perpetual inventory" system to accurately know what inventory is on the pharmacy's shelves. This helps track not only what drugs are in stock but also when drugs need to be reordered. Pharmacy technicians may be placed in charge of overseeing the inventory management process and may have regular responsibilities to maintain the accuracy of the information in the inventory management software.

■ **Billing Software**
Although this may be integrated into the EMR software, some situations require stand-alone billing software. This can especially be true if the pharmacy is billing for services other than dispensing drugs (such as immunization administration, dispensing medical equipment or medication therapy management (MTM) services). Pharmacy technicians typically are the billing experts of the pharmacy and will likely be the ones to interact most with billing software, either stand-alone or integrated software.

Beyond the hardware and software, there are many features that are still emerging into regular use. Electronic prescribing is slowly becoming the norm as more and more prescribers and pharmacies adopt the necessary software. All states allow some degree of electronic prescribing; though, each state has set unique restrictions on what constitutes a valid electronic prescription. In 2010, the DEA issued rules that allow prescriptions for controlled substances to be electronically signed by prescribers, transmitted to a pharmacy and received by a pharmacy electronically as soon as both the pharmacy software and prescriber software are certified as having met the security requirements set forth in the DEA rules and if State rules allow for electronic prescribing of controlled substances. Electronic prescribing eliminates errors caused by confusing or illegible handwriting, prescriptions altered by patients en route to the pharmacy and generally helps prevent common errors (such as indicating more refills on a prescription than are allowed by law). A new set of errors must be guarded against, however, as interface options such as drop-down lists make the possibility of selecting the wrong drug a new reality. Among the other benefits, though, of electronic prescribing are that most software can screen for drug interactions, screen for insurance restrictions before the prescription reaches the pharmacy and provide convenience for patients to have prescriptions often prepared before reaching the pharmacy.

Claim Rejections from Third Parties (Insurance Companies) and Common Billing Errors

Although every pharmacy software will handle and display rejections differently, and each third party will craft the wording of rejections differently, there are a few common rejection types that a pharmacy technician must know how to handle. There are two types of rejections. Hard rejections are those that prevent the pharmacy from dispensing the drug to the patient if that insurance plan is to be used. Soft rejections are those that provide useful information to the pharmacy or patient but that do not prevent the patient from receiving the drug after the rejection is received. Some of the more common rejections are as follows:

■ **Refill Too Soon**
This rejection appears when the patient has requested a refill of the medication earlier than the limits of the patient's plan allows. If nothing has changed about the patient's therapy, if the patient does not have any special life events (like a vacation) to justify the early fill and if there is no good medical reason to fill the prescription early, a refill too soon rejection means that the patient must consume more of the medication they already have at home before returning to the pharmacy for a refill. If a prescriber increases the dose or frequency, if the patient has lost their medication or if the patient is going on a vacation that will prevent them from picking up a refill in the normal time frame, then most insurance plans will allow for an override of the rejection.

■ **Prior Authorization Required**
Some insurance plans require that a prescriber obtain authorization from the insurance company before initiating a therapy. Generally, this is because the therapy is costly and less-expensive alternatives exist. The insurance company seeks to ensure that the more expensive therapy is truly the best choice for that patient when less expensive options exist. When the pharmacy receives this rejection, the prescriber must be informed that a prior authorization is required. It is considered a professional courtesy to provide the contact information and contract information for the patient's insurance to the prescriber when informing his or her staff that the prior authorization is required. Since the drug claim has not been approved by the insurance, a patient must wait until the drug is approved unless the patient elects to purchase the drug without using his or her insurance plan.

■ **Plan Limitations Exceeded**
Most plans have some restriction on either the quantity of drug that can be dispensed at one time or the length of therapy a patient may receive at one time. Some insurances limit the quantity for each fill, regardless of how often the patient is using the medication, to a static number (e.g., some plans allow only 100 tablets or capsules to be dispensed regardless of how long that will last the patient). Another common limit is in the "days supply" of the medication; some insurance plans allow patients to receive a maximum of one month of a drug at each visit to the pharmacy (one month can be anywhere from a 28-day supply to a 34-day supply depending on the plan), while other plans allow a patient to receive three months

(three months can be anywhere from an 84-day supply to a 100-day supply depending on the plan) of a drug at each visit. Although exceptions exist, generally, a "plan limitations exceeded" rejection requires that in order for the insurance company to accept the claim, the patient must receive less of the drug at each visit than was prescribed by his or her physician (though, the overall amount of drug that the patient will receive over the life of the prescription is not altered because of this rejection).

■ **NDC Not Covered**
This generally means that either the drug is not covered by the insurance company or that specific manufacturer's drug is not covered by the insurance company. This exclusion may be for a number of reasons including the manufacturer has been restricted from selling drugs in the United States by the FDA; the drug is considered an elective therapy (rather than a required therapy); the drug is not FDA-approved; the patient (or the person/company that selected the plan) chose to exclude that class of drugs from their plan (e.g., some plans exclude weight loss drugs, oral contraceptives, wrinkle reducers and/or cosmetic therapies).

■ **Submit Bill to Primary Payor**
This patient has more than one active insurance that must be billed in the proper order, and that has not been done. Upon determining the patient's primary payor, the claim must be submitted to the primary payor. This may be because the patient has an assistance program that helps in covering copays left after billing the primary payor. Generally, the secondary insurance is a government-sponsored plan (e.g., Medicaid) or a manufacturer's discount card.

■ **Member Not Found/Patient Not Covered**
This can be a tricky rejection to overcome. This could actually be because the patient does not have active insurance coverage with the plan that is being sent the claim. It may, however, mean that the pharmacy's information does not match what is on file with the insurance company. Simple typographical errors can result in genders being incorrect, birthdays not matching, names not being spelled correctly and identification numbers being entered incorrectly. Although having the patient's insurance card is a good start, a direct contact (either by Web site or by phone) to a patient's insurance company may be necessary to root out the difference between the pharmacy's file and the insurance company's file. If it is a typographical error, correcting the erroneous information generally resolves this rejection.

■ **DUR Rejection**
This is generally a more clinical rejection. DUR stands for Drug Utilization Review, and the reason for the rejection is that the insurance company has a reason to believe that this therapy may be inappropriate and wishes a pharmacist to take a closer look at the prescription before filling it. This may be because the patient has received an interacting drug (possibly from another pharmacy), because the patient is pregnant and the drug is not recommended for pregnant patients, or any number of reasons based on claim data available to the insurance company. These rejections generally require a pharmacy technician to seek the expertise of a pharmacist before proceeding.

Although many more and varied rejections will be handled by a pharmacy technician in a single day, these more common rejections are seen hundreds of times per week by pharmacy staff. A pharmacy technician must learn to navigate through the billing requirements for each insurance plan, noting that each plan may have slightly different text for their rejection notices. Pharmacy technicians who do not properly handle such rejections can cost the pharmacy during an audit and can prevent patients from getting medications that they should have access to; it is essential that claims be billed correctly.

Common errors that arise during the billing process can lead to costly findings on an audit. Strategies to minimize billing errors are generally established in each pharmacy because it is far less costly to do it right the first time than have a billing error found during an audit. The most common errors are as follows:

■ **Incorrect Days Supply**

In many pharmacy EMR software, the pharmacy technician must calculate how long a drug will last a patient based on the quantity of drug being dispensed and the directions prescribed. If this calculation is done incorrectly, it can lead to an incorrect day supply being submitted to the insurance company. For most prescriptions, this is straightforward (e.g., the patient is receiving 30 tablets and taking one per day, a 30-day supply); however, some regimens get more complicated (e.g., the patient is receiving 24 tablets and taking three tablets twice weekly for the first two weeks and then two tablets twice weekly until gone, a 35-day supply). This calculation must also be made for eye drops, ear drops, creams, ointments and any other product being dispensed. Every insurance plan has slightly different rules for how many drops are found in a single milliliter of eye and ear drops or how long a standard tube of cream must last. This process becomes very tricky for topical creams or ointments because estimating exactly how much the patient will use to cover the body area where the drug is being applied can be quite difficult. Eye drops and ear drops must be converted from drops to milliliters for billing; although each insurance provider has a preferred conversion formula, 15 drops per milliliter is a common conversion factor used for billing.

■ **Incorrect Date Written**

Nothing requires a patient to bring a prescription to the pharmacy on the day that the prescription is written. If a patient presents a prescription well after the day that the prescription is written, the pharmacy must still record the day that the prescription was written because the prescription will expire at an interval based on when it was written. Pharmacy technicians must be careful to find the date on the prescription rather than entering the date that the prescription is being filled into the "date written" field in the EMR software.

■ **Incorrect DAW Code**

In most states, the lowest-cost, FDA-approved option must be dispensed when filling a prescription unless the prescriber or the patient indicates otherwise. Specifying a particular manufacturer for a product is referred to as "DAWing" a prescription. DAW stands for "dispense as written" and when it appears on a prescription from a prescriber (in the manner specified by state law), it prevents the pharmacist from making any substitutions to a different manufacturer's product. A patient also has the right to request that a particular manufacturer's product be used. In this case, it is called a "patient DAW" because the patient (rather than the prescriber) has requested the particular brand. Because the chosen brand in a DAW is generally more expensive than the default (least-expensive) option, the insurance company is told, in the claim, who requested that more-expensive brand. Depending on whether the prescriber or the patient issues the DAW request, the patient may be charged a significantly different copay or there may be restrictions from the insurance that prevent the patient from using their insurance at all for that drug. Ensuring that the proper code (physician DAW or patient DAW) on a DAW prescription is essential.

■ **Incorrect Origin Code**

Some insurance companies, including Medicare Part D and Medicaid, generally require the pharmacy to submit to them how the prescription arrived at the pharmacy. Partly, this is because some insurance companies will pay physicians to use electronic prescribing software, and this is a way to verify their usage. Submitting the incorrect code can result in a pharmacy losing money during an audit. The hardest to distinguish are fax and electronic, as both can print out on a fax machine (in some instances). There are four possible codes:

1. **Telephone** – When the prescription is telephoned into the pharmacy or if the pharmacy must call to clarify any information on the prescription
2. **Written** – When the prescription is written in the prescriber's office and is physically brought to the pharmacy on paper
3. **Fax** – When the prescriber prints or writes out the prescription (on paper) in the office and then puts that paper onto a fax machine and sends it to the pharmacy (the original paper is retained by the prescriber)
4. **Electronic** – When the prescriber transmits the prescription from his/her computer directly to the pharmacy (either to the pharmacy computer or the pharmacy fax machine, depending on the software and laws involved)

■ Incorrect Prescriber

It is important that the correct prescriber appear on the label being typed. Sometimes this is difficult to do. If pharmacy staff are unfamiliar with a prescriber's signature and cannot identify the proper prescriber based on the signature or if a prescriber is new to the area, then the pharmacy staff must verify the identity of the prescriber with the prescriber's office. It is important to identify the correct prescriber in case later contact with the prescriber is required. Further, many patients expect to see their physician's name on their prescription vial. A common error is to simply pick the first physician that appears preprinted on the prescription blank rather than calling the office to identify the prescriber.

■ Incorrect Directions

Translating the directions from the written prescription to the label is one of the most complex parts of filling a prescription. First, most prescriptions are presented in "sig codes" or Latin abbreviations that must be both translated into their meaning but also fit into the context of a complete sentence. Often directions are incomplete, and therefore incorrect, because they are either not specific enough to ensure proper use of the medication or because they lack essential information. A common error is to omit the route of administration (e.g., by mouth, topically, into the eyes).

■ Incorrect Product Selection

There are two main types of errors that occur here. First is selecting the correct drug and strength but the wrong manufacturer. This happens when the pharmacy software lists multiple manufacturers for the same product as being available at the pharmacy, and the one selected is not the one that is intended to be dispensed to the patient. The NDC submitted to the insurance company must match the product being dispensed. Second, this happens when drugs with similar names are confused and the wrong drug is typed (e.g., Toprol® and Topamax®).

■ Incorrect Patient

If a prescription is presented to the pharmacy with only a name to identify the patient, it is common practice to obtain the date of birth (or another identifier such as the address or phone number) from the person presenting the prescription. It is important when entering a prescription into a patient's chart that all available information be used to identify the correct patient's chart. A mix up is more likely when a single person brings in prescriptions for multiple patients (such as their spouse and their child) at the same time. It is a good idea to treat each prescription as a totally new process (and verify the patient name at the start of each new prescription processing) to ensure that the right chart is selected every time.

The Prescription Label—The Essentials

Each product that is dispensed from a pharmacy must be properly labeled. Each state has slightly different rules on what must be on the label; however, the following are generally universal characteristics of a prescription label.

[1] East River Pharmacy 231.591.7227 Ph. 231.591.7228 Fax 4455 Town Blvd. Laketown, MN 55425 www.easteriverpharmacy.com **[2]** 765890 **[3]** 08/09/2013 **[4]** Mary Jane Harshbarger 5325 Northern Heights Road Laketown, MN 231.591.8899 **[5]** Synthroid / **[6]** Levothyroxine 125 mcg **[7]** Take one tablet, by mouth, every morning on an empty stomach (at least 30 minutes before food or other medications). **[8]** Qty: 90	**[11]** James Nathaniel, N.P./ Dr. Selena Ndebe, D.O. 231.594.9857
	[12] Take on an empty stomach
	[12] Take 30 minutes before all other medications
	[12] Do not take with antacids or iron-containing supplements. Separate by at least four hours.
	[12] Take in the morning
	[13] NDC: 00378-1809-01 **[14]** "M" "L|8" yellow oblong scored tablet **[15]** Mylan Pharmaceuticals **[16]** HB/DH/BR
[9] Refills: 1 before 12/22/2013 **[10]** Caution: Federal Law prohibits the transfer of this drug to anyone other than to whom it was prescribed.	

[1] **Pharmacy Information**

Although exactly what is required will change based on the state where the pharmacy is located, generally the pharmacy's name and telephone number are required to appear on the label.

[2] **Prescription Number**

Every prescription is assigned a number at the pharmacy. Each pharmacy will choose a numbering system that works for that pharmacy; numbers are generally issued sequentially, though some systems assign different sets of numbers to different types of prescriptions (e.g., prescriptions for Schedule 2 controlled substances all begin with a 2).

[3] **Dispensing Date**

This is the date that the prescription is prepared for dispensing.

[4] **Patient Information**

Universally, the patient's name will appear; some states require specific information (such as an address or phone number) to appear along with the patient's name.

[5] Drug Written

This is the name written on the prescription presented to the pharmacy. In this case, the prescriber indicated Synthroid® on the prescription.

[6] Drug Dispensed

This is the name of the product actually dispensed. In this case, a substitution has been made from original brand Synthroid® to Mylan's levothyroxine because it is less expensive. Both the originally written name for the drug and the name of the drug being dispensed must appear on the label.

[7] Directions or Sig

These are the directions for the patient on how to use the medication. Notice that the directions form a complete sentence, including how many to take (one), what to take (tablet), what route to take it by (by mouth), how often to take it (every morning) and any additional information included on the prescription.

[8] Quantity to be Dispensed

In this case, this is the number of tablets to be put into the vial. If this were a prescription for a liquid, cream, etc., then this would be the metric volume (mL) or weight (g) to dispense.

[9] Refills

Notice that after the number of remaining refills that the expiration date for those refills is also specified. Again, each state has slightly different rules; but, most prescriptions for noncontrolled substances, and controlled substances in Schedule 5, expire one year after they are written (even if the patient has not taken advantage of all of the originally written refills). Prescriptions for controlled substances in Schedules 3 and 4 are valid for six months, and prescriptions for controlled substances in Schedule 2 vary by state.

[10] Caution Statement

This statement must appear on all prescription labels for controlled substances; however, many pharmacies have this pre-printed onto their labels and so it appears on all prescriptions.

[11] Prescriber Information

Although the name of the prescriber is generally required, some pharmacies also include a phone number for the physician. Further, when a mid-level prescriber (such as a nurse practitioner) writes a prescription, it is sometimes required that the physician who coordinates with the mid-level practitioner also appear on the label.

[12] Auxiliary Labels

These are sometimes printed when the prescription is processed and sometimes are separate stickers applied by the pharmacy technician (or pharmacist) during the filling process. These provide information on how to properly use the medication that goes beyond the information included on the prescription. Each pharmacist will have directions for their pharmacy technicians on how to apply auxiliary labels.

[13] National Drug Code (NDC)

This is a unique number that identifies exactly which drug is to be dispensed. This is generally not required; however, it is essential to the process used by most pharmacies and so it is nearly always present on the label.

[14] Product Description

Although not required, many pharmacy systems now print a description of the product on the label. This helps both pharmacy staff and patients to ensure that the correct product reaches the intended patient.

[15] Manufacturer

This is the name of the manufacturer of the product being dispensed. This is generally required, and there are often stiff penalties if this information is incorrectly reported on a pharmacy label.

[16] Pharmacy Staff Initials

Depending on how the pharmacy software used by the pharmacy tracks who is involved in the filling process, there may be many sets of initials present on the label. Generally, at least the pharmacist's initials will appear; often, the person who entered the prescription (or refill request) into the pharmacy computer system will have their initials on the label as well. Some systems include the pharmacy technician who counts the prescription.

Drug Information Dissemination

Patients receive information in many forms when they visit a pharmacy. Most prescriptions are accompanied by a monograph (drug information handout) that highlights the most important information a patient would need to know about a drug. Further, some drugs have a medication guide that is required to be dispensed at each fill of the drug. Although neither of these written ways of distributing drug information are a substitute for a pharmacist's counseling, they provide a foundation of information that is used to educate patients. Pharmacy technicians can always provide the pharmacy's monograph (or medication guide when appropriate) to a patient, but should always refer specific questions about a drug's function, use or interactions to a pharmacist. It is generally accepted that anything found in the drug monograph, in the medication guide or on the label found on a drug dispensed to the patient can be read to the patient by a pharmacy technician if the patient is unable (or struggling) to read that information; however, any question that involves interpreting this information, applying this information to the specific patient or providing other clinical information to patients is reserved only for pharmacists. Answering such questions may not be delegated to a pharmacy technician.

Administration of a Pharmacy and the Role of Pharmacy Technicians

A pharmacy is a complex machine with many moving parts. Pharmacy technicians can take on many administrative roles to free up pharmacists to spend more time talking with patients. Pharmacy technicians commonly have a role in ordering supplies (vials, labels, printer cartridges, etc.) for the pharmacy, ordering drugs for the pharmacy (under the supervision of a pharmacist), processing received orders and managing the pharmacy's inventory. Inventory management can include everything from preparing and sending expired drugs to the pharmacy's reverse distributor for destruction to helping review reports of a product's dispensing history and deciding to carry more or less of that drug on the shelf. Other tasks often delegated to pharmacy technicians include filing, document storage, report generation, data entry and compilation, stocking shelves, cleaning and many other tasks that assist a pharmacist to spend more time with patients. Some pharmacy technicians are also expected to run a cash register, prepare a daily bank deposit and handle other transactions involving money. The possibilities are nearly endless for what a pharmacy technician can expect to do in the course of practice; the needs of the particular pharmacist will determine the scope of exactly how the pharmacy technician may assist.

Conclusion

Although the only way to truly learn the process of filling prescription is to participate in a functioning pharmacy, a pharmacy technician who begins with an understanding of the overall process, and common pitfalls, of working in a pharmacy, will be well on her or his way to being a competent assistant to their pharmacist(s). After reviewing this chapter, a pharmacy technician is expected to be able to describe the basic work flow of a pharmacy, navigate a prescription, navigate a dispensing label, discuss the common errors encountered when filling a prescription and discuss some of the technologies employed to make a pharmacy more efficient.

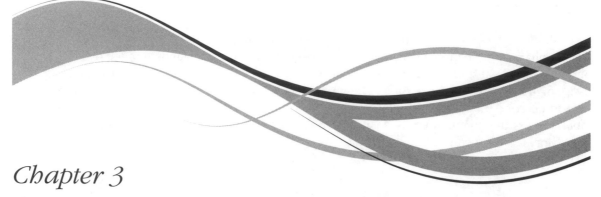

Chapter 3
REVIEW QUESTIONS

1. Schedule I controlled substances are:
    a. powerful narcotics that a physician may prescribe for pain.
    b. street drugs that have been determined to have no medicinal value.
    c. sometimes available with a pharmacist's prescription and sometimes with a physician's prescription.
    d. not regulated by the federal government.

2. Unless prohibited by state law, emergency oral contraceptives (Plan B®, et al.) are available without a prescription to those:
    a. 17 years old and older.
    b. seven years old and older.
    c. 18 years old and older.
    d. 21 years old and older.

3. Which of the following professionals are generally not allowed to prescribe?
    a. M.D.
    b. D.O.
    c. D.C.
    d. O.D.

4. What is missing from the following prescription?

608.892.4385 Phone 608.892.4386 Fax	Rex Exempli, M.D. 8822 Portage Road Portage, IN 46368	NPI 1124049176 DEA FE8043159
Rhonda Kingslight, P.A. NPI 8763019287 DEA MK6561876	Jeff Jamerson, N.P. NPI 6532856987	JoAnne Langdon, C.N.M. NPI 1121134523 DEA ML8888543

Patient:_____Heather Allen_____   D.O.B.: __10/18/1952__
Address: __6909 West Q Avenue West LaFayette, IN 47907__

Date: ___07 May 2013___

Zovirax® 800 mg Capsules

Dispense: __40 (forty) tablets__   Refills: ___5 (five)___

DAW*: _____   Signature: _____JoAnne Langdon_____

*If manufacturer specification is medically necessary, then "DAW" must appear in the prescriber's own handwriting.

a. Name of the patient
b. Quantity of medication to dispense
c. Strength of the drug
d. Directions for use of the medication

5. What is wrong with this prescription?

608.892.4385 Phone 608.892.4386 Fax	Rex Exempli, M.D. 8822 Portage Road Portage, IN 46368	NPI 1124049176 DEA FE8043159

Patient:_____Heather Allen_____   D.O.B.: __10/18/1952__
Address: __6909 West Q Avenue West LaFayette, IN 47907__

Date: ___07 May 2013___

Lisinopril 10 mg Tablets by
Mylan
Sig: ꝉ PO QAM

Dispense: _____90 tablets_____   Refills: ___PRN___

DAW*: _____DAW_____   Signature: _____Rex Exempli_____

*If manufacturer specification is medically necessary, then "DAW" must appear in the prescriber's own handwriting.

Note: Lisinopril is used to manage high blood pressure.

a. Prescriber is outside the scope of his practice
b. Quantity is too high
c. Refills are not allowed on this prescription
d. Drug may not be written generically with a DAW

6. Prescriptions for controlled substances can be transmitted electronically to a pharmacy if allowed by state law.
    a. True
    b. False

7. For medications with a MedGuide, the MedGuide is required to be dispensed at:
    a. only the first dispensing from a new prescription.
    b. every refill.
    c. only at the request of the patient.
    d. only at the request of the prescriber.

8. Counseling a patient on the proper use of a medication, including describing the common side effects, is a common function for a pharmacy technician.
    a. True
    b. False

9. Which of the following must appear on the dispensing label for morphine (a Schedule 2 controlled substance)?
    a. Caution: Federal Law encourages the transfer of this drug to anyone other than to whom it was prescribed.
    b. Manufacturer's telephone number
    c. Quantity dispensed to the patient
    d. Pharmacy's DEA registration number

10. Prescriptions telephoned into the pharmacy may be directly entered into the EMR without first creating a written record of the transmitted prescription.
    a. True
    b. False

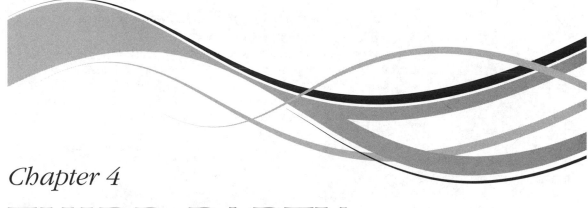

Chapter 4

THIRD PARTY INSURANCE ISSUES

By Franz Neubrecht, Pharm.D.

Learning Objectives

This chapter seeks to prepare a pharmacy technician to:

- understand the standard terminology associated with billing third party insurance programs.
- differentiate between Medicare and Medicaid.
- review the basics of entering prescription claims into a pharmacy's electronic medical record system and billing such claims electronically.
- discuss best practices for the Health Insurance Portability and Accountability Act (HIPAA); fraud, waste and abuse (FWA); and pseudoephedrine regulations.

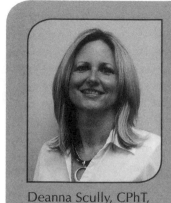

Why are technicians often utilized to communicate with third party payers and process plan claims?

"The education and skills of a pharmacist are better utilized to counsel patients and perform clinical duties. Therefore, they often rely on pharmacy technicians to perform administrative duties related to the billing of pharmacy claims. Technicians have become the experts in understanding insurance requirements, and managing the challenging role of coordinating billing issues related to prior authorizations and coverage limitations imposed by the third party payers."

Deanna Scully, CPhT, pharmacy contract coordinator, HealthPlus of Michigan, Flint, Mich.

What is the technician's first priority in submitting insurance billings?

"The most important priority is accuracy. All of the required fields that are submitted on an insurance claim must accurately portray each pharmacy event. The quantity and days supply submitted must be able to stand up in an audit. Due to the tremendous cost of medications, insurance companies are challenged to reduce the cost of the prescription drug benefit and have instituted coverage limitations as one means of controlling skyrocketing costs. It is important that every prescription filled and billed is done according to the rules communicated by each health plan."

Introduction

Health care is a major industry, employing millions of health care providers and supportive personnel. In the United States, health care is provided through a mixture of public and private plans. Consequently, the financing and delivery of health care is complex. Patients may have prescription drug programs that are entirely private, sponsored by a state (or local) government, sponsored by the federal government, or a hybrid of these options. Examples of private prescription drug programs would be those offered by large corporate manufacturers to all full-time employees. State programs include Medicaid (**Medicaid** is a hybrid that is sponsored by a state with some regulation and collaboration by the federal government) and disability insurance programs. Federal programs include Medicare and worker's compensation. It is also possible to have a combination of prescription programs (e.g., both Medicare and Medicaid), further complicating the billing process for pharmacy technicians and pharmacists.

This chapter includes a brief description of the terminology associated with third party insurance billing, followed by the steps a pharmacy technician takes when a prescription claim is electronically billed to the patient's insurance company or companies. As part of the examination of this process, pitfalls and barriers to proper claim processing will be discussed. The final section of this chapter will include a brief description of the federal **Health Insurance Portability and Accountability Act (HIPAA)**; the FWA prevention efforts initiated by the **Centers for Medicare and Medicaid Services (CMS)**; and the federal laws relevant to the regulation of pseudoephedrine.

Terminology

- **Average Wholesale Price**

  Average wholesale price (AWP) is a theoretical drug price determined by the drug manufacturer and First DataBank, Inc., which provides a national drug pricing database to providers; however, there is no standard among the various drug manufacturers for determining this price. The value that AWP is supposed to represent is the average price that a pharmaceutical company charges wholesalers wishing to purchase the product; this is not the reality, as no standard exists for listing an AWP.

  Many insurance contracts still define the cost that will be paid to a pharmacy for a medication that the pharmacy bills as a formula involving AWP. Generally, the formulae take the form of: AWP – X% + Dispensing Fee. The percentage reduction from AWP varies for each contract from each insurance company or pharmacy benefit manager (PBM), and is often different for generic, brand name and expensive (specialty) drugs. The range of discounts from AWP specified in insurance contracts can vary widely. Since AWP is a published value, updated regularly by First DataBank, Inc., insurance companies and PBMs are required to update their AWP file regularly. There have been multiple lawsuits, brought by pharmacies against PBMs, due to insurance companies not updating AWP files properly. Although AWP continues to be used, it is being phased out due a court ruling mandating that it stop being used (due to the long history of law suits relating to AWP issues).

- **Bank Identification Number and Processor Control Number**

  Each insurance company, and PBM, has a **Bank Identification Number (BIN)** that is used to route claims to the correct insurance company. Each plan offered by an insurance company has a specific **Processor Control Number (PCN)** that is used to route claims to the specific area within the insurance company that is responsible for that plan. The BIN is a six-digit numerical code. Some PBMs process claims for many different insurance companies, so there may be many different insurance companies using the same BIN. The PCN does not have a consistent format and may not be required for successful claim transmission (some pharmacy software will insert a placeholder (e.g., 00000) when a PCN is not required). A PCN may contain both letters and numbers. Along with the BIN and PCN, a patient's insurance card will also generally list the patient's identification number and group number, which will be necessary for submitting a claim to the patient's insurance company. Unfortunately, there are no standards for insurance cards and some insurance companies will not put all of the necessary information on the card.

- **Copayment or Copay**

  A **copay** is the out-of-pocket cost paid by the patient in addition to the cost paid by the insurance company to provide the total reimbursement to the pharmacy for the drugs and services provided. Each insurance plan will have a specified copayment structure that may require a patient to pay a flat fee (e.g., $5 for generic drugs and $10 for brand-name drugs) or a percentage of the total price. The patient's health plan determines the copayment amount that is owed to the pharmacy; the pharmacy does not control the patient's copayment and is generally not allowed to collect more or less from the patient for the service or product provided.

- **Dispense as Written** *on test*

  A dispense as written (DAW) designation on a prescription compels a pharmacist to dispense a prescription exactly as it was written by the physician. Prescribers designate DAW mostly on prescriptions written for brand name medications when, in their judgment, substitution to an equivalent generic is inappropriate. A prescriber may indicate DAW on a prescription written for a generic medication (if a manufacturer is supplied) when a patient is stable on a particular manufacturer's product and the prescriber wishes the patient to remain on that particular manufacturer's product. When billing an insurance company for a prescription, an indication must be submitted for whether or not a DAW was included on the prescription.

Generally, the values eligible for submission in the DAW field on an insurance claim are 0-9 with the following corresponding to each number:

0 = No product selection indicated – generic or lowest-cost option dispensed

1 = Substitution not allowed by provider (prescriber designated DAW on the prescription)

2 = Substitution allowed – patient requested the more expensive product be dispensed

3 = Substitution allowed – pharmacist selected the more expensive product to be dispensed

4 = Substitution allowed – generic drug not in stock

5 = Substitution allowed – brand drug dispensed as generic (used when brand is less expensive than the available generic drugs)

6 = Override

7 = Substitution not allowed – brand drug mandated by law (usually state law when applicable)

8 = Substitution allowed – generic drug not available in marketplace (e.g., due to recall, legal action against the generic manufacturer or manufacturing problems)

9 = Other[1]

In many instances, a DAW designation (other than 0) will increase the patient's copay amount because the lowest cost option is not being dispensed. Generally, DAW codes 3, 4, 6 and 9 are never used and 5, 7 and 8 are used very rarely; DAW codes 0, 1 and 2 are used routinely as either no DAW is specified, the prescriber requests a specific product or the patient requests a specific product. Finally, each state may specify the manner in which a DAW is properly designated on a prescription; a pharmacy technician must know his or her state's requirements for a prescriber (or patient) to request that specific product be dispensed.

■ **Formulary System**

The **formulary system** is a method for evaluating and selecting suitable drug products for an organized health setting (e.g., a hospital or a community pharmacy). Most community pharmacies are not required to adhere to a formulary; therefore, they stock and dispense those medications that are commonly prescribed by physicians in the local area. In the ambulatory setting, a patient may be limited to a specific formulary of medications that are covered by his or her insurance plan; or, as an alternative, nonformulary medications may be covered by the patient's insurance plan but at a significantly higher copayment than that for formulary medications. Generally, PBMs incentivize patients to use the lowest-cost options within a drug class and those brand name drugs for which the PBM receives monetary rebates from pharmaceutical manufacturers. PBMs may also use a tiered system where the cheapest drugs, generally generic drugs, have the lowest copayment; drugs for which no generic equivalent is available have a moderate copayment and drugs for which a generic is available (but the patient elects to use the higher-cost drug) have the highest copayment.

Medicaid

Medicaid became law in 1965 as a jointly-funded cooperative venture between the federal and state governments, to assist states in the provision of adequate medical care to eligible needy persons. Medicaid is the largest program providing medical and health-related services to America's poorest people. The federal statute identifies more than 25 different eligibility categories for which federal funds are available. These statutory categories can be classified into five broad coverage groups: children, pregnant women, adults in families with dependent children, individuals with disabilities and individuals age 65 and older. Medicaid coverage varies considerably from state to state. Within broad federal guidelines, each state establishes its own eligibility standards; determines the type, amount, duration and scope of services offered; sets the rate of payment for services; and administers its own program. Medicaid recipients may obtain coverage for things like nursing home care, home health care and outpatient prescription drugs that aren't covered by Medicare. Title XIX of the Social Security Act requires that, in order to receive federal matching funds, certain basic services are offered to the categorically needy population in any state program.

Medicare

In 1965, the Social Security Act established both Medicare and Medicaid. **Medicare** is health insurance for people age 65 or older, under 65 with certain disabilities and of any age with end-stage renal disease (ESRD).[2] ESRD is permanent kidney failure requiring dialysis or a kidney transplant. In 1977, the Health Care Financing Administration (HCFA) was created under the Department of Health, Education and Welfare (HEW) to effectively coordinate Medicare and Medicaid. In 1980, HEW was divided into the Department of Education and the **Department of Health and Human Services (HHS)**. In 2001, HCFA was renamed the Centers for Medicare and Medicaid Services (CMS). CMS is the federal agency that administers the Medicare program. As of 2010, Medicare provides coverage for approximately 47.5 million Americans.[3]

Medicare Part D

The **Medicare Prescription Drug, Improvement and Modernization Act (MMA)** of 2003 introduced **Medicare Part D** prescription drug coverage. This voluntary benefit began Jan. 1, 2006. Medicare prescription drug coverage is insurance that covers prescription drugs at participating pharmacies. Medicare prescription drug coverage provides protection for people who have very high drug costs or unexpected prescription drug bills in the future. Everyone with Medicare is eligible for this coverage regardless of income and resources, health status or current prescription expenses. Patients may sign up, without penalty, when they first become eligible for Medicare (for most, that means three months before your 65th birthday). If patients are entitled to Medicare due to a disability, they can join from three months before to three months after their 25th month of cash disability payments without penalty. Patients who are eligible for Medicare Part D, but elect not to sign up when benefits become available to them, may incur fines and penalties if they elect to sign up for benefits at a later date.

Medication Therapy Management Services

MMA mandates that **medication therapy management services (MTMS)** are provided to patients to ensure that drugs covered by Medicare Part D plans are being appropriately used to their maximum benefit with a minimization of adverse effects experienced by the patient. Although MMA does not specifically require that a pharmacist, rather than other health care professionals, administer MTMS, it does allow pharmacists, and any qualified professional providing MTMS, to bill the patient's Medicare Part D plan for such services. This is a change for pharmacists who are traditionally billing only for drugs being dispensed. So, to assist with billing for this clinical service, pharmacists have been assigned **Current Procedural Terminology (CPT) codes** that are specific to MTMS administered by pharmacists (CPT codes are generally reserved for health care providers furnishing a service, such as a physician seeing patients in his or her office, respiratory therapists training patients to use oxygen or a chiropractor performing chiropractic services in her or his office.)

Not every patient qualifies under the program to have MTMS provided (and therefore billed to their Medicare Part D plan); the patients who qualify for MTMS in 2011 include those with multiple diseases (e.g., diabetes, asthma, hypertension, hyperlipidemia and congestive heart failure) using multiple drugs with annual drug costs that exceed $3,000. The annual cost threshold will be revised by CMS each year to reflect the costs of covered Medicare Part D drugs.

For the first time in many decades, thanks to MMA, a public document states that pharmacists are essential for improving the health outcomes of elderly patients. MTMS has provided an opportunity for pharmacists to be paid for patient services instead of just dispensing a drug product. This is a much-needed paradigm shift that will dictate the clinical future of community pharmacy and the continued importance of pharmacy technicians. Examples of the types of activities included in MTMS include the following:

- Assessing a patient's health status
- Providing comprehensive medical chart reviews (with a focus on the drugs that the patient is using)
- Formulating/monitoring/adjusting prescription drug treatment plans
- Educating patients on drug therapy management in collaboration with physicians and other health care professionals
- Providing the patient with special packaging to assist in consistent medication use
- Providing patients with reminders to refill their prescriptions

■ **National Association of Boards of Pharmacy/**
National Council for Prescription Drug Programs
The National Association of Boards of Pharmacy (NABP) is an impartial professional organization that supports the state boards of pharmacy in creating uniform regulations to protect public health.[4] Pharmacies are issued a NABP/NCPDP (National Council for Prescription Drug Programs) number that allows them to process electronically transmitted third party insurance drug claims.

■ **National Drug Code**
The **National Drug Code (NDC)** is a unique 10-digit number separated into three segments. A typical NDC number looks like this: 1234-5678-90, where the first four or five digits identify the manufacturer, the next three or four digits identify the product code of a specific drug, and the last two digits identify the package size or dosage form of the product. An NDC is assigned by the manufacturer, in collaboration with the FDA, and is used in pharmacy third party billing to identify the manufacturer, drug and package size being dispensed by the pharmacy. It is essential that the correct NDC be submitted when billing an insurance company because the pharmacy's reimbursement is based on exactly which NDC was dispensed to the patient.

■ National Provider Identification

All health care providers (including physicians, nurses and pharmacists) must apply to the National Plan and Provider Enumeration System (NPPES) for a National Provider Identification (NPI) if they are billing third parties for services provided to a patient. Further, each medical facility, including each pharmacy, must have a NPI to identify where services are rendered. The 10-digit NPI from the prescriber, the pharmacy and sometimes the pharmacist, must appear on all insurance claims for prescription drugs. A provider's or facility's NPI can be obtained from https://nppes.cms.hhs.gov/NPPES/Welcome.do.

■ Pharmacy Benefit Manager

Private companies may elect to provide their employees with insurance for prescription drugs that are obtained through the use of a **pharmacy benefit manager (PBM)** or insurance company. Some of the largest PBMs are shown in Table 1. PBMs are companies under contract with managed care organizations, self-insured companies and government programs to manage pharmacy networks, drug utilization reviews, outcomes management and disease management. The goal in utilizing a PBM is to contain health care costs by incentivizing or mandating cost-effective behaviors. A PBM may, for example, require patients to use a mail-order pharmacy owned by the PBM as part of a corporate health insurance plan. In order for patients to utilize a pharmacy, and have the cost of their prescription drugs billed directly to their PBM, pharmacies must sign a contract with their specific PBM. PBMs provide management techniques, such as formularies, drug utilization reviews, disease management services and mail services at a negotiated price to the employer group; to benefit the employer, this negotiated rate must be lower than the cost of receiving these services under "normal conditions."

Table 1

Top 25 PBMs by Annual Prescription Volume, as of Third Quarter 2010[5]

Company	Total Rx / Year	Market Share
Medco Health Solutions, Inc.	695,000,000	18.20%
CVS / Caremark Rx, Inc.	658,500,000	17.25%
Argus Health Systems, Inc.	504,000,000	13.20%
Express Scripts, Inc.	449,300,000	11.77%
Prescription Solutions	274,920,504	7.20%
ACS, Inc.	250,000,000	6.55%
MedImpact Healthcare Systems, Inc.	170,400,000	4.46%
First Health Services Corporation	148,500,000	3.89%
Prime Therapeutics LLC	114,000,000	2.99%
HealthTrans	90,102,300	2.36%
Aetna Pharmacy Management (APM)	89,709,989	2.35%
Walgreens Health Services Division	84,105,927	2.20%

Table 1 *cont.*

Top 25 PBMs by Annual Prescription Volume, as of Third Quarter 2010[5]

Company	Total Rx / Year	Market Share
Catalyst Rx	64,879,964	1.70%
CIGNA Pharmacy Management	51,108,000	1.34%
RESTAT, LLC	25,046,964	0.66%
SXC Health Solutions, Inc. / informedRx	22,800,000	0.60%
ScriptSave	17,000,000	0.45%
FutureScripts	15,503,019	0.41%
RegenceRx	15,325,432	0.40%
Pharmacy Data Management, Inc. (PDMI)	14,100,000	0.37%
Navitus Health Solutions, LLC	10,500,000	0.28%
National Pharmaceutical Services	10,000,000	0.26%
PerformRx, LLC	9,771,216	0.26%
BioScrip	7,735,710	0.20%
NovoLogix	4,800,000	0.13%

■ **Pharmacy Override Codes**[6]

For certain rejections, there is a procedure to manually override a rejected prescription claim without calling the pharmacy help desk at the insurance company. These rejections usually contain clinical information (such as "drug interaction found" or "lower-cost option exists") or information regarding when a prescription can be filled (such as "refill too soon" or "next refill available on [date]"). By the use of a set of override codes, a pharmacy technician, with the expressed permission of a pharmacist, may be able to override these rejections when a valid reason is present. This reason, along with the codes used, must be clearly documented on the prescription so that the reason for the override is clear if an audit of that prescription is ever performed by the insurance company. The codes accepted by each insurance company are different; a list of acceptable codes is available from each insurance company and many pharmacies have notebooks of "cheat sheets" with the codes listed.

■ **Prior Authorization**

An insurance company or PBM may add certain drugs to a restricted list of medications on its formulary. These designations are assigned to medications that have a potential for serious side effects, are of a particularly high cost, are considered lifestyle drugs (e.g., wrinkle-reducing creams, weight-loss drugs) or have less advantageous manufacturer rebates for the PBM. When a medication requires a **prior authorization (PA)**, the prescriber must contact the insurance company and submit all of the required documentation before the pharmacy may bill the insurance company for the drug on behalf of the patient; since pharmacy billing must be done before dispensing a product, if a PA has not been obtained prior to the prescription being written, then a patient will be delayed in receiving medication unless they elect to pay the pharmacy's usual and customary price (U&C) and not use the prescription insurance that is requiring the PA. When a prescription is presented to a pharmacy that requires a PA and the pharmacy contacts the prescriber to notify him/her that PA is required, this is called a **prior authorization request**, or PAR.

■ **Usual and Customary Pricing**

The price that pharmacy would charge a patient, without any help from an insurance company or other source, is called the **usual and customary price (U&C)**, or cash price. The U&C price must reflect all advertised discounts, special promotions or other programs initiated to reduce prices for product costs available to the general public or to a special population.[7] This pricing would also include senior citizen pricing or discounts offered to any special group. When submitting a claim to a third party, the U&C is generally submitted because insurance companies will not generally reimburse a pharmacy more than the U&C provided by the pharmacy (the insurance company is not going to pay more for a product or service than a person without insurance would pay). It is up to each pharmacy to set the U&C for each product and service being furnished and this price may vary greatly between pharmacies (even in the same geographical area).

■ **Wholesale Acquisition Cost**

Due to the phasing out of AWP, **wholesale acquisition cost (WAC)** is quickly becoming the standard in formulae presented by insurance companies in contracts for reimbursement with pharmacies. Theoretically, this is the price that the wholesaler paid for the product (in purchasing it from a drug manufacturer). It is, unfortunately, also a list price that may or may not represent the actual price paid by a wholesaler. Generally, formulae involving WAC are in the format: WAC + X% + Dispensing Fee. The percentage increase from WAC varies for each contract from each insurance company (or PBM) and is often different for generic, brand and specialty drugs.

Third Party Prescription Claim Billing Procedures

A necessary, though sometimes tedious, part of working in a community pharmacy is billing insurance companies for the services and products furnished to patients. Pharmacists are medication experts, not necessarily insurance experts, so most pharmacists rely heavily on pharmacy technicians to be the insurance experts for the pharmacy. A basic knowledge of how to bill a pharmacy claim to an insurance company is vitally important for every pharmacy technician. Third-party billing is essential for most patients to receive medication, as many would not be able to pay the entire cost of their prescription drugs at each visit. Pharmacists delegate the bulk of this billing work to pharmacy technicians in order to spend more time interacting directly with patients and performing their clinical duties.

Due to the high cost of today's medications, most patients choose to pay for medications through an insurance company or PBM. Those who do not have adequate insurance coverage are faced with a myriad of issues, such as going without medication, being inconsistent in their therapy or trying to research and find other available resources to make their medication affordable. Pharmacy technicians can also play an active role in helping these patients by assisting in the research for coupons and discount programs available to help patients better afford their medications. Many brand name pharmaceutical manufacturers have coupons available on their Web sites or participate in needs-based assistance programs for patients.

Information to Collect from Each Patient

In addition to the information required by the pharmacy for processing a prescription (such as the patient's name, date of birth, allergies, etc.), the patient's insurance card must be requested. Possession of an insurance card is not a guarantee of insurance coverage; however, it contains the necessary information (usually) to submit a claim to that insurance to determine the patient's eligibility and coverage terms. The information that is needed to submit a claim, which can usually be found on the insurance card, includes the following:

- **BIN and PCN**
  As was mentioned previously in the chapter, each insurance company and PBM has a BIN that is used to route claims to the correct insurance company. Each plan offered by an insurance company also has a specific PCN that is used to route claims to the specific area within the insurance company that is responsible for that plan. Along with the BIN and PCN, a patient's insurance card will generally also list the patient's identification number and group number, which will be necessary for submitting a claim to the patient's insurance company. Unfortunately, there are no standards for insurance cards and some insurance companies will not put all of the necessary information on the card.

- **Patient Identification (ID) Number**
  This number can be any combination of letters and numbers (some are all numbers, some all letters and some are mixed). If there is no ID number on the card, then the cardholder's social security number may suffice. Each insurance company, and each PBM, lists the patient's ID number differently on their insurance cards. For example, some insurance cards always have an ID that begins with a letter or set of letters; however the letters are never used for prescription billing (but are used for medical billing, which is why they are present on the card). Others use a 10-digit format, but the provided card often only has eight digits; then the pharmacy technician submitting the claim must add two zeros to the front of the eight-digit number. Such information can be obtained by calling the pharmacy help desk for the specific insurance, but generally this information is learned "on the job" through experience in billing pharmacy claims.

- **Group Number**
  Most insurance companies reference a specific group on the insurance card. Specifically, the pharmacy group number may be required for successful claim submission; however, the pharmacy group number may not be the only group number on the patient's insurance card. For example, some insurances have two group numbers, one for medical billing and one for prescription billing. The pharmacy billing group is designated as the "Rx Group." In other cases, there is no referenced group number on the patient's card.

As previously mentioned, there are no standards for producing insurance cards; thus, this information may be difficult to locate or may be buried within other information on the card. Some of this information may be on the back of the card while the ID number is on the front. Further, some cards do not list an ID number at all and instead read "cardholder's social security number" and, therefore, the pharmacy technician submitting the claim must ask the patient for the cardholder's social security number (not necessarily the patient's social security number). Still, other cards are not kind enough to list all of the required information on the card; only by calling the insurance company's pharmacy help desk can the complete information be obtained.

Other information that is necessary for billing pharmacy claims, that is often not listed on the card, includes the following:

- **Relationship**

  The information on the card is generally for the cardholder (the person who holds the policy or works for the company providing the insurance), but this may not be the patient. The claim must, therefore, identify the relationship between the patient and the cardholder. There are one or two fields to accomplish this identification: a relationship field and/or a person code field. In the relationship code field, a "1" designates that the patient is the cardholder, a "2" designates that the patient is the cardholder's spouse and a "3" designates that the patient is a dependent (usually a child) of the cardholder. In the person code field, the cardholder is usually designated as either "00" or "01" depending on the insurance company. Then, the cardholder's spouse is one number higher than the cardholder, and the cardholder's dependents (e.g., children) are listed in successive numbers after the spouse. In some instances (such as a family taking care of an elderly parent or an unmarried couple with domestic partner benefits), a cardholder may have adult dependents with or without a spouse and so these numbers may be adjusted to account for these situations.

- **Prescription Origin Code**

  Most insurance companies, including Medicaid and Medicare Part D, require the manner in which the prescription was received by the pharmacy be identified on the prescription claim. The ways in which a prescription can be received are: written, telephone, fax and electronic. Not all prescriptions may be received in all of these ways (e.g., Schedule 2 controlled substance prescriptions may not be faxed in most instances). Further, many states and insurance companies require that original written prescriptions must be written on tamper-resistant prescription pads, and those created from phone, fax or electronic transmissions must be created and maintained in printed form.

All of the above-mentioned information must be obtained during the intake of a new prescription because processing of that prescription cannot occur without complete billing information. View Figure 2 for an example of a patient information form that can be used to ensure that all of the necessary information is obtained. When all of the patient and insurance information is successfully entered in to the pharmacy electronic medical record system, a claim can then be electronically submitted to the insurance company for adjudication and payment. The pharmacy technician submitting the claim will receive a nearly-instantaneous response from the insurance company indicating whether the claim was paid or rejected. If the claim was paid, the pharmacy technician submitting the claim may be asked to ensure that the reimbursement received was greater than the pharmacy's cost for the drug (depending on the pharmacy's procedures). Upon receiving a paid claim, most pharmacy software will generate a label that is printed in the pharmacy. This label will be used on the container in which the medication will be dispensed. Further, a portion of the label will be placed on the back of the hard-copy prescription; this sticker often contains information about how much the insurance company paid for the submitted claim. Attached to the label is also usually a receipt showing the patient's copayment. If the submitted claim is rejected, then the insurance company provides a reason for the rejection that usually displays on the claim-submission screen of the pharmacy software.

Figure 2
Patient Information Form

Patient Information Form

Name ——————————————————————————————————————

Address —————————————————————————————————————

City ————————————————————— State ——— Zip ———————

Telephone ———————————————— E-mail ————————————————

Date of Birth ——— / ——— / ———

Driver's License # —————————————————————————————————

Allergies ————————————————————————————————————

Current Supplements, Vitamins, OTC Medications and Prescription Medications:

——

——

——

——

——

Any additional information you think we should know:

——

——

——

——

Please give your current prescription card and this form to the technician or pharmacist. All information helps us serve you better and is kept confidential.

The following are some of the most common reasons that prescription claims are rejected or denied by insurance companies, with some strategies for handling the rejections.

■ **Patient Not on File / Missing/Invalid Patient ID / Patient Not Found**
  - Check that the patient ID, group and PCN have been entered correctly from the insurance card
  - Verify the patient's date of birth, sex, zip code and cardholder relationship code.
  - Using the BIN, check that the correct insurance company is being billed.
  - Call the pharmacy help desk for that specific insurance if the submitted information matches the information provided by the patient.

■ **Refill Too Soon**
  - Ask the patient how they are currently taking the medication. If they indicate that they are using more than the prescription on file, ask if their physician authorized the increased usage. If the physician authorized the increase but neglected to inform the pharmacy, contact the prescriber for a new prescription indicating the current directions.
  - Ask the patient if there is a reason that they are requesting an early refill:
    - If the patient is going on a vacation, many insurance policies allow for a one-time override to refill a prescription early in the case of a vacation. Be sure to document that the patient indicated that they were going on a vacation and the date that the patient is scheduled to leave the area before submitting the override codes for a vacation supply.
    - Has the medication been lost or destroyed? Some insurance companies will allow an override for this predicament. Be sure to document that the patient indicated that they lost the medication and how they lost it before submitting the override codes for a lost medication override.
  - If this information is not contained in the rejection, ask the patient if this prescription was recently filled at another pharmacy. If this has occurred, the patient may not be eligible for an early refill; this will let the pharmacy know the reason for the rejection. The patient may simply be asking for the refill before his or her plan allows for it. Each insurance company uses a different formula for determining how soon a patient may refill a medication; most require a certain portion of the medication from the last fill to be consumed before a refill is dispensed. Commonly, these formulae lead to a five- to seven-day window where a patient may refill their medications before completely using the previous fill; some plans, and certain drugs, like narcotic pain relievers, require patients to have only one day of medication remaining before allowing a refill.

■ **Therapeutic Duplication**
  - This means that the insurance company has received claims for other drugs to treat the same condition. Before approving the claim, the insurance company wants a pharmacist to ensure that it is appropriate to fill this medication knowing that another drug for the same condition may also be used by the patient.
  - Ask a pharmacist if the prescription may be filled. Only after obtaining approval, enter the proper override codes and resubmit the claim. The pharmacist may request that you document his or her approval on the back of the prescription; documentation must be maintained that a pharmacist approved filling this prescription after being made aware of the potential duplication of therapy.

■ **Drug/Drug Interaction**
- Ask a pharmacist if the prescription may be filled. Only after obtaining approval, enter the proper override codes and resubmit the claim. The pharmacist may request that you document his or her approval on the back of the prescription; documentation must be maintained that a pharmacist approved filling this prescription after being made aware of the potential drug interaction.

■ **Drug Not Covered or NDC Not Covered**
- This means that the insurance company does not cover the specific drug submitted. Sometimes, this means that PA must be obtained before the drug is covered. Sometimes, this means that switching to a less-expensive drug that acts in a similar fashion will be covered but this particular drug is not. Further, sometimes this simply means that the patient will need to pay the entire cost themselves in order to obtain the drug.
- Ensure that the NDC submitted matches the NDC on the product being dispensed.
- Determine if the NDC submitted is listed as being obsolete or discontinued. If so, change the NDC, document why the NDC on the product in the pharmacy does not match the NDC being submitted and resubmit the claim.
- Ask a pharmacist if there is a lower-cost medication in the same class that could be used. With approval of the pharmacist, contact the prescriber to request that change be made to the drug recommended by the pharmacist.
- Some prescription drug insurance programs will not cover certain classes of medications such as birth control, weight-loss drugs, injectables or chemotherapy. The patient is responsible for the entire cost if he or she wishes to obtain the drug.

■ **Step Therapy Required[8]**
- Rather than require a PA for a medication, an insurance company may provide a pathway to coverage for a medication that includes trying other (usually less expensive) options first. If the patient either fails to respond to the alternatives, or has a medical reason not to use those alternatives, then the patient may use the originally requested drug. Going through these steps to get to a drug therapy is called utilizing **step therapy**.
- Generally, this comes up when a claim is submitted to an insurance company and it rejects with the message that the drug submitted is part of a step therapy program and that other drugs must first be tried before this drug will be covered. Some insurance companies require patients to try (and/or fail) certain medications before allowing a more costly medication to be covered.
- Contact the prescriber's office and inform the prescriber's assistant or nurse of the step therapy requirement. It is the physician's responsibility to contact the insurance company; however, the pharmacy can assist with this process by providing the insurance company's pharmacy help desk phone number (or the phone number provided in the rejection) and a list of less expensive alternatives in the same class (sometimes provided in the rejection from the insurance company). Ask the physician's office to contact the pharmacy when a determination has been made regarding a new medication; no override code will be necessary.

■ **Prior Authorization Required**
- Contact the prescriber's office and inform the prescriber's assistant or nurse that a PA will be required before the prescriber therapy can be provided to the patient. As with the step therapy rejection, it is the prescriber's responsibility to contact the insurance company, obtain the necessary forms, submit the necessary documentation and obtain the authorization.

- To speed up the process, provide the office personnel all of the patient's insurance information (pharmacy help desk phone number or the phone number provided in the rejection, the name of the company, the patient's ID number and any information from the rejection that seems relevant). Ask the assistant or nurse to contact the pharmacy when the PA is issued.

■ **Plan Limitations Exceeded**
- This rejection may occur for a variety of reasons. Most commonly, the quantity being dispensed exceeds the maximum allowed by the plan. The plan may only allow a certain quantity or a certain length of therapy to be dispensed at one time. Adjust BOTH the quantity being dispensed and corresponding day supply (length of therapy) to match the maximum allowed by the insurance company while maintaining the correct proportion based on the directions.
- Examples:
    ■ The prescription is written for a 90-day supply of a medication taken twice daily (quantity=180). The insurance allows a 34-day supply. The quantity being dispensed must be reduced from 180 to 68 and the day supply must be reduced from 90 to 34.
    ■ The prescription is written for 300 tablets of a medication taken twice daily. The insurance allows a maximum quantity of 100 tablets to be dispensed at each fill. Reduce the quantity dispensed from 300 to 100 and reduce the day supply from 150 days to 50 days and resubmit the claim.
    ■ The patient may only receive a limited number of fills at a local pharmacy and has already received that number of fills, and must now use a mail-order pharmacy owned and operated by the insurance company to continue receiving medication. This must be verified, over the phone, with the insurance company's pharmacy help desk before a patient is told that this is the case.
    ■ The patient's insurance only allows a limited number of fills each year (or ever). Example: a patient receives a prescription to help quit smoking; the insurance company will only pay for three months of therapy. The patient and physician determine that fourth month is required for complete therapy; the patient must pay for the fourth month without any insurance help.

Health Insurance Portability and Accountability Act of 1996

Pharmacy technicians play an enormous role in the daily functioning of the busy pharmacy. They, often times, are the first pharmacy employee to greet each patient and are often involved in giving refills (after being review by a pharmacist) to the patient. The following information will introduce a pharmacy technician to the basics of HIPAA as it applies to pharmacy practice in order for them to become sensitive to the far-reaching scope of this legislation and how it impacts the practice of pharmacy and everyone's everyday life. See Chapter 11 for a further discussion of HIPAA.

- ■ **Common Sense and Practical HIPAA Applications in the Community Pharmacy**
  - • Be discreet when discussing patients, their disease(s) and drug(s). Never discuss patient **protected health information (PHI)** with family or friends or in public places (such as elevators, restaurants or outside the pharmacy).
  - • Use private consultation areas or booths when speaking with patients.
  - • Only call out a first or last name (not both) to alert a waiting patient that their prescription is ready for pick-up at the pharmacy.
  - • Ensure that prescription receipts on prepared prescriptions are not visible to anyone but pharmacy staff.
  - • Shred old labels, receipts and prescription vials.
  - • Restrict access to patient files to only those engaged in treating patients.

- ■ **HIPAA Compliance "To-Do" List**
  - • Appoint a privacy official for the company.
  - • Conduct a company privacy assessment to determine the pharmacy's level of compliance.
  - • Adopt policies and procedures, including privacy rules.
  - • Conduct ongoing employee privacy training.
  - • Prepare and distribute a notice of privacy practices (NOPP).
  - • Prepare and use a patient consent document before initiating care.
  - • Prepare and implement a policy by which patients may request access to their information (including an account of all disclosures of their information to those not employed by the pharmacy).
  - • Design and use a marketing statement that complies with the privacy rules.

Fraud, Waste and Abuse Prevention

Fraud is defined in Title 18, United States Code (U.S.C.) §1347, as knowingly and willfully executing or attempting to execute a scheme or artifice to defraud any health care benefit program or to obtain (by means of false or fraudulent pretenses, representations or promises) any of the money or property owned by, or under the custody or control of, any health care benefit program.[9] Typically, abuse is unintentional, whereas fraud is intentional. Abuse is a practice that either directly or indirectly results in unnecessary costs to the Medicare program including improper payment, payment for services that fail to meet professionally recognized standards of care or payment for services that are medically unnecessary. Waste is a form of abuse that uses resources unwisely or inefficiently.

FWA prevention training in the pharmacy needs to be conducted at the time of contracting, when new personnel are hired and annually for all personnel. Pharmacists and pharmacy technicians are responsible for detecting and preventing FWA. Training records must be retained for 10 years. Examples of Medicare FWA include charging patients in excess of approved copays for services or supplies furnished to patients, billing Medicare beneficiaries a higher price than nonMedicare recipients, or submitting claims to Medicare and another plan sponsor for the same services or supplies. A comprehensive FWA program in the pharmacy includes written policies and procedures, a compliance officer and committee, plus the training and education of all staff.

Federal Pseudoephedrine Law

On March 9, 2006, President George W. Bush signed into law the USA Patriot Act, Title VII, which includes the Combat Methamphetamine Epidemic Act of 2005. This federal law applies to all cough and cold products (including combination products) that contain the methamphetamine precursor chemicals ephedrine, pseudoephedrine (PSE) or phenylpropanolamine. All such products, regardless of dosage form, are subject to the law. Products reformulated so that they no longer contain these precursors may be sold without regard to the new statutory provisions. Although all three chemicals are restricted, generally, these products are referred to as PSE products because pseudoephedrine is the most commonly used of these chemicals.

The following requirements are currently in effect:

- Sales to a patient may not exceed 3.6 g/day of PSE from a given store (regardless of the number of transactions engaged in with that store)
- Thirty-day purchase limit: Patients are prohibited from purchasing more than 9 g within a 30-day period
- Non-liquid forms: All non-liquid forms (including gelcaps) of PSE products must be sold in blister packs with no more than two dosages per blister or in unit-dose packets or pouches.
- Mail-order limits: Mail-order companies may not sell more than 7.5 g to a customer within a 30-day period
- Must not sell to any individual under the age of 18

The following requirements went into effect Sept. 30, 2006:

- Behind-the-counter placement: All PSE products must be placed behind a counter (any counter, not necessarily the pharmacy counter) that is not accessible to purchasing consumers or in a locked display case that is located on the selling floor. Retailers must give the product directly to the purchaser; therefore, a retailer without a pharmacy may still sell the combination PSE products from behind a counter or locked display case.

- Logbook: Retailers must maintain a logbook of information detailing the sale of PSE products. The logbook may be maintained in either written or electronic form. The logbooks must capture the following information:
  - Purchaser's signature
  - Purchaser's name and address
  - Date and time of sale
  - Description of the product sold
  - Quantity sold
  - Description of the identifcation used to make the purchase (ex: driver's license, including license number)

Logbooks must provide notice to purchasers that entering false statements or misrepresentations in the logbook may subject purchasers to criminal penalties under Title 18 United States Code §1001. The purchaser must sign the logbook and enter his or her name and address, as well as the date and time of the sale. The retailer must check the information entered by the purchaser against a government-issued photo ID and enter the name and quantity of the product sold. Logbook requirements do not apply to purchases of single sales packages that contain no more than 60 mg of PSE. Each entry must be maintained for two years following the date of entry. Information entered into the National Precursor Log Exchange (NPLEx) satisfies the requirement to maintain a log or some form of record detailing sales. The seller shall require the purchaser to sign the log at the time of the sale. If the pharmacy does not have an electronic signature capture system, and they utilize NPLEx for data reporting, this would allow them to maintain a written log and tie the data back to NPLEx at a later time.

■ Photo ID: In conjunction with the logbook requirement, retailers will be required to ask for photo identification (ID) issued by either a state or the federal government.

■ Training and certification: Retailers must train applicable sales personnel to ensure that they understand the requirements of PSE product sales and submit self-certifications to the U.S. Attorney General to this effect. The Drug Enforcement Administration has issued regulations on the training criteria.

Many states have enacted additional sales restrictions of PSE products and, therefore, pharmacy technicians will want to be knowledgeable and understand those requirements. This includes possible requirements to check the NPLEx prior to completing sales of products containing methamphetamine precursor chemicals. A summary of this Act's requirements can be found on the United States Drug Enforcement Administration's (DEA) Web site at www.DEAdiversion.usdoj.gov/meth/cma2005.htm.

Conclusion

This chapter introduced the key components of the third party billing process and provided an explanation of the main differences between federal and state prescription insurance programs, such as Medicaid, Medicare and private insurance plans.

The modern-day pharmacy technician is involved in a complex array of duties and functions. These duties include receiving the prescription, determining a patient's insurance eligibility, processing the prescription and notifying a pharmacist of any system messages that might affect the filling or billing process.

Being able to assess whether the patient is paying cash or is covered by insurance, whether the insurance information on file is active, and whether the patient needs to be asked for new insurance information is critical to the pharmacy running smoothly. Pharmacy technicians are also counted on to provide accurate information to patients on the message received from insurance companies and to follow through and ensure that these messages are handled appropriately.

Medicare Part D prescription drug coverage for seniors eligible for Medicare offers some opportunities for cognitive services reimbursement for pharmacists. If the concept continues to expand, a pharmacy technician's role and professional standing will reach new heights of responsibility in the pharmacy workplace. This chapter concluded with a brief explanation of the federal laws associated with HIPAA, FWA and PSE. These laws are in the forefront of pharmacy practice regardless of the practice setting for a pharmacy technician.

Acknowledgement

The author wishes to acknowledge pharmacy technicians Helen Thompson, CPhT, and Susan Wilson for their assistance in the writing of this chapter.

References

1. NCPDP Letter of Response to the National Committee on Vital and Health Statistics, www.ncvhs.hhs.gov/970416w2.htm, April 10, 2010.

2. U.S. Centers for Medicare and Medicaid Services, Office of the Actuary, CMS Statistics Medicare Enrollment, "National Trends."

3. 2011 Annual Report of the Boards of Trustees of the Federal Hospital Insurance and Federal Supplementary Medical Insurance Trust Funds, https://www.cms.gov/ReportsTrustFunds/downloads/tr2011.pdf, Aug. 7, 2011.

4. National Association of Boards of Pharmacy, www.nabp.net.

5. Pharmacy Benefit Management Institute, "Top 25 Pharmacy Benefit Management Companies and Market Share By Annual Prescription Volume, as of 3rd Quarter 2010," www.pbmi.com/PBMmarketshare2.asp.

6. Medco Health Solutions, Inc., Pharmacy Manual, www.medcohealth.com.

7. Michigan Medicaid Provider Manual, p. 23, April 1, 2010.

8. Blue Cross Blue Shield of Michigan, "Prior Authorization and Step Therapy," www.bcbsm.com/member/prescription_drugs/prior_auth_step_therapy.shtml.

9. Jason, B., "CMS Requirements for a Part D Program to Control Fraud, Waste and Abuse," *Michigan Pharmacist*, pp. 13-19, May/June 2008.

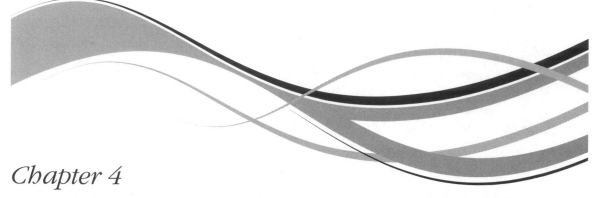

Chapter 4

REVIEW QUESTIONS

1. The federal health insurance provided to people over the age of 65 is typically covered under which health care program?
    a. Medicaid
    b. Medicare
    c. Blue Cross/Blue Shield
    d. Managed care

2. The federal-state health insurance, which provides for the basic health care services of needy persons, is covered under which health care program?
    a. Medicaid
    b. Medicare
    c. Blue Cross/Blue Shield
    d. Managed care

3. CMS is the federal agency that administers the Medicare program. As of 2010, Medicare provided coverage for approximately:
    a. Medicare does not provide any coverage to the elderly.
    b. 400,000 Americans.
    c. 47.5 million Americans.
    d. 4.52 million Americans.

4. The Medicare Part D prescription program provides medications for the following persons except:
    a. enrollees over age 65.
    b. enrollees with high drug costs and several disease states.
    c. enrollees with disabilities.
    d. only enrollees who are government employees.

5. Medication therapy management services will reimburse health professionals for all of the following activities except:
    a. patient education and training.
    b. patient health status assessments.
    c. all over-the-counter medications.
    d. formulating/monitoring/adjusting prescription drug treatment plans.

6. Pharmacy benefit managers provide the following services except:
    a. manage pharmacy networks.
    b. drug packaging supplies.
    c. mail-order options.
    d. outcome management.

7. AWP is the abbreviation for:
    a. ain't what's paid.
    b. average wholesale price.
    c. average warehouse price.
    d. awful wholesale price.

8. Reasons for electronic prescription claims to be rejected online include all of the following except:
    a. the pharmacist's initials were missing on the prescription.
    b. the quantity of medication prescribed exceeds the limits set by the prescription plan.
    c. the patient's card/coverage has expired.
    d. the patient had Medicaid prescription coverage.

9. If an electronic prescription claim adjudication provides a message to the technician that a prescription will be dispensed and billed below cost, he or she should:
    a. bill the difference on the next claim submission by increasing the quantity of drug.
    b. not worry about it, as the software will find the error and rebill automatically.
    c. transmit another claim to make up for the difference.
    d. contact the pharmacist immediately.

10. A pharmacy technician would run a BIN search if he or she would like to:
    a. determine which wholesaler was billed for the drug.
    b. determine which container the drug came from.
    c. determine if the medication was billed too soon.
    d. determine if the correct insurance company was billed.

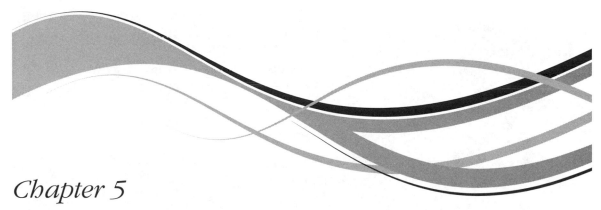

Chapter 5

PHARMACY COMPOUNDING

By Kenny R. Walkup, R.Ph., FIACP

Learning Objectives

This chapter seeks to prepare a pharmacy technician to:

- define pharmacy compounding.
- explain the role of the United States Pharmacopeia.
- explain the difference between pharmacy compounding and manufacturing.
- explain the role of the Pharmacy Compounding Accreditation Board.
- explain the triad as it relates to medication delivery.
- discuss the various pieces of equipment used in pharmacy compounding.
- discuss the various dosage forms prepared in compounding pharmacies.

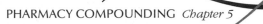

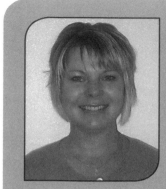

What challenges do technicians face in compounding?

"I'm currently a Certified Pharmacy Technician (CPhT) and have been working in a compounding pharmacy for the last three years. When I started, I had very minimal experience and, as technicians, we face many challenges. I have found that I needed to develop an organized system to run an efficient compounding lab. My training came from pharmacists and CPhTs, as well as hands-on experience.

In order to meet our patients' needs, a good rule of thumb is to set expectations during initial contact. This involves communicating the time frame and cost issues associated with making a precise compounded product.

Personally, my gratification has come from providing service to customers who need unique medications that are not available from a noncompounding pharmacy. I encourage any of you to further your professional capabilities by exploring compounding techniques."

Dawn Meder, CPhT,
Medicap Pharmacy,
Urbandale, Iowa

Introduction

According to Merriam-Webster's dictionary, "compound" is a transitive verb meaning "to put together (parts) so as to form a whole," as in to combine ingredients or "to form by combining parts," as in to compound a medication.

In pharmacy, compounding could be defined as "the art of customizing medications to fit individual needs." In collaboration with physicians, pharmacists may provide medications in the proper strengths and easy-to-administer doses even when those strengths and doses may not be commercially available. This becomes important when dealing with certain populations. Please refer to Table 1 for examples of patient populations where compounding could play an integral role in drug therapy. For example, pediatric patients may need a medication that only exists in an adult form; geriatric patients may no longer be able to swallow tablets or capsules; and animals may need medications only available in human doses or forms. Hospice patients may no longer be able to swallow or absorb medications after oral ingestion. Compounding allows the medication and delivery route to be individualized to the patient.

Table 1
Populations Where Compounding Plays an Important Role

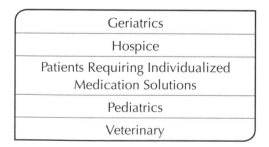

Geriatrics
Hospice
Patients Requiring Individualized Medication Solutions
Pediatrics
Veterinary

The Basis of a Profession

Pharmacy compounding is the basis for the beginning of the profession of pharmacy. In 1823, the state of Louisiana licensed the first pharmacist in America, Louis J. Dufliho.[2] This was in response to an 1804 law requiring a licensing examination for pharmacists wishing to distribute and sell pharmaceuticals. The site of that first pharmacy is a museum today where a visitor can walk through the store and into the botanical garden and see where many of the ingredients were grown that eventually were made into compounded medications. In the beginning of medicine, one patient would visit one physician and then present a prescription to a pharmacist to be filled. This prescription would contain a recipe for a medication that the pharmacist would then have to make, or compound. Many times these were special mixtures that a physician had worked with the pharmacist to create. This was a time before large scale manufacturing of medications existed and the only access to medicine was from drugs or ingredients being compounded by a pharmacist. This was also the beginning of the triad relationship between a physician, a patient and a pharmacist. This triad relationship is vitally important in pharmacy compounding. As patients present to physicians with unique challenges, it becomes vital for a pharmacist to be able to develop a medication working with that physician. Collaboration between these three individuals on doses and dosage forms could be the difference between a therapeutic success or failure.

The Role of the United States Pharmacopeia

The **United States Pharmacopeia (USP)** is a nongovernmental, official, public, standards-setting authority for prescription and over-the-counter medicines and other health care products manufactured or sold in the United States. The USP was founded in 1820 when state medical societies were invited by Dr. Lyman Spaulding to send delegates to the first meeting of the USP Convention. In all, 11 delegates attended that first meeting, which was held in the U.S. Capitol building in Washington, D.C. At that first meeting, the delegates created the framework for a "*Pharmacopoeia of the United States,*" which was published later in 1820. The first Pharmacopoeia of the United States included formulas (recipes) for 217 of the "most fully-established and best understood" substances available at the time. This collection of recipes allowed pharmacists to consistently compound products based on a standard followed nationwide. This was becoming more important as people continued to move from one location to another, from one physician to another and from one pharmacist to another. The delegates also decided to meet every 10 years to update the Pharmacopoeia. In 1830, pharmacists began to get involved with USP and eventually became dominant contributors. As the pharmaceutical industry emerged and grew, USP transitioned from a book of recipes for medicines to become a compendium of quality tests and manufacturer specifications. In 1975, USP purchased the National Formulary (NF) from the American Pharmaceutical Association (now the American Pharmacists Association). The NF now includes excipient standards, which regulate inactive substances that serve as a medium for a drug or other substance. Today, the Pharmacopeia is published as the USP-NF, and has several line extensions (including the Dietary Supplements Compendium and the Pharmacists' Pharmacopeia). The USP-NF includes monographs for drug substances, drug products, excipients, dietary supplements, compounded preparations and more.

The USP-NF also includes general chapters, which are used for general tests and assays that apply broadly to a large number of monographs. These general chapters are numbered to reflect whether or not they are mandatory (below <1,000>) or informational (above <1,000>). The two USP General Chapters that have the most impact on pharmacy compounding today are General Chapter <795>, Pharmaceutical Compounding – Nonsterile Preparations, and General Chapter <797>, Pharmaceutical Compounding – Sterile Preparations. Many state Boards of Pharmacy adopt all or part of these standards into their state pharmacy rules.

All pharmacy personnel who are going to be involved in compounding must read and understand General Chapter <795>, and those engaging in sterile compounding must read and understand both chapters. There must also be processes in place to address competency in both areas. While General Chapter <795> covers nonsterile compounding processes, it also covers the following general areas: the responsibility of the compounder, the compounding environment, the stability of compounded preparations, beyond-use labeling (expiration date determination), ingredient selection, the compounding process, records and documents, quality control and patient counseling requirements. A good understanding of General Chapter <795> is essential as a foundation for all compounding personnel. General Chapter <797> covers issues directly relating to the compounding of sterile preparations. The following are a partial list of covered topics: microbial contamination risk levels, personnel training and evaluation in aseptic manipulation skills, immediate use CSP, single- and multiple-dose containers, as well as hazardous drugs, radiopharmaceuticals and allergen extracts as CSP. As with General Chapter <795>, all pharmacists and pharmacy technicians who engage in sterile compounding must be familiar with this general chapter.

Compounding Versus Manufacturing

It is important to distinguish between two facets of pharmacy that, although apparently close from the outside, are completely different in their scope. Those two facets are pharmacy compounding and commercial manufacturing.

The **National Association of Boards of Pharmacy® (NABP®)** defines compounding as the preparation of components into a drug product:

1. as the result of a practitioner's prescription drug order or initiative based on the practitioner/patient/pharmacist relationship in the course of professional practice.
2. for the purpose of, or as an incident to, research, teaching or chemical analysis and not for sale or dispensing. Compounding includes the preparation of drugs or devices in anticipation of receiving prescription drug orders based on routine, regularly observed prescribing patterns.

NABP® defines "manufacturing" as the production, preparation, propagation, conversion or processing of a drug or device, either directly or indirectly, by extraction from substances of natural origin or independently by means of chemical or biological synthesis. Manufacturing includes the packaging or repackaging of a drug or device, or the labeling or relabeling of the container of a drug or device for resale by pharmacies, practitioners or other persons.[3]

Compounding pharmacies, just like other retail pharmacies, are under the regulation and oversight of the individual Board of Pharmacy for the state in which the pharmacy is physically located. Compounded medications are provided under the direction of a physician, via a written prescription, acting on behalf of a specific patient. Compounded medications are not made in anticipation of a prescription unless the applicable state Board of Pharmacy specifically allows anticipatory compounding. In contrast, manufacturers and manufacturing are under the jurisdiction of the Food and Drug Administration (FDA). Manufacturers prepare medications in large volumes for distribution to wholesalers or directly to pharmacies. Based on the scope of practice for a manufacturer, medications are generally produced without receiving prescriptions and are not produced for patients with whom the manufacturer has a direct relationship. All pharmacists and pharmacy technicians are encouraged to know the regulations of their state Board of Pharmacy and act in accordance with all applicable rules when compounding.

Compounding Equipment: Then and Now

As the triad of patient care and the need for personalized medicine has remained constant over the years, the ways to deliver that care have evolved with the times. That change is clearly evident in the use of equipment in the compounding process. Over the years, as technology has advanced, so has the equipment found in today's pharmacies. It wasn't that long ago that in pharmacy practice the standard equipment was graduated cylinders, flasks, mortars and pestles, and a torsion balance. Actually, one can find all of these in a modern pharmacy, but those that actually compound medications will also have much more advanced tools.

■ **Mortars and Pestles**

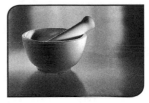

Mortars and pestles come in a wide array of sizes, shapes and materials. The **mortar** is the bowl shaped mixing dish, and the **pestle** is the bat shaped object used to mix, crush and grind. Knowing which mortar and pestle to use is very important, as using the wrong one may result in damage to the mortar or may result in a low-quality product. Glass mortar and pestles are very useful in triturating or mixing items. A glass mortar and pestle is a good choice when one needs to mix two (or more) powders or to make creams and suspensions. It is very important that a glass mortar and pestle not be used for crushing or grinding. Crushing and grinding are highly abrasive and will lead to pitting the glass; pits in the glass become a place where materials will collect and make mixing ineffective, make cleaning the mortar and pestle more difficult and could weaken the glass to the point where the grinding action could crack or shatter the glass. Ceramic and wedgewood mortars and pestles are a much better choice for crushing and grinding. The inside of the mortar is rougher, enabling the technician or pharmacist to crush a tablet and grind it to a fine powder. There are other substances used to make mortars and pestles, like wood, brass, marble and steel, but they are seldom used in pharmacies.

■ **Flasks, Graduated Cylinders and Pipettes**

Flasks, graduated cylinders and pipettes are useful tools for measuring or holding liquids. Of the three, the pipette is most useful for measuring small quantities with the most accuracy. A **pipette** is a slender graduated cylinder with a bulb at one end. The bulb is used to draw liquid up into the cylinder for measurement. A properly calibrated pipette is one of the most accurate tools for measuring small volumes of liquid. **Graduated cylinders** can measure small volumes of liquid (e.g., 10 mL) or large volumes of liquid (1 L). Graduated cylinders are generally made of clear plastic or glass and have accurate markings (called graduates) to measure the contained volume of liquid. To properly read a graduated cylinder, the liquid inside must be at rest (e.g., the cylinder is sitting on a table or other flat, level surface) and then the line closest to the bottom of the **meniscus** (the curved "half bubble" that appears at the top of the liquid when viewed through the graduated cylinder) is used to read the volume. Flasks commonly come in two shapes; round bottom (Florence flasks) and flat bottom (Erlenmeyer flasks) are the most commonly used flasks in pharmacy practice. **Flasks** are used for storing or holding liquids, rather than measuring a liquid's volume (with the exception of a volumetric flask). A volumetric flask, when used correctly, is a highly accurate way of measuring medium to large volumes of fluid; however, such accuracy is usually not required and, therefore, these are only used when extreme accuracy is necessary, otherwise a graduated cylinder is used.

■ **Beakers**

Beakers come in a wide range of sizes starting as small as 5 mL and ranging to larger than 2,000 mL. Beakers are especially useful for mixing suspensions and emulsions. It is important to know that the markings on beakers are generally not reliable measurement graduates but are there to provide an estimate of the volume. Using a graduated cylinder to verify all markings on the beaker before the first use would be a recommended step.

■ **Torsion Balance**

Torsion balances use a bar suspended on a fulcrum with weigh boats on each end. Accurate weights are placed in one weight boat, while the substance being weighed is in placed in the other. When the indicator shows equal weight on both sides of the fulcrum, the desired weight has been achieved. The weights used on a torsion balance are special weights with their known weight printed on

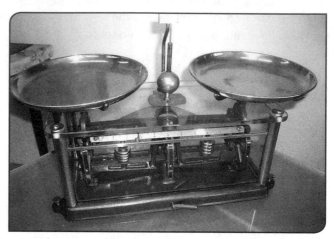

them. It is important that the technician or pharmacist never touch the weights with their bare hands, as oil can transfer to the weights and render them inaccurate. Most weight sets will come with a glove or forceps to handle the weights and cleaning instructions in case of contamination or accidental contact.

■ **Digital Balance**

The torsion balances of yesterday have been replaced in many pharmacies by highly-accurate **digital balances**. Digital balances can weigh down to the milligram with a high degree of accuracy. Digital balances come in a wide array of sizes and styles and must be chosen to meet the specific needs of the pharmacy where they will be used. Additional options, such as air flow shields, will help to keep air flow from disturbing the readings. Many balances also offer the ability to plug in an external printer so that measured weights can be recorded without relying on a human to read the scale and transfer the number by hand (potentially creating errors). Printing the weights will allow the readings to be kept on file with the prescription in

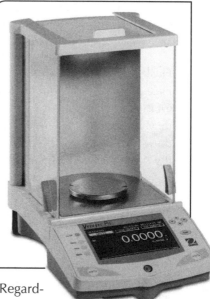

case there is a need to retrieve that information later. Regardless of the type of digital balance used, all balances must be calibrated on a daily basis and a log of that calibration must be kept in the pharmacy's quality assurance (QA) file. It is also recommended that all digital balances be validated on a yearly basis by an outside scale company, and those records also be kept in the pharmacy's QA files.

■ Mixing Equipment

The **Electronic Mortar and Pestle (EMP)** gives the pharmacist a tool for producing a pharmaceutically elegant ointment, cream or gel. The same machine can be used to compound suspensions. To use the machine, all ingredients are weighed in the EMP jar and the jar is transferred to the machine. Working like an inverted drill press, the machine mixes the ingredients at the predetermined speed for a predetermined amount of time. When mixing is complete, the product can be dispensed in the EMP jar, eliminating compounding time, clean-up and waste.

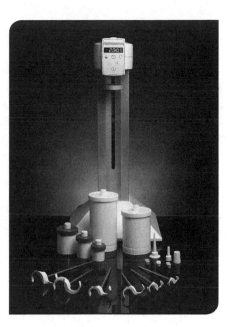

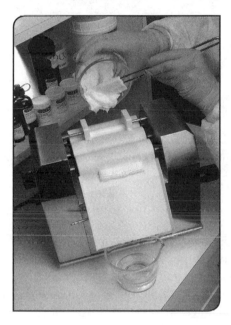

An **ointment mill** is a very useful tool for the reduction of particle size and incorporation of the active ingredient into a cream or ointment base. The machine is made of three ceramic rollers that the compound passes through. After several passes through the rollers, the product can be collected and placed into a dispensing container or run through the EMP for additional mixing.

The **homogenizer** is another piece of equipment with a specific, but very important, place in the compounding lab. A homogenizer is a high-performance dispersing and emulsifying instrument. Homogenizers are primarily used to reduce particle size in suspensions and lotions. The dispersing parts can be sterilized and used in the preparation of sterile compounds.

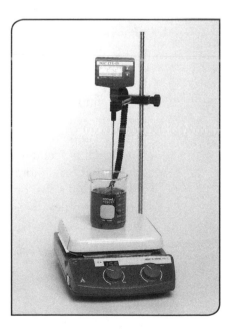

A standard kitchen stand mixer is also a very useful tool in the pharmacy. Large batches of creams, gels and suspensions can be combined and set to mix over a period of time.

Capsule Machine

The filling of empty capsules has long been an important, yet tedious, task for a compounder; however, the introduction of the **capsule filling machine** has made that chore much easier and quicker. Today's pharmacy has the option to choose from a variety of companies that produce capsule filling devices. The most common configurations are 100-count and 300-count options. Both devices are comprised of a base, interchangeable plates and a top plate to separate and secure the tops of the capsules. Once the capsules are in place, the tops can be removed and the powder mixture can be poured onto the device. A powder scraper and tamper are used to move the powder and pack it into the bottoms of the capsules. Once the capsules are full, the tops are returned and then pressed together by hand. An experienced technician can make 100 capsules in a matter of a few minutes using a 100 count capsule machine.

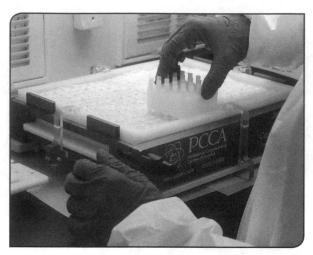

Today's Dosage Forms

Just like in Louis J. Dufliho's day, today's pharmacy technicians and pharmacists are called upon to make unique creams, ointments, suspensions, emulsions, elixirs and even more formulations. Unlike those days, we have very unique dosage forms to treat patients with various needs.

Implantable pellets start as powder weighed on balances that measure down to the milligram. After being weighed, they are prepared using a pellet press. The pellet press uses a lever to form a pellet under high pressure. Pellets are weighed and pressed individually. After pressing, they are packaged and sterilized. Once sterilized, the pellet is inserted under the skin of the patient by a physician using a special needle.

Lollipops are a unique dosage form with multiple uses. Lollipops with a numbing agent can be used by dentists for numbing the oral cavity before dental procedures. This is a great application for children. Dentists can also use lollipops on patients with a bad gag reflex to aid them having dental procedures. Nicotine lollipops are also useful to control the hand-to-mouth habits of those wishing to end nicotine addictions.

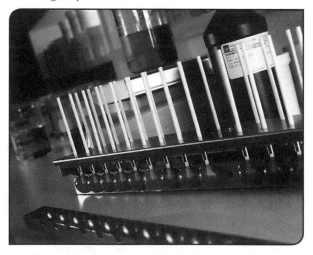

Troches are gelatin or glycol compounds that are placed in the buccal cavity (between the cheek and gum inside the mouth) to dissolve. They have a wide array of uses, including dentistry, wound management and hormone replacement.

Effervescent packets originated with Alka Selzer®. Today, pharmacies have the ability to make their own effervescent packets. This is a great application for patients needing doses that would be too large for a single capsule or for medications that have an unpleasant taste. The effervescing can act as an aid to mask the taste.

Unique formulations of **sterile products** have become a mainstay for many physicians. Compounding pharmacies that are equipped with sterile facilities can compound a number of sterile dosage forms. Commonly compounded sterile products include otic preparations, ophthalmic preparations, injectables, intravenous medications and parenteral nutrition. It is imperative that pharmacies that provide compounded sterile products follow USP Chapter <797> guidelines. It is also imperative that steps be taken to ensure the compound is tested to prove sterility and potency and that the preparation passes endotoxin testing. More detailed information on sterile compounding is available in the Aseptic Technique chapter of this Manual.

These are just a few of the unique dosage forms that innovative pharmacists have compounded. Other examples of unique dosage forms include suppositories, transdermal gels, animal biscuits and even popsicles. The compounding pharmacist has a unique ability and position to come up with creative solutions to address the patient's unique and complex problem.

Quality Assurance

Regardless of the type or size of the pharmacy, all pharmacies engaging in compounding need to institute a quality assurance (QA) program. A good QA program will consist of employee training procedures and detailed programs to assure that finished products are of the highest quality. A good starting point would be the random testing of finished products on a monthly basis. The use of a third party laboratory is highly recommended for this, and there are a number of companies that specialize in testing pharmacy compounds. It is important that your pharmacy's testing program be outlined in your standard operating procedures and followed.

Accreditation for Compounding Pharmacies

In 2004, eight pharmacy organizations came together to form the **Pharmacy Compounding Accreditation Board (PCAB™)**. Please see Table 2 for a list of the founding organizations of PCAB™. PCAB™ was formed to provide quality standards for compounding pharmacies through a voluntary accreditation program. PCAB™ assesses those pharmacies that voluntarily apply and awards the PCAB™ Seal of Accreditation to those pharmacies that accept the PCAB™ requirements, meet the criteria and comply with the Rules and Terms of the PCAB™ program (including adherence to PCAB™ Standards). The PCAB™ Seal of Accreditation provides evidence of adherence to quality standards and to principles of the profession of pharmacy compounding.[4]

Table 2
Founding Organizations of the Pharmacy Compounding Accreditation Board (PCAB™)

American College of Apothecaries
American Pharmacists Association
International Academy of Compounding Pharmacists
National Association of Boards of Pharmacy
National Alliance of State Pharmacy Associations
National Community Pharmacists Association
National Home Infusion Association
United States Pharmacopeia

Conclusion

Pharmacy compounding played an important role in the origins of the profession of pharmacy. Today, advancements in equipment, dosage forms and technology continue to advance pharmacy compounding, and medicine is constantly changing. Patients are looking for personalized medicine. Physicians are looking for individualized treatment plans. Pharmacists and technicians working with physicians and patients are creating unique, individualized solutions to complex medical challenges, and pharmacy compounding is at the forefront of those changes.

Acknowledgement

The author wishes to acknowledge the following individuals for their review of this chapter: Dr. Lloyd Allen, Ph.D., R.Ph., from the International Journal of Pharmaceutical Compounding; Dr. Eileen Lewalski, Pharm.D., JD, from the National Association of Boards of Pharmacy®; and Rick Schnatz, Pharm.D., from the United States Pharmacopeia. The author also wishes to acknowledge the Professional Compounding Centers of America, Houston, Texas, for their contribution of photos to this chapter.

References

1. Merriam-Webster Online Dictionary and Thesaurus, www.merriam-webster.com, July 14, 2010.
2. New Orleans Pharmacy Museum, www.pharmacymuseum.org, July 12, 2010.
3. *Model State Pharmacy Act and the Model Rules of the National Association of Boards of Pharmacy*, August 2009.
4. Pharmacy Compounding Accreditation Board, www.pcab.info, July 12, 2010.

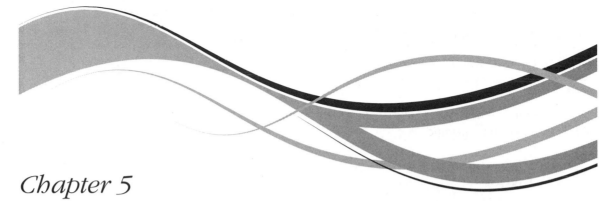

Chapter 5
REVIEW QUESTIONS

1. The triad of patient care includes all of the following except the:
    a. patient.
    b. physician.
    c. pharmacist.
    d. nurse.

2. The United States Pharmacopeia is a governmental agency that writes standards and guidelines for pharmacy compounding.
    a. True
    b. False

3. USP chapters below _____ are considered enforceable.
    a. 500
    b. 750
    c. 797
    d. 1,000

4. Which of the following USP chapters contain information regarding nonsterile compounding?
    a. 575
    b. 685
    c. 795
    d. 797

5. Which of the following USP chapters contain information regarding sterile compounding?
    a. 575
    b. 685
    c. 795
    d. 797

6. Which is the best type of mortar and pestle to use when triturating powders?
   a. glass
   b. ceramic
   c. wedgewood
   d. brass

7. Which is the best type of glassware to use when measuring small amounts of liquids?
   a. graduated cylinder
   b. pipette
   c. flask
   d. beaker

8. Digital balances should be calibrated _____ and validated _____.
   a. daily, monthly
   b. daily, yearly
   c. weekly, monthly
   d. monthly, yearly

9. Which piece of equipment is used for reducing particle size while incorporating an active ingredient into a cream or ointment base?
   a. EMP
   b. brass mortar and pestle
   c. ointment mill
   d. kitchen stand mixer

10. A good QA program for a compounding pharmacy:
    a. includes employee training.
    b. is incorporated into the pharmacy's standard operating procedures.
    c. includes random testing of finished products.
    d. All of the above.

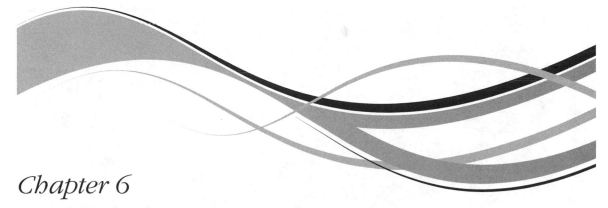

Chapter 6

HEALTH-SYSTEM PHARMACY PRACTICE

By Jim M. Lile, Pharm.D.

Learning Objectives

This chapter seeks to prepare a pharmacy technician to:

- provide an overview of hospital pharmacy practice.
- outline the steps in a medication order.
- describe the distributive and administrative roles of a pharmacy technician in health-system practice.
- describe the nontraditional opportunities for pharmacy technicians in health-systems.

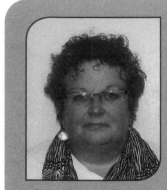

Introduction

Institutional pharmacy practice typically refers to the provision of distributive and clinical services to patients in hospitals, home care, long-term care and hospice, as well as activities of palliative care. The focus of this chapter is on health-system pharmacy practice. The structure of a hospital pharmacy department varies with the size of the institution where it is located; however, all departments are led by a director or chief of pharmacy. There may be one or more assistant directors and clinical pharmacists. Staff pharmacists and pharmacy technicians complete the pharmacy team. Large hospitals may have more than 100 pharmacists and technicians on staff. The smallest hospitals may have only two part-time pharmacists and no technicians. Regardless of the size of the hospital or department, it is critical for the pharmacy staff to function as a team to provide safe and effective medication management for hospitalized patients.

Background

■ **Regulation and Oversight**

Hospitals must be surveyed and accredited by **The Joint Commission (TJC)**, the American Osteopathic Association (AOA), state inspectors or Det Norske Veritas (DNV) Healthcare. There are written standards that a hospital must adhere to when providing care to patients. The standards generally include provisions on patient care, medication management, environment of care, medical staff, leadership and competency of all staff. Without accreditation by one of these organizations, institutions will not be paid for charges submitted to the **Centers for Medicare and Medicaid Services (CMS)**. Other third party insurers may deny claims for nonaccreditation, as well.

The **Drug Enforcement Administration (DEA)** is a component of the federal Department of Justice. The primary focus of the DEA is avoiding diversion of controlled substances (both legal drugs and illegal drugs). Officers have the authority to seize contraband, investigate individuals and groups under suspicion of violating the law, and enforce the provisions of the federal Controlled Substances Act. The DEA is responsible for assigning DEA numbers to appropriately qualified physicians, hospitals and clinics, manufacturers, distributors, pharmacies and others to carefully track the manufacture, distribution and use of controlled substance. Recently, the DEA has taken on a role providing educational materials to adults, children and schools related to the dangers of drug diversion and abuse.

■ **Internal Oversight**

There is an important multi-disciplinary committee structure in most hospitals. The most active committees are generally the **Pharmacy and Therapeutics (P&T) or Formulary Committee, Infection Control Committee and Institutional Review Board (IRB)**.

The P&T is comprised of physicians, nurses, pharmacists, administrators and other representatives. Among the functions of the P&T are selecting drug products for use in the hospital, reviewing medication errors and adverse drug reactions, and evaluating standing order forms.

The Infection Control Committee studies bacterial resistance trends and infection rates, evaluates antimicrobial use, and educates the hospital staff on topics related to infection control. Composition of the Infection Control Committee is broader than the P&T. Members include physicians, nurses, pharmacists, microbiologists, administrators, engineers and housekeepers.

If an institution performs clinical research, it must have access to an IRB. The IRB has the responsibility of approving human research studies that are performed in the hospital. All research protocols are carefully reviewed for safety and appropriate documentation and are monitored for ongoing approval. The IRB is charged with protecting research subjects from unwanted, unethical or unsafe research. This multi-disciplinary committee has members of the hospital staff as well as community members such as clergy, lawyers and other volunteers from the local community.

The **Medical Executive Committee (MEC)** oversees all medical staff committees and practice departments (e.g., internal medicine, family practice, surgery) and reports to the Board of Directors of the institution. The MEC ensures the professional conduct of the physicians who practice in the institution and also distributes information on accreditation to the medical staff.

Finally, the Board of Directors is a group of internal and external (community) leaders who authorizes the institution's budget, sets the clinical direction of the hospital and reviews all reports from the clinical committees. The Board appoints senior leadership for the hospital. State and federal laws, and any applicable standards from accrediting bodies, regulate the Board of Directors.

Overview of Institution Medication Use Process

The pharmacy department is responsible for the provision of safe medication use for all patients who come to the institution for care. Depending on the size of the hospital and the services provided, the pharmacy department may be open for only a few hours each day or it may be continuously open 24 hours per day. Any time the pharmacy is open, a pharmacist must be on duty. Most medications are dispensed directly from the pharmacy. However, if the pharmacy is closed, nurses are given access to an **automated dispensing cabinet (ADC)** or nonautomated storage cabinet outside the pharmacy. The nonautomated cabinet is commonly referred to as the night cart. The **night cart** or ADC is replenished the next day when the pharmacy opens.

The basic steps of the medication use process start and end with the patient. Medications are used for the treatment, diagnosis or prevention of a disease or symptom. The patient's physician, or mid-level provider (physician's assistant or advance practice registered nurse/nurse practitioner), makes a decision regarding what medication to prescribe to a specific patient. A **medication order** (prescription) is written into a patient's medical record or is entered electronically into the electronic medical record or chart. The medication may be removed from an ADC, or the order is sent to the pharmacy for the medication to be entered into the patient's profile, dispensed and delivered to the patient. The medication is then administered to the patient by a nurse, or by the patient themselves, and the patient's response to the medication is measured. During each component of the medication use process, pharmacists and technicians work closely together and with the rest of the medical team to assure the safe processing of each medication order and in monitoring the clinical benefit and adverse effects of each administered medication.

Medication orders may be designated as "**stat**" or regular priority. "Stat" orders generally refer to orders needed in 15 minutes or less. "Stat" medications are needed for acute changes in the patient's condition, and delay in administration may result in patient harm. An example of a "stat" medication is nitroglycerin sublingual tablets for a patient with new onset chest pain (**angina**). "Now" orders are less urgent than stat orders; however, the desired turn-around is still expected to be quick (less than 30 minutes). A "now" order could be an oral pain medicine that is not routinely stocked in the automated dispensing cabinet. Routine orders usually have a one to two hour turn-around time. These prescriptions are typically new orders or modifications of old orders for chronic conditions like **hypercholesterolemia** or **hypertension**.

Medication administration in hospitals generally occurs at what is termed "standard times." The goals of standard times are to streamline workflow for the nursing and pharmacy staffs, and provide consistency from one patient care area to another. Patient preference for administration time may come into play in some situations; however, standard times are followed in the majority of instances. A sample of standard administration times can be found in Table 1.

Table 1
Standard Administration Times

Daily, empty stomach	7:30 a.m.
Daily	9 a.m.
Twice daily, empty stomach	7:30 a.m. and 4:30 p.m.
Twice daily, with food	8 a.m. and 5 p.m.
Twice daily or every 12 hours	9 a.m. and 9 p.m.
Three times a day	9 a.m., 1 p.m. and 9 p.m.
Three times a day, with food	8 a.m., noon and 5 p.m.
Every eight hours	5 a.m., 1 p.m. and 9 p.m.
Every six hours	5 a.m., 11 a.m., 5 p.m. and 11 p.m.
Every four hours	1 a.m., 5 a.m., 9 a.m., 1 p.m., 5 p.m. and 9 p.m.

The **medication profile** is a list of all medications the patient is receiving in the hospital. A medication may be scheduled, or given regularly, for an ongoing condition or as needed based on an acute symptom such as pain or nausea. The profile may be printed on paper or available electronically. The physician uses the profile as a point of reference for monitoring and modifying drug therapy. The nurse uses the profile to document medication administration by making this document into a **medication administration record (MAR)**. The pharmacist uses the medication profile for monitoring drug therapy. The MAR is a communication tool for the medical team so that everyone knows what drugs have been given, how much was given and when they were given.

Distributive Roles of a Pharmacy Technician

Traditional roles of pharmacy technicians are primarily distributive. Pharmacy technicians are involved in a wide variety of activities that range from ordering and storing medications to preparing medications to delivering medications to the patient care areas.

■ **Preparation of Parenteral Products**

Pharmacy technicians prepare medications for intravenous and intramuscular (i.e., parenteral) administration using sterile technique, usually in an environment that is compliant with USP Chapter <797> (see Chapter 7). The room where parenteral products are made is divided into three areas: the sterile preparation area, an ante area and a storage area. Parenteral products may be intravenous solutions, antibiotics, nutrition, electrolytes or other medications. Cancer chemotherapy agents are prepared by pharmacy technicians in a separate room with special hoods to protect the pharmacy technician from possible harmful effects of the drugs.

■ **Automated Dispensing Cabinets**

ADCs are specially designed devices that allow for the secure storage and the safe dispensing of medications in a patient care area. Each nurse has his or her own access code and password that allows access to the medications inside the cabinet. In some circumstances, the nurse is able to view the patient's profile on a computer screen and select the medication from a list. In other situations, the nurse may "override" the profile to obtain emergency, "stat" or "now" medications. Many hospitals store narcotics and other controlled substances in ADC to improve control and documentation through the electronic network of the hospital. Selected other "as needed" (pro re nata or **PRN**) medications are stored in the ADC.

On at least a daily basis, reports are generated that indicate low levels of medications that need be restocked. A pharmacy technician assembles the medications indicated on the report to be checked by a second technician or a pharmacist. Then, a pharmacy technician takes the medications to the cabinet, signs in and restocks the drugs in the appropriate drawers and secure areas. A follow-up report may be generated that compares what was restocked to what was required.

■ **Robotics**

Pharmacy dispensing robots are machines that are capable of storing and retrieving medications from pegs along the robot's interior walls. The robot is programmed to move a dispensing arm to the peg where a specific dose of a specific medication hangs. The robot scans the barcode on the packaging, removes the correct number of doses from the peg, and places the medication in an envelope or bin for checking. If the barcode is incorrect or lacking, the robot will unload the medication in a reject bin. Robots may be used for first doses of medications as well as cart fill. Cart fill refers to filling bins of medications to be taken to a patient care area for distribution to patients in that area on a regular basis.

■ **Repackaging**

Medications that are delivered to patient care areas of hospitals are typically packaged in unit-of-use (single-dose) containers. Instead of a 30-day supply that a patient may receive from their community pharmacy, a patient will receive a 24-hour supply of their medication in their nurse's medication cart. Most oral, solid, dosage forms are available in unit-dose packaging; however, other medications are available only in bulk bottles, and pharmacy technicians may be assigned to repackage these medications into smaller units.

Repackaging medications takes one of three broad forms: manual, semi-automated or automated. Manual repackaging involves a technician placing individual doses of a medication into an appropriately sized container (e.g., small plastic bag for vials or injection syringes, oral syringe for liquids, mini-cups for tablets and capsules). The individual doses are labeled at a minimum with the generic and brand name, strength, expiration date and lot number. Semi-automated repackaging involves some manual manipulation of the dose forms or packaging equipment by the pharmacy technician. Fully-automated systems require very little handling by the technician. The machine may have small bins of bulk medication that are funneled to the packaging material to be individually sealed and properly labeled.

Some repackaging systems allow for a barcode to be placed on the packaging. The barcode may serve as additional identification for the medication at the patient's bedside. In some electronic systems, the nurse would scan the patient's wristband identification, scan his or her badge, and scan the barcode on the package. The pharmacy information system compares what was scanned to the patient's medication profile. If the correct medication is in the correct dose for the correct patient at the correct time via the correct route, then the nurse proceeds with the administration step. The dose is charted electronically. If any one of the five components of the administration is incorrect, the nurse receives an alert and must investigate possible causes of the alert before administering the medication.

■ Dose Preparation and Compounding

Once new orders are received and processed, a pharmacy technician gathers the medication(s) from stock and assembles the medication label, medication and physician order for a pharmacist to verify that the order is appropriate, that the pharmacy technician has gathered and labeled the product correctly, and that the medication is ready to be sent to the patient. Further preparation may be required for an oral antibiotic suspension, bulk liquids poured into smaller containers and other dosage forms. A number of products are not commercially available in liquid formulation, and pharmacy technicians may play a role in preparing these medications. Some products are compounded from special recipes (e.g., Magic Mouthwash, Miles Mixture or Hawaiian Punch), which involve mixing two or three individual ingredients together for their combined therapeutic benefit.

■ Cart Fill

As noted above, a hospitalized patient receives a 24-hour supply of most medications once each day. A few hospitals use the ADC in the patient care areas for most of the 24-hour supply of scheduled doses, but the majority of hospitals provide medications in drawers labeled with the patient's name. The drawer will contain most of the oral solid and liquid dose forms, injectable medications and topical products that the patient is scheduled to use that day. Once each day, a new cart containing the upcoming day's medications is exchanged for the old cart. Any unused and returnable medications in the old cart are credited to the patient's account. The empty carts are stored until the cart fill begins again.

■ Floor Stock

Selected medications may be available as floor stock; such systems do not assign a drug specifically to a patient. These medications in floor stock are available for general patient use and are not stored in an ADC. Pharmacy technicians are responsible for checking floor stock medications to make sure they are unexpired, intact and properly stored. There may be a minimum and maximum number of a specific floor stock drug that the pharmacy technician would assure is accurate. Pharmacy technicians typically check floor stock on a monthly basis.

■ Recalled and Expired Medications

Pharmacy technicians play an important part in reviewing pharmacy stock for medications that are recalled by pharmaceutical manufacturers. Medications may be recalled for any number of reasons including poor dissolution, subpotency, contamination, incomplete documentation, device malfunction, etc. In the event of a recall, a pharmaceutical manufacturer sends a letter or e-mail to the pharmacy department with the specific lot numbers involved in the recall. If the recalled medication is currently stocked by the pharmacy, it is segregated from the rest of the stock and handled according to the manufacturer's instructions.

Periodically, the entire pharmacy department must be swept looking for expired medications. Typically, this activity occurs on a monthly basis. Technicians and pharmacists may be assigned to a specific area (e.g., the refrigerator in the IV room) to look through the items for outdated medications. The expired drugs would be segregated from the other products and sent to a reverse distributor for destruction, according to the hospital's policy, or returned to the manufacturer (as allowed by the specific manufacturer). Controlled substances require special documentation, including when they expire or are destroyed.

■ Emergency Medication Sources

Within the hospital, critical-need medications are stored in a mobile cart commonly known as a crash cart. The crash cart generally contains drugs to support a patient's blood pressure, drugs to restore a patient's heart rhythm, antidotes to common poisons/toxins and drugs to correct a patient's acid-base balance. If a drug tray from a crash cart drawer is used, it is immediately replaced or replenished.

Emergency Medical Technicians (EMTs) and paramedics carry a specially designed box with specific emergency medications. The emergency medication sources (EMS) box is a crash cart tray that the first-responders can carry to the scene of an emergency. The EMS box may also have intravenous fluids and catheters, respiratory drugs, cardiac drugs, controlled substances and anti-emetics.

■ Charge and Credit

Charging for medications and services assures that the department receives reimbursement for goods and services. Most charges are done through the pharmacy information system; however, some manual billing may need to be done. Unused and reusable medications that are returned to the pharmacy are credited to the patient's account. Pharmacy technicians and pharmacists are responsible for this task to assure accurate and complete billing. The credit function may be completed electronically through the pharmacy information system or through a paper system.

Administrative Roles of a Pharmacy Technician

■ **Technical Supervisor**

The technical supervisor is the administrative leader of the pharmacy technicians. This individual may be responsible for training newly hired staff, evaluating the performance of current staff and serving as an arbitrator during conflict. Special education and training may be required for a position with this level of responsibility.

■ **Maintenance of Technology**

ADC, pharmacy robots and other equipment require both regular and emergency maintenance to function properly and safely. Pharmacy technicians may take on some of this responsibility to assure these investments operate well. An experienced pharmacy technician, with the appropriate training and background, may save the institution expensive service calls from manufacturer representatives when technology needs basic maintenance.

■ **Scheduling**

Pharmacy technicians may be involved in scheduling other pharmacy technicians and/or pharmacists to meet department needs. Scheduling requires a careful balance between available staff and requests for time off. The pharmacy technician responsible for coordinating the schedule may be involved in approving or denying days off.

■ **Technician Training Programs**

Hospitals, colleges and universities have, or are developing, structured academic and experience-based pharmacy technician training programs. Technicians may be involved in the classroom as instructors and in the hospital as preceptors and mentors. Well-trained pharmacy technicians are critical to the proper functioning of a pharmacy department, and technician training programs are one component of pharmacy technician education.

Nontraditional Roles of a Pharmacy Technician

■ **Purchasing and Inventory Control**

Pharmacy technicians may be responsible for purchasing and inventory control. Maintaining an adequate inventory is critical to supplying medication to the hospitalized patients. At the same time, excess inventory creates budget issues for the director of pharmacy. Identifying minimum and maximum quantities of stock is an important duty of the purchasing pharmacy technician. When drugs are in short supply or on back-order, the purchasing pharmacy technician works closely with their pharmacists to identify other sources for the product or strategies for substitution with a similar agent.

■ **Medication Histories**

When a patient enters a hospital or health-system, it is the institution's responsibility to collect a complete and accurate list of the patient's current medications including prescription drugs, nonprescription drugs, herbal products and medical devices. Some institutions have stationed pharmacy technicians in emergency departments, pre-admission departments and in patient care areas to collect this important information. Pharmacy technicians are in a unique position to help sort through a patient's outpatient medication list and ensure that physicians and pharmacists have the complete information they need to best care for hospitalized patients. A physician determines which of the drugs he or she wants to continue while the patient is in the hospital.

■ Medication Reconciliation

An extremely important activity that is particularly necessary in the elderly, but certainly extends beyond this population, is medication reconciliation. TJC has included the concept of medication reconciliation in its National Patient Safety Goals (NPSG). **Medication reconciliation** is a process designed to ensure adequate review of a patient's drug list at any transfer point in the health care system. The drug list ideally contains prescription drugs, nonprescription medications, vitamins and herbal supplements, along with doses, directions and indications. Medication reconciliation should occur upon admission to and discharge from a hospital and upon transfer between different levels of care (for example, between a critical care setting and a medical floor setting). The patient's drug list needs to be reviewed for appropriateness of indication, dose, frequency and route of administration; then, the entire health care team (including at least a pharmacist and a physician) must determine if each drug will be continued, or modified, between different transfer points. Initial collection of a patient's medication list is one of many points during this process that may be delegated to a pharmacy technician from a pharmacist.

■ Clinical Data Technician

Pharmacy technicians may assist pharmacists in the task of collecting patient laboratory data. Specially trained pharmacy technicians use the patient's medical record and the laboratory information system to gather monitoring parameters necessary for managing drug therapy. This may include results from bacterial cultures used to determine appropriate antibiotic therapy, results from blood draws that include drugs levels, blood cell counts, electrolyte levels and many other results.

■ Medication Safety

Medication safety can be ensured with the "five rights" of medication use:
1. RIGHT Patient
2. RIGHT Medication
3. RIGHT Dose
4. RIGHT Route
5. RIGHT Time

Pharmacy technicians have an important role in medication safety. Upon a patient's entry into the institution, pharmacy technicians may take medication histories, which is the first step in a safe medication use system. Assuring that the correct dose of the correct medication has been prepared is determined in collaboration with the pharmacists on duty. Minimizing distractions and maintaining a clutter-free work environment is everyone's responsibility, and pharmacy technicians can play an important role in sustaining a safe work area. Pharmacy technicians play a critical part in barcode technology, ADC and USP <797> compliance. These vital duties all play an important role in medication safety and are just some examples of how pharmacy technicians help keep patients safe.

Conclusion

Pharmacy technicians can take on a wide variety of roles in a pharmacy department. Distributive, administrative and nontraditional roles exist in many institutions. In the complex world of health-system pharmacy practice, pharmacy technicians play an important part in safe and effective medication use.

Acknowledgement

The author wishes to acknowledge the pharmacy technicians of McLaren Regional Medical Center and Mid-Michigan Medical Center-Midland for their assistance in the preparation of this chapter.

Bibliography

- American Society of Health-System Pharmacists, "ASHP statement on bar-code-enabled medication administration technology," *American Journal of Health-System Pharmacy*, Vol. 66, pp. 588-590, 2009.

- American Society of Health-System Pharmacists, "ASHP guidelines on the safe use of automated dispensing devices," *American Journal of Health-System Pharmacy*, Vol. 67, pp. 483-490, 2010.

- Bates, D.W., "Preventing medication errors: A summary," *American Journal of Health-System Pharmacy*, Vol. 64, Suppl. 9, S3-9, 2007.

- Helmons, P.J., Wargel, L.N., Daniels, C.E., "Effect of bar-code-assisted medication administration on medication administration errors and accuracy in multiple patient care areas," *American Journal of Health-System Pharmacy*, Vol. 66, pp. 1202-1210, 2009.

- The Joint Commission, www.jointcommission.org, Aug. 3, 2010.

- Knight, H., Edgerton, L., Foster, R., "Pharmacy technicians obtaining medication histories within the emergency department," *American Journal of Health-System Pharmacy*, Vol. 67, pp. 512-513, 2010.

- Meller, R.D., Pazour, J.A., Thomas, L.M., Mason, S.J., Root, S.E., Churchill, W.W., "Third-party repackaging in hospital pharmacy unit dose acquisition," *American Journal of Health-System Pharmacy*, Vol. 67, pp. 1108-1114, 2010.

- Pedersen, C.A., Schneider, P.J., Scheckelhoff, D.J., "ASHP national survey of pharmacy practice in hospital settings: Dispensing and administration – 2008," *American Journal of Health-System Pharmacy*, Vol. 66, pp. 926-946, 2009.

- Rouse, M.J., "White paper on pharmacy technicians 2002: Needed changes can no longer wait," *American Journal of Health-System Pharmacy*, Vol. 60, pp. 37-51, 2003.

- Rubino, M., Hoffman, J.M., Koesterer, L.J., Swendrzynski, R.G., "ASHP guidelines on medication cost management strategies for hospitals and health systems," *American Journal of Health-System Pharmacy*, Vol. 65, pp. 1368-1384, 2008.

- Skibinski, K.A., White, B.A., Lin, L.I.K., Dong, Y., Wu, W., "Effects of technological interventions on the safety of a medication-use system," *American Journal of Health-System Pharmacy*, Vol. 64, pp. 90-96, 2007.

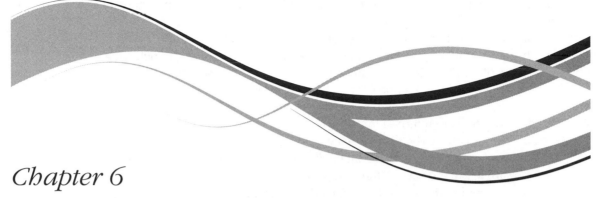

Chapter 6

REVIEW QUESTIONS

1. Which of following committees is primarily responsible for the safety of research subjects?
    a. P&T Committee
    b. Institutional Review Board
    c. Medical Executive Committee
    d. Infection Control Committee

2. Which of the following statements is true?
    a. All pharmacy departments have a director of pharmacy.
    b. All pharmacy departments have full-time technicians.
    c. All pharmacy departments have clinical pharmacists.
    d. All pharmacy departments have an assistant director.

3. Which of the following is not one of the five "rights" of medication safety?
    a. Right patient
    b. Right drug
    c. Right nurse
    d. Right route

4. Which of the following requires the fastest turn-around time?
    a. Routine orders
    b. "Stat" orders
    c. "Now" orders
    d. None of these

5. ADCs:
    a. may be used to access medications when the pharmacy is closed.
    b. reduce the amount of paper documentation for controlled substances.
    c. are restocked daily.
    d. all of these

6. If a pharmacy technician discovers an expired medication in a crash cart, he or she is expected to:
   a. leave the medication in the cart for another month.
   b. move the medication to a nearby automated dispensing cabinet.
   c. replace the medication and segregate it from the rest of the stock.
   d. give the drug to a nurse for administration to a patient.

7. Medications that are returned in the medication cart:
   a. should always be thrown away.
   b. are credited back to the patient if they can be reused.
   c. are left in the cart for the next patient.
   d. are returned to stock without crediting the patient.

8. A pharmacy technician taking a medication history from a patient in an emergency department is expected to:
   a. collect prescription, nonprescription and herbal product information.
   b. disregard scheduled medications on the patient's profile.
   c. disregard as needed medications on the patient's profile.
   d. collect only the names and doses of the herbal products.

9. The three components of a clean room include the:
   a. sterile preparation, compounding and storage areas.
   b. compounding, ante and storage areas.
   c. storage, compounding and labeling areas.
   d. sterile preparation, ante and storage areas.

10. Repackaged medication labels must include:
    a. drug name, expiration date and lot number.
    b. date repackaged, color of medication and drug dose.
    c. expiration date, lot number and color of medication.
    d. drug name, person repackaging and lot number.

Chapter 7

ASEPTIC TECHNIQUE AND STERILE PRODUCT PREPARATION

By Allen R. Doan, Pharm.D., ARRT

Learning Objectives

This chapter seeks to prepare a pharmacy technician to:
- list four major routes of parenteral administration.
- define aseptic technique.
- define compounded sterile products (CSPs).
- describe primary engineering controls.
- describe laminar air flow.
- list four examples of critical sites.
- define ISO Class 5, 6, 7 and 8 air quality environments.
- describe low, medium and high-risk microbial compounding levels.
- list the visual checks that must be made on a parenteral solution.
- describe the proper cleaning and disinfection procedure for various primary engineering control (PEC).
- determine beyond use dating of CSPs made under low, medium and high microbial risk levels.
- describe how to withdraw a solution from an ampule or vial.
- describe how to reconstitute a sterile powder.

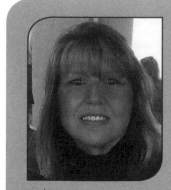

What is a traditional role for technicians in sterile product compounding and preparation?

"The traditional role for technicians in compounding and preparation of sterile products is to free up the pharmacist for more clinical duties in patient care. Technicians are an invaluable asset to the pharmacy setting because they take on the hands-on and technical aspect of pharmacy practice. The preparation of sterile products involves knowledge of pharmaceutical calculations, proper use of equipment, safe handling of chemotherapy and other hazardous products, as well as safety techniques, aseptic technique and knowledge of reconstitution of medications, correct diluents, and solutions needed for each medication, and the correct amount of solution for the strength of the medication being used."

In establishing a proper aseptic technique, in what ways can a technician serve as an educational resource for other health care professionals?

"The first and most important maneuver in aseptic technique is hand washing. This is the single most important factor in reducing contamination. As a technician moves around the hospital, it becomes even more important to be aware of the need for aseptic technique in preparing sterile product, as well as the day-to-day contact that we have with other professionals, clients, patients, peers and visitors. Establishing a proper aseptic technique starts with establishing proper hand washing techniques; this is information that is useful to everyone, not just other health care professionals, in helping to reduce the occurrence and the spread of germs. Correct hand washing should take at least 15 seconds with a good antibacterial soap, making sure to wash the backs of the hands, the palms and in between the fingers, washing from the elbows down, and then using paper towels to dry."

Robin Summers
CPhT, RPT
James A. Haley Veterans
Administration Hospital
Tampa, Fla.

Introduction

Aseptic processing of **compounded sterile products (CSPs)** is intended to prevent harm, including death, to patients, from any of the following: microbial contamination, excessive bacterial endotoxins, variability in the intended strength and unintended physical or chemical contaminants. CSPs can be given either parenterally or topically (generally topical CSPs are only used in the eyes). Parenteral products are given by injection and, therefore, bypass the gastrointestinal (GI) tract. Drugs needed in emergency situations and those inactivated or destroyed by the GI tract can be given by the parenteral route of administration. Patient characteristics, such as inability to swallow, uncooperativeness or unconsciousness can also necessitate the parenteral route of administration.

The United States Pharmacopeia (USP) is a nongovernmental, nonprofit agency that sets official public standards for prescription and over-the-counter medicine, food ingredients, medical devices and other health care products. The standards cover strength, quality, purity and consistency of these products and are published on a yearly basis. These standards are published under the title The United States Pharmacopeia (The USP) so pharmacy technicians must be careful to distinguish between the organization and the standards. The USP is organized in numbered chapters, each pertaining to a different process; the chapter covering compounding of sterile preparations is *USP General Chapter*

<797> Pharmaceutical Compounding – Sterile Preparations, first released in January 2004. These guidelines apply to all health care professionals who prepare CSPs. The final changes to this chapter were published in December 2007, and the official 2nd Supplement of Chapter *<797>* was published June 31, 2008.

Parenteral Routes of Administration

There are multiple routes of administration for parenteral products, the most common parenteral routes of administration being intravenous, intramuscular, subcutaneous, intradermal and intra-arterial. Other less common parenteral routes of administration are listed at the end of this section.

■ **Intravenous Route**

The **intravenous (IV)** route of administration is used for drugs that must be injected directly into the venous system. This route of administration gives a rapid effect with a predictable response. The IV route of administration can be given by bolus, continuous or intermittent infusion. The bolus route of IV administration is used when a relatively small volume of medication is given. This route of IV administration is most often used for emergency situations when rapid effect of the medication is needed. Some examples of medications given by this route of administration are epinephrine, amiodarone and various narcotics. These products are typically prepared in syringes. Continuous infusions are used for large volume parenterals (LVP); these products are typically prepared in bags or bottles. LVP can be used with or without other medications added to them. Some common uses of LVP include: the correction of electrolyte and fluid balance disturbances; to provide nutrition when enteral feeding is not possible; and as a vehicle for administering other drugs. An example of a common LVP is 0.9% NaCl (normal saline) in a 1,000 mL bag. Intermittent infusions are used to administer smaller volumes of medications at specified times or over a defined time interval. A few of the most common medications given by intermittent infusion include antibiotics, narcotics and nonsteroidal antiinflammatory drugs (NSAIDs).

■ **Intramuscular Route**

The **intramuscular (IM)** route of administration is used when medication must be injected deep into a large muscle (e.g., a thigh, the buttocks or the upper arm). After IM injection, the injected medication is absorbed slowly, through the muscle tissue, acting more quickly than medications given by the oral route but slower than drugs given by IV administration. The typical maximum volume to be administered by this route of administration is 2.5 mL as a solution or a suspension. IM injections are typically painful and reversing any adverse effects from the injected medication can be difficult. Examples of medications sometimes given by this route of administration steroids, antibiotics, vaccines, narcotics and NSAIDs.

■ **Subcutaneous Route**

The **subcutaneous (SC or SQ)** route of administration is used when medication must be injected just beneath the surface of the skin layers. A medication administered by this route can be either a solution or suspension. It is usually not absorbed as well and has a slower onset of action than either the IV or IM routes. The maximum volume given by subcutaneous injection is 2 mL due to the relatively small space available for injection. A medication commonly given by this route of administration is insulin.

■ **Intradermal Route**

The **intradermal (ID)** route of administration is used when a drug needs to be injected just underneath the top layer of the skin. Medications given by this route of administration reside between the top two layers of the skin. The most common medications given by this route are for diagnostic purposes (such as a tuberculin skin test and common allergy tests). The volume administered to this space is limited to 0.1 mL. The onset of action for medications given by this route tend to be the slowest of all routes previously mentioned.

■ **Intra-arterial Route**

The **intra-arterial** route of administration is used to inject a drug directly into an artery. This route of parenteral administration is most commonly used for radio-opaque medications (dye that can be seen on x-ray) that can be used to diagnose disease.

■ **Other Less Common Routes of Parenteral Administration**
  - **Intra-articular:** injected into a joint, such as a knee or ankle
  - **Intracardiac:** injected directly into the muscle of the heart
  - **Intraperitoneal:** injected into the peritoneal or abdominal cavities
  - **Intrapleural:** injected into the sac surrounding the lungs
  - **Intraventricular:** injected directly into the ventricle of the brain
  - **Intravesicular:** instilled into the urinary bladder
  - **Intravitrial:** injected into the fluid filled space in the eye
  - **Intrathecal:** injected into the space around the spinal cord

Intravenous Bottles and Bags

Intravenous solutions can be supplied in three types of containers:

1. A glass container with an air tube, sometimes referred to as an **open system** because unfiltered air enters the container, requiring a nonvented administration set (see Figures 1 and 2).
   - The closure of an open system has two openings: one is the airway tube and the other receives the spike from the administration set. The closure is covered with a thin rubber diaphragm. Small indentations in the seal over the holes indicate that a vacuum is present in the bottle. If the bottle has lost its vacuum, it should be discarded immediately. Medications can be added to the bottle by injecting them through the additive injection port or through the seal covering the hole for the spike. Medication should never be added to the air tube. The seal on the closure is removed just before the bottle is spiked.

Figure 1
Open System

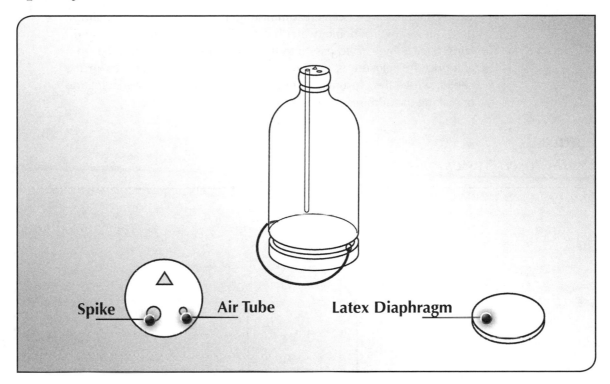

Spike   Air Tube   Latex Diaphragm

Figure 2
Nonvented Set

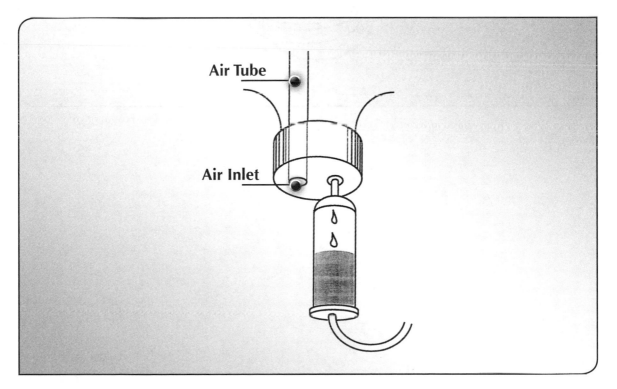

Air Tube

Air Inlet

2. A glass container without an air tube and containing a vacuum is sometimes called a **semi-closed system**, because the air that enters the container is filtered (see Figure 3).

    ▪ This system requires a vented administration set. The air vent contains a 0.20 micron hydrophobic (water-hating) filter (see Figure 4). The sterilizing filter allows air to pass into the bottle but prevents bacteria from entering. The closure is a solid rubber stopper. The target area in the center, where the closure is thinner, allows the injection of medication or spiking the administration set through this area.

Figure 3
Semi-Closed System

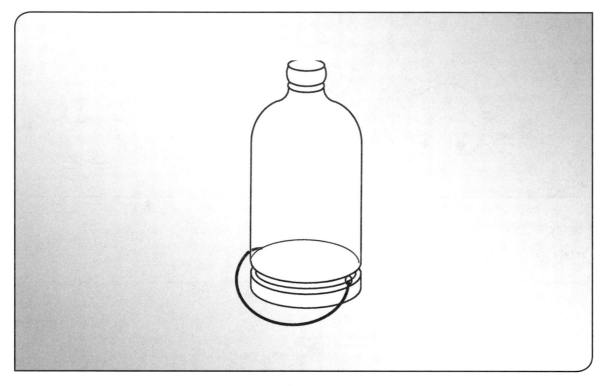

Figure 4
Vented Set

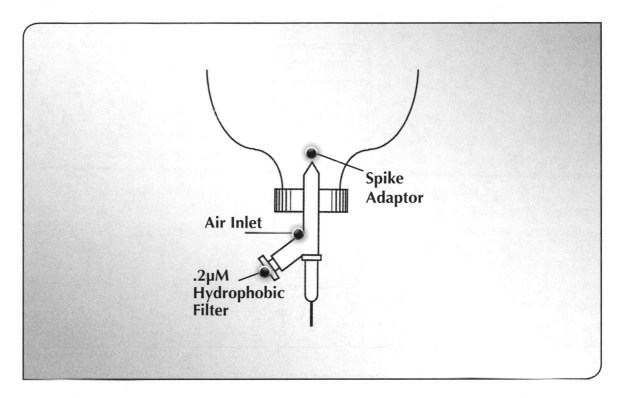

3. A flexible plastic bag is referred to as a **closed system** because the bag collapses to prevent air from entering the system (see Figure 5).
   - There are two ports on the bag. If the system is designed to be needle-less, one port will have a plastic cover that is removed to accept the spike of the administration set. The other port is the adapter (not requiring a needle) used for the attachment of medication to the bag (e.g., Mini Bag Plus®, ADD-Vantage®). The flexible bags that are not designed to be needleless will also have two ports. One port has a plastic cover that is removed to accept the spike of the administration set. The other port has a gum rubber covering used for the addition of medication to the bag using a syringe with a needle. Both of these types of flexible bags will require a nonvented IV set.

Figure 5
Closed System

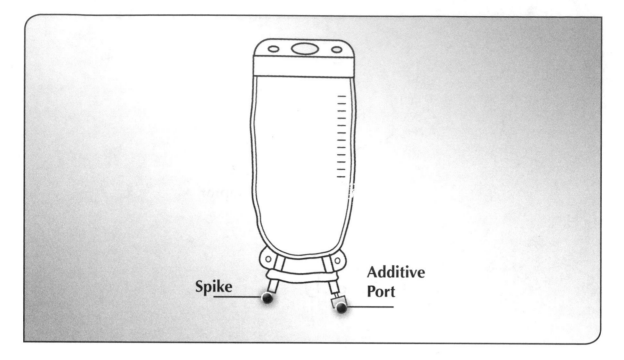

Spike

Additive Port

Sterilization by Filtration

Filtration is the most common method of sterilization in a pharmacy. Filters come in various pore sizes and configurations; however, a sterilizing filter pore size must be 0.2 microns. A sterilizing filter is one that, when challenged with a solution of *Brevundimonas diminuta* at a concentration of 107 CFU/cm² (colony-forming units per centimeter squared) of filter surface area, will give a sterile effluent. A larger pore size filter (e.g., 0.45, 0.8, 1.2 and 5 microns) is used for clarification of solutions. When selecting a filter, it is important to know if the solution is aqueous or nonaqueous and the volume of the solution being filtered. An aqueous solution requires a hydrophilic (water loving) filter, and a nonaqueous solution needs a hydrophobic filter. When selecting a filter, one must consider the pore size, the compatibility of the solution with the filter membrane and filter housing, the volume of solution to be filtered and the size and amount of particulate present in the solution. Filter suppliers are a great source of help in filter selection.

Other methods of sterilization for products and devices include cold sterilization and heat sterilization. **Cold sterilization** uses chemicals (e.g., ethylene oxide gas), radiation or an ultrasonic process. **Heat sterilization** uses steam and pressure (as with an autoclave) or hot air oven (in which high temperatures sterilize products or devices).

Pyrogens

Like bacterial contamination, pyrogen contamination is a concern when preparing products for parenteral administration. **Pyrogens** are substances that produce a fever. One type of pyrogen, a bacterial endotoxin, is a lipopolysaccharide (a large molecule consisting of a lipid and multiple sugars joined by chemical bonds) shed from a gram-negative bacteria cell wall. An endotoxin can also be released when bacteria die. Pyrogens are not removed with a 0.2 micron filter and are not destroyed

Chapter 7 ASEPTIC TECHNIQUE AND STERILE PRODUCT PREPARATION

by autoclaving. Products contaminated with pyrogens must be thrown away. The **bacterial endotoxin test** determines the amount of endotoxins in a parenteral product. When commercially prepared sterile products are used and aseptic technique is observed, pyrogens will not be a concern; however, if a sterile product is being compounded from a nonsterile product, one should check for pyrogens before releasing the product.

Aseptic Processing Glossary

■ **Admixture**

A parenteral dosage form made from combining several drug products for administration as a single entity.

■ **Ante Area**

An ISO Class 8, or better, area where high-particulate-generating activities are appropriate (e.g., hand hygiene, garbing, order entry, CSP labeling). It can also be used as a transition area into the clean room/buffer, usually separated by some type of barrier. This barrier can be a wall or curtain. A properly designed ante area will provide assurance of a constant pressure relationship between clean room and outside environment and reduce the need for heating and ventilation systems to respond to large air disturbances.

■ **Aseptic Processing**

A mode of processing pharmaceutical and medical products that involves manipulating a sterile product without contaminating it. This type of processing is done in at least an ISO Class 5 environment.

■ **Beyond-use Date**

The **beyond-use date (BUD)** is the date and time after which a CSP shall not be stored or used

■ **Biological Safety Cabinet**

A **biological safety cabinet (BSC)** is ventilated for use in making CSPs. A BSC has an open front with inward airflow that is designed for personnel protection. BSC are most commonly used to process hazardous CSPs (e.g., biologics).

■ **Buffer Area**

Provides at least an ISO Class 7 environment and is the area in which the primary engineering control (e.g., horizontal laminar flow workbench, vertical laminar flow workbench and BSC) is located. It is the area in the pharmacy that is second in cleanliness to the primary engineering control (PEC).

■ **Clean Room**

A room in which the airborne particle concentration is controlled to meet a specified ISO Class, most commonly ISO Class 7 or better.

■ **Compounding Aseptic Containment Isolator**

A **compounding aseptic containment isolator (CACI)** provides worker protection from hazardous materials being handled during the aseptic transfer process. Similar to a Class II BSC, but this is totally enclosed and air exchange does not occur with outside room air. All exhausted air must be filtered before being vented directly to the outside environment to ensure that none of the volatile hazardous drugs being prepared are released into the environment.

■ **Compounding Aseptic Isolator**

A **compounding aseptic isolator (CAI)** is designed for the aseptic compounding of pharmaceutical ingredients. It is designed to maintain an ISO Class 5 environment or better throughout the compounding process. Air exchange may occur with the room as long as it is passed through a **High-Efficiency Particulate Air (HEPA)** filter first. All exhausted air will be passed through a HEPA filter in order to provide protection for the operator before being put back into the room.

■ **Critical Area**

An area designed to maintain at least an ISO Class 5 environment

■ **Critical Site**

An opening or surface that can provide a pathway between the sterile product and the environment. Examples of a critical site are the hub of a needle, the tip of the syringe, the open neck of an ampule, the top of the vial closure and the ribs of the plunger on a syringe. The risk of microbial contamination of critical sites will increase with an increase in the size of the site or an increase in the time of exposure.

■ **Direct Compounding Area**

Direct compounding areas (DCAs) are located within the ISO Class 5 primary engineering control (PEC) where critical sites are exposed to unidirectional HEPA filtered air, also known as first air.

■ **First Air**

This is the first air to exit the HEPA filter in a unidirectional flow that is essentially particle free.

■ **Hazardous Drugs**

Substances classified as hazardous to humans or animals

■ **High-Efficiency Particulate Air**

High-efficiency particulate air (HEPA) is air that is produced by a specialized filter called a "HEPA filter" consisting of banks of filter-medium pleats. The separators direct air in a laminar flow. The HEPA filter is 99.97 percent efficient at removing particles 0.3 microns and larger. To put this in perspective, the smallest particles visible to the human eye are about 40-50 microns in size.

■ **Horizontal Laminar Flow Workstation**

A **horizontal laminar flow workstation (HLFW)** provides an ISO Class 5 environment in which the air is blown across the work surface toward the operator (see Figure 6).

Figure 6
Horizontal Laminar Flow Workstation

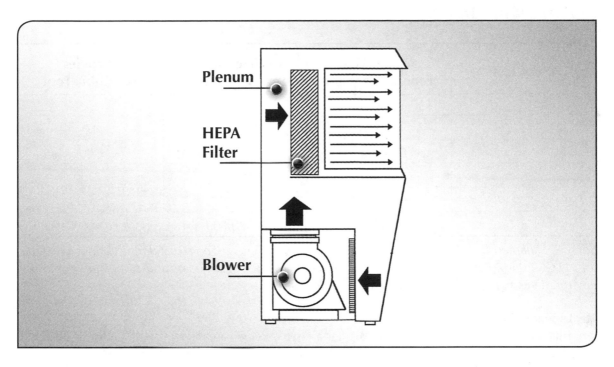

- **ISO Class 5 Area**

  This is an area in which the air has a count of no more than 3,520 particles, 0.5 microns or larger, per cubic meter of air. It is equivalent to the **Class 100 area** in which the air has a count of no more than 100 particles, 0.5 microns and larger, per cubic foot of air. This is the quality of air required for sterile product preparation (see Table 1).

- **ISO Class 6 Area**

  This is an area in which the air has a count of no more than 35,200 particles, 0.5 microns or larger, per cubic meter of air. It is equivalent to the **Class 1,000 area** in which the air has a count of no more than 1,000 particles, 0.5 microns and larger, per cubic foot of air (see Table 1).

- **ISO Class 7 Area**

  This is an area in which there is no more than 352,000 particles, 0.5 microns or larger, per cubic meter of air. It is equivalent to a **Class 10,000 area**, which is an area that has no more than 10,000 particles, 0.5 microns and larger, per cubic foot of air (see Table 1).

- **ISO Class 8 Area**

  This is an area in which there is no more than 3,520,000 particles, 0.5 microns or larger, per cubic meter of air. It is equivalent to a **Class 100,000 area**, which is an area that has no more than 100,000 particles, 0.5 microns and larger, per cubic foot of air (see Table 1).

Table 1

International Organization for Standardization (ISO) Classification of Particulate Matter in Room Air

ISO Class	Former U.S. Federal Standard	Particle Counts Per Cubic Meter	Particles Per Cubic Foot
3	Class 1	35.2	1
4	Class 10	352	10
5	Class 100	3,520	100
6	Class 1,000	35,200	1,000
7	Class 10,000	352,000	10,000
8	Class 100,000	3,520,000	100,000

Source: Adapted by USP from Federal Standard 209E, General Services Administration, Washington, D.C., 20407 (Sept. 11, 1992) and ISO 14644-1 1:1999 Cleanrooms and associated controlled environments-part 1: Classification of air cleanliness.

■ **Laminar Flow**
This is also known as unidirectional air. It is air in a confined area moving with uniform speed along parallel lines. Airflow in a laminar flow workbench (LFW) must have a velocity of 90 feet/minute +/- 20 percent. An LFW can be a horizontal flow (HLFW) where the air flows toward the operator or a vertical flow (VLFW) where the air flows down toward the bench.

■ **Media Fill Test**
This is a test used to qualify aseptic technique of compounding personnel or processes.

■ **Primary Engineering Control**
The **primary engineering control (PEC)** is a room or device that provides an ISO Class 5 environment for the exposure of critical sites (e.g., clean room, VLFW, HLFW, BSC, CAI and CACI).

■ **Vertical Laminar Flow Workbench**
The **vertical laminar flow workbench (VLFW)** is similar to an HLFW in that air is drawn in through a pre-filter, pressurized in the plenum and pushed through the HEPA filter (see Figure 7). Unlike a HLFW, however, the air is blown down from the top of the workstation onto the work surface rather than across it. Working in vertical laminar flow (VLF) requires different techniques than working in HLF. In VLF, the hands of the operator or any object must not be above an object in the hood. In HLF, the hands of the operator or any object must not be in back of another object. The hands of the operator must never come between the HEPA filter and the object. The critical site must always be protected.

Figure 7
Vertical Laminar Flow Workbench

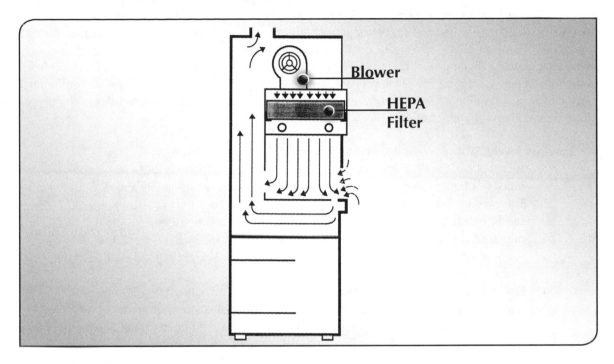

- **Secondary Engineering Control**

  A room, or segregated area, in the pharmacy that provides a location to place the PEC. Secondary engineering controls can have a different ISO Class air quality; most commonly they are ISO Class 7 or 8 depending on what will be located there and the functions that will be performed. Examples of secondary engineering controls are ante rooms, buffer areas and segregated compounding areas.

- **Segregated Compounding Area**

  A space designated by either a line of demarcation or a separate room that is restricted to preparing low-risk level CSP with a 12-hour maximum BUD. This area shall contain a PEC to provide unidirectional airflow of ISO Class 5 or better.

- **Sterility**

  This is the state of being "free of all living microorganisms." It does not mean that the solution is free from pyrogens or viruses. Compounding sterile products takes place in an ISO Class 5 area. Usually the ISO Class 5 area is only in the LFW; however, some institutions have an ISO Class 5 room.

- **Validation**

  This is establishing documented evidence that provides a high degree of assurance that a specific process will consistently produce a product that meets predetermined specifications. In other words, validation is documentation or evidence that you are producing what you say you are producing.

Microbial Risk Levels of Compounded Sterile Products

There are five risk levels to characterize the processing of CSPs. They are assigned according to the potential, or probability of, contamination occurring from (1) microbial contamination (e.g., endotoxins, microbial organisms) and (2) physical or chemical contamination (e.g., physical matter, foreign chemicals). There are many sources of contamination: personnel and objects; nonsterile components incorporated into a final product before sterilization; and solid or liquid matter present in the restricted compounding environment. The risk levels only apply to the quality of CSPs immediately after the final aseptic mixing and filling, or immediately after final sterilization, unless the characteristics of the preparation deem otherwise (refer to Table 2 for a summary).

■ **Low-risk level CSP** must comply with all of the following four conditions:
   1. All aseptic manipulations involved in the preparation are done in ISO Class 5 conditions or better using only sterile ingredients, products, components and devices
   2. The preparation involves the use of not more than three commercially prepared sterile products and not more than two entries into any one sterile container to prepare the CSP
   3. All processes require aseptic manipulations of ampules, vials, packages and sterile containers
   4. Beyond use dating (BUD), without passing a sterility test, cannot be more than 48 hours at controlled room temperature (20° to 25° Celsius), for more than 14 days at cold temperature (2° to 8° Celsius), and 45 days in a solid frozen state (between -25° and -10° Celsius). Examples of low-risk compounding include single volume transfers and simple aseptic measuring and transferring involving not more than three commercially prepared sterile components.

■ **Low-risk level CSP with 12-hour or less BUD** result if the PEC (e.g., BSC, VLFW, HLFW) cannot be located in at least an ISO Class 7 environment or if the compounding is being conducted in a CAI or CACI that meets ISO Class 5 conditions within the isolator at all times but that does not provide isolation from less than ISO Class 7 conditions. CSPs made in this manner must be pursuant to a physician's order; be prepared for a specific patient; have a 12 hour, or less, BUD (or as recommended in the manufacturer's package insert, whichever is less); and meet the following four criteria:
   1. PEC shall be certified and maintain at least an ISO Class 5 environment for exposure of critical sites and be located in a segregated compounding area with restricted access
   2. The segregated compounding area will have no outdoor access, be located in a low-traffic area of the pharmacy and not be adjacent to construction sites or food preparation areas
   3. Personnel shall be properly trained and validated prior to performing compounding activities. Sinks will not be located adjacent to the ISO Class 5 environment.
   4. All specifications with respect to cleaning, disinfection and personnel training and evaluation will be followed according to USP <797> guidelines

■ **Medium-risk level CSP** are produced when low-risk conditions are aseptically followed and one or more of the following four conditions apply:
   1. Multiple small or individual preparations of sterile products are combined to produce one or more products for patient use
   2. Compounding includes complex aseptic manipulations other than single volume transfer

3. Compounding process is unusually long (e.g., long dissolution time)
4. Without passing a sterility test, the BUD cannot be more than 30 hours at controlled room temperature (20° to 25° Celsius), more than nine days at cold temperature (2° to 8° Celsius) and more than 45 days in a solid frozen state (between -25° and -10° Celsius).

Examples of medium-risk compounding include total parenteral nutrition, filling reservoirs or injection devices and transfer from multiple ampules or vials.

- **High-risk level CSP** are products produced under any of the following five conditions:
  1. When nonsterile ingredients are incorporated into the final product
  2. If the following are exposed to less than ISO Class 5 air for more than one hour: sterile contents of commercially prepared products, CSPs not containing antimicrobial preservatives, and sterile devices and containers used in the preparation of CSPs
  3. When improperly garbed personnel are present in the restricted compounding area during the compounding process
  4. When water-containing preparations that are nonsterile are stored for more than six hours before sterilization
  5. When not verifying the chemical purity and content of ingredients being used in the compounding process before opening packages

Once sterilized, high-risk level preparations have BUD of not more than 24 hours at controlled room temperature (20° to 25° Celsius), not more than three days at cold temperature (2° to 8° Celsius) and 45 days in a solid frozen state (between -25° and -10° Celsius). Examples of high-risk conditions include dissolving nonsterile bulk drug to be sterilized later, exposing sterile ingredients to less than ISO Class 5 air for more than one hour, using nonsterile devices to mix sterile ingredients and using unverified bulk products.

- **Immediate-use CSP** must meet all of the following six criteria:
  1. The compounding process involves only simple transfer of not more than three commercially available sterile products, is conducted using only original containers and does not have more than two entries into any one container
  2. The compounding process is continuous and does not exceed one hour unless required by preparation
  3. Aseptic technique is followed and the product, if not immediately administered, is under constant supervision
  4. Administration must begin no later than one hour following the start of preparation
  5. Unless completely used, the product will be labeled with proper patient identification, preparer identification and an exact one hour BUD
  6. If administration cannot commence within one hour of preparation, the product shall be discarded and not used. Examples of immediate-use CSPs are emergency medications, diagnostic agents (such as radiopharmaceuticals) and critical therapies that if administration is delayed could cause harm to the patient.

Table 2
Summary: Microbial Risk Classification of CSPs

Classification	Conditions	BUD at Controlled Room Temp.	BUD at Cold Temp.	BUD in Solid Frozen State	Requires the Use of PEC
Low-Risk Level CSP	Only sterile ingredients, components and devices are used	48 Hours	14 Days	45 Days	Yes
	Not more than three commercially prepared products are used to make final preparation				
	Not more than two entries into any one sterile vial, package or container occurs				
	PEC must be located in ISO Class 7 or better environment				
Low-Risk Level CSP with 12-hour or Less BUD	Must have a physician's order and be made for a specific patient (no batch compounding)	12 Hours	12 Hours	12 Hours	Yes
	Have a 12-hour or less BUD				
	PEC is located in a segregated compounding area that may have less than ISO Class 7 air quality				
Medium-Risk Level CSP	Multiple small or individual sterile products are combined	30 Hours	9 Days	45 Days	Yes
	Complex aseptic manipulations occur				
	Compounding process is unusually long				

Classification	Conditions	BUD at Controlled Room Temp.	BUD at Cold Temp.	BUD in Solid Frozen State	Requires the Use of PEC
High-Risk Level CSP	Nonsterile ingredients are incorporated into final product	24 Hours	3 Days	45 Days	Yes
	Sterile contents are exposed to less than ISO Class 5 air for more than one hour				
	Improperly garbed personnel are in the compounding environment during compounding				
	Nonsterile water containing preparations are not sterilized within six hours of compounding				
	Inability to verify the chemical purity or content of products used in final preparation				
Immediate-Use CSP	Not more than three commercially available sterile products are used	1 Hour	1 Hour	1 Hour	No
	Only single transfer is conducted while preparing				
	Compounding is continuous and does not exceed one hour				
	Product is under constant supervision				
	Administration to patient begins no later than one hour from the beginning of preparation				

Primary Engineering Controls

Primary engineering controls (PECs) can be devices (e.g., clean room, VLFWs, HLFWs, BSCs, CAIs and CACIs) or an entire room as long as qualification as an ISO Class 5 air quality environment is documented and maintained. To ensure its proper working condition, a PEC must be certified every six months, every time the HEPA filter is wetted or every time the device is moved (for summary, refer to Table 3).

Table 3
Summary of Primary Engineering Controls

PEC	Characteristics	ISO Class 7 Required
Vertical Laminar Flow Workbench (VLFW)	■ Air is blown down from the top onto the work surface ■ In order to prevent disruption of laminar flow, objects should not be above the critical site ■ All items needed for compounding are introduced into workstation at one time. ■ All aseptic manipulations should be conducted at least six inches inside of workstation ■ Used for general drug compounding	Yes
Horizontal Laminar Flow Workbench (HLFW)	■ Air is blown across the work surface toward the operator ■ In order to prevent disruption of laminar flow, objects should not be placed behind the critical site ■ All aseptic manipulations should be conducted at least six inches inside of workstation ■ Items are placed either to the left or right of work area in the first six inches of workstation ■ Used for nonhazardous drug compounding	Yes
Biological Safety Cabinet (BSC)	■ All air exhausted from cabinet is HEPA filtered in order to protect personnel and environment ■ Come in three classes; Class II is most commonly used in pharmaceutical compounding ■ All aseptic manipulations should be conducted at least 12 inches inside of cabinet ■ Used for hazardous drug compounding or biological hazard sample manipulations	Yes*

PEC	Characteristics	ISO Class 7 Required
Compounding Aseptic Isolator (CAI)	■ All air exhausted is HEPA filtered in order to protect personnel and environment ■ Air exhausted can be vented into room or to the outside ■ Unlike VLFW and HLFW, can be placed in less than ISO Class 8 environments** ■ Exchange of air may occur between isolator and surrounding environment ■ Used for general drug compounding; great option for small institutions with low volume compounding needs ■ Dose doesn't require direct venting to outdoor environment	No**
Compounding Aseptic Containment Isolator (CACI)	■ All air exhausted is HEPA filtered in order to protect personnel and environment ■ Unlike VLFW and HLFW, can be placed in less than ISO Class 8 environments ■ Must be vented to the outdoor environment requiring HVAC modifications ■ Exchange of air does not occur between surrounding environment ■ Used for hazardous drug compounding ■ Unlike VLFW and HLFW, can be placed in less than ISO Class 8 environments**	No**
Clean Room	■ Can be designed to provide any of the six ISO Class environments; must be Class 5 to be considered a PEC ■ All air entering room is HEPA filtered, with air entering at the ceiling and exiting at the floor ■ Has a positive pressure as compared to all surrounding rooms ■ Highest level of cleanliness as compared to surrounding rooms ■ Restricted access only to personnel trained and properly garbed for aseptic manipulations	Yes

* Only for Class I and II because Class III BSCs are an entirely closed environment, similar to CACIs, except much larger

** CAIs and CACIs can be placed in less than ISO Class 8 air quality as long as ISO Class 5 air quality inside isolator is met at all times even during dynamic compounding processing

Types of Primary Engineering Controls

The **Horizontal Laminar Flow Workstation (HLFW)** draws air in through a pre-filter (see Figure 6). The pre-filtered air is pressurized in the plenum for an even distribution of air to the **HEPA filter**. The **plenum** of the hood is the space between the pre-filter and the HEPA filter. The air is blown across the work surface toward the operator. The pre-filter in the laminar flow workstation protects the HEPA filter from premature clogging. Pre-filters are similar to furnace filters and must be checked regularly. This type of workstation is commonly used to prepare nonhazardous CSP because any spills that occur during compounding will be blown directly toward the operator.

When an item is in the HLFW, it disturbs the laminar flow of air. The air flow is disturbed downstream of the object, for approximately three times the diameter of the object. If the item is flush with the side wall, it will disturb the laminar flow for approximately six times the diameter of the object (see Figure 8). Any nonsterile object has the potential to contaminate articles downstream with particles. It is very important that a direct path exists between the HEPA filter and the critical site.

Vertical Laminar Flow Workbench (VLFW) is similar to an HLFW in that air is drawn in through a pre-filter, pressurized in the plenum and pushed through the HEPA filter (see Figure 7). However, the air is blown down from the top of the workstation onto the work surface, not across it. Working in vertical laminar flow (VLF) requires different techniques than working in HLF. In VLF, the hands of the operator or any object must not be above an object in the hood. In HLF, the hands of the operator or any object must not be in back of another object. The hands of the operator must never come between the HEPA filter and the object. The critical site must always be protected.

Figure 8
Downward View of a Laminar Airflow Hood

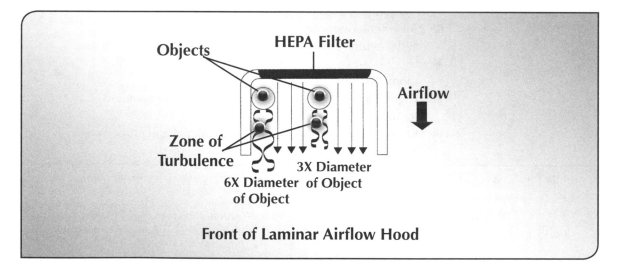

Preparation of Laminar Flow Workbench

The blower to the LFW remains continuously in operation. If the hood is shut off, it must be turned on for at least 30 minutes (or according to the manufacturer recommendations) before use. The hood is wiped with a sanitizing agent, such as sterile 70% isopropyl alcohol. The bar should be wiped first, using a no-shedding wipe soaked with the sanitizing agent, followed by the sides of the hood. Wiping should commence at the end closest to the filter, working outward from the top edge of the side to the bottom. The bench top is cleaned last, starting closest to the filter, wiped from side to side, from the filter to the outside. Work should be from the cleanest part outward. The LFW is wiped at the beginning of the shift and, at a minimum, after any spill. Spraying the sanitizing agent increases the chances of wetting the HEPA filter. The sanitizing agent should not be sprayed into the hood; it is better to pour the agent from a bottle onto the wiping material. A wet HEPA filter could easily develop a pinhole.

In a VLFW, supplies are placed so that the operator may work without placing a hand or object above the critical site. Movements in and out of the hood must be minimized. All items needed for the aseptic manipulation are introduced into the work area at one time. Articles to be thrown away may be dropped over the edge of the hood into the trash or they may be left in the first six inches of the hood until the manipulations are complete, and then thrown away in the trash or container for sharp contaminated objects.

Compounding Aseptic Isolators

Compounding aseptic isolators come in two types and many configurations; all types provide ISO Class 5 air quality or better using HEPA filtration. The first type of isolator is classified as a **compounding aseptic isolator (CAI)**. In this case, in order to provide ISO Class 5 air quality, air exchange may occur with the room in which the isolator is located by methods very similar to how a HLFW and VLFW produce HEPA filtered air. **Compounding aseptic containment isolators (CACIs)** are configured in a manner to prevent the exchange of air between the isolator and the room in which it is placed. Generally, this requires specialized heating, ventilation and air conditioning (HVAC) modifications and can be costly. All the air that is exhausted from a CAI, be it a containment unit or not, is HEPA filtered to prevent contamination of personnel and the environment.

Both CAIs and CACIs come in configurations allowing more than one person to work in the compounding environment at the same time, depending on the amount of compounding that is done at the site. Generally, CAIs are required to be placed in an ISO Class 7 air quality environment; but, one advantage of the CAI over laminar flow workbenches is that they can be placed in less than ISO Class 8 air quality environments as long as they meet the following three requirements:

1. They must provide isolation from the room and maintain an ISO Class 5 environment, or better, even during dynamic aseptic compounding processes
2. They must maintain particle counts six to 12 inches upstream of the critical site and maintain ISO Class 5 air, or better, even during dynamic aseptic compounding processes
3. When certified, not more than 3,520 particles of a size 0.5 microns/m³, or larger, are counted, even during aseptic processing with a measurement probe located as close to the transfer as possible without obstructing it

Documentation to support that each of these requirements have been met must be provided by the manufacturer. If the CAI or CACI meets or exceeds these requirements, it can provide a much cheaper alternative to other secondary engineering controls or a fully functioning clean room and are considered a good option for smaller institutions with lower compounding needs. The CACI in particular is a good option even for larger institutions having an off-site cancer treatment center providing compounded antineoplastic agents.

Biological Safety Cabinets

Biological safety cabinets (BSCs) protect the operator, and the surrounding environment, from pathogens and hazardous materials. All the air that is exhausted from a BSC is HEPA filtered to prevent contamination of personnel and the environment. There are three types of BSC: Class I, Class

II and Class III. Class I BSCs provide protection to the personnel and the environment but do not protect the product from contaminants that may come from the environment. For this reason, Class I BSCs are generally used to enclose equipment used in processing samples that are not exposed (e.g., centrifuges). Class II BSCs are the most common and protect both the environment and the product being manipulated. Class II BSCs may be used to prepare chemotherapeutic agents. The last type of BSC, Class III, is designed to work with highly pathogenic agents. They are typically custom-made and installed in specialized microbial laboratories. This type of protection would not be needed for pharmaceutical compounding applications. Unlike LFW, aseptic manipulations must be performed at least 12 inches inside the cabinet.

Maintenance of Primary Engineering Controls

To ensure proper working condition, a PEC must be certified every six months, every time the HEPA filter is wetted or every time the PEC is moved. A reputable testing company may be used to test the velocity of the laminar flow and the integrity of the HEPA filter. The velocity of the air from the HEPA filter is checked using a **velometer**. The average air velocity is 90 ft/min (linear feet per minute), +/- 20 percent. No one measurement may be less than 72 ft/min. The integrity of the HEPA filter is checked by introducing aerosolized Emery 3004 or a similar agent into the plenum or air intake of the PEC while monitoring for penetration of the Emery 3004 on the downstream side of the HEPA filter. The aerosol has an average particle size of 0.3 microns. No more than 0.01 percent of the upstream concentration may be detected downstream of the HEPA filter.

Secondary Engineering Controls

Secondary engineering controls can be rooms or locations within the pharmacy that provide an environment for specific pharmacy functions. The functions could be placement of PEC for aseptic compounding (e.g., buffer area or clean room). The secondary engineering control could also provide a place for garbing, unpacking supplies and prescription entry (as in anterooms). The air quality can still be controlled to a specific standard in any of these environments depending on the intended use and the guidelines set forth by USP <797>.

Clean Room

Clean rooms are defined as a controlled environment in which the number of particles circulating in the air is controlled to a specified standard (e.g., ISO Class 8, ISO Class 7 or ISO Class 5). Microbial contamination is monitored by the use of microbial air, surface and personnel sampling conducted at specified intervals based on the purpose of the room and the microbial contamination risk level.

Buffer Area

The buffer area, which is second in cleanliness to the PEC, is enclosed from other pharmacy operations (preferably with walls); soft-wall rooms are acceptable. The buffer area provides a place to locate the PEC. The PEC must be located away from excess traffic, doors, air vents or anything that could produce air currents that may introduce contamination into the PEC. Any air currents, or movements greater than the velocity of the airflow from the HEPA filter, may introduce contaminants into the PEC (e.g., coughing or sneezing into the PEC and quick movements in and out of the PEC).

Surfaces in the buffer area should be smooth, nonporous, nonshedding and easily cleaned or disinfected. Cracks, crevices and seams must be avoided. Cracks and crevices are hard to keep clean and are a perfect place for microorganisms to flourish. Ledges or other places where dust may collect should also be avoided. The buffer room should meet the requirement of at least ISO 8 (Class 100,000) clean room; in some cases, an ISO Class 7 (Class 10,000) clean room is recommended. This room must have positive pressure in relationship to the rest of the pharmacy to prevent dirty air from entering the clean room. Access to the buffer area must be restricted to only qualified personnel who must be properly scrubbed and gowned. Housekeeping of the buffer area must be kept at high standards. The cleaning tools and supplies must be kept separate and only used in the buffer area. The cleaning personnel must be trained in the appropriate procedures.

Anteroom

The anteroom is an area of high cleanliness separated from the buffer area by a barrier. This barrier is preferably a wall, but in some cases a curtain is acceptable. The anteroom is used to decontaminate supplies, equipment and personnel. Hand washing, gowning and unpacking supplies from cardboard boxes is done in the anteroom to reduce the number of particles in the buffer area. Clean and sanitized supplies can also be stored in this area. Like the buffer area, the anteroom is constructed from nonshedding, easily cleaned material. Ideally, this room is less positive pressure than the buffer area, but still positive to the rest of the pharmacy.

Segregated Compounding Area

The segregated compounding area is a location within the pharmacy that is separated from other noncompounding activities and contains the PEC. The air quality in this location is not controlled to a standard; therefore, only low-risk level CSPs with 12 hour or less BUD may be prepared here. This location can be either a room or just a line of demarcation that separates the area from the rest of the pharmacy. This area must have restricted access and a have a higher level of cleanliness then the rest of the pharmacy.

Compounding Supplies

■ **Needles**

Sterile needles are wrapped in rigid or semi-rigid plastic covers. This wrap must be inspected before using the needle; tears or pinholes in the wrap will compromise the sterility of the needle. Needles come in a variety of sizes. The **gauge** of the needle refers to the outer diameter of the needle; the larger the number, the smaller the bore (hole) of the needle. The smallest used for CSPs are 27-gauge and the largest are 13-gauge. Most facilities use an 18-gauge to 21-gauge needle. Needle length is measured in inches. Commonly used are 1-inch and 1.5-inch lengths.

The basic parts of a needle include the hub, the needle shaft, the bevel heel and the tip (see Figure 9). The needle shaft is encased in a rigid plastic sheath by which the needle is handled. This sheath is left on until the needle and syringe are used. The needle shaft is never swabbed with alcohol, as it is usually coated with silicone to allow for easy penetration of rubber. The critical sites on a needle are the needle hub and the tip.

Figure 9
Basic Parts of a Needle

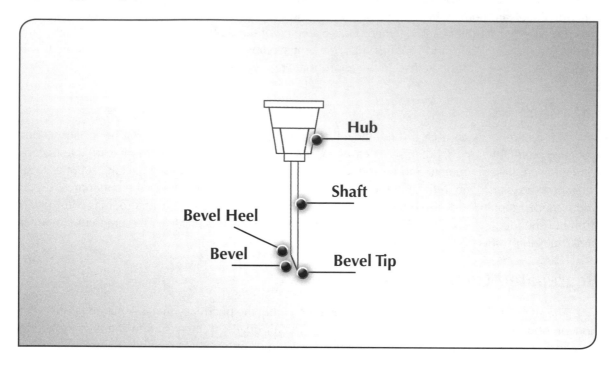

- **Syringes**

Syringes can be made of plastic or glass. Disposable plastic syringes are now used most often in the preparation of sterile products. They are sterile, pyrogen-free and packaged in either paper or a rigid plastic container. The syringe wrap must be inspected carefully to assure that the syringe is intact and sterile. The basic parts of a syringe are the barrel, the plunger, the rubber tip of the plunger and the tip (see Figure 10). The critical sites on the syringe are the ribs of the plunger and the tip of the syringe.

Syringes have either a Luer-Lok® tip or a slip (friction fit) tip (see Figure 10). The Luer Lok® tip is threaded and the needle is tightened on the threaded tip. The friction tip needle simply slides onto the tip of the syringe. It is held in place by friction. A protective cover is usually on the tip of the syringe. This cap remains on until the needle is attached.

Calibration marks are on the barrel of the syringe. Larger syringes have greater increments on the barrel of the syringe. These marks are accurate to one-half of the interval marked on the syringe. For the sake of accuracy, the operator should use the smallest syringe available to hold the amount of solution needed. To deliver a given volume in a syringe, the final edge of the rubber tip of the plunger that comes in contact with the syringe is lined up with the calibration mark that corresponds with the volume of fluid desired (see Figure 11).

Figure 10
Basic Parts of a Syringe

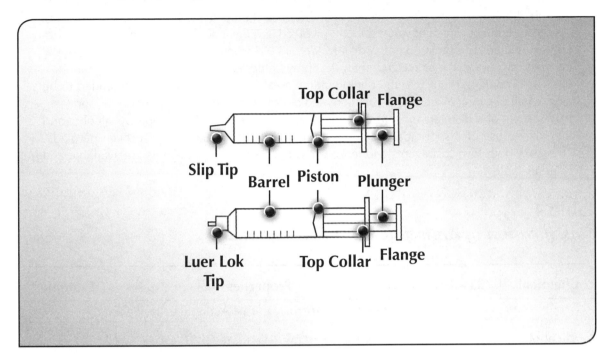

Figure 11
Syringe Markings on the Barrel with 2 mL Withdrawn

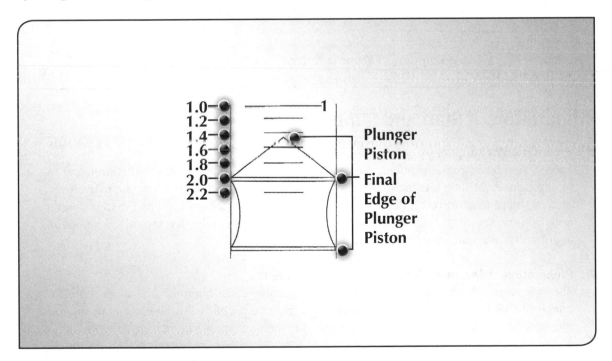

■ Disinfectants and Antiseptics

Disinfectants and antiseptics provide a means for cleaning and sanitizing the work environment. The effectiveness of these agents depends on a number of factors, including the microbial-killing activity, the concentration, the contact time, the nature of the surface being disinfected, the hardness of water diluents involved and the amount of dirt on the surface being disinfected. The most common disinfectant is 70% isopropyl alcohol because it rapidly destroys bacteria in the active growth cycle. Spray bottles can be used to decontaminate supplies before taking them into the compounding area, but they are not recommended to be used when cleaning a PEC due to the increased risk of wetting the HEPA filter during spraying. An example of a disinfectant program would be the daily use of 70% isopropyl alcohol and the weekly use of a sporicidal (bacterial spore killing) agent like 10% hydrogen peroxide. These are both low-cost agents and leave very little residue. Other agents are available and listed in Table 4.

Table 4
Classification of Antiseptics and Disinfectants

Chemical	Classification	Properties				Example
		Residue	Corrosive	Fast Acting	Irritating	
Alcohols	General Purpose	No	Low	Yes	Low	70% Isopropyl Alcohol
Chlorine and Sodium Hypochlorite	Sporicidal Agent	Yes	High	Yes	High	10% Bleach, 0.5% Sodium Hypochlorite
Hydrogen Peroxide	Sporicidal Agent	No	Medium	Yes	High	10% Solution, 3% Solution
Quaternary Ammonium Compound	General Purpose	Yes	Low	Yes	Low	Benzalkonium Chloride

Preparation of Staff and Supplies

■ Preparation of Supplies

Large volume parenteral products (volume of 100 mL and greater) and small volume parenteral products (volume less than 100 mL), devices and other supplies must not be in the buffer area in shipping cartons. Cardboard sheds many particles. Supplies must be unpacked in the anteroom on the dirty side, wiped with a non-lint producing wipe soaked with a sanitizing agent and placed on a cart for transfer into the buffer area.

■ Preparation of Pharmacy Technicians and Pharmacists

The operators (pharmacy technicians and pharmacists) must minimize the introduction of contaminants into the buffer area. The operator must be properly scrubbed and gowned before entering the buffer area. Proper preparation of the operator is a critical key to maintaining a controlled environment. The greatest source of contamination in a clean room is the people in the area. A person sitting down releases 100,000 particles per minute. A person moving at two miles per hour releases five million particles into the air each minute.

Operators scrub from the elbow to hands for an appropriate amount of time with antimicrobial skin cleanser. Hands are dried using a forced air dryer or disposable, nonshedding towels. After scrubbing, frequent use of a foamed sanitizing agent or sterile 70% isopropyl alcohol during the shift and before entering the hood is essential.

The operator should not wear jewelry or makeup when working in the buffer area. Before entering the buffer room, the operator dons a hair cover; shoe covers; a clean, knee-length, nonshedding gown or coverall; and sterile gloves. The sterile gloves are put on aseptically, with the cuffs of the gown inside the gloves. Once the gloves are out of the package they are no longer sterile. The purpose of the gloves is to contain the particles shed from the operator's hands, not to replace good aseptic technique. To maintain glove surfaces as free from contamination as possible, the glove must be rinsed frequently with a sanitizing agent. Before working in the hood, the operator dons a face mask.

Only pharmacy technicians and pharmacists highly skilled in aseptic technique may enter the buffer area. Before compounding sterile products, an operator must be validated by successfully completing one process simulation test with growth promotion media. After completing the initial validation, revalidation occurs at least annually for low- and medium-risk compounding and semi-annually for high-risk compounding. Media is used to compound the sterile product instead of drug and diluent. The process is as complicated as the most complex item being compounded now or to be compounded in the future. The media is incubated for 14 days and then inspected for growth. One container with growth constitutes a media fill failure. If a media fill fails at any time, the operator must successfully revalidate with one successful media fill.

■ Working in the PEC

An operator must always use good aseptic technique to compound sterile products. Working in a PEC may give the operator a false sense of security concerning the sterility of the products prepared. Products and supplies not in an overwrap are first wiped with 70% isopropyl alcohol before being placed in the compounding area. A PEC does not remove microbial contaminants from the surface of containers or other items placed in the workstation. PEC is not a sterilization process.

Any items not in a protective overwrap (e.g., ampules, vials, IV bags and bottles) must be wiped with a non-lint producing wipe soaked with sterile 70% isopropyl alcohol before being placed in the PEC. All containers must be checked for cracks, tears and particles before they are used to compound IV admixtures. If an item is in a protective overwrap, it may be taken from the overwrap at the edge of the hood and placed in the hood. One exception to this practice is the needle, which is not removed from its overwrap until immediately before its use. Needles are placed in the first six inches of the hood until they are ready to be removed from their wrap and used. Items in an HLFW are placed to the left or right of the critical work area. The critical sites must be in laminar flow at all times. The operator in an HLFW must work without placing a hand or object behind a critical site.

All work conducted in the HLFW must be done at least six inches inside the hood. Room air can be carried into the front of the hood from the turbulence created as the laminar flow air passes around the person working at the hood. It must be remembered that an HLFW is not a means of sterilization; it only maintains an area free of microorganisms, contaminants and particulate matter when it is properly maintained, prepared and used by operators with good aseptic technique. An HLFW will not compensate for bad aseptic technique.

■ Gowning

First, a clean hair cover is selected and donned with little or no touching of the hair (see Picture 1). The hands and forearms must be scrubbed to the elbow with a sanitizing soap and a brush for at least 30 seconds (see Picture 2). The arms must be rinsed and the hand dryer started with the elbow (see Picture 3). Two clean shoe covers must be selected while sitting on the bench with feet on the "dirty side." The shoe cover must be opened using three fingers of each hand to protect the clean fingers as the cover is placed on the shoe (see Pictures 4 and 5). Once the shoe cover is on, the foot must be swung over the bench to the clean side. This is repeated for the other foot. A clean, non-lint producing coat is selected, put on and zipped all the way (see Picture 6). The appropriate-sized gloves are opened, removed from the package and the inner package unfolded. The first glove must be picked up by the folded down cuff of the glove (see Picture 7). The hand must be touching the inside of the glove. The ungloved hand must never touch the outside of the glove (see Picture 8). The cuff of the glove must not be fully pulled off at this time. Two fingers of the gloved hand must be inserted into the cuff of the other glove. The gloved hand must now be touching the outside of the glove (see Picture 9). The glove is pulled on and the cuff pulled up over the sleeve of the gown. The cuff of the second glove must then be pulled over the coat (see Picture 10). Before working in the hood, a face mask must be donned. The top inside of the mask (wire band) must be placed over the bridge of the nose. The mask must be fitted to the head (see Picture 11). The top strings are tied tightly in a bow at the crown of the skull (see Picture 12). The lower edge of the mask is pulled down gently and the bottom strings tied loosely (see Picture 13).

Chapter 7 ASEPTIC TECHNIQUE AND STERILE PRODUCT PREPARATION

Pictures 1-13

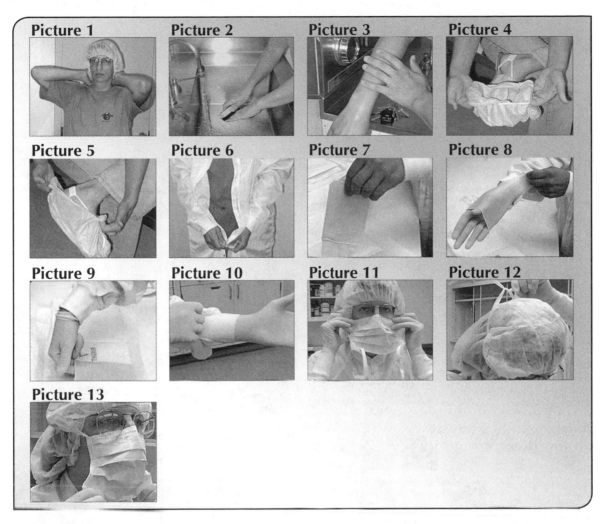

Picture 1	Picture 2	Picture 3	Picture 4
Picture 5	Picture 6	Picture 7	Picture 8
Picture 9	Picture 10	Picture 11	Picture 12
Picture 13			

■ **Preparing the Horizontal Laminar Flow Workbench**

The hood is sanitized with sterile 70% isopropyl alcohol. Isopropyl alcohol is poured on the stainless steel counter in the hood (see Picture 14). The sterile, nonshedding, urethane wipe is wet with isopropyl alcohol. The bar of the hood is wiped first (see Picture 15). Next, the side walls are wiped. They are wiped up and down, from front (closest to the HEPA filter) to back, not going over any previously wiped surfaces (see Pictures 16 and 17). The last thing to be wiped is the counter, starting in the back corner by the HEPA filter and wiping all the way across the bench (see Picture 18). Wiping is done from side-to-side working from the HEPA filter to the edge of the counter (see Picture 19).

■ **Putting a Needle on a Syringe**

A syringe large enough to accommodate the volume required must be selected. The integrity of the outer wrap must be inspected for defects, such as holes or tears in the package. At the edge of the hood, the paper must be peeled from the syringe and the syringe placed in the hood (see Picture 20). The syringe must not be pushed through the paper wrap, because tearing the paper generates many particles. A needle is selected and the package is examined for defects. While pointing the hub of the needle toward the HEPA filter, the wrap is peeled back (see Picture 21).

The following instructions are given for a right-handed person. If the technician or pharmacist is left-handed, the directions are reversed. The needle is held between the thumb and first finger on the left hand (see Picture 22). The syringe is held in the right hand and the protective tip of the syringe is taken with the thumb and first finger of the left hand (see Picture 23). The syringe is twisted to remove the protective tip. The left hand is rotated, and the hub of the needle is attached to the tip of the syringe (see Picture 24). The plunger is pushed down to the tip of the barrel while keeping the needle cover on to unlock the syringe (see Picture 25).

Pictures 14-25

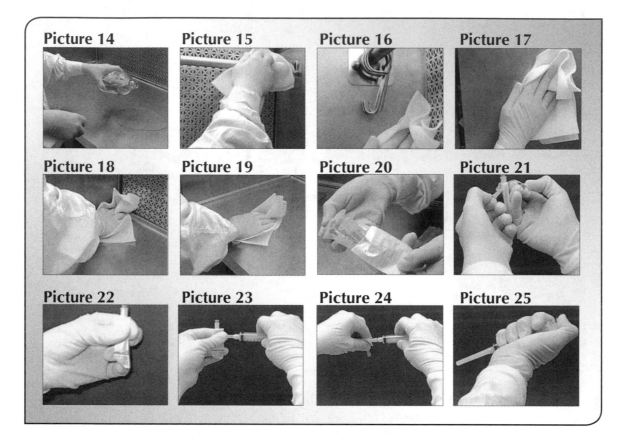

Performing Compounding Activities

■ **Withdrawing from an Ampule**

Ampules are single-dose containers. Once the tip is broken open, the ampule is an open system with air passing freely in and out of the container. The ampule must be wiped with sterile 70% isopropyl alcohol before being placed in the HLFW (see Picture 26). With the ampule in an upright position, the neck is tapped to release solution trapped in the end of the ampule. The neck of the ampule is wiped with a sterile alcohol pad to further clean the neck of the ampule as glass particles will fall into the solution when the ampule is broken (see Picture 27). The ampule must be dry so the operator's hands do not slip while attempting to break it open. The thumbs are positioned about one-half inch apart on either side of the constricted neck of the ampule to apply pressure with the fingers as if breaking a pencil in half (see Picture 28). The ampule is broken toward the side of the hood and not toward the HEPA filter. Glass particles and drops of fluid are dispersed when the ampule is broken. If the ampule does not break easily, it must be rotated one-half turn and tried again. The top is placed to the side of the bench, and the ampule placed in laminar air flow (see Picture 29). The needle cover is removed from the needle and syringe and placed either between the ring finger (see Picture 30) and little finger or placed on a sterile alcohol prep pad pointing toward the HEPA filter.

The ampule is picked up and the needle bevel inserted into the shoulder of the ampule (see Picture 31). The ampule is tilted at an angle to keep the tip of the needle in the solution. When inserting the needle into the ampule, the needle must not touch the outside edge of the ampule. If this does happen, the contaminated needle must be replaced with a new needle on the syringe. The opening of the ampule and the tip of the needle are critical sites; therefore, care must be taken to keep them in uninterrupted laminar air flow.

The syringe is held by wrapping the fingers around the barrel and pulling back the plunger with the thumb (see Picture 32). The ribs of the plunger must not be contaminated by being touched. Another safe method is to use the index finger to push the plunger out and withdraw the fluid from the ampule. Any unused solution in the ampule must be discarded.

If air is in the syringe, the syringe is held with the needle up and tapped firmly to allow air bubbles to rise (see Picture 33). The plunger is drawn back to get the drop of fluid out of the hub of the needle, then the plunger gently pushed up to expel all the air from the syringe (see Pictures 34 and 35). To adjust the volume in the syringe to the correct amount, the edge of the rubber plunger closest to the tip is moved to the correct calibration mark. Any excess solution is put back into the ampule (see Picture 36).

Any solution taken from an ampule must always be filtered because glass particles can fall in the ampule when it breaks open. The solution is filtered when withdrawing from an ampule using a filter needle, a filter disk or filter straw. The filter is discarded and replaced by a clean needle before injecting.

Pictures 26-36

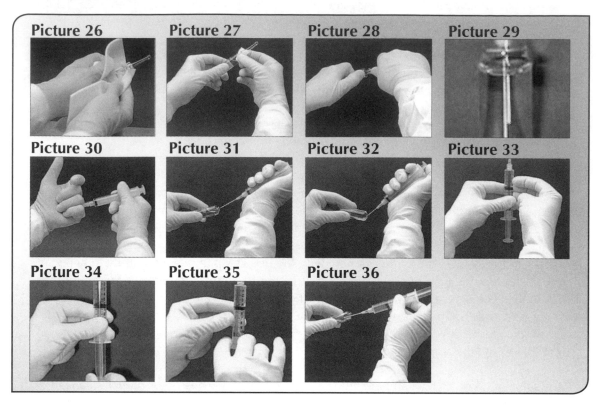

Picture 26   Picture 27   Picture 28   Picture 29

Picture 30   Picture 31   Picture 32   Picture 33

Picture 34   Picture 35   Picture 36

■ **Withdrawing Solution from a Vial**

Vials are molded glass or plastic containers with rubber closures secured in place with an aluminum seal. Vials can be filled with dry powders, sterile solutions or lyophilized (freeze dried) medications; a vial could also be an empty, evacuated container. Vials may be single-dose or multiple-dose containers. A multiple-dose vial contains preservatives and can be entered more than once. Usually each practice site has a written policy about the use of multi-dose vials after the initial entry. Generally, the standard is that multiple-dose vials may be used for up to 28 days after their first use. Because single-dose vials contain no preservatives, pharmaceutical manufacturers recommend entering each vial only once. Generally, the standard of practice is that a single-dose vial may be used for six hours after the initial entry as long as the vial remains in the laminar flow workstation. It is imperative that the first person opening and using a single-dose vial labels the vial with the date and time of initial entry and his or her initials.

Using a non-lint producing wipe soaked in 70% isopropyl alcohol, the vial is wiped before being placed in the hood (see Picture 37). The flip-top seal is removed from the vial and the closure is swabbed with a sterile alcohol pad, wiping in one direction with several strokes (see Pictures 38 and 39). Wiping the closure with the sterile 70% isopropyl alcohol helps clean and sanitize the surface of the closure. While the alcohol on the surface of the closure is drying, the needle and syringe are assembled.

The needle cover is removed and placed between the ring finger and little finger or on a sterile alcohol pad with the opening pointing toward the HEPA filter. Air must be injected into the vial so fluid may be withdrawn because the vial is a closed system. An amount of air equal to the volume of the solution needed is drawn in (see Picture 40).

The base of the vial is grasped in one hand. The syringe is held at an angle of approximately 60 degrees with the bevel of the needle up (see Picture 41). As the closure is penetrated, the needle is elevated to a vertical position while lateral pressure is exerted on the needle. The critical sites must be in direct laminar flow (see Picture 42).

The vial and syringe are inverted and air is injected into the vial by depressing the plunger (see Pictures 43 and 44). The solution must be allowed to run back into the syringe as air is injected into the vial. The flat top of the plunger is held with the middle finger and thumb, and the collar of the syringe is pushed against with the index finger to pull back on the plunger. The amount withdrawn is slightly larger than desired (see Picture 45).

The syringe is tapped firmly to dislodge any air bubbles (see Picture 46). The plunger is pushed to dispel any air and the plunger adjusted until the appropriate amount of solution is in the syringe. The inverted vial is held with one hand and the syringe barrel with the other, and the vial and syringe are turned over (see Picture 47). When turning the syringe, care must be used to keep the hand away from the HEPA filter and the critical site. The needle and syringe are then withdrawn from the vial.

Pictures 37-47

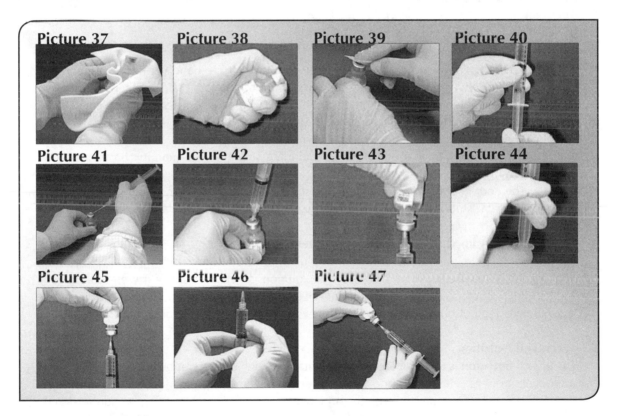

Picture 37 Picture 38 Picture 39 Picture 40
Picture 41 Picture 42 Picture 43 Picture 44
Picture 45 Picture 46 Picture 47

■ **Reconstitution of a Sterile Powder**

Medication may be in powder form because it has limited stability in solution. A **diluent** is a fluid solvent that is added to a solid to turn it into a solution. **Reconstitution** is the process of adding a diluent to the powdered solid to yield a solution and is not considered pharmaceutical compounding. The label must always be read to determine the proper diluent, and volume of diluent, needed before reconstitution.

The correct amount of diluent is withdrawn from an ampule or vial using aseptic technique (see Picture 48). The diluent is then injected into the vial of powder. The air must be allowed to re-enter the syringe, so the vial will contain positive pressure (see Picture 49). If this is not done, some of the vial content may blow out of the vial due to the positive pressure in the vial when the needle is removed. The vial must be shaken to make sure that the medication is completely dissolved before the necessary amount of drug solution is withdrawn (see Picture 50). The reconstituted solution does not need filtering unless, upon inspection of the vial, a particle or a rubber core is floating in the solution.

Pictures 48-50

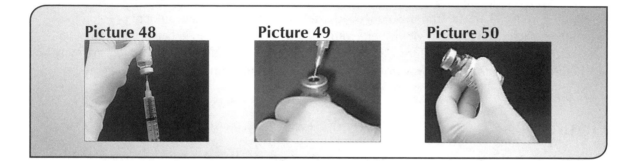

Picture 48   **Picture 49**   **Picture 50**

■ **Visual Inspections of Parenteral Solutions**
Each completed parenteral admixture solution must be inspected and verified by a pharmacist before it is delivered to the nursing unit for administration to a patient. The operator also checks the completed admixture immediately after it is prepared. The following checks for accuracy must be made on every completed admixture:
  • The label is complete and free from errors
  • The correct intravenous solutions, including strength and quantity, have been used
  • The correct drug additives, including strength and quantity, have been given
  • The admixture is clear and free from particulate matter, crystals and precipitation

■ **Viewing an IV Admixture for Particulate Matter**
When checking for particulate matter, the solution is inverted and swirled gently. Vigorous shaking may produce some air bubbles. The solution is held in front of a well-illuminated light and dark background to detect particles of different colors. It is sometimes hard to distinguish between air bubbles and particles; however, air bubbles will rise and particles will sink.

■ **Parenteral Nutrition**
Parenteral nutrition is an intravenous food containing high concentrations of dextrose, amino acids, electrolytes, vitamins, trace elements and sometimes insulin. A lipid (fat) emulsion may be mixed in the same bag with the amino acids and dextrose, or it can be administered separately. Lipids provide calories and help to treat or prevent essential fatty acid deficiency. The parenteral nutrition solution is designed to provide adequate caloric intake while keeping the volume of solution administered to a minimum. The nutrition solution is administered through a large vein, such as the subclavian (by the base of the neck), over eight to 24 hours. Parenteral nutrition is used when a patient cannot tolerate an oral feeding or when it is necessary to bypass the gastrointestinal tract. A full discussion of compounding parenteral nutrition solutions is beyond the scope of this chapter.

■ **Chemotherapeutic Agents**

Concern exists that handling, preparing and administering chemotherapeutic (antineoplastic) agents may constitute an occupational hazard. When handling chemotherapeutic agents, individuals need to be concerned about using good aseptic technique to keep the product sterile and must take measures to minimize unnecessary exposure to these agents.

Pharmacy technicians and pharmacists working with antineoplastic agents must receive special training and be informed of the potential risks involved. All mixing of antineoplastic drugs must be performed in a certified Class II BSC or CACI. No other IV admixtures may be prepared in the BSC or CACI designated for the mixing of antineoplastic drugs. The viewing window in the BSC is lowered when compounding antineoplastic drugs. Disposable gloves and protective barrier garments with a closed front, long sleeves and closed cuff are worn for all procedures. Syringes and IV sets with Leur-Lok® fittings are used. A sterile, plastic-backed, absorbent drape is placed on the work surface of the safety cabinet or isolator during mixing procedures. It is exchanged after significant spillage or at the end of each production sequence.

Vials must be vented with hydrophobic filters. Many compounding devices now prevent the buildup of positive pressure inside the vial. Final medication measurement must be performed before removing the needle from the stopper of the vial. Because the medication is contained, it decreases the operator's exposure to the medications. Written special procedures must be followed in case of a major spill or acute exposure. All disposable items that have a potential contact with antineoplastic drugs during compounding or administration must be disposed of in specifically designated containers displaying a biohazard symbol. All of these hazardous waste containers must be disposed of using proper methods.

Conclusion

Compounded sterile products used for any of the four major routes of parenteral administration (intravenous, intradermal, intramuscular and subcutaneous) are an important part of medication therapy for patients. It is essential that health care professionals continually strive to provide patients with the best product possible. Aseptic technique, manipulation of sterile products without contaminating them, is a means to provide CSPs that are sterile, free of undesired contaminants and of the highest quality and purity as possible. All of this would be difficult without the use of primary engineering controls, laminar flow, ISO Class air quality environments, proper cleaning and disinfection, and competent staff.

Bibliography

■ United States Pharmacopeia Chapter <797> Pharmaceutical Compounding: Sterile Preparations, www.usp.org , August 2010.

■ USP Chapter <797> Pharmaceutical Compounding: Sterile Preparations Potential Impact on Handling Radiopharmaceuticals, Vol. 13, No. 6.

■ Clean Room and Work Station Requirements, Controlled Environment, Federal Standard 209E, Government Printing Office, Washington, D.C., September 1992.

■ American Society of Health-System Pharmacists, "ASHP Guidelines on Quality Assurance for Pharmacy-Prepared Sterile Products," *American Journal of Health-System Pharmacists*, Vol. 57, pp. 1150-1169, 2000.

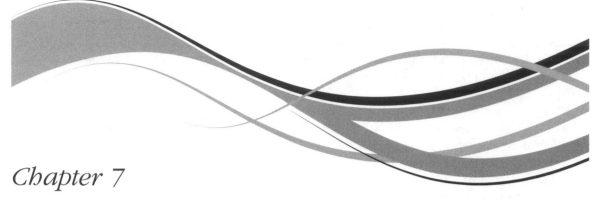

Chapter 7
REVIEW QUESTIONS

1. A properly-functioning and maintained primary engineering control will filter out all particles that have a diameter of ___ or larger.
    a. 1 micron
    b. 0.5 microns
    c. 0.2 microns
    d. 0.8 microns

2. When preparing a parenteral preparation for the following routes of injection, match the maximum recommended volume to each route provided.
    a. 2.5 mL   Subcutaneous_____
    b. 0.1 mL   Intravenous_____
    c. 2.0 mL   Intradermal_____
    d. no limit on volume   Intramuscular_____

3. Which of the following is not an example of a closed system?
    a. ADD-Vantage®
    b. Flexible IV bag
    c. Evacuated glass vial
    d. Mini Bag Plus®

4. If you suspect that your CSP has been contaminated with pyrogens, which of the following methods can be used to remove them?
    a. Filtration using a 0.2 micron filter
    b. Autoclaving for 60 minutes
    c. Exposure of CSP to a radioactive source of Cs-137 for 24 hours
    d. None of the above

5. Which of the following places the ISO Classes in the order of the least to the most particles present circulating in the air?
    a. ISO Class 5, ISO Class 8, ISO Class 7, ISO Class 6
    b. ISO Class 5, ISO Class 6, ISO Class 7, ISO Class 8
    c. ISO Class 8, ISO Class 7, ISO Class 6, ISO Class 5
    d. ISO Class 5, ISO Class 6, ISO Class 8, ISO Class 7

6. A sterile product is one that is:
    a. free from all viruses.
    b. free from all pyrogens.
    c. free from all living microorganisms.
    d. All of the above

7. When cleaning a PEC, where is the best place to start?
    a. From the outside and work inward
    b. From the top down
    c. Wherever is the most convenient location
    d. From the cleanest area (closest to HEPA filter) to the dirtiest

8. Antineoplastic medications can be compounded under which of the following conditions?
    a. In a compounding aseptic containment isolator vented to the outside that is also used for the preparation of parenteral nutrition
    b. In a Class I Biological Safety Cabinet
    c. In a compounding aseptic isolator that is vented inside of the room
    d. None of the above

9. Of the following, which leads to the greatest risk of contamination inside of a clean room environment?
    a. The syringes and needles used in the compounding process
    b. The air flowing into the room from the heating ventilation and air conditioning system
    c. Properly garbed and trained staff conducting compounding activities
    d. The cracking of ampules in order to get the medication out

10. What are the critical sites of a syringe?
    a. Barrel of the syringe and the plunger
    b. Plunger and the tip of the syringe
    c. Ribs of the plunger and the tip of the syringe
    d. Tip of the syringe and the barrel

Chapter 8

CONSULTANT AND LONG-TERM CARE PHARMACY PRACTICE

By Cynthia Peitzsch, R.Ph.

Learning Objectives

This chapter seeks to prepare a pharmacy technician to:

■ explain the role of the pharmacy technician in a long-term care pharmacy.

■ identify requirements for a medication order for a skilled nursing facility, assisted living facility and a group home.

■ explain the differences between anniversary, cycle and on-demand methods of medication supply to facilities.

■ describe the role of a pharmacy technician in various phases of long-term care pharmacy practice, including data entry, billing, medical records, emergency dispensing kits, therapeutic interchange and intravenous therapy.

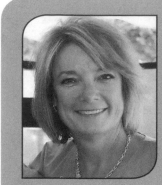

With the ever-growing number of individuals in long-term care, why is it important to have a variety of pharmacy personnel on staff, including pharmacy technicians?

"If the facility has staff pharmacy personnel, the pharmacy staff would serve in a variety of roles. Their roles would range from picking up prescriptions from each unit, to processing prescription orders within the pharmacy operating system, preparing medications and maintaining medication carts. Additionally, the staff pharmacist would be utilized to confirm prescription medications, preserve stock and have direct communication with the staff on the units for any possible counseling situations."

Robyn Parker, CPhT,
Diplomat Pharmacy,
Flint, Mich.

Introduction

As in many other areas of pharmacy, the consultant and long-term care field has many commonly used abbreviations. Table 1 provides a short list of those a pharmacy technician must be familiar with, and able to use, on a regular basis when working in a long-term care pharmacy. These abbreviations will also be used through the rest of this chapter.

Table 1
Commonly Used Abbreviations in Consultant and Long-term Care Pharmacy Practice

Term	Abbreviation	Explanation
Assisted-living Facility	ALF	An ALF is a living arrangement whereby those who need assistance with activities of daily living, but who do not need round-the-clock nursing care, may reside.
Emergency Dispensing Kit (or Stat Kit)	EDK	An inventory of drugs that can be administered by a nurse, on the order of a physician, when time is critical. A maintenance medication that is being initiated for a patient may first be dosed from the EDK and then the pharmacy will be given an order to dispense all future doses.
Facility	Not Available	Any SNF, ALF or GH
Group Home	GH	A GH is a residence for individuals in need of supervision, care or assistance in some way (e.g., developmentally disabled persons and foster children).
House Stock	Not Available	Over-the-counter (OTC) medications kept in bulk by a facility for distribution to residents when requested.
Long-term Care	LTC	LTC is a setting where nonacute care is provided that includes rehabilitative, restorative and ongoing maintenance care for patients in need of assistance performing activities of daily living.

Term	Abbreviation	Explanation
Medication Administration Record	MAR	An MAR generally is a calendar, or schedule, of when medications are to be given to a patient. As medications are given, the person who gave the medication to the patient indicates as such on the MAR.
Physician Order Sheet	POS	A list of physician orders for a patient that may include many different types of orders (e.g., medication orders, dietary restrictions and orders for therapy, like physical therapy or respiratory therapy, to be administered).
Skilled Nursing Facility	SNF	A SNF is a health care institution that meets federal criteria for Medicaid and Medicare reimbursement for nursing care. These criteria include the supervision of care for patients by a physician, the employment of full-time registered nurses (RNs), round-the-clock availability of nursing care, and appropriate facilities to store and dispense drugs to patients.
United States Pharmacopeia	USP	Both an organization and a book (published by that organization) that provides standards for preparation of drug products for dispensing to patients in the United States.

What is Long-term Care Pharmacy?

LTC pharmacies dispense medications to SNFs, ALFs, hospices and GI Is. Although stand-alone hospital pharmacies and stand-alone retail pharmacies have traditionally serviced this population, a proper LTC pharmacy requires a hybrid of both hospital and retail pharmacy. This possesses challenges for regulations and laws that distinguish between inpatient and outpatient pharmacies, since LTC pharmacies are often both at the same time. Nursing homes are one of the most highly regulated industries, second only to nuclear power, and even these regulations often fail to properly address the unique nature of the LTC pharmacy. Pharmacies that are dedicated to LTC generally do not have an ambulatory, walk-in, pharmacy dispensing area for the public to present prescriptions to be filled; also, pharmacies that are dedicated to LTC generally do not provide medications to patients housed in a hospital. A single LTC pharmacy may service many facilities and receive orders for medications from many different prescribers for a single patient in a given facility. Upon filling these orders, the LTC pharmacy generally delivers medications, and medical devices when appropriate, to the facilities or directly to the patients, depending on the type of living arrangement. The services required for these patients cover the complete spectrum; the LTC pharmacy may provide IV drugs, total parenteral nutrition (IV food), compounded preparations, vaccines, daily aspirin, blood glucose testing supplies and many other medical items. To adequately service its patients, the LTC pharmacy may make routine deliveries to a facility multiple times each day, and then make emergency deliveries any time of the day or night when a medication or device is urgently needed. Beyond needing pharmacy technicians to help prepare all of these orders for delivery, and delivering them, pharmacy technicians may also assist pharmacists in their direct patient care activities. A pharmacist is required by law to conduct a monthly drug regimen review for each resident in an SNF. A pharmacist will review the patient's chart (focusing on the MAR) and make recommendations to the patient's physician to modify the patient's therapy when needed. The pharmacist who practices in this way is called a **consultant pharmacist**. Although the same degree and license is required to be a consultant pharmacist as to practice in any other common pharmacy setting, many consultant pharmacists specialize in **geriatrics** (care for the elderly). A pharmacy technician may assist a consultant pharmacist in many ways, including: preparing charts for review, transcribing the pharmacist's recommendations for presentation to physicians, presenting therapy change recommendations to physicians, interviewing and assessing patients to provide the pharmacist with more information to base recommendations, and updating pharmacy computer systems to reflect order changes approved by physicians. The role of pharmacy technicians in this setting will continue to expand as pharmacists also continue to increase their role in these patients' care.

Data Entry

Although computer systems used in hospital pharmacies and retail pharmacies may be similar to those used in LTC pharmacies, there are some unique elements of orders sent to an LTC pharmacy that are not found in other settings. Unlike a retail prescription or an hospital order to dispense a medication, the LTC order may include much more information about the patient because the pharmacy will not have any contact with the patient, and sometimes the patient's chart at the facility, until after the first doses of medication are prepared.

The required elements on a physician's order in the LTC setting include the following:
- Facility name
- Patient room and bed
- Patient payer source
- Patient birth date or age
- Patient allergies
- Medication name
- Medication strength
- Medication dose form (i.e., tablet, IV, topical, etc.)
- Medication administration frequency
- Medication administration route
- Signature of the nurse processing the order
- Date and hour the order was written
- Duration of therapy (when applicable)

Additional information may be included as to when the medication is needed or even not to send the medication until it is specifically requested.

Original orders are to remain in the resident's chart. When an electronic charting system is not being used to communicate orders to the pharmacy, orders may be communicated to the pharmacy by a nurse via telephone or fax, or may come directly from a prescriber. Each order must be documented in the patient's chart; even if a prescriber gives a verbal order, a record of that order must be entered into the chart. Orders for noncontrolled medications may lack a physician's signature because physicians are often not in the building with the patient when the order is issued. Generally these orders are verbally communicated from the prescriber to a nurse to transcribe the order into the patient's chart. Such orders are valid orders, and a pharmacist may dispense drugs to a patient based on such orders. Schedule 3-5 controlled substance orders, however, must either be verbally communicated directly to the pharmacy by the prescriber, or the prescriber's designated agent, or as a written order signed by the prescriber. Schedule 2 controlled substance orders must be written orders unless an emergency need arises. Unlike in the outpatient setting, a Schedule 2 controlled substance order that is complete and signed may be faxed to a LTC pharmacy for dispensing to a patient who is terminally ill or who is in a LTC facility, as long as the original order is maintained in the patient's chart at the facility. If the patient is not terminally ill, and is in an ALF or GH, an original written prescription must be obtained before drugs may be dispensed, and the faxed Schedule 2 controlled substance order is considered invalid. Only in an emergency may a prescriber communicate a verbal order for up to 72 hours worth of a Schedule 2 controlled substance to a pharmacy; however, a complete written prescription must be issued to the pharmacy within seven days to substantiate the verbal order.

Another difference between a LTC medication order and those issued in hospitals or in the outpatient setting is the inclusion of delivery schedules. Many factors determine how much of a medication will be provided for a patient in each delivery and when the delivery will occur. In some cases, the patient's insurance company will dictate how much medication may be dispensed at one time (e.g., Medicare may only approve a seven-day supply to be dispensed at any time for any medication). Further, some facilities have a preference for how they prefer medications to be delivered. Certain medications may also have special protocols due to lab monitoring requirements or other factors that may require short fills to be routinely dispensed to prevent waste when doses are adjusted frequently (e.g., the anticoagulant warfarin is routinely adjusted based on the results of a blood test, called an INR, that may be drawn as often as every five days). Sometimes, an order will specify that the medication is used only "as needed," and so the patient's requests for the medication are observed over time to try to determine the expected need.

There are two ways to handle deliveries of regularly-used medications. One way is called **anniversary filling**; with this method, a regular delivery schedule is established using the day that the order is first written as the "anniversary" of when the delivery will be made. For example, if the patient is always provided with a seven-day supply of every medication and medication A is ordered on Monday and medication B is ordered on Thursday, then medication A will always be delivered every Monday and medication B will always be delivered every Thursday. Another method is called **cycle filling**; with this method, a specific day of the week, or month, is selected for the patient to receive all of their medications and the first fill is adjusted so that all future fills will fall in line with all other medications. For example, if a patient's delivery day is Wednesday and a new drug is ordered on Friday then an emergency supply is delivered to carry the patient from Friday through Wednesday, and then the drug is filled for a full seven-day supply, along with all of the patient's other medications for delivery on Wednesday. Some medications are only delivered by **on-demand filling**; generally, these are "as needed" medications, new medications or short-term use medications (e.g., antibiotics) that are only delivered if a nurse calls and specifically asks for a certain length of therapy to be delivered.

Each facility will have established times for medication administration that will also affect when deliveries will need to be made. For example, a once-daily dose of a medication may be given in one building at 8 a.m., and in another facility once-daily dosing is done at 10 a.m. These times need to be communicated to the pharmacist to not only ensure that the right medications are delivered at the right times but also so that the pharmacies can check for those drug interactions that occur when two medications are given at the same time of day. To ensure that the delivered medications are administered at the correct time of day, it is important for the pharmacy to include administration times on all medication administration instructions provided to the nursing staff. Although a pharmacist is ultimately responsible for all of these data elements being entered correctly into the pharmacy's electronic medical record system, entering all of this information is done almost exclusively by pharmacy technicians.

Dispensing and Packaging

Rather than dispensing larger quantities of drugs to patients in vials, as is done in the retail pharmacy setting, LTC pharmacies often prepare patient-specific medication packages that combine all of a patient's medications into a single package that makes it easier for the patient to be sure that all of their prescribed medications have been taken. Studies show that these systems increase resident safety by reducing errors in administration. They are particularly critical when patients are taking multiple drugs. Solid oral medication forms (tablets and capsules) are usually dispensed in unit-dose packaging, punch cards, cassettes or other specialized dispensing systems. All unit-dose medications are labeled with a lot number, an expiration date, the product's name, the product's strength and any other information required by state or federal regulations. Medications packaged by the pharmacy are done so in accordance with USP standards and state and federal guidelines.

Medications that require packaging other than in unit-dose packs include medications requiring refrigeration, liquid medications, injectable medications, eye drops, nasal sprays, externally applied medications (ointments, patches), and oversized or irregularly shaped medications or containers. Blister packs (see Figure 1) are generally sealed with an application of heat to the sealing film that causes it to shrink slightly and create the sealed blister. Some drugs will not tolerate the heat that must be applied to seal such blister packs. For such medications, blister packs exist with a peel-and-stick seal; however, these packages are more expensive and labor-intensive to use.

Figure 1
Blister Pack

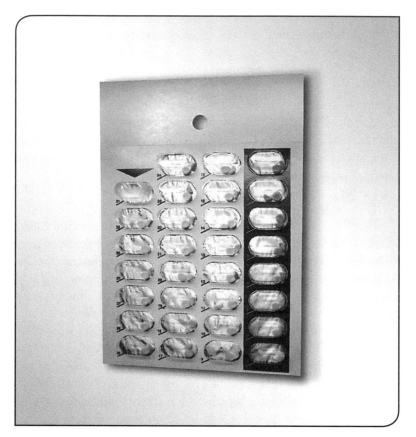

LTC pharmacies design their dispensing systems with multiple quality checkpoints to prevent potentially adverse drug interactions. The pharmacy will generally have a specialized record system that allows documentation of a quality check at each point along the dispensing system pathway. This rigorous quality assessment culture is essential to preventing errors and drug interactions and for keeping patients safe. Technology has also played a huge role in these dispensing systems. Bar-code scanner technology has improved accuracy by helping to catch when the wrong drug is about to be dispensed. It is still the responsibility, though, of every person in the chain to check their own work to ensure that they have done everything they can to prevent errors. A properly-designed dispensing system will balance procedures and technology so that a pharmacy technician can be confident that when a finished order is presented to a pharmacist for a final review that all potential errors have already been caught by the system. After a final review by a pharmacist, filled orders must then be packaged for delivery. Sealed delivery boxes (totes) are generally used to prevent diversion of drugs by delivery personnel and so that nursing staff and patients can feel confident that the drugs being delivered are exactly as they were when the pharmacist last checked them. Along with the medications, invoices and other records pertaining to the delivery are also generally included in the totes.

Emergency Dispensing Kits or Stat Kits

In a SNF, a supply of medication is often available to the nursing staff for administration to a patient on short notice. This stock of medication is often called an EDK or stat kit. EDK are not allowed for ALFs/GHs. An EDK is prepared by an LTC pharmacy with an inventory of the entire contents of the kit including each medication's expiration date. When a medication is removed from the kit to be dispensed, the nurse records exactly how much medication was administered and to whom it was administered. As the stock becomes depleted, or on a regular schedule, the pharmacy will collect the EDK that is in use and validate that all of the medications dispensed from the EDK have a corresponding prescriber's order and that these orders are appropriately recorded in the patient's chart. Since a pharmacist is generally not reviewing the order prior to the EDK being accessed, physicians and nurses must be instructed to take extra precautions to prevent medication misuse (e.g., a patient's allergies must be screened and the potential for drug interactions must be screened before initiating the therapy). These kits are generally portable boxes, carts or cabinets that are sealed and secured to prevent diversion or tampering with the medications inside. Inside the kit, medications are in unit-dose packages in the smallest quantity that can be reasonably packaged. Generally, the contents of such a kit are selected to allow for dosing of the drugs without significant manipulation of the dose form. This helps prevent waste and errors in administration (e.g., warfarin in an emergency kit may contain 1 mg and 0.5 mg tablets. This provides the ability to administer an order for warfarin 2.5 mg without splitting tablets. Levaquin in 250 mg tablets allows for dosing orders for 250 mg, 500 mg or 750 mg. Nitroglycerin in bottles of 25 tablets, rather than 100 tablets, reduces waste). Common medication in EDKs include antibiotics, treatment for hypoglycemia, pain medication, nitroglycerin and anti-hypertensive drugs. Pharmacy technicians are utilized to track the usage, expiration dating, proper storage and condition of these medications when restocking each kit for return to a facility. The expectation is to have the listed medications available at all times. The restocking schedule, quantities and contents are subject to review. Organization and attention to detail are needed to monitor and track these emergency kits.

Infusion Therapy

As previously mentioned, a LTC pharmacy may be involved in dispensing nonoral medications, such as IV infusions. Generally, when an IV preparation is delivered to a facility, it needs to be completely ready to administer to the intended patient. In the event that a product cannot be prepared ahead of time and must be delivered to the facility with instructions for onsite preparation, the pharmacy technician delivering the medication to the facility must be prepared to instruct the nursing staff on exactly how that medication is to be prepared (and this instruction must match the provided, written instructions). Pharmacy technicians are also vital to the preparation process of these products. Special training and attention to detail are required for the technician who chooses to assist in IV therapy preparation and management. More information on preparing IV admixtures can be found in this Manual in Chapter 7 on Aseptic Technique and Sterile Product Preparation.

Pharmacy Billing

The process of obtaining, dispensing and delivering a medication order can be derailed due to problems in billing the associated payer. With literally hundreds of insurance companies throughout the country, each with their own rules and requirements, it can be quite a challenge determining exactly what must be done to satisfy each payer's requirements. The process may be as simple as entering the right standardized codes into the correct fields in the claim. It may also be as difficult as needing to obtain a prior authorization or using a **step-therapy** protocol. A step-therapy protocol is a requirement by a payer that a particular agent, or class of agents, be tried before a more expensive agent, or class of agents, is tried. For instance, if a prescriber writes for the blood pressure lowering medication Diovan®, which is only available as a branded product, the patient's insurance company may require that lisinopril, another blood pressure-lowering medication, be used first because it is generically available and much less expensive. If the prescriber believes that the less-expensive options are medically inappropriate for the patient, the physician may fill out the insurance company's forms to obtain authorization to circumvent the step-therapy process. Because this authorization must be obtained prior to the pharmacy dispensing the drug, it is called a **prior authorization**. Some drugs are not part of a step-therapy protocol; however, due to cost, or because they may be used for certain conditions that are not covered by the insurance company, a prior authorization must be obtained before the drug may be dispensed. Also, an insurance claim may require more information from the prescriber than was originally included. This may include the diagnosis that leads to the use of the medication, lab values that justify the use of the drug or the dose of the drug, and previous therapies that have been tried and information on their success or failure to treat the condition.

Formularies

The pharmacy, medical director, administrator, director of nursing and pharmacy consultant may also collaborate to determine a list of preferred products for a facility or group of facilities. House stock lists are developed for OTC medications, and formularies are developed for prescription drugs. A **formulary** is a list of drugs, selected from within the commonly-used classes of drugs, that will be stocked and dispensed. Reducing the number of drugs that must be stocked by the pharmacy can lead to a considerable savings for the pharmacy and can be used to prevent medication errors. An example of a formulary selection would be to select levofloxacin as the formulary agent from the class of antibiotics called the fluoroquinolones and then only carry levofloxacin (and, therefore, not carry ciprofloxacin, gatifloxacin, gemifloxacin, moxifloxacin, norfloxacin or ofloxacin). The application of having a formulary is that a pharmacist may need to make a **therapeutic substitution** from one agent to another; that is, a prescriber may write for a drug that is not on the formulary and the pharmacist may need to switch that order to the formulary agent. In some states, a pharmacist can enter into a **collaborative practice agreement** with the physicians at a facility to allow the pharmacist to make this substitution without calling the physician for specific permission. This process, called a therapeutic substitution, must be done by a pharmacist to ensure that the correct agent at the correct dose is selected. An example of how this would work is as follows: a physician writes an order for the pharmacy to dispense moxifloxacin; however, the formulary fluoroquinolone is levofloxacin. The pharmacist converts the moxifloxacin order into a levofloxacin order, calculates the appropriate conversion dose and dispenses levofloxacin to the facility with a note explaining that the therapeutic substitution occurred to be in compliance with the facility's formulary. The nurse then updates the patient's chart to indicate the change. In some circumstances, for some drugs, and in some states, the pharmacy must obtain the prescriber's specific approval each time such a substitution needs to be made.

Field Work

Pharmacy technicians working for LTC pharmacies may have the opportunity to get out of the pharmacy and work in the facilities. Pharmacies that supply medication carts, IV pumps and EDKs may find it more convenient to send a pharmacy technician capable of addressing these devices rather than sending a courier to retrieve the device and return it to the pharmacy for processing. A pharmacy technician is often responsible for the maintenance, repair and stocking of medication carts, EDKs and other medication storage areas. Pharmacy technicians may also be utilized as the facility's resident expert on laws and regulations surrounding medication use, storage, administration, disposal and other medication use topics. Working at the facilities requires the willingness to travel and a good driving record. As "the face of the pharmacy" to the patient and other health care providers, impeccable communication skills, both verbal and written, are necessary, along with ability to problem solve. This can be a rewarding practice area with significant interaction with patients and other health care professionals and para-professionals.

Conclusion

The pharmacy services provided in nursing care facilities focus on multiple chronic diseases in patients who are dependent on others for their care. Each individual involved in delivering this care must place the safety of these residents before any other consideration. Open communication between pharmacy staff and other health care providers becomes absolutely necessary to ensure safe patient care. With LTC pharmacy technicians often serving as the pharmacy's first contact with the patient for the rest of the health care team, they are in a unique position to shape quality care and ensure safe medication use.

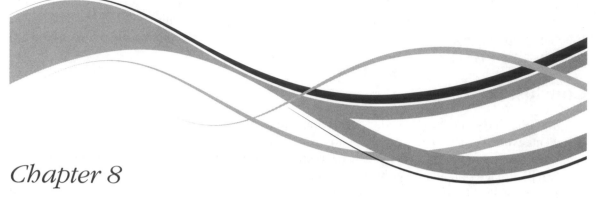

Chapter 8

REVIEW QUESTIONS

1. A POS in the context of long-term care pharmacy refers to the point-of-sale system used to track payments from facilities to the pharmacy.
    a. True
    b. False

2. An ALF nurse receives an order for an antibiotic. The medication is removed from the EDK for first-dose administration until the complete order is sent from the pharmacy. Is this scenario plausible?
    a. Yes
    b. No

3. Who must be aware that a medication order is not a covered benefit by the patient's insurance plan?
    a. The pharmacist
    b. The nurse caring for the patient
    c. The prescriber
    d. All of the above

4. Which of the following orders for aspirin is complete?
    a. Aspirin 1 daily
    b. Aspirin 81 mg
    c. Aspirin 81 mg chewable one daily
    d. Aspirin 81 mg chewable one tablet by mouth daily

5. Medication orders in a LTC pharmacy setting require all of the following elements, except:
    a. the patient's name.
    b. the prescriber's name.
    c. the route of administration.
    d. the frequency.
    e. the duration of therapy.

6. Cycle fill medications are refilled upon request.
   a. True
   b. False

7. An order for a Schedule 2 controlled substance to a SNF can be communicated by all of the following, except a:
   a. signed prescription sent to the pharmacy from the prescriber via fax.
   b. 72-hour emergency supply through a verbal order from the prescriber to the pharmacist, as long as written follow-up is received within seven days by the pharmacy.
   c. verbal order from the nurse to the pharmacist.
   d. signed prescription sent to the pharmacy via a courier service.

8. Each resident in a SNF is required by law to have their medications reviewed monthly by a pharmacist.
   a. True
   b. False

9. Where would a nurse retrieve over-the-counter medications available in bulk quantities in a LTC facility?
   a. EDK
   b. EMK
   c. House stock
   d. STAT kit

10. A pharmacist may always substitute a formulary drug for a prescribed drug under his or her therapeutic substitution powers.
    a. True
    b. False

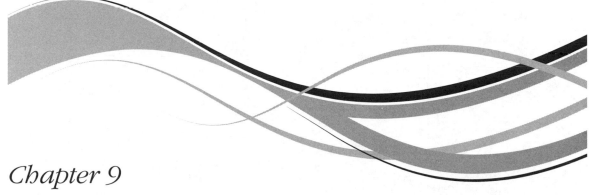

Chapter 9
MEDICAL EQUIPMENT

By   D. Joshua Potter
     John Watkins, MBA

Learning Objectives

This chapter seeks to prepare a pharmacy technician to:

- define durable medical equipment, prosthetics, orthotics and supplies (DMEPOS) and discuss how dispensing DMEPOS differs from dispensing drugs.
- discuss requirements for billing Medicare Part B, Medicaid and private medical insurance for DMEPOS.
- discuss accreditation, requirements to become and stay accredited, and the role of an accreditation provider.
- discuss the role of pharmacy technicians in fitting or setting up DMEPOS and training patients to use DMEPOS.

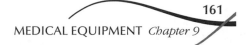

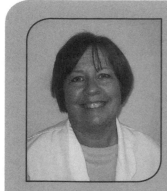

In your current position, how did you become familiar with the medical equipment in your environment?

"I have worked for an independent community pharmacy for the last several years. We have seen an increased need in the medical equipment line. As the need increases, I have learned a lot by asking questions and relying on the expertise of our durable medical equipment billing department. I have also stayed up-to-date on Medicare policies and procedures. In addition, I have also attended seminars and classes when they are offered, including a three-day class on diabetes education and one on fitting compression garments."

Patricia Gomolak, CPhT
The Prescription Shop,
Traverse City, Mich.

In what practice setting do technicians most frequently interact with medical equipment and why?

"I think that community pharmacy is the setting most likely to deal with medical equipment. I think that it is a good thing to offer our patients a place to get their prescriptions and other medical needs in one convenient place. I also like the diversity it offers me in my job."

Introduction

The pharmacy technician's role in providing DMEPOS goes above and beyond what the technician would typically do in the drug dispensing world. With the uncontrolled nature of the vast majority of DMEPOS items, technicians will often perform the set-up, training and answering of questions about a specific piece of DMEPOS; however, as always, pharmacy technicians must refer clinical and disease state questions, that a patient or caregiver may have to a pharmacist. In pharmacies that have larger DMEPOS departments, and have received DMEPOS accreditation, pharmacy technicians are typically the individuals who are responsible for the development and implementation of the pharmacy's DMEPOS Accreditation Compliance Program.

In recent years, pharmacies have been adding specialty services (e.g., compounding, chemotherapy preparation, respiratory therapy and DMEPOS) to fill niches that exist in their community. The potential in these specialty services and the overall growth of health care in the past two decades because of the aging population are providing community pharmacies with a tremendous opportunity to expand their DMEPOS and other specialty services.

With this growth, it is important for pharmacy technicians to understand the potentially complicated world of DMEPOS. There are several key areas that are important to any endeavor in DMEPOS:

- DMEPOS prescriptions (orders are not always as straight forward as pharmaceuticals)
- Documentation requirements
- DMEPOS accreditation
- DMEPOS accreditation exemption
- Payers with rules (Medicare, Medicaid, private third parties)
- Dispensing process differences (compared to pharmaceuticals)
- Training, setup and fitting of DMEPOS

DMEPOS Overview

DMEPOS includes **durable medical equipment (DME), prosthetics, orthotics and supplies**. Each state defines these terms, though most states have definitions that are very similar. For instance, in Michigan, the Medicaid Provider Manual defines DME as, "those items that can stand repeated use, are primarily and customarily used to serve a medical purpose, are not useful to a person in the absence of illness or injury, and can be used in the beneficiary's home." Prosthetics are defined by the manual as, "devices that artificially replace a portion of the body to prevent or correct a physical anomaly or malfunctioning portion of the body." In addition, it defines orthotics as devices that, "assist in correcting or strengthening a congenital or acquired physical anomaly or malfunctioning portion of the body."[1]

Compared to the prescription requirements of a medication, which are set forth in state Public Health Codes and Administrative Rules of the state Board of Pharmacy, the prescription requirements for DMEPOS vary based on who is paying for the DMEPOS.

Medicare Prescription and Documentation Requirements

One of the main areas in the DME world that causes the most deficiencies during a Medicare audit is the lack of a proper Detailed Written Order (prescription) and documentation. Medicare requires specific handouts and forms to be generated for each new DME order, and this paperwork must remain in a patient's chart.

A **Medicare Detailed Written Order** must contain key information in order for a supplier to submit a claim to Medicare. This information includes the following:

- Patient's name
- Description of the product being prescribed
- Any accessories, upgrades or options
- Signature of the prescriber
- Start date
- Quantity (if for supplies)
- Instructions for use: for supplies, it is important to understand that Medicare does not accept "as directed." The instructions must clearly define the frequency (e.g., twice per day)
- Duration of need (if for supplies and rental items)

Before submitting a claim to the DME **Medicare Administrative Contractor (MAC)**, the supplier (pharmacy or business) must have the following documentation on file:

- A verbal/dispensing/preliminary order
- Detailed written order
- Certificate of Medical Necessity (CMN) (if applicable)
- DME Information Form (DIF) (if applicable)
- Proof of delivery
- Beneficiary authorization
- Advance Beneficiary Notice of Non-Coverage (ABN) (if applicable)
- Information from the treating physician concerning the patient's diagnosis (if an ICD-9-CM or ICD-10 code is required on the claim; these codes are used to indicate diagnosis for all patient encounters. ICD-10 is a diagnosis code revision to ICD-9-CM)
- Any information required for the use of specific modifiers, or attestation statements, as defined in certain DME policies

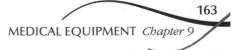

The supplier must also obtain as much documentation from the patient's medical record as they determine is needed to assure that coverage criterion for an item has been met. If the information in the patient's medical record does not adequately support the medical necessity for the item, the suppliers are liable for the dollar amount involved unless a properly executed ABN has been obtained for possible denial. Documentation must be maintained in the supplier's files for seven years.[2]

Medicaid Prescription Requirements

While the requirements of a Medicare DMEPOS order go above the typical requirements of a pharmaceutical, Medicaid DMEPOS orders follow the same basic principles of a pharmaceutical prescription. Check your state's requirements for specific details. Below outlines what is required in Michigan, as an example:

A prescription must contain all of the following:

- Beneficiary's name
- Beneficiary's date of birth (DOB)
- Beneficiary ID number or Social Security Number (SSN) (if known)
- Prescribing physician's name, address and telephone number
- Prescribing physician's signature (a stamped or co-signature will not be accepted)
- The date the prescription was written
- The specific item prescribed
- The quantity of items and supplies to be provided and the duration of therapy
- The date of the order if different from the physician's signature date

The prescription must meet the following timeframe:

- For medical supplies, refills are allowed for up to one year from the original physician's signature date on the prescription
- For oxygen, ventilators and other long-term use items, refills/use up to one year from the original physician signature date
- For the purchase of DME, the original physician signature date must be within the last 180 days
- For orthotics and prosthetics, the original physician signature date for an initial service must be within the last 60 days. For replacement of an orthotic or prosthetic, the physician signature date must be within the last 180 days.

A new prescription will be required when there is a change in the beneficiary's condition causing a change in the item or the frequency of its use.[1]

Private Third Party Payers

The individual documentation and prescription requirements are different for every third party payer. To determine what is required, the pharmacy must contact the third party to validate and authorize the order. They will also vary if the third party requires the pharmacy to be accredited. If so, the pharmacy would be required to maintain its accreditor's required documentation.

Dispensing Process

When dispensing DMEPOS, the pharmacy will go through a two-step process: the intake and dispensing. These steps are broken down into several intermediary processes. While this can be time consuming, it does ensure that claims are clean, paid and that the pharmacy has all the proper

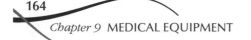

documentation to ensure that any audits that may occur by the payer will not find significant deficiencies that could require the pharmacy to return payment to the payer.

The **intake process** itself is more of a fact-finding task. During the intake process, the pharmacy will verify that the claim will be paid by calling the private third party payer to validate and authorize payment. During the validation and authorization process, the pharmacy inquires as to whether or not they are contracted with the payer, if the patient is eligible for physician-ordered benefits, any co-payment amounts to be collected and if there is any documentation requirement for the claim to be submitted.

During the **dispensing process**, the pharmacy will take care of all the tasks that are required to ensure the patient or caregiver will be able to properly utilize the piece of equipment. Depending upon the item, this could entail setting up the DME per the physician's and manufacturer's protocols, fitting the patient, training and educating the patient and finally dispensing the product to the patient. The individual aspects of the dispensing process will be discussed later in the chapter.

Possibly the most important aspect of the entire intake and dispensing process is to document, document, document. This is how the pharmacy can protect itself from future audits. Remember, if an event is not documented, then it did not happen.

DMEPOS Billing Requirements and Processes

Several government agencies, and contracted agencies, oversee and enforce DMEPOS billing requirements and administer payment.

The Centers for Medicare and Medicaid Services (CMS) is the branch of the Department of Health and Human Services (HHS) that is responsible for Medicare and has oversight of state Medicaid programs. CMS contracts most of its functions that are important to Medicare Part B supplies to two agencies: the National Supplier Clearinghouse (NSC) and the DME-MAC.

National Supplier Clearinghouse

The NSC has been contracted by CMS to administrate the Medicare Part B enrollment process. It acts as a conduit to receive and approve the Medicare Enrollment Application (otherwise known as the CMS-855S form). Once it approves a pharmacy's application, the pharmacy may begin submitting DMEPOS claims to Medicare. If a pharmacy is billing for Medicare Part B pharmaceuticals, it does not need to be accredited; however, if it is billing DMEPOS and the accreditation exemption (discussed later in the chapter) is not met, the pharmacy must be accredited by one of the CMS-approved accreditation organizations.

Durable Medical Equipment Medicare Administrative Contractor

Durable Medical Equipment Medicare Administrative Contractors (DME-MAC) are contracted by CMS to administer Medicare claims. They are responsible for handling all DMEPOS Medicare claims and to be the point of contact for DMEPOS Medicare suppliers. Currently, there are four DME-MACs and each is responsible for different CMS jurisdictions of the United States. View contact information for each DME-MAC in Table 1.

Table 1
DME-MAC Contact Information

DME-MAC	Jurisdiction Area	Interactive Voice Response System	Toll-Free Number	Written General Inquiries
CIGNA Government Services	Jurisdiction C (Alabama, Arkansas, Colorado, Florida, Georgia, Louisiana, Mississippi, New Mexico, North Carolina, Oklahoma, Puerto Rico, South Carolina, Tennessee, Texas, U.S. Virgin Islands, Virginia and West Virginia)	(866) 238-9650	(866) 270-4909	P.O. Box 20010 Nashville, TN 37202
National Government Services, Inc.	Jurisdiction B (Illinois, Indiana, Kentucky, Michigan, Minnesota, Ohio, and Wisconsin)	(877) 299-7900	(866) 590-6727	P.O. Box 6306 Indianapolis, IN 42606
NHIC, Corp.	Jurisdiction A (Connecticut, Delaware, Maine, Maryland, Massachusetts, New Hampshire, New Jersey, New York, Pennsylvania, Rhode Island, Vermont and Washington, D.C.)	(866) 419-9458	(866) 590-6731	P.O. Box 9146 Hingham, MA 02043
Noridian Administrative Services	Jurisdiction D (Alaska, American Samoa, Arizona, California, Guam, Hawaii, Idaho, Iowa, Kansas, N. Mariana Islands, Missouri, Montana, Nebraska, Nevada, North Dakota, Oregon, South Dakota, Utah, Washington and Wyoming)	(877) 320-0390	(866) 243-7272	P.O. Box 6727 Fargo, ND 58108

With the responsibilities required of a DME-MAC, they have become an important and vital source of information and education for DMEPOS suppliers. They provide news, forms and other information that Medicare suppliers must be familiar with to ensure they are properly billing DMEPOS.

Some of the most important items that are maintained by the DME-MAC are: the DME-MAC Supplier Manual, the local coverage determinations (LCD) and policy articles. The Supplier Manual provides detailed information, and necessary links to relevant information, for submitting clean claims that meet Medicare policies. The LCD and policy articles define coverage criteria, payment rules and documentation that are applied to DMEPOS claims processed by the DME-MAC. The policies are a combination of national and local decisions. National policies are established by CMS, and the DME-MACs are required to follow national policy where it exists; however, when there is no national policy on a subject, the DME-MAC has the authority and responsibility to establish local policy.[3]

Medicare DMEPOS Supplier Standards

The Medicare DMEPOS Supplier Standards is a document of 30 standards with which a pharmacy must be in compliance if they wish to obtain, or retain, Medicare billing privileges. These standards must also be provided by the pharmacy to all Medicare beneficiaries.

Accreditation

As part of the Medicare Modernization Act of 2003, Congress required suppliers (including pharmacies) of DMEPOS to meet Medicare Part B Quality Standards. To handle this, Congress asked the Secretary of Health and Human Services to designate accreditation organizations to review supplier's compliance with the Medicare Part B Quality Standards.

Congressional action in March 2010 exempted certain pharmacies and extended DMEPOS accreditation deadlines for other pharmacies to Jan. 1, 2011.

Supplier Quality Standards

In August 2006, CMS released the DMEPOS Quality Standards, not to be confused with the Medicare DMEPOS Supplier Standards. These Quality Standards were used by the accreditation organizations to create and/or amend their own accreditation standards. This is an important distinction; while a pharmacy is complying with the CMS Quality Standards, it must also meet the accreditation standards of the accreditation organization the pharmacy has selected. The following are different areas where the Quality Standards are applied:

■ **Administrative**
The Administrative Standards are designed as the form and the foundation of the organization, starting with ownership, leadership and compliance with state and federal laws.

■ **Financial Management**
The Financial Management Standards are designed to ensure the supplier has a keen sense of its financial standing. These Standards require the supplier to have an annual operating budget that is routinely monitored through the year to help diagnose financial problems before they become a hindrance to quality of care and service. The Financial Management Standards also require a supplier to reconcile their Medicare DME claims.

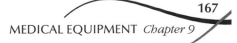

■ **Human Resources**

The next section of the Quality Standards reflects on the organization's human resources department. To comply with this section, the pharmacy needs to create, implement and document the pharmacy's overall processes related to its employees. These processes relate to the hiring and training of new employees and the continual training, on a regular basis, of employees in subjects relating to their job functions.

■ **Consumer Services**

The Consumer Services Standards reflect on the activities of dispensing DMEPOS. These standards cover the handling of the patient as they bring their order into the pharmacy; equipment set-up, whether it is at the pharmacy or the patient's residence; patient training and education; and other necessary tasks.

■ **Performance Management**

To better ensure the overall quality of care and services provided by an organization, CMS requires accredited facilities to monitor key aspects of its operation. The Performance Management Standard requires the pharmacy to track patient satisfaction, patient complaints, adverse events, billing and coding errors, and the impact of business changes.

■ **Product Safety**

The Product Safety Standards require the pharmacy to implement a program that promotes the safe use of equipment and item(s) and minimizes safety risks, infection and hazards both for its staff and patients. These standards include maintenance and repair of the DMEPOS that the pharmacy has provided to patients.

Accreditation Organization

The chief responsibility of the accreditation organization (AO) is to ensure that suppliers are meeting the AO interpretation of the CMS Supplier Quality Standards. Based on the Supplier Quality Standards, the AO creates its own accreditation standards. Suppliers then contract with an AO and create policies, procedures and practices to meet the AO accreditation standards. The AO will then visit the pharmacy and conduct a survey of the location. From that point, the location will either pass or fail inspection and be accredited or not. In the case of a pass, the location will be awarded an accreditation certificate for a specific period of time (often three years). In the event of a fail, the pharmacy must create and implement a Corrective Action Plan (CAP). Once the CAP is implemented, the pharmacy will notify the AO, and the AO will make a decision if the implemented CAP corrects the deficiencies found during the initial survey. If it does, the pharmacy will be granted full accreditation status again. Generally, unless major violations of standards are observed on survey, once a pharmacy is accredited, it will retain accreditation even if a CAP is required by the AO for successful approval for accreditation.

Pharmacy DMEPOS Accreditation Exemption

By the accreditation deadline in 2009, more than 35,000 pharmacies in the nation had received DMEPOS accreditation. Then, as part of the Healthcare Reform Act of 2010, Congress provided pharmacies with an exemption provided they meet a few simple criteria. As an industry, this exemption was viewed by many as a blessing; however, in reality, pharmacies in many cases were not properly maintaining the documentation needed to comply with Medicare Manuals and LCD. Fortunately, when pharmacies were preparing for accreditation, it gave them a chance to educate themselves on the Medicare documentation requirements.

All pharmacies that wish to be considered exempt from DMEPOS accreditation must meet all of the following criteria:

1. The total billings by the pharmacy, for DMEPOS, are less than 5 percent of total pharmacy sales for the previous three calendar years
2. The pharmacy has been enrolled as a supplier of DMEPOS, and has been issued a provider number, for at least five years
3. No final adverse action has been imposed on the pharmacy in the past five years
4. The pharmacy submits an attestation, in the manner and at the time frame to be determined, that the pharmacy meets the criteria listed in 1-3
5. The pharmacy agrees to submit materials, as requested, during the course of an audit conducted on a random sample of pharmacies selected annually

Total DMEPOS billings are considered as less than 5 percent of the total *pharmacy* revenue. For example, if a pharmacy is part of a larger location, such as a grocery store that also has a pharmacy, or a pharmacy that sells other items, the DMEPOS sales would be less than 5 percent of the pharmacy sales not that of the total grocery/store receipts.[4] All pharmacies that bill Medicare for DMEPOS must still be in compliance with the 30 Medicare DMEPOS Supplier Standards.

Licensure and Certification

Some states require that a DMEPOS supplier be licensed by the state before DMEPOS may be dispensed to patients. For pharmacies, this right may be inherent in their pharmacy license but it may be a separate license that must be maintained by the pharmacy. Some states have no such requirements and do not license or register DMEPOS suppliers; pharmacy technicians must know their state's requirements before engaging in any activities related to DMEPOS. Further, some training and education related to fitting and setting up certain DMEPOS grants a pharmacist, or pharmacy technician, a certificate that must be held before providing such DMEPOS to a Medicare or Medicaid beneficiary (e.g., a fitter's certificate may be required before fitting a patient for diabetic shoes that will be billed to Medicare).

DMEPOS Training, Education and Fitting

In certain circumstances, a DMEPOS product must be prepared, set-up, fitted and/or customized to meet the requirements of the physician's order and the manufacturer's protocols. In these cases, a pharmacy technician and/or pharmacist must be educated by the manufacturer. In many cases, this could be online or by other means. In either case, make sure there is documentation of this training being completed and passed by anyone providing training to patients.

Privileging

Privileging is the process used by health care organizations to grant to a specific practitioner the authorization to provide specific patient care services. Privileging ensures that the individual requesting clinical privileges is capable of providing those patient care services in accordance with the standard of care of the facility granting the privilege. In many cases, pharmacy technicians are not among the personnel trained or educated to provide a piece of DMEPOS; however, they may work under the supervision of someone who has certification or licensing (e.g., another pharmacy technician, a pharmacist or a respiratory therapist).

Set-up

In some cases, a pharmacy technician will be responsible for setting up the DME product. This could be as simple as ensuring a cane, walker or crutch is set at the proper height for the patient or it could be ensuring that a more complex piece of equipment, like a Continuous Positive Airway Pressure (CPAP) machine has been set to the appropriate pressure settings.

Training

To go along with the set-up, it is the pharmacy's responsibility to ensure adequate training of the patient or caregiver(s) on how to use each provided device. To properly train a patient, or caregiver, the pharmacy must ensure the patient understands the proper use and maintenance of an item. Additionally, the pharmacy must ensure the patient understands any potential hazards that may exist and that the patient is aware of any infection control protocols that need to be in place to prevent infections from spreading due to the use of the product.

Fitting

Some DMEPOS, such as therapeutic shoes and orthotics, require special fitting. This fitting must be performed by someone who has been trained and educated to perform the fitting properly. Fitting is one of the most important functions that a pharmacy technician can provide as it relates to DMEPOS. For example, improperly fitted diabetic shoes could lead to poor circulation and pressure ulcers.

Conclusion

Why pharmacy and DMEPOS? Being a practitioner of medicine, pharmacists have a unique position to provide a patient's drug therapy and DMEPOS. Looking at one disease state population, diabetics are one of the patient groups that often need many medications and tend to require more DMEPOS over the years. The DMEPOS a diabetic is likely to require over the years include blood glucose monitors and supplies (to monitor their glucose levels), therapeutic footwear (to help prevent foot ulcerations) and Respiratory Assist Devices (to help treat apnea).

Because of the different devices a pharmacy could offer, documentation is key, regardless of accreditation status. Auditing arms of Medicare, Medicaid and third party payers must have proper documentation, and pharmacy technicians can play a key role in that process. DMEPOS has potential as a profit center for the pharmacy provided a proactive individual, such as a pharmacy technician, is in place to direct and grow a pharmacy's DMEPOS business. A quality pharmacy technician can take the extra time to learn the paperwork so the business can realize the higher profit margins associated with many of the DMEPOS items and services.

References

1. Michigan Department of Community Health, www.mdch.state.mi.us/dch-medicaid/manuals/MedicaidProviderManual.zip, Nov. 1, 2010.
2. Noridian Administrative Services, LLC, www.noridianmedicare.com/dme/news/manual/chapter3.html, Nov. 1, 2010.
3. Noridian Administrative Services, LLC, www.noridianmedicare.com/dme/news/manual/chapter9.html, Nov. 1, 2010.
4. Centers for Medicare and Medicaid Services, www.cms.gov/MedicareProviderSupEnroll/Downloads/DMEPOSAccExemptForCertainPharmaciesFactSheet.pdf, Nov. 1, 2010.

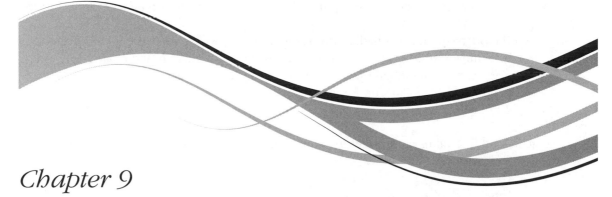

Chapter 9
REVIEW QUESTIONS

1. Pharmacy technicians can dispense DMEPOS items to patients if:
    a. they are supervised by a pharmacist.
    b. they have been properly trained on products being dispensed.
    c. they are certified.
    d. they are employed by an accredited pharmacy.

2. One of the most important items maintained by the DME-MAC is:
    a. patient eligibility criteria.
    b. DMEPOS set-up instructions.
    c. accreditation manuals.
    d. supplier manuals.

3. The DMEPOS Supplier Standards (30) must be:
    a. followed only if the pharmacy obtains DMEPOS accreditation.
    b. furnished to every prescribing physician who writes an order for DMEPOS.
    c. adhered to if the pharmacy wishes to obtain and maintain a Medicare billing number and provide to Medicare beneficiaries.
    d. reviewed once per year.

4. If a pharmacy wishes to obtain DMEPOS accreditation, it needs to:
    a. comply with the standards of a CMS-approved AO by having a written, and implemented, policy and procedure manual.
    b. comply with all 30 supplier standards.
    c. comply with CMS standards and incur a survey from a CMS official.
    d. supply all product categories for which Medicare reimburses.

5. When a pharmacy is accredited for DMEPOS, it can:
    a. supply DMEPOS products and services to Medicare and Medicaid beneficiaries and bill Medicare and/or Medicaid for the DMEPOS.
    b. supply any DMEPOS product to Medicare or Medicaid beneficiaries.
    c. bill premium reimbursement rates on DMEPOS items.
    d. modify or change DMEPOS prescriptions.

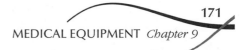

6. Pharmacies are exempt from the Medicare DMEPOS accreditation if they meet which of the following criteria?
   a. The pharmacy has not had actions taken against its Medicare Part B Supplier Number.
   b. Its annual Medicare DMEPOS sales are less than 5 percent of the pharmacy's annual sales with an attestation to this being submitted to Medicare.
   c. It has had a Medicare Part B supplier number for more than five years.
   d. All of the above

7. Medicare Part B requires pharmacies to maintain their patient files for how many years?
   a. Six
   b. 10
   c. Three
   d. Seven

8. Proper training for a patient who has received DMEPOS includes:
   a. training and education of proper use of a piece of DMEPOS.
   b. proper maintenance of the DMEPOS.
   c. understanding any potential hazards that may exist and any infection control protocols that must be followed.
   d. All of the above

9. New pharmacies must become accredited to obtain their Medicare Part B Supplier Number for DMEPOS.
   a. True
   b. False

10. If a pharmacy has question about Medicare coverage criteria, payment rules and documentation requirements, what action must be taken?
   a. Review the LCD
   b. Contact the NSC
   c. Contact Medicare
   d. Contact the physician

Chapter 10

PATIENT AND MEDICATION SAFETY

By Mary E. Burkhardt, M.S., R.Ph., FASHP

Learning Objectives

This chapter seeks to prepare a pharmacy technician to:

- list three medication safety tools in use today in the health care environment.
- describe the value of close call reports to safety.
- describe the basics of root cause analysis and its use in health care safety.
- explain The Joint Commission's role in medication safety.
- give three examples of good topics for an failure mode and effects analysis (FMEA) project.

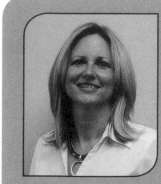

What is a technician's role in medication error prevention?

"Technicians play an important role in preventing medication errors. They provide an extra set of eyes and have the opportunity to stop a potential error before it reaches the patient. Unlike other industries, the consequences of mistakes made in a medical setting can be severe and may result in injury, or even death."

What are some ways that technicians can promote patient safety?

"First, recognize the importance of asking questions, and following your intuition if you have any doubts or concerns about the task you are performing; never guess. If you are at all uncertain of something, get clarification. You are an important part of the health care team. A good pharmacist or physician will appreciate and respect your diligence in making sure the right patient, gets the right medication, in the right dose, at the right time.

In a hospital setting, make sure you get adequate training and fully understand the importance of aseptic technique. Often the product you are mixing will go directly into the vein of another human being; there is no chance to recall it.

Don't become complacent, and always read the label. Never select a product based on habit; because it looks the same, has the same shape, size or color, or was placed in a particular spot on the shelf. Consider moving drugs with similar labels or packaging to different locations to prevent incorrect product selection.

My final check before completing a task is to ask myself this question: 'would I hang this I.V. (or deliver this medication, etc.) to my loved one.' If not, I start over."

Deanna Scully, CPhT, pharmacy contract coordinator, HealthPlus of Michigan, Flint, Mich.

Introduction

Long before the landmark Institute of Medicine (IOM) report was released in 1999, pharmacists and other health care providers had been concerned with the safe care of patients.[1] Patient safety is not a new concept. The literature about medication error prevention spans decades, and medication safety is a core philosophy of pharmacy practice. So why is there so much discussion about safety recently? What has changed is organized health care's approach to safety. Numerous forces in health care, including The Joint Commission (TJC), and various state and national regulations have worked to encourage organizations to take a more systematic approach. Health care organizations across the country are using lessons learned from other industries, such as aviation, nuclear power and engineering, to make patient safety a part of the daily tasks of health care rather than a separate focus.

Medication safety and medication error prevention are not strictly the domain of pharmacists. They are fundamental parts of work processes in pharmacy practice. The process of formalized pharmacy technician education and certification began, in part, out of a need for well-trained and technically competent pharmacy technicians ready to help reduce the likelihood that medication errors would occur. The skill level required for many pharmacy technician positions exceeded that which could easily be taught on the job. There was also a need to standardize the approach to technician education. More clinical and workload demands put on pharmacists increase their reliance on pharmacy technicians, and specifically well-trained and qualified pharmacy technicians.

Pharmacy technicians are in a key position to recognize and report safety issues because they are often the first to notice look-alike medications, sound-alike drug names and packaging/

labeling that is confusing. Pharmacy technicians are often the first to see new medications coming into a pharmacy from wholesale or warehouse orders, and they are responsible for removing medications from pharmacy shelves and for selecting drugs to be dispensed based on information presented from a pharmacy's dispensing software. Pharmacy technicians are exposed to almost every potential failure in the medication system that could occur. Therefore, it is imperative for pharmacy technicians to have a solid background in the principles of medication safety in order to work with pharmacists in preventing patient harm. Because many pharmacists are not specifically trained in pharmacy school on the underlying science involved in medication safety, by virtue of completing this chapter, a pharmacy technician may actually have more training in medication safety than his or her coworkers. Dedicated and courageous pharmacy technicians who take the initiative to speak up about unsafe conditions or hazards have made numerous first-time discoveries that contribute to the profession's understanding of safe medication practices.

Systems Approach

Medicine has traditionally treated quality problems and errors as failings on the part of individual providers, support personnel or single factors. The **systems approach**, by contrast, takes the position that most errors reflect predictable human failings in the context of poorly designed systems (e.g., expected lapses in human vigilance in the face of long work hours, predictable mistakes on the part of relatively inexperienced personnel faced with situations requiring complex thinking, or unregimented procedures that do not promote an unfocused and repetitive execution of tasks). Rather than focusing corrective efforts on reprimanding individuals or pursuing remedial education, the systems approach seeks to identify situations or factors likely to give rise to human error and implement systems changes that will reduce the occurrence of errors or minimize their impact on patients. This view holds that efforts to catch human errors before they occur, or block them from causing harm, will ultimately be more fruitful than those that seek to somehow create flawless providers.

Reporting Systems

One feature of a well-designed medication safety system is a **medication event reporting system**. Often referred to by different names (e.g., medication error reports, variances, incident reports, etc.), the focus remains the same: collect information on errors that occur in order to develop tweaks to the system to prevent the same, or a similar, error from occurring again. Various methods exist to report an event, ranging from online reporting, paper reporting and anonymous reporting to hotlines using phone mailboxes. No matter how the information is gathered, there are some general principles that can be followed to help make the collection program more successful.

- Safety reporting systems are based on a belief that employees do NOT come to work to hurt patients. The vast majority of safety issues are systems-based rather than caused by individuals trying to do the wrong thing on purpose. Even with violations of procedures, the safety system asks why the employee has trouble following the procedures and does not see the lack of following a procedure as the true root cause of an event. In other words, there must be something deeper than the obvious procedure violation, such as a lack of appropriate training, exhaustion of the person, etc.
- Good systems accept information from all sources. It can be conversation in a hallway, a phone report or an official incident form, but all information is considered important.
- A good system is nonpunitive to the reporter and the employee(s) involved. The information is used to make things safer; it is not used to punish employees, otherwise, no one will report events and any safety efforts are stymied. Punitive

work environments are counter-productive to safety improvement because employees can be fearful of being shamed or disciplined for their involvement in an adverse event.

■ In order to sustain the system, follow-up must be initiated with the reporter to alert him or her to what was learned and how the information was used to improve care. This encourages reporting because reporters see that there is value in making reports of errors.

Spontaneous reporting systems (e.g., medication error reports) are not a numbers game. Receiving more actual event reports (and perhaps more close call information) is not necessarily a bad thing. It could reflect an improved culture for reporting what is really going on rather than a reduction in the safety of care. The **National Coordinating Committee for Medication Error Reporting and Prevention (NCC MERP)** of the United States Pharmacopoeia issued a press release that does an excellent job of explaining the perils of using medication error reporting rates to benchmark organizations against each other.[2] This release is available online at www.nccmerp.org/council/council2002-06-11.html.

Safety Culture and Leadership

There is no question that the leadership in an organization sets the tone for the safety culture. If insufficient safety resources exist, there is punishment for reporting unsafe situations or purchases and policies focus only on short-term economics, not safety or quality, then the overall functioning of the health care system is adversely affected. With a leadership team that is conscious of fostering a culture of safety, a safety program can become part of standard practice rather than a burdensome addition to daily routines. One mindset that can cause trouble for an organization is declaring that safety is a priority; this may sound like a reasonable initiative, but it misses the reality of how safety needs to be viewed if patients are to be protected. Saying it is a priority assumes you can juggle it around and put something else first, and that it is a separate line item on an agenda. In order to be a true safety-minded organization, safety must be of value to the organization and integrated into everything that the organization does, rather than declaring it a priority.[3] Those things that a person or an organization declares to be of value are those things that form their core belief system. These beliefs are immovable, and it is expected that the person or organization that holds such beliefs will be uncompromising in the pursuit of such beliefs. Creating a system of values, and learning how to work with one's values, is not an overnight process; organizations and people must work for years to develop and refine not just their values, but how holding those values translates into decision making.

Swiss Cheese Theory

James Reason developed what is known as the **Swiss Cheese Model of System Accidents** that can be seen in Figure 1.

Figure 1
James Reason's Swiss Cheese Theory of Organizational Accidents

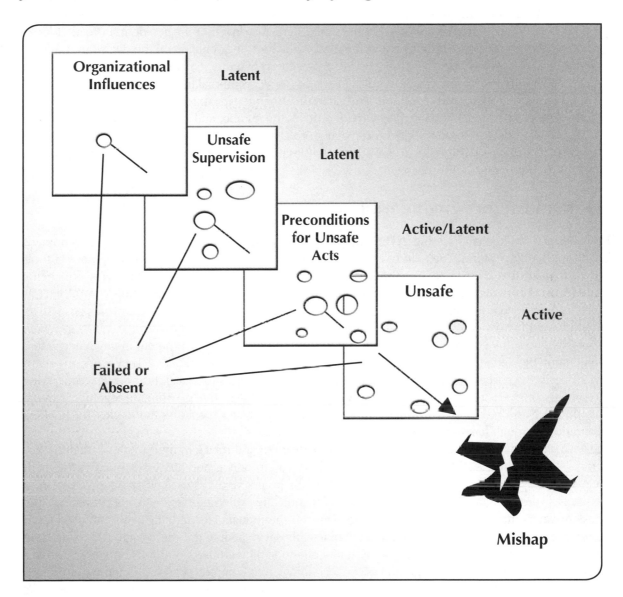

This theory illustrates the chance of multiple errors by examining the factors contributing to organizational accidents.[4] Imagine that there are many slices of Swiss cheese sliding past each other. The holes in the cheese have to line up just right in order for an event to cascade from a hazard to an actual accident. These pieces of cheese are systems and the holes are accidents waiting to happen. The slices of cheese represent systems, procedures and tasks within an organization. Each slice includes two types of holes: both latent (or passive) conditions that promote errors and active failures that occur because the conditions were right for the error to occur. A latent condition is a condition that is not itself an accident but that dooms the system to failure because of its passive presence. Latent conditions are system defects, such as a poorly maintained physical plant, a workplace culture that does not foster openness and transparency, or a technology that is implemented without proper training of all relevant staff members. In and of itself, there is no direct hazard in these situations existing; however, with the right trigger, these conditions lead to disasters. An active failure is any action that goes awry because of a latent condition. For example, icy roads are a latent condition because they do not create accidents; however, they do contribute to accidents when people try to carry out their normal driving procedures in an environment with icy roads. If there were no drivers, then the icy roads would just be icy roads. A driver attempting to operate a car in such conditions is required in order for the accident to happen.

A well-implemented safety program does not blame the driver for the accident; instead, it looks at the accident and asks questions about the road conditions, the vehicle and the decisions made by the driver that seemed appropriate but led to the accident. Further, each organization must decide how much of its resources will be spent addressing the decision-making processes of the "drivers" and how much of its resources will be spent in addressing the "icy roads." Back in the Swiss cheese model, spending time addressing the icy roads reduces the number and size of the holes in each slice of cheese; spending time on the decision-making processes is more about preventing the holes from lining up to allow an error to occur as each slice slides past the other slices. A well-designed program focuses on both parts of the cheese model.

Human Factors Engineering

Human factors engineering (HFE) is a discipline in science that studies the interaction of humans with and within systems. The field of HFE involves the study of factors and the development of tools that facilitate the achievement of the goals of reducing errors, increasing productivity, enhancing safety and improving comfort.[5] Just as microbiology is the core science for infection control, HFE is the "-ology" for patient safety.

Human factors engineering professionals are employed in aviation, aerospace, nuclear power, Web site and software development companies, and with the federal government in any place where interaction between the human and the system is critical for safety or efficiency. They work on equipment design (e.g., battleship control panels, cockpits, medical instruments), task design (e.g., trying to prevent workers from work-related injury), environmental design (e.g., bringing together lighting, temperature and noise control concepts) and training (e.g., better preparing the worker for working conditions through teaching, instructional design and policies).

Until recently, very few medical professionals learned about HFE in their medical training programs. This training is still not commonplace. Health care products and processes, such as the medication-use system, medical devices (like intravenous pumps and glucose meters) and information systems, were designed using the best efforts of technically-skilled professionals and designers. The design was completed based on what made sense to the individual(s) familiar with that product or the design engineer. In essence, many technologically-savvy people did the design and focused on features using the latest technology rather than collaborating with users of the technology to ensure safe, user-friendly, intuitive integration of the technology into common practice. Often those designs did not consider the learning curve to become familiar with the system or the challenge of integrating rotating employees and students into the process and then out of the process. The design often did not factor in the appearance of buttons, labels and controls or the consistency of the new product with other products already in use. For example, those who have ever had difficulty programming or using a video cassette recorder (VCR), home theater system or cell phone have probably been the victim of a design that is focused on technology rather than on usability. User-centered design (a design centered on humans and their capabilities and limitations) demands a more consistent, and simplified, approach to all tasks within a system. If everything had a user-centered design, then all VCR's would be configured similarly, as would all cell phones and home theater systems. There might be models that only have basic features, but these basic features, regardless of the model, would always function the same way and be in the same place to ensure that anyone trained to use one VCR, mobile phone or home theater system basically would be able to use them all. Taking this idea to a more complex system, can you imagine the safety hazards if all airplane cockpits were designed differently? The aviation industry (through its analysis of safety events) has employed human factor design concepts into aircraft and cockpit design. Now, think of an intensive care unit in a hospital and observe the technical complexity. Buttons flash, monitors beep and printouts spew from the machines; but, if each of these processes and machines is designed with a user-centered model in mind, then any trained nurse, physician or pharmacy technician can know at least how to basically operate each of these machines. Unfortunately, health care has been slower than other industries to see the value in such designs, and so each intensive care unit functions differently than most others; one must be completely retrained to work in each new unit when going between facilities. Someday, a nurse will be able to work in any intensive care unit after being trained to work in a single unit, much like people walk up to automated teller machines almost anywhere in the world and know exactly what to do because they all function in a similar way. In a well-designed system, the user just knows what to do based on the simple and obvious design of the machine. Such systems are often multilingual and even include Braille so that no matter how one communicates, they can interact with these simply designed devices.

HFE can serve as a valuable tool in improving the medication use process. Areas where HFE could be useful include:

- the design of labels and packaging;
- the design of workflow;
- the design of the computer system to mimic the natural work processes of filling a prescription;
- the layout of screens in the computer system so that the correct patient, or medication is easier to select within menus; and
- the human computer interface for automated dispensing equipment, such as robots and counting devices, designed to be intuitive for the human rather than intuitive for the machine.

A comprehensive discussion of HFE in the medication use process can be found in a publication from the American Society of Health-System Pharmacists entitled, "Medication Safety: A Guide for Healthcare Organizations." This publication contains an entire chapter on HFE in medication use and is a valuable resource for any pharmacy technician seeking to be a more effective part of a safe medication use system.[6]

Root Cause Analysis

One way that HFE is used in health care is in the process of conducting **root cause analysis (RCA)**. RCA is the systematic and organized analysis of a safety event in order to determine what happened, why it happened and what can be done to prevent it from happening again.[7] Often occurring after catastrophic events in health care and other industries (e.g., plane crashes, chemical plant explosions and nuclear incidents), RCA is a formalized way to investigate the systems issues that contribute to an event. It is the backbone of most safety programs; however, industries that are safety-wise don't wait to analyze actual events. They realize that systems learning and improvements can come from the analysis of events that almost happened but, by happenstance, never came to be. These events are often referred to as near misses but are more accurately termed close calls. Analysis of these events puts the safety learning in place without waiting for accidents or the death of a patient to encourage changes.

RCA is a "retrospective" look at an event; it occurs after the event does. It involves the formation of an interdisciplinary team to thoroughly analyze the event and determine exactly what happened, why it happened and what can be done to prevent it from happening again. Such teams generally interview witnesses, interview the patient and interview relevant staff members. Further, the team often visits the site of the accident to get a sense of the environment in which the accident occurred. Then, the team will prepare a report discussing the system, how it failed to prevent the error from occurring and how the system can be strengthened to prevent the error from recurring.

RCA reports are generally kept confidential; however, some organizations chose to disclose their events and subsequent analysis so that others may learn from their work. As part of the accreditation process, discussed elsewhere in this manual, TJC has the right to review RCA documents on selected events known as "reviewable sentinel events," such as inpatient suicide, serious medication errors leading to permanent harm, patient falls leading to permanent injury or death and surgeries performed on the wrong patient or the wrong part of the patient.[4] Table 1 is an example of the common elements included in an RCA report.

For further information, there are examples of RCA reports posted on the Internet and published in many journals. There are also training courses available, and materials from various organizations available, to the novice. Pharmacy technicians who find themselves in a position to interact with an RCA team are encouraged to look further into this topic.

Table 1
Elements of RCA Reports

Element	Description
Event Descriptions and Flow Charts	A description of what is known initially and the final understanding after a thorough analysis (time lines are often included)
Immediate Actions Taken	A description of what was done to contain the situation or help the patient right away before the analysis can occur
Resources Used	What sorts of records and documents need to be reviewed for information
References Consulted	A search of the literature to determine how often this has been reported and various methods of prevention of further events
Lessons Learned	Knowledge gained along the way that may or may not have direct applicability to the event but is important to pass on to others
Root Cause / Contributing Factors Identified	A listing of those things that failed to prevent the event and those things that enabled the event to occur (this is one area where HFE is helpful)
Action Plans that Facilities will Implement	These are the organization's detailed plans to prevent future occurrences. Action plan design is another area where HFE is useful. Emphasis must be placed on hard fixes (like physical plant changes or redesigns vs. policy and procedure updates or more training).
Outcome Measures that Evaluate the Effectiveness of Each Action	The method to measure and evaluate how effective those fixes have been

Failure Mode and Effect Analysis

Organizations interested in preventing events prospectively often conduct what is known as **failure mode and effect analysis (FMEA)**. FMEA is a proactive, prospective technique used to prevent process and product problems before they occur. This safety tool looks not only at what problems could occur, but also at how severe the effects of the problems could be and how often they could occur. FMEA is not new. It has been used since the mid-1960s in aerospace. By the 1970s and 1980s, FMEA had gained widespread use in other fields, including nuclear and chemical power, electronics and food processing. The automotive industry also began using FMEA and has relied upon that process as an integral part of improved vehicle quality and safety.

FMEA in health care has become more commonplace since the TJC requirement to prospectively perform risk assessment was implemented in July 2001. FMEA is one method of proactive risk assessment that can be used by organizations to meet that TJC standard. FMEA is well suited to analyze the following situations:

- Implementation of a new computer system
- Patient identification in outpatient pharmacy
- Allergy information processing
- Telephone (verbal) orders from physician offices
- Restocking the robot with oral solid medications
- Patient-controlled analgesia

These topics are complex systems and tend to be problem-prone for most organizations. The emphasis is not on elimination of errors (although that is a lofty goal), but rather the prevention of harm to the patient. Systems can be made safer by reducing the frequency of errors, making errors more obvious and reducing the severity of an error. Many safety systems in place in everyday life (such as seat belts, baby safety devices and traffic safety interventions) capitalize on those factors. Typical steps in a FMEA are shown in Table 2. An example of one page of a medication-related FMEA is included in Figure 2.

Table 2
Typical Steps in a FMEA[8]

Step	Description
1. Select a High-Risk Process and Assemble a Team	A topic is picked by the organizational leadership and an appropriate multidisciplinary team is selected (three to eight individuals)
2. Diagram the Process	The steps of the process, as they actually occur, not how the procedure says they should be, are outlined in a flow chart
3. Brainstorm Potential Failure Modes and Determine their Effects	Team members postulate how the process could fail no matter how off the wall the failures seem. Each failure mode developed must have a resultant effect of that failure mode. This portion examines what could happen.
4. Prioritize Failure Modes	Each failure mode is hazard scored for: ■ severity. (How severe is this failure to the system?) ■ detectability. (How easy is it to identify it before it happens?) ■ occurrence, probability or frequency. (How often would this failure occur?) These factors are scored from 1-10 and multiplied together to determine a criticality score. The higher the score, the more critical the failure mode.
5. Identify Root Causes of Failure Modes	For each failure listed, there is an accompanying cause or causes of that failure. This step identifies why the particular failure occurred.
6. Redesign the Process	Using HFE concepts and systems theory, the system is redesigned to decrease the criticality
7. Analyze and Test the New Process	The team completes steps 2, 3 and 4 of the new process and then pilot tests the changes. The criticality must be lower for the redesigned process.
8. Implement and Monitor the New	The new process is implemented, and its success is regularly measured

Figure 2
Sample FMEA Data Collection Sheet

FMEA Subject:								
Process Step:					**Process Step Number:**			
Potential Failure Mode	Single Point Weakness?	**Potential Effect(s) of Failure**	**Potential Cause(s) of Failure**	**Effective Control Measures in Place**	Severity	Frequency	Detection	Risk Priority Number

Medication Safety Self-Assessment

Another valuable tool in the medication safety toolbox is the task of doing a self-assessment. The **Institute for Safe Medication Practices (ISMP)**, a nonprofit safety agency, has produced several medication safety self-assessment (MSSA) documents. The first was for hospitals in 2000. Subsequently, the ISMP produced an outpatient pharmacy tool and one for assessing the readiness of an organization to implement bar code drug distribution. In 2004, there was a follow-up survey for hospitals; and in 2005, a self-assessment for anti-thrombotic care (covering anticoagulant use) was released. Experts in the field of medication safety develop these MSSA tools and the questions come from known safety practices and a collection of events and close calls that have occurred in health care around the world. The process to complete a MSSA includes the formation of a multidisciplinary team. The team goes through the MSSA document question by question. It rates the organization on each facet covered by the question. The questions state the concept that represents the safest practice and the team decides if this is applicable to that organization; if it is, the team decides how close the organization is to having a full implementation of the practice. For example, an item such as "Medication orders cannot be entered into the pharmacy computer system until the patient's weight has been entered (weight is a required field)," is discussed among the team members and then scored as follows: no activity to implement; considered, but not implemented; partially implemented in some or all areas; fully implemented in some areas; or fully implemented throughout. Pharmacy technicians are valuable members of the assessment team given their day-to-day exposure to the exact conditions being assessed. Pharmacy technicians may also read the assessment tools to find out what constitutes best practices in medication safety and use this information to suggest positive changes in the work environment.

Once the team scores the various items, the scores are entered into a Web site and then collected and compared to other organizations based on similar demographics. The MSSA is designed to weigh certain items more heavily, and the total results are scored electronically. The participating organization can review how it does against the national average, any other organizations in its own system and how it is doing against itself over time as the assessments are repeated. Generally, organizations do a "gap analysis" to find out which areas have the biggest gaps between ideal situations for safety and the actual conditions of that organization. From the gap analysis, the organizations usually develop an action plan to close those gaps identified. More information can be found on the ISMP Web site at www.ismp.org.

Teamwork and Communication

Many studies on the factors contributing to safety events have pointed to communication failures and the erosion of teamwork. In fact, communication failure has been implicated in as many as 80 percent of safety-related events. This has long been recognized by the military and aviation industries, where such failure can lead to catastrophic events. To counteract these vulnerabilities, the concept of **crew resource management (CRM)** evolved. Health care organizations are now beginning to use similar methods, such as **medical team training (MTT)**, to reduce communication failure and teamwork erosion related events. There are many different methods to conduct MTT, but several have common elements. First, an entire workplace is trained simultaneously. The training of an entire staff is a large commitment of resources because often the normal workplace is closed or operates under reduced services while the workers are being trained. The theory is that after the training and repeated use, behaviors in the coursework will become more automatic. Second, MTT is aimed at teaching health care professionals how to communicate with each other in a more organized and structured way. They introduce the concepts of briefings and debriefings and also teach individuals how to better state their portion of information that contributes to patient care. An important factor is teaching people how to accurately and succinctly challenge another person, even though that person might be in a higher position, or of a higher rank, than the employee challenging them. It also involves employees and physicians taking team responsibility for the care of patients and constantly checking each other to make sure that no one has strayed off course (lost situational awareness). By this constant checking and adjusting (course corrections), the theory is that the care of the patient will be better and safer.

Areas that typically utilize MTT include intensive care units (ICUs), emergency departments, operating rooms and ambulatory clinics; but, almost any workplace in health care would benefit from the program. Within pharmacy practice, a pharmacist might be involved in MTT for the ICU or any other area where that pharmacist is a part of the medical team. Within the pharmacy itself, the MTT could be useful in those areas where there are hand-offs and high stress levels or highly technically complex areas (such as dosing services, during shift changes and the intravenous admixture area). Pharmacy technicians can and must be part of this training if the opportunity for that training exists.

Measuring Medication Safety[9]

The organization that makes system changes for safety has the added challenge of measuring what has changed to see if there is improvement. There are whole organizations that function around implementation and measurement of change, but it is important for pharmacy technicians to have a basic grasp of the principles. Often, a pharmacy technician may be asked to collect the information needed to assess the success of the change.

There are several types of measures in complex systems.

- **Outcome measures** can be thought of as the end-of-the-road effect of a change. Has the change resulted in a better outcome for the patient such that the change reduced the overall harm to patients from adverse drug events? Think of this as the destination on a trip. Did you get where you wanted to go?
- **Process measures** are the steps taken to make changes in systems and subsystems in the hopes that those improved steps will lead to a better outcome. When you measure a process change, it is generally measuring the steps utilized to perform tasks were done correctly (you can do all the steps right and still not have a

good outcome). Think of this as measuring how you did on a long-distance trip. Filling the car with gas, keeping air in the tires and driving the speed limit can be measured and increase the likelihood that a traveler would arrive at a destination safely.

■ **Balance measures** are performed to determine if an improvement in one part of the process had negative consequences somewhere else. In the example of driving across the country, a traveler might choose to drive safely but take a longer route. If the individual was absent from his or her job for an additional week to get to the destination, the balance measure would be to measure if he or she was also following the work rules of his or her job. This individual might get to the destination, but may get fired in the process.

Examples of outcome measures related to medication use could include the percentage of admissions to the hospital that had an adverse drug event or the presence or absence of bleeding events during anticoagulation care.

Examples of process measures related to medication use could include the number of pharmacy interventions (clarifications or therapy changes made by pharmacists) per 100 admissions or per day and the number of times an action step was taken (as part of a procedure), such as identifying the patient using two identifiers, collecting allergy information for patients, etc. Benchmarking facility to facility or one unit against another with their spontaneous medication error reporting is NOT a good idea for a number of reasons. A higher number of reports are not necessarily a bad thing, and the reporting rate going down may be a reflection of a negative change in culture rather than a positive improvement in safety. NCC MFRP has a position statement that covers this antiquated view of medication error reports. This position statement is available online at www.nccmerp.org/council/council2002-06-11.html.

The Joint Commission

This nonprofit organization accredits almost 20,000 health care organizations and programs in the United States. While TJC is not a governmental agency, having its accreditation is as important as having a government-issued license to practice. Health care organizations reviewed by TJC are expected to have programs addressing any form of adverse incident that occurs. Pharmacies in organizations surveyed by TJC are particularly interested in events involving medications. If an event involves the death, or serious physical or psychological injury, a **sentinel event** has occurred. The health care organization where the sentinel event occurs may be required to notify TJC and may have additional requirements to investigate the system failure that led to such an event. TJC also requires hospitals to develop and use an **adverse drug reaction (ADR)** reporting system and use the data obtained to improve the quality of care offered in the hospital. ADRs encompass both side effects and allergic reactions. Some of these reactions are mild, but some of them may be life-threatening.

TJC also establishes **National Patient Safety Goals (NPSGs)** that are specific programs or processes aimed at improving safety. These are safety ideas that are generally new. Once these ideas are vetted nationally, they may eventually be incorporated into the main standards manual. Examples of NPSG include methods for dealing with look-alike/sound-alike drugs, the use of two patient identifiers (e.g., name and date of birth) before administering medication and specific processes aimed at improving the safety of verbal and telephone orders.

Drug utilization evaluations are performance improvement studies used to evaluate and improve drug therapy outcomes for patients. These concurrent or retrospective projects are a valuable part of the oversight of medication use.

Safety vs. Quality vs. Risk

Many organizations do not have separate medication safety resources and, as such, have integrated medication safety activities into performance improvement (quality) activities or risk management activities. Safety is a dimension of quality, but the primary focus of risk management, quality improvement and safety assurance is different. Quality improvement focuses on the performance of the organization as a whole and may look at factors other than safety. Risk management focuses on reducing risk (via reduced malpractice claims) for the organization, but it may not look at safety as a primary focus. What distinguishes patient safety assurance is the focus on the safety of the patient rather than having the focus be on the organization. Ideally, these areas work cooperatively with the end result of making things better for everyone; but, too often, the organization forgets to weigh the needs of the patient above the needs of the organization. Quality improvement, by nature, is based on measurement of actual events, while safety assurance is based on preventing events from occurring. To quote Dr. James Bagian, MD, director of the Veterans Health Administration National Center for Patient Safety, "Not everything that matters can be measured; and, not everything that can be measured matters." For example, rare safety events are often the once-in-a-lifetime confluence of events, not something that happens with any regularity. To say that the organization will "measure" to be sure month after month that the event has not happened again is nonsensical since, even by leaving the situation as is, it might not recur for five or 10 years. It doesn't mean that you don't fix what is known to be broken, but outcome measurement may not be a useful tool in that circumstance. Imagine a large organization, with high prescription volume, that aims for a "safety goal" of no more than 3.4 errors per one million prescriptions filled. One of the ways that an organization can determine such a goal is to find an average error rate for similar conditions and then try to be better than that average. A particular scheme for doing this is called the **Six Sigma method**; to achieve Six Sigma means that the organization's level of performance is an adjusted six standard deviations from the mean performance. The traditional symbol used in statistics for standard deviation is the Greek letter sigma (σ). Although the computation of standard deviation is complex, and not applicable to this chapter, one must understand that the more standard deviations away from the average one gets, the more exceptional one gets. Further, to be six adjusted standard deviations away from the average (under normal conditions) translates to having only 3.4 errors for every million events. This is a great quality goal; however, if the organization fills three million prescriptions each week, then they could be harming 10 patients each week with a 3.4 errors/million rate. Achieving a Six Sigma level of performance does not assure all patients are safe because, while the organization is performing remarkably well as an organization, from the patient safety perspective, 10 patients would tell you there are still improvements to be made.

Look-Alike/Sound-Like Drug Names (Confused Drug Names)

One of the most common factors in medication errors are problems with look-alike and sound-alike drug names and packages. Look-alike medication names can be problematic because humans often have trouble regularly discerning one name from the other when only a few characters differ. This is problematic for drug names within a class of medications, such as benzodiazepines that often end in –am, or beta blocker medications that often end in –olol, or the myriad of drugs beginning with chlor- or meth-.

In the science of language and communication, there are fields of study that evaluate the similarity between words. **Phonology** is the study and measurement of the similarity of words. **Orthography** is the study of the similarity of the spelling of words. Those who study these topics are generally called upon to help industries, including health care, develop tools to minimize the impact of sound-alike/look-alike names. Further, most drug companies will design a brand name for newly-developed products that attempt to avoid such errors. Occasionally, these efforts fail and a drug is forced to change its name due to errors that happen at an unacceptably high rate. One such example is the drug now known as Lovaza®. It was once known as Omacor®; however, that sounded and looked too close to Amicar®. So, the manufacturer successfully changed the product's name in collaboration with the FDA.

Packaging also plays a large role in drug mix-ups. Some companies produce products that are so similar that it makes it very difficult to discern one product from another. ISMP continues to work with the pharmaceutical industry and the FDA to improve the readability of the drug package labels. Further, ISMP has helped to create innovative ways to make packaging distinct for each drug and strength of drug available. Although the pharmaceutical industry has made great strides in recent years to assist in preventing mix-ups due to packaging, the ultimate responsibility for preventing these errors lies with each health care organization. Pharmacy technicians are in a unique position to identify those drugs that are most prone to error and work with the entire pharmacy team to minimize errors related to these drugs. One strategy is to make sure that these drugs are physically separated from each other on pharmacy shelves. Another is to flag both drugs with a bright-colored sign alerting staff to the higher possibility of an error. One safety strategy that is already being employed by some pharmaceutical companies is the use of "tall man" letters on commercial labels. The name "tall man" refers to highlighting differences between commonly confused words by writing the letters that are different in all capital (tall) letters and leaving the similar parts in lower-case letters (e.g., topAMAX vs. topROL XL, DOBUTamine vs. DOPamine).

High-Alert Medications

Year after year there are a number of medications that continue to be involved in medication errors that cause harm to patients. The ISMP has established a list of those medications that are continually involved in injury-related medication errors. Those medications are called "high-alert" medications to signify that the consequences of a medication error with these drugs more often result in an injury. The actual incidence of error is <u>not</u> more common with high-alert medications, but the result is more severe than errors with other drugs. Additionally, because some high-alert medications are also frequently used medications, several therapeutic categories appear as most frequently involved in injury. The usual top three most common ones are insulin products, anticoagulants and narcotics.

The high-alert medication list, which is updated every few years, is established through data drawn from reporting systems and through professional consensus. An updated list of these medications can be found on the ISMP Web site at www.ismp.org. The list began with medications commonly used in acute care hospitals, but there is ongoing work to develop a separate list more applicable to ambulatory care. If an ambulatory care list is released, it would be located on the ISMP Web site as well.

Medication Safety Organizations

The National Patient Safety Foundation (NPSF) is not only a patient safety organization itself, but it has compiled links to nearly all active and relevant patient safety organizations that exist. A sampling of the organizations recognized by NPSF can be found in Table 3. For additional information, visit www.npsf.org.

Table 3
Select Medication Safety Organizations

Organization	URL	Description
American Society of Health-System Pharmacists (ASHP)	www.safemedication.com	This site includes information on medication safety geared toward consumers.
Food and Drug Administration (FDA)	www.fda.gov	This web site is a comprehensive source of information about drug safety. Any recall information and actions by the FDA (such as seizure or counterfeit medications) can be found here. Additional detailed information can be obtained via a Freedom of Information Act (FOIA) request.
Institute for Safe Medication Practices (ISMP) Also visit their consumer medication safety page: www.consumermedsafety.org	www.ismp.org	This web site includes the ISMP's newsletters and some of hte most complete reference sources for information about medication errors.
National Coordinating Committee for Medication Error Reporting and Prevention (NCC MERP)	www.nccmerp.org	This group includes representatives from a number of organizations. It publishes statements and information and it is linked to the United States Pharmacopeia, which is a drug standards organization.

The Pharmacy Technician's Role

Because pharmacy technicians are so crucial to the medication-use system, pharmacy technicians are crucial to the medication safety system. As illustrated throughout this chapter, medication safety impacts everyone involved in the medication use process. Pharmacy technicians are often the first in a pharmacy to encounter potential problems and they are in a unique position to recommend strategies to minimize the risk of errors. Some simple ideas that can be used to improve medication safety can be found in Table 4.

Table 4
Ideas for Improving Medication Safety

- **Speak up.** If unsafe working conditions are noticed or if orders/procedures do not seem to keep the patient's safety as the main focus, alert management and continue to pursue them until all concerns are addressed.

- **Communicate with patients.** Although the entire health care team is part of the safety net intended to keep patients safe, patients themselves are the last line of defense in preventing harmful medication errors. Encourage patients to ask questions, to be aware of changes to their medications and to consistently tell the entire health care team about all of their medications.

- **Listen.** The entire health care team, not just pharmacists and pharmacy technicians, are part of safe medication delivery. Be sure that safe medication practices include input from the entire team.

- **Volunteer.** Rather than leave the work of improving current procedures to someone else, volunteer to work on safety issues.

- **Read and distribute.** Whether it's through the ISMP Newsletter or one of the many other publications on medication safety, stay up-to-date on ideas for keeping patients safe and share them with colleagues.

- **Be proactive.** Always be on the lookout for new look-alike and sound-alike medications and be prepared to implement strategies to minimize errors involving these medications.

- **Rest well.** Come to work rested and healthy and take breaks. Exhausted workers are much more likely to make mistakes.

- **Don't give up.** If a work environment is unsafe, find one where safety is considered more important or keep working with management until the environment is safe.

Conclusion

Pharmacy technicians are in a position to participate in medication safety activities regardless of their area of practice. The first step is being aware that, as a pharmacy technician, there exists a responsibility to be aware of potential errors and how to avoid them. This awareness will help foster a work culture that is rooted in patient safety and that encourages everyone to participate in keeping patients safe. Although the ideas in this chapter do not represent the entirety of the information available on patient safety, this chapter is a starting point that can be used to begin to transform workplaces into ones with patient safety built into every health care decision.

References

1. Institute of Medicine, "To Err Is Human: Building a Safer Health System," IOM Report, 1999.
2. National Coordinating Committee for Medication Error Reporting and Prevention, "The Use of Medication Error Rates to Compare Health Care Organizations is of No Value," June 2002.
3. The Institute for Safe Medication Practices, "Patient Safety Should NOT Be a Priority in Healthcare," ISMP newsletter, Sept. 23, 2004.
4. Reason, J.T., "Human Error: Models and Management," *British Medical Journal*, London, England, Vol. 320, pp. 768-770, March 18, 2000.
5. Wickens, C., An Introduction to Human Factors Engineering, New York, NY, 1997.
6. Gosbee, L., Burkhardt, M., "Human Factors Engineering in Equipment and Process Design," Medication Safety: A Guide for Health-Care Organizations, American Society of Health-System Pharmacists, Bethesda, MD, 2005.
7. Joint Commission Resources, Root Cause Analysis in Health Care: Tools and Techniques, Oakbrook Terrace, IL, 2000.
8. Joint Commission Resources, Failure Mode and Effects Analysis in Health Care: Proactive Risk Reduction, Oakbrook Terrace, IL, 2002.
9. The Institute for Healthcare Improvement, www.ihi.org/IHI/Topics/PatientSafety/MedicationSystems/Measures, Aug. 28, 2005.

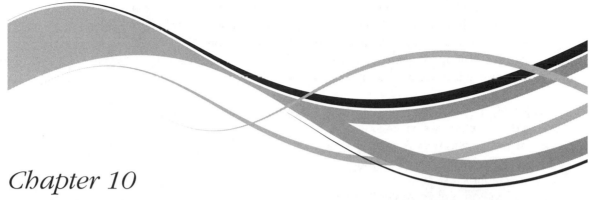

Chapter 10

REVIEW QUESTIONS

1. Which of the following type of investigation must be performed by a hospital, accredited by TJC, after a reviewable sentinel event occurs?
    a. Failure mode and effect analysis (FMEA)
    b. Medication safety self-assessment (MSSA)
    c. Root cause analysis (RCA)
    d. Medical team training (MTT)

2. Which of the following is the science that studies the interaction of humans with and within systems?
    a. Psychometrics
    b. Human factors engineering
    c. Sociology
    d. Genetics

3. Which industry is most often used as a good example of safety improvements?
    a. Aviation
    b. Law enforcement
    c. Metallurgy
    d. Food manufacturing

4. Which patient safety organization listed below has published self-assessment tools that a pharmacy can use to determine, not only how their current practices compare to ideal safety practices, but also what a pharmacy can do to move toward implementation of these goals?
    a. The National Quality Forum
    b. The National Council on Patient Education
    c. The Institute for Safe Medication Practices
    d. The Institute of Medicine

5. Which of the following is one way a pharmacy technician can improve medication safety?
   a. Not telling anyone about dispensing errors that never reached the patient
   b. Scouting for look-alike and sound-alike medications
   c. Not listening to patient complaints
   d. Doing jobs for which you received no training

6. Which of the following potential drug mix-ups might be prevented if tall-man letters are employed on each drug's packaging?
   a. Apresoline® vs. Atarax®
   b. Oxycodone vs. Oxycontin®
   c. Lipitor® vs. Zestril®
   d. Metoprolol vs. Amlodipine

7. All of the following drugs are considered high-alert medications by ISMP, except:
   a. Warfarin
   b. Lantus®
   c. Morphine
   d. Azithromycin

8. In relation to quality measure and evaluation, to achieve a Six Sigma, the error rate must be at (or be better than):
   a. one error per 1000 events.
   b. 3.4 errors per 10,000 events.
   c. 3.4 errors per 1,000,000 events.
   d. one error per 1,000,000 events.

9. Which of the following combinations is at greatest risk for a "sound-alike" error?
   a. Xanax® vs. Zantac®
   b. Zocor® vs. Cozaar®
   c. Amoxicillin vs. Cephalexin
   d. Mirtazepine vs. Fluoxetine

10. An adverse event reporting system in a hospital captures data on which of the following?
    a. Side effects experienced by patients
    b. Allergic reactions experienced by patients
    c. Both of the above
    d. None of the above

Chapter 11

LAW AND ETHICS FOR PHARMACY TECHNICIANS

By Jesse C. Vivian, R.Ph., J.D.

This chapter is based on federal laws and nationally accepted ethical standards. Consult your state pharmacy association or Board of Pharmacy for the laws and professional standards applicable in your state.

Learning Objectives

This chapter seeks to prepare a pharmacy technician to:

- understand how legal and ethical principles interact to regulate and guide behavior in pharmacy practice.
- list the entities covered by the Health Insurance Portability and Accountability Act of 1996 (HIPAA) Privacy Rules.
- define protected health information (PHI).
- identify the uses and disclosures of PHI permitted by the Privacy Rule.
- discuss the role of the pharmacy technician in maintaining patient confidentiality.
- name two federal agencies that develop and enforce drug product regulations.
- explain the difference between a prescription-only (legend) and nonprescription (over-the-counter) drug.
- describe the role of the Food and Drug Administration (FDA) with regard to ensuring drug efficacy and safety.
- describe the classes of drug recalls.
- define each class of controlled substances and give examples.
- list the recordkeeping requirements for controlled substances.
- define tamper-resistant packaging.

- define child-resistant packaging and give examples of exempted drugs.
- describe the main provisions of the Prescription Drug Marketing Act.
- define the prospective drug use review requirements under the Omnibus Budget Reconciliation Act of 1990 (OBRA '90).
- describe different acts of negligence by a pharmacist or pharmacy technician that can lead to a malpractice lawsuit.
- explain how professional ethics establish normative behavior and provide guidelines for resolving ethical dilemmas.
- cite relevant codes of ethics for pharmacists and pharmacy technicians.
- name and discuss the most common ethical principles used in analyzing ethical issues in pharmacy practice.
- describe and utilize a problem-solving technique for resolving ethical conflicts.

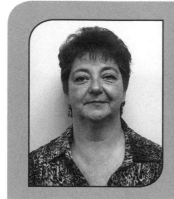

What influence do regulations and laws have on technician practice?

"Knowing the laws pertaining to pharmacy technicians in your state is critical. Technicians must keep up with current laws that affect them. We all need to know what we can legally do when it comes to performing our job duties."

Linda Branoff, CPhT,
Baker College, Flint, Mich.

Introduction

In the United States, there are two similar but very distinct systems of regulating human conduct. The most common sets of standards are found in laws. Laws can be legislatively enacted or determined from principals associated with the common law (judge-made) rulings. Rules may be promulgated by administrative agencies, such as a board of pharmacy, that have the effect of law. The function of laws, wherever they are derived from, is to tell the citizens within the society what the minimal standard of conduct is. Laws tell us what we can do and what we cannot do. People who disobey laws may be subject to criminal punishments, statutory fines or administrative penalties, like the revocation of a license. Examples of criminal acts that may apply to pharmacy technicians include violation of the patient's privacy rights, making false claims to Medicare/Medicaid and stealing narcotics from the workplace. Civil law covers various disputes between people in society. The remedy in a civil lawsuit is monetary damages. Examples of civil liability that may apply to pharmacy technicians include negligence and intentional torts, such as false imprisonment and assault and battery. Some actions (such as assault and battery) can lead to both civil and criminal liability.

Pharmacy is regulated by numerous state and federal laws designed to protect the public from harm that may occur as a result of taking medications. Even so, laws, no matter how comprehensive they may be, do not dictate all behaviors for pharmacists and pharmacy technicians. Likewise, the law does not provide answers to many questions encountered in daily practice. Nonlegal standards are also part of the professional discretion afforded practitioners.

It is in the nonlegal realm that ethical standards interject a second form of regulating conduct. Ethics is a branch of philosophy that studies and describes right and wrong conduct. It also suggests explanations or justifications for the moral choices that people make. The values and principles that individuals follow in making moral decisions are founded in their upbringing, education, religion and environment. All social groups, whether a nation, an ethnic division, a small fraternity or just a group of friends, exhibit normative behavior that suggests what kinds of conduct within the group are acceptable and what are unacceptable. Unlike legal standards, which are enforced by a governmental entity, ethical norms within a group are followed voluntarily. With some exceptions, these ethical behavioral patterns are not formally enforced. Individuals who do not conduct themselves within the behavioral expectations of the group may be ostracized or shunned. Using codes of ethics adopted by professional organizations is discussed at the end of this chapter.

The third method of regulating conduct is usually called something like "standards of care" or the "prevailing standards of practice." These can be a bit more confusing because they often fall into a gray area somewhere between legal and ethical methods of regulating behavior. Many standards of care have the same ramifications as the laws described above do, especially if they are accepted as legally binding by a court of law. Other standards of care are more recognized as ethical precepts, telling pharmacists and pharmacy technicians what they should and should not do. These issues are most likely to arise in civil cases where a patient claims that a pharmacy and its staff should have or should not have done something after a patient is harmed as a result of an act of commission or omission.

An example might help explain the differences. Assume a patient with a known history of allergies to penicillin brings a prescription for imipenem into a pharmacy. The pharmacy technician notes from the medication history on file in the pharmacy that the patient has listed an allergy to penicillin, noting the patient states that it causes a rash, and notifies the pharmacist. The pharmacist decides to fill the prescription as written. Assume next that the patient takes the imipenem and has an anaphylactic allergic reaction to the medication, resulting in severe damage to several organ systems. If she sues the pharmacy for malpractice, she would have to claim that the pharmacy knew of her penicillin allergy and that it was negligent to fill the imipenem prescription because it should have been foreseeable that there is a cross sensitivity between the two drugs. Whether or not the pharmacy will be legally responsible to pay for the patient's damages will depend on whether the alleged standard of care, that is, knowledge of allergic cross-sensitivity potential to the two medications, is a legally recognized standard or prevailing practice of pharmacy. Some experts in this field would argue that potential harm from cross-sensitivity is a known problem and the pharmacy should have taken steps to prevent its occurrence. Other experts would argue the opposite, that allergic cross-sensitivity to these drugs is not well-known or is extremely rare, such that a reasonable pharmacist acting under these circumstances would not be expected to foresee a problem. Whether these arguments are accepted or not would be up to the judge and/or jury deciding the case and would depend upon the quality or persuasiveness of the evidence presented at the trial. In situations such as these, it is usually better to err on the side of caution and do whatever is reasonable to best protect the interests of the patient.

Standards of care can be ethical, legal or both in nature. Often the pharmacist's professional discretion, based on education, training and experience, will be the guiding factor in deciding how to handle standard of care issues.

Federal Laws and Regulations

There are generally two legislative sources for laws that govern the practice of pharmacy. One is found in the enactments of state legislatures and state administrative bodies. The other source is found in the laws adopted by the federal Congress and the federal agencies that adopt regulations designed to implement the statutes passed by Congress. This chapter focuses primarily on federal laws. Readers must be aware of state laws governing the practice of pharmacy because these state laws may affect or even modify the federal statutes and rules. Where there are interactions between state and federal regulations, the stricter of the two must be followed. However, if a state law or regulation conflicts with a valid federal law or regulation and does not require at least what the federal law requires, the state law must yield to the federal law. Pharmacies in health care institutions are subject to regulations from federal and state laws, national and state organizations, such as the Joint Commission on Accreditation of Health Care Organizations (JCAHO), state public health departments and other local agencies that have a direct influence on health care institutions.

The major federal laws affecting pharmacy practice are the **Health Insurance Portability and Accountability Act (HIPAA)**, the **Food, Drug, and Cosmetic Act (FDCA)**, the **Controlled Substances Act (CSA)**, the **Poison Prevention Packaging Act (PPPA)** and the **Omnibus Budget Reconciliation Act of 1990 (OBRA '90)**. State laws affecting pharmacy are found in the state Public Health Code and pharmacy practice laws.

Patient Confidentiality

A patient's medical record is a confidential, legal document. Most states consider the pharmacy prescription record to be a medical record, and laws protecting medical records also generally apply to pharmacy prescription records. Information gained in a pharmacy-patient relationship is also considered confidential within the context of ethical standards.

HIPAA is a federal law that requires, among other things, the **Department of Health and Human Services (HHS)** to establish national standards to protect the privacy of patient health information. These standards were published by the HHS in a regulation entitled the Standards for Privacy of Individually Identifiable Health Information (Privacy Rule). These standards apply to health care providers, health plans and health care clearinghouses (**covered entities**).

The **Privacy Rule** creates a class of patient knowledge called **protected health information (PHI)** that places limits on how PHI may be used by health care practitioners. The Privacy Rule defines PHI as oral, written or electronic information created or received by a health care provider, health plan or health care clearinghouse that relates to the patient's physical or mental health or condition, the provision of health care to the patient or the payment for the provision of health care to the patient and identifies the patient or provides a reasonable basis for identifying the patient. Examples of PHI include oral patient counseling, a verbal copy of the patient's prescription to another pharmacy, the patient's computer profile, the patient's prescription records and the patient's prescription payment records.

Generally, the Privacy Rule permits a pharmacy to use and disclose a patient's PHI for purposes of providing treatment, obtaining payment and performing the pharmacy's health care operations. For example, the pharmacy will use information obtained from the patient's prescription to dispense the prescribed medication, and the pharmacist may then disclose that information to a new pharmacy technician to train him or her on how to process the prescription through the pharmacy's computer. Finally, the pharmacy may disclose information related to the medication dispensed to the patient's prescription insurer to obtain payment.

A pharmacist or pharmacy technician, subject to certain restrictions, may also use his or her professional judgment to disclose PHI to persons involved in the patient's health care, such as relatives, friends and caregivers, relevant to that individual's involvement with the patient's health care. In addition, when the patient is not present at the pharmacy or otherwise available, a pharmacist or pharmacy technician may, exercising professional judgment to determine the best interests of the patient, disclose PHI to a person involved in the patient's health care or payment for health care. As an example, the pharmacist may, using professional judgment, determine that it is in the patient's best interest to allow a friend or family member acting on behalf of the patient to pick up a filled prescription.

The Privacy Rule also permits the pharmacy to disclose PHI in other circumstances, including disclosures required by law, for health oversight activities, for judicial and administrative proceedings, for law enforcement purposes, for reporting victims of abuse and to comply with workers' compensation laws. The pharmacy could disclose PHI for health oversight activities to a Board of Pharmacy inspector investigating a possible violation of state pharmacy laws by the pharmacy or a pharmacist.

The pharmacy must obtain the patient's written authorization before using or disclosing PHI for purposes other than those permitted by the Privacy Rule. This includes obtaining a written authorization from the patient before disclosing PHI for most marketing purposes. For example, a pharmacy must first obtain written authorization from the patients if it wants to sell a list of the names of its diabetic patients to a company that sells blood glucose monitors and then uses that information to send the pharmacy's patients brochures on the benefits of purchasing and using the monitors. However, the Privacy Rule carves out exceptions to the definition of marketing that permits, among other things, the pharmacy to send refill reminders to its patients and the pharmacist to recommend to the patient a particular brand of an over-the-counter product.

As a general rule, the pharmacy must limit the amount of PHI it uses or discloses to the "minimum necessary" to carry out treatment, payment and health care operations, or other use or disclosure permitted by the Privacy Rule. There are some exceptions to this rule, however, such as communications with the patient, communications between the pharmacy and other health care providers for treatment purposes and disclosures made pursuant to an authorization. A pharmacist or pharmacy technician may, as part of the pharmacy's health care operations, announce the patient's name, but not the name of the medication, when his or her prescription is ready. When the patient arrives at the pharmacy to pick up their prescription, the pharmacist or pharmacy technician may freely discuss the patient's health condition and prescription. On the other hand, if a friend or family member comes into the pharmacy to pick up the patient's prescription, the pharmacist or pharmacy technician may only disclose to the person that PHI which is directly relevant to that person's involvement in the patient's health care. The pharmacist or pharmacy technician may disclose to a friend the prescription receipt for payment purposes, whereas a pharmacist may counsel the patient's spouse, who is also the patient's caregiver, about the safe and effective use of the medication dispensed for treatment purposes.

The Privacy Rule generally requires that the pharmacy verify the identity and authority of persons requesting PHI about a patient. If the identity and authority of the person are already known to the pharmacy, no further verification is required. If the identity and authority of the individual are not known to the pharmacy, the pharmacist or pharmacy technician may request written identification or ask questions to determine whether the person is who he or she claims to be (e.g., the patient or the patient's personal representative). The fact that a friend arrives at a pharmacy and asks to pick up a specific prescription for an individual effectively verifies that the friend is involved in the individual's care, and the rule allows the pharmacy to give the filled prescription to the friend. The Privacy Rule contains additional verification requirements for disclosures to public authorities such as law enforcement officials.

The most common breach of patient confidentiality is caused by verbal slips. These can occur in the elevator, cafeteria or lobby of a hospital. When interviewing or counseling patients about their medications, care must be taken that other patients cannot hear the discussion. Use of speakerphones must also be discouraged to prevent others from overhearing a conversation. Another type of confidentiality breach includes discussing patients with family and friends. A recent pre-HIPAA Michigan case illustrates this problem. A man with HIV/AIDS sued a chain pharmacy because he claimed a pharmacy technician employee told her son that the man had HIV/AIDS. The patient had not yet told his children about his illness, but claimed the technician's son taunted his children at school, calling one of them an AIDS baby. The case settled for an undisclosed amount of money. Under HIPAA, the pharmacy technician would also be subject to federal penalties for knowingly disclosing PHI in violation of the Privacy Rule standards.

The pharmacy must make a **good faith effort** to obtain the patient's written acknowledgment of receipt of the pharmacy's Notice of Privacy Practices (NOPP) no later than the date the pharmacy first provides service to the patient (e.g., fills the patient's prescription). The pharmacist or pharmacy technician may hand the privacy notice to the patient and ask the patient to sign the pharmacy's acknowledgment form or other form of acknowledgment. The patient is not required to sign or acknowledge the pharmacy's privacy notice. Therefore, the pharmacy may fill prescriptions for a patient who refuses to sign the acknowledgment after being asked to do so.

Finally, the importance of protecting PHI from inappropriate uses and disclosures is emphasized by the federal penalties for noncompliance with the Privacy Rule standards. Failure to make a good faith effort to comply with the Privacy Rule can result in a fine of $100 for each Privacy Rule standard violated and up to $25,000 in a calendar year for all violations of the same standard. A person who knowingly violates the Privacy Rule standards may be subject to fines ranging from $50,000 to $250,000 and/or one to 10 years imprisonment.

Food, Drug, and Cosmetic Act

In 1938, Congress passed legislation known as the Food, Drug, and Cosmetic Act (FDCA) to protect citizens from drugs that were not considered to be safe for human consumption. That Act has been amended a number of times to meet the changing needs of society and to recognize technological and scientific developments of the products it affects. The date that this law was adopted is significant because it grandfathered drugs on the market before the law became effective. Put another way, if the manufacturer of a drug had it in the marketplace in advance of the effective date of the FDCA, the manufacturer did not have to submit data to prove the drug was safe for human consumption. All drugs introduced to interstate commerce in the United States after 1938 became subject to the New Drug Application (NDA) requirements mandating that the manufacturer of a new drug prove that it is safe. Now a pharmaceutical manufacturer must prove a new drug to be not only safe, but also effective, before an NDA is granted by the **Food and Drug Administration (FDA)**. The FDA is the administrative agency, under the auspices of the Health and Human Services Department, that oversees the marketing of products under its jurisdiction.

It is important to understand what is meant by the terms food, drugs, cosmetics and dietary supplements, because often manufacturers market a product in a manner that could put its product into any one or two of these categories and cause it to be governed by different sets of rules. In this context, a **cosmetic** is defined under the FDCA as any substance applied externally to the human body for cleansing, beautifying or affecting appearance. **Food** is defined as any substance used for food or drink by man and animals, and includes chewing gum. The term **dietary supplement** includes vitamins, minerals, herbs and nutritional supplements. Dietary supplements are regulated as a special class of foods. Unlike cases involving drugs, the FDA must prove a dietary supplement unsafe before it can be removed from the market. Dietary supplements cannot make health claims of treating a specific disease (e.g., may alleviate depression) on a label without prior review by the FDA, but they can indicate how they may affect the normal structure or function of the human body (e.g., helps stabilize mood). The advertising of dietary supplements is governed by the **Federal Trade Commission (FTC)**.

A **drug** is defined as a substance used in diagnosis, cure, mitigation treatment or prevention of disease in man or animals. A drug affects the structure or function of the body of humans or animals. Before a drug can be distributed in the United States, the manufacturer must prove to the satisfaction of the FDA that the drug is both safe and efficacious for its intended use. This is generally characterized as the pre-market approval process. When approved, the FDA grants the manufacturer an NDA certificate that means the product may be sold in this country. The FDA has the authority to regulate the sale, promotion and advertising of drugs, whether they are available over-the-counter (OTC) or by prescription only. Note that dietary supplement advertising is not regulated by the FDA. All drugs (but not dietary supplements) distributed in the United States must be manufactured under a set of regulations called the Current Good Manufacturing Practice guidelines (often referred to as the GMPs or CGMPs). The FDA requires manufacturers to include a summary of information, such as side effects, contraindications and effectiveness, in all advertising of a prescription drug. Advertising can occur in journals, magazines, newspapers, and on the radio, television and Internet.

Over-the-Counter and Prescription Drugs

The FDCA created two categories of drugs: prescription and nonprescription. Nonprescription drugs or OTCs are those believed by experts in the field to be safe and effective when used as labeled without medical supervision. Prescription drugs are also safe and effective when used as intended, but because of potential harmful effects, require medical supervision. All prescription drugs require specific labeling (called a legend or caution statement). For many years, prescription-only drugs had to bear a label containing the following statement: "Caution: Federal law prohibits dispensing without a prescription." This labeling requirement was simplified, and now drugs in this class must bear a label stating: "Rx only," meaning "prescription only." The FDA also approves the drug package insert labeling that accompanies a prescription drug product, irrespective of whether it is on the market as an OTC or prescription-only drug. Another distinction between OTC and prescription-only drugs has to do with the labeling. Both categories of drugs must be labeled with "adequate directions for use" when they leave the manufacturer and upon arrival in a pharmacy. Prescription-only drugs do not have to be labeled with the manufacturer's original adequate directions for use if they are dispensed pursuant to a valid prescription. In this situation, the label generated by the pharmacy will be used instead of the manufacturer's labeling. The method of labeling a drug becomes a bit more complicated when a prescriber issues a prescription for an OTC drug that is dispensed as if it were a prescription-only drug. State laws and prescription drug insurance benefits rules could affect these labeling issues.

Investigational New Drugs

In addition to its authority to regulate drugs on the market in the United States, the FDA also has authority to regulate **Investigational New Drugs (INDs)** after a manufacturer applies to the FDA for an IND. INDs are drugs that are being used for experimental or investigational use. Physicians must generally seek approval to do research using an IND at a health care facility through the facility's Institutional Review Board (IRB). It is noteworthy that an approved drug (i.e., a drug already on the market with an NDA) may also be classified as a new drug requiring IND status if it is being used in a different way or by a different method of administration than was approved during the original NDA process. If a manufacturer is seeking new labeling indications for an approved drug or deviation from the routes of administration than were originally investigated, it will apply for a **Supplemental New Drug (SND)** application. The SND is a unique procedure because the manufacturer does not have to resubmit the original data supporting the conclusion that the drug is safe and efficacious for its intended uses or methods of administration.

Investigational drugs are studied using humans under **Phase I**, **Phase II**, **Phase III** and **Phase IV**, which are defined in Table 1.

Table 1
Investigational Drug Phases

Phase	Description
I	Clinical investigation in a small number of patients to determine the preferred route of administration and safe dosage
II	Clinical investigation on a limited number of patients for a specific disease treatment or prevention of disease to further determine the drug's safety
III	Clinical trials are expanded to further test for safety and efficacy of the drug
IV	Post-marketing surveillance continues after a drug is marketed. The manufacturer must report to the FDA all serious adverse drug reactions, along with other information, including additional drug safety and efficacy data. The FDA may withdraw its approval of a new drug upon review of post-marketing information.

Generic Drugs

Before a manufacturer of a new drug seeks approval for its use in humans, it will seek a patent from the United States Patent and Trademark Office. A patent gives the inventor of a product, such as a drug, the right to exclusive marketing for a period of time. There is usually a long lag period between the granting of a patent and approval of an NDA. After the exclusivity period runs out, manufacturers of a generic version of the drug may begin marketing it after obtaining an Abbreviated New Drug Approval (ANDA). The generic version has to contain the exact same active chemical ingredient(s) as the innovator or brand name drug. An ANDA differs from an NDA—as obtained by the manufacturer of the brand name version—because the generic company does not need to submit any of the safety and efficacy data already on file with the FDA from the manufacturer of the brand-name version as long as the manufacturer seeking the ANDA can prove that its product is bioequivalent to the innovator drug. There are complex methods available to make the bioequivalence determination. Once the manufacturer satisfies the FDA that its generic version drug will act very much like the previously approved branded drug, the FDA approves the ANDA. At that point, the generic manufacturer may start marketing the drug in competition with the brand-name version produced by the innovator company. The usual motivation for marketing generic drugs is that they are produced and sold at significant savings compared with branded drugs. The FDA maintains a list of generic drugs that have been compared to brand-name drugs marketed with an NDA. The list is published annually and may be accessed online at www.fda.gov/cder/orange/default.htm. Generic drug entities are assigned a two-letter coding system in the FDA publication "Approved Drug Products with Therapeutic Equivalence Evaluations," also known as the "Orange Book." Looking only at the first letter of the two-letter symbol, an "A" rating indicates drug products considered therapeutically equivalent; a "B" rating indicates that the FDA considers the drug products not to be therapeutically equivalent. Many states require a drug product to be "A" rated before it can be substituted as a generic equivalent for a brand name drug.

Federal Recall of Drug Products or Devices

The FDA cannot order a product recall, but it can ask a manufacturer to voluntarily recall a product rather than be forced to cease making the product or have the FDA confiscate the product. The manufacturer must notify sellers of the recall. Sellers are notified of a recall through letters, telegrams, e-mail, sales representatives and listings in pharmacy publications. The three classes of recalls are described from most serious to least serious in Table 2. They are **Class I, Class II** and **Class III drug recalls**.

Health care institutions, such as hospitals, must document and maintain records on action taken with drug recalls. Recall classes and controlled substance schedules should not be confused. Precautionary note: It is easy to confuse drug recall and investigational drug rating systems because they use a similar numbering scheme.

Table 2
Drug Recall Classifications

Class	Description
I	Reasonable probability that the product will cause serious adverse health consequences or death
II	Product may cause temporary or medically reversible adverse health consequences; probability of serious adverse consequences is remote
III	Product not likely to cause adverse health consequences

Omnibus Budget Reconciliation Act of 1990

Pharmacy practice has been influenced by major provisions under OBRA '90. Congress recognized the pharmacist as a health care professional who can improve the quality of drug therapy and, therefore, save health care costs. The most important area of OBRA '90 for pharmacy is **drug utilization review (DUR)** for all Medicaid patients. Almost all states have expanded OBRA '90 requirements under their pharmacy practice statutes to all patients, not just Medicaid patients. Some states may require DUR for all Medicaid patients and varying levels of DUR to other patients. Other insurance companies may also require DUR as part of the provider contract. The DUR process has three parts: retrospective review, educational programs and prospective review. Retrospective review is done in each state by a DUR board. Large amounts of data on drug use by Medicaid patients are reviewed to identify areas of improvement. From this, topics for educational programs may be established. Educational programs for pharmacists and physicians are the second area necessary for compliance under OBRA '90. The programs are focused on improvement of medication use and can be face-to-face visits by an expert with the pharmacist or physician, large educational meetings or written materials sent to the pharmacist or physician. Prospective DUR is the area required by each pharmacist when dispensing a prescription to a Medicaid patient. Prospective review includes: (1) a review of a patient's prescription drug therapy before dispensing, (2) patient counseling by the pharmacist and (3) pharmacist documentation of patient information. Any changes made for the patient are best documented in the patient's medication use profile. Pharmacists review a patient's drug therapy before dispensing by screening for the following potential drug therapy problems:

- Therapeutic duplication (two drugs being used for the same purpose)
- Drug-disease contraindications (certain drugs not appropriate because of a patient's disease state)
- Drug-drug interactions (including interactions with nonprescription and dietary supplement drugs)
- Wrong drug dosage or length of drug therapy
- Clinical abuse/misuse (underuse or overuse of a drug)

To enhance patient compliance with medication use, a pharmacist must offer to counsel each Medicaid patient on the use of a dispensed prescription. Some states allow a nonpharmacist, such as a pharmacy technician, to offer counseling; however, a pharmacist must do the actual counseling. Although not mandatory, a patient signature can be obtained when the patient refuses counseling. Information discussed during patient counseling is left to the professional discretion of the pharmacist under OBRA '90. Suggested information for discussion during counseling includes:

- the name and description of the medication.
- the dosage form, dose, route of administration and duration of drug therapy.
- special directions and precautions for preparation, administration and use by the patient.
- common severe side effects, adverse effects or interactions and therapeutic contraindications that may be encountered, including ways to prevent them and the action required if they do occur.
- techniques for self-monitoring drug therapy.
- proper storage.
- prescription refill information.
- action taken in case of a missed dose.
- how to contact the pharmacist for questions or concerns.

Giving the patient written information about a prescription without an oral consultation does not meet the counseling requirement under OBRA '90.

The last requirement pharmacists must comply with under OBRA '90 is to attempt to obtain patient-specific information. States may allow nonpharmacist personnel, such as pharmacy technicians, to help the pharmacist in obtaining information from the patient. The minimum information obtained and recorded is: (1) name, address, telephone number, date of birth (or age) and sex; (2) individual histories where significant, including disease state or states, known allergies and drug reactions and a complete list of current medications and relevant devices; and (3) pharmacist comments about the individual's drug therapy.

Prescription Drug Marketing Act

The Prescription Drug Marketing Act (PDMA) was passed by the federal Congress to further prevent misbranding and adulteration of prescription drug products by giving the FDA authority to prevent the resale, relabeling or adulteration of any prescription drug product sold outside normal channels. While the PDMA contains several sections and addresses several matters, the two most important measures involve manufacturer drug samples and purchases and resale of drugs by hospitals and health care facilities. Drug samples cannot be sold, traded or purchased. Samples may only be distributed to practitioners licensed to prescribe or to pharmacies of hospitals or health care entities (e.g., a hospital inpatient pharmacy) at the written request of the prescriber. The PDMA requires certain information in the request and several recordkeeping requirements after receipt of the samples. A community pharmacy (ambulatory, chain, corporate or retail) cannot receive any sample prescription drugs. The law creates a presumption that any sample drugs found in a community pharmacy are there in violation of the PDMA. Fines for violation of this law are significant. Hospital pharmacies may receive and store samples if requested by a prescriber without violating the law. The PDMA prohibits the sale, purchase or trade (or offer to do so) of prescription drugs purchased by a hospital, health care entity or charitable organization. Hospitals and some health care entities can purchase drugs at large discounts. This may lead to the illegal resale of drugs from hospitals to other entities. Drugs sold in this manner are often improperly stored or labeled where the integrity of the drug product may be uncertain. The purchase of drugs outside normal purchasing channels leads to unfair competition by the pharmacies purchasing the drugs at discounted prices. Some exceptions in the PDMA are:

- purchases by a hospital from a group purchasing organization for its own use.
- sales or purchases to nonprofit affiliates.
- sales or purchases for emergency medical reasons (e.g., a transfer between hospitals and from a hospital to a community pharmacy if there is a temporary drug shortage).

Food, Drug, and Cosmetic Act Enforcement

The FDA can force a violator of the FDCA to cease illegal activity and can begin criminal proceedings (fines and/or imprisonment) against a violator. The FDA may also, with court approval, seize any **adulterated** (contaminated or not manufactured appropriately) or **misbranded** (mislabeled) food, drug or cosmetic. The FDA's authority over dietary supplements is much more limited and complicated. Suffice it to understand that the FDA can order a manufacturer to stop marketing a dietary supplement after it assembles convincing evidence that the product is harmful for use in humans.

Controlled Substances

In addition to the OTC and prescription-only classifications used by the FDA, another federal agency, the Drug Enforcement Administration (DEA), has jurisdiction to determine whether a drug is treated as a **controlled substance** or a noncontrolled substance. Note that the DEA has authority to regulate substances without regard to whether the substance is or is not considered to be a drug. For example, heroin is not considered to be a drug in the United States because it has no generally recognizable medical use; nevertheless, heroin is a Schedule 1 controlled substance. It is also important to remember that drugs may be controlled substances in DEA terms, yet not restricted to prescription-only status in FDA terms. For example, there are Schedule 5 cough suppressants that are available as over-the-counter drugs. State laws frequently require a pharmacy to obtain information about these OTC narcotic sales in logs that may be referred to as an "exempt narcotic" book or something similar. Another factor to consider about controlled substances is that there are a number of other state-based laws that affect dispensing and distribution of drugs classified as controlled substances. This situation exists because the federal Controlled Substances Act allows states to also regulate these drugs. This is an area where the state and federal governments have concurrent jurisdiction. This is also an area where state laws might differ from federal laws. In instances such as this, remember that the stricter law will govern the actions of pharmacy practice. For example, if federal laws require a pharmacy to keep controlled substance inventories for two years and a state law requires them to be retained for five years, the longer retention policy must be followed.

The DEA has classified certain substances, including several drugs, by abuse potential and has made regulations based on this classification under the Controlled Substances Act (CSA). The regulations cover buying, inventorying, prescribing, dispensing, storing, using and destroying these drugs. The DEA administers the CSA; coordination with the FDA is frequently required.

Controlled substances are classified into five schedules shown in Table 3.

Table 3
Controlled Substance Classifications

Classification	Description	Examples
Schedule 1 (C-I)	Drugs having no accepted medical use in the United States and having a high abuse potential	Heroin, lysergic acid diethylamide (LSD), mescaline, peyote and tetrahydrocannabinol (THC, marijuana)
Schedule 2 (C-II)	Drugs having an accepted medical use and a high abuse potential with severe psychic or dependence liability	Amobarbital, amphetamines, cocaine, codeine (not in combination with other drugs), hydromorphone, meperidine, methadone, morphine, oxycodone, pentobarbital and secobarbital
Schedule 3 (C-III)	Drugs having an accepted medical use and an abuse potential less than those in Schedules 1 and 2	Barbiturates not in Schedules 1 or 2; paregoric, combination narcotics (e.g., acetaminophen with codeine #2, #3, #4, etc.) and anabolic steroids
Schedule 4 (C-IV)	Drugs having an accepted medical use and an abuse potential less than those listed in Schedule 3	Alprazolam, chloral hydrate, diazepam, dextropropoxyphene, flurazepam, lorazepam, meprobamate, phenobarbital and phentermine
Schedule 5 (C-V)	Drugs having an accepted medical use and an abuse potential less than those listed in Schedule 4	Cough preparations containing narcotics (e.g., guaifenesin with codeine), diphenoxylate and atropine sulfate

Electronic Prescribing

In June 2010, the DEA began allowing the electronic transmission (basically over the Internet) of Schedule 2-5 prescriptions. This is an optional method of communicating a prescription drug order from a properly licensed and DEA registered physician to a properly licensed and DEA registered pharmacy. Neither the physician nor the pharmacy is required to use an electronic means for communicating prescriptions.

If a prescription for a controlled substance is electronically transmitted, both the pharmacy and the physician must meet specific security certification requirements. The pharmacy's system of receiving prescriptions must be approved by an independent auditor or certification vendor approved by the DEA. The prescribing physician must also have an approved system for transmitting controlled substance prescriptions and must use a two step method of applying an electronically verifiable signature that lets the pharmacy receiving the prescription know that it originated from a legitimate and authorized prescriber.

Refills

Schedule 2 drugs may not be refilled. However, partial fillings are allowed under some circumstances where it would not be prudent to have a large quantity of these drugs in a patient's home. Schedule 3 and 4 substances may be refilled, if authorized by the prescriber, up to five times within a six-month period from the date the prescription was issued. The date of issuance controls the length of time that the prescription is valid, even if the patient waits a few days or weeks or even months to get the prescription filled. Schedule 5 drugs may be refilled as authorized by the prescriber. While the federal law does not specify a time limit for refilling Schedule 5 drugs, many state laws generally have a one-year limitation for dispensing any prescription-only drugs.

Labels and Labeling

Bulk containers of controlled substances must be labeled with symbols for each class (e.g., C-II, C-III, etc.). All controlled substance prescriptions must contain the full name and address of the patient and the name, address and DEA registration number of the prescribing practitioner. When controlled substance prescriptions are filled, the number of units or volume dispensed, the date of dispensing and a handwritten or typewritten name of the dispensing professional must be included. Pharmacists may enter missing information on the prescription if state law or DEA regulation does not prohibit this activity.

Documentation

Record-keeping requirements are very important under the CSA. Records must be kept for inventory, drugs received and drugs dispensed. An initial inventory of controlled substances must be taken when a pharmacy opens and again every two years. In some states, a controlled substance inventory is required every year. Since this is a more stringent requirement than the federal law, pharmacists in those states must comply by performing an annual inventory. Schedule 2 (C-II) controlled substances must be ordered by a pharmacy on a special DEA form (DEA Form 222-C) and C-II records must be kept separate from C-III, C-IV and C-V records. Violation of recordkeeping requirements can lead to imprisonment and/or fines.

Registration

The pharmacy where a pharmacist practices must be registered with the DEA. With the exception of sole proprietorships, individual pharmacists do not need to be registered with the DEA. Pharmacists may also have to obtain a controlled substance license in addition to a pharmacist license under certain state laws. Individual practitioners, such as physicians, dentists, veterinarians and others allowed by the state (e.g., nurse practitioners, physician assistants), must be registered with the DEA and obtain a DEA number in order to prescribe controlled substances. Physician assistants and others who prescribe controlled substances using "delegated authority" from a physician need to obtain a "mid-level practitioner" registration from the DEA. Exceptions to this include practitioners who are employed by a hospital or other health care facility and prescribe controlled substances only for inpatients at that institution; these practitioners use the institution's DEA number.

Pharmacists dispense controlled substances under an individual controlled substance state license. Pharmacy technicians, student pharmacists and other ancillary personnel may dispense controlled substances under the supervision of a pharmacist only if allowed by state law. Under federal law, pharmacists are required to assure that a controlled substance is prescribed for a "legitimate medical purpose" for a patient in the usual course of professional practice.

Tamper-Resistant Packaging

The FDA has established requirements for **tamper-resistant packaging**. A tamper-resistant package provides a barrier to entry that clearly indicates to a consumer if some kind of tampering has occurred with the package. A tamper-resistant package may involve an immediate container-and-closure system, a secondary container or carton system or any combination of systems intended to provide a visual indication of package integrity. These regulations were established after the tampering of nonprescription products led to at least seven deaths. However, some products, such as dermatological, dentifrice, insulin or throat lozenge products, are exempt from these packaging requirements.

Child-Resistant (Safety) Packaging

In April 1974, the FDA issued regulations regarding child-resistant containers to comply with the Poison Prevention Packaging Act (PPPA). The regulation requires that all prescription medications dispensed from a pharmacy or a hospital be dispensed in child-resistant containers. This includes drugs dispensed from outpatient clinics and emergency rooms, or medications given to patients upon discharge. **Child-resistant packaging** requirements do not apply to medications administered within an institution. Unit-dose packaging does not qualify as safety packaging.

Several nonprescription drugs are covered under the PPPA. Both acetaminophen and aspirin-containing products intended for oral administration must be sold in child-resistant packaging (with some exemptions). Other examples of substances covered by the PPPA include furniture polish, methyl salicylate (oil of wintergreen), turpentine, methyl alcohol (methanol), ethylene and ethylene glycol. Additionally, some iron-containing drugs and dietary supplements are listed in the PPPA.

Certain drugs are exempt from safety packaging. Patients may request that their prescription be filled in a nonchild-resistant package. In these cases, it is recommended that a pharmacist should require the patient's signature for permission to dispense in a nonchild-resistant package. Preferably, the signature is obtained each time the prescription is filled. Examples of exempted prescription drugs that do not have to comply with the requirements of child-resistant packaging are listed in Table 4.

Table 4
Exemptions from Child-Resistant Packaging

- Sublingual dosage forms of nitroglycerin and isosorbide dinitrate

- A potassium supplement in unit-dose forms, including individually wrapped effervescent tablets, unit-dose containers of liquid potassium and powdered potassium in unit-dose packets

- Medically-administered oral contraceptives in manufacturers' calendar-reminder dispensing packages.

- Conjugated estrogen and norethindrone tablets when dispensed in mnemonic (memory-aid) dispenser packages

- Medroxyprogesterone acetate tablets

Federal Hazardous Substance Act

Under the **Federal Hazardous Substance Act (FHSA)**, a **hazardous substance** is one that can cause injury or illness and potential danger, especially to children, if mishandled. Federal legislation covering hazardous substances does not include drugs, but regulates household items, such as bleach, cleaning fluids, antifreeze and drainpipe cleaners. Pharmacies selling hazardous substances covered by the FHSA must do so only in the original containers labeled by the manufacturer or supplier or label the product as outlined in the FHSA.

State Laws and Regulations

State law, not federal law, regulates professionals practicing in each state. Regulation is accomplished through professional licensure. Beyond the responsibility as an employee in any given situation, licensed professionals are also accountable to the state board that regulates their license to practice as professionals. Pharmacy practice statutes contain the state laws that regulate the practice of pharmacy. In most states, a Board of Pharmacy is the administrative agency designated to protect the public through enforcement of the pharmacy practice statutes, especially in granting licenses to pharmacists and pharmacies. Some states also provide regulations for pharmacy technicians that may be administered by the Board of Pharmacy.

Utilization of Pharmacy Technicians

States regulate many details of the practice of pharmacy, and regulations vary from state to state. Some examples of differing state regulations include the dispensing label of the prescription product, required controlled substance prescription forms, the pharmacist-to-technician ratio and the functions a pharmacy technician is allowed to perform. Pharmacy technicians are utilized for as many functions as legally possible under state and federal law to allow pharmacists time to do screening, counseling and monitoring functions. To comply with OBRA '90 counseling requirements, some states allow a pharmacy technician or other designated person to offer to counsel the patient, as long as the pharmacist does the actual counseling.

Several states are recognizing certified pharmacy technicians in various ways. Kentucky allows certified technicians to have a higher level of responsibilities than noncertified technicians. Tennessee allows a higher pharmacist-to-technician ratio if technicians are certified. Some states, such as Texas and Utah, require technicians to be certified in order to work as a pharmacy technician in their states. Since state laws are very different, as discussed above, the reader is urged to consult the state pharmacy association or state Board of Pharmacy for the laws applicable in his or her state.

Malpractice

Malpractice falls under tort law, a type of civil liability. A tort involves causing injury or damage to another through negligence or intentional action. Anyone can be considered negligent if he or she does or does not perform an act that a reasonable person would have done in a similar situation, and that action or inaction causes some type of harm.

Malpractice, or professional negligence, involves the following elements: (1) a duty owed by the defendant (health care professional); (2) the defendant (health care professional) has to breach (or not adhere to) the duty, (3) the plaintiff (patient) has to be injured and (4) the injury has to be caused by the breach of the duty. A duty by the defendant (health care professional) is determined by state and federal law, professional group standards and expert witness testimony. Courts of law have traditionally made the pharmacist responsible only when committing a dispensing error that causes patient harm. Examples of dispensing errors include giving the patient the wrong drug, the wrong strength of the drug or incorrect directions on how to take the drug. New requirements under OBRA '90 and state law have courts expanding the responsibility of pharmacists to include a duty to recognize potential drug therapy problems and warning the patient and/or physician of the potential problem. An example of this type of error includes not warning the patient and/or physician of a possible severe drug interaction between two drugs that are dispensed together. Pharmacists can be responsible for malpractice, and the state board can take disciplinary actions against their license for the same act.

Since pharmacy technicians are not generally licensed by the state, their primary accountability is to their employer as supervised by licensed pharmacists. Employers are responsible for their employees (and their negligent acts) as long as the employee is acting within the scope of their employment. It is important for the pharmacy technician to follow policies and procedures and not act in place of a pharmacist. Pharmacy technicians are frequently asked to testify in medication error and other types of pharmacy lawsuits. Several insurance companies now provide malpractice insurance policies for pharmacy technicians. The issue of having malpractice insurance is a personal one, and a pharmacy technician is recommended to seek out legal advice if there is uncertainty of need in this area.

Ethics

As discussed in the introductory materials of this chapter, the practice of pharmacy and our nation's system of drug distribution are the subjects of intense legal regulation. Of all the health professions, pharmacy is, without doubt, the most highly regulated. However, even with this complex set of legal requirements, the law does not address all desirable modes of behavior for pharmacists and pharmacy technicians. Likewise, the law does not provide answers to many questions encountered in daily practice. Occasionally, a well-intended, but erroneous, application of the law will cause an undesirable outcome for a patient. The use of common sense and adherence to ethical values might even suggest that unlawful conduct will provide a better result for the patient's well-being. For example, consider the situation when a patient's prescription refill expires for a medication that she takes regularly to prevent angina (heart-related chest pain), and the physician is not available to extend or renew the prescription. In the vast majority of states, the law prohibits the pharmacy from dispensing the medication under these circumstances. Failure to provide the medication, however, will result in significant discomfort or even harm for the patient. The compassionate response would be to deliver at least some of the medication to her until the physician can be contacted. The argument in favor of breaking the law in order to protect the patient's well-being might not be as compelling if the expired refills were for something like birth-control or Viagra®. In either case, there are different laws, beyond the scope of this chapter, which would protect the pharmacist making a discretionary judgment to protect the best interest of the patient.

More commonly, pharmacy practitioners are faced with multiple alternative behaviors and find almost no guidance in vague laws that are subject to differing interpretations. As an example, consider what may be done when a husband asks for a copy of his wife's prescription records. This seemingly innocent request has multiple implications and consequences. This request may facilitate an income tax deduction or make a claim for reimbursement on an insurance policy. There could, however, be a more sinister motivation for the request. The couple might be divorcing or engaged in a child custody battle that might be affected by the wife's use of psychotropic drugs. Or it could be that the husband is concerned that the wife is being treated for a sexually transmitted disease. In any event, does the wife have an expectation that her prescription records are confidential, even against her own husband's request? Does a husband have the legal or moral right to know the medications his spouse is using? Does your state law clearly address these kinds of questions or are there several ways to interpret the law? Does the pharmacy profession have any guidelines for helping make decisions with this type of request? As discussed under the HIPAA laws, disclosure of this protected information could result in a violation of federal law. Confidentiality laws and standards of care may also be violated. While laws may have some application to these situations, there are often no clear answers.

The Changing Environment of Pharmacy Practice

Pharmacy practitioners might dismiss these dilemmas as not the kind of moral questions that should be addressed by pharmacy technicians. After all, if a pharmacy technician is only there to assist a pharmacist, are not the decisions on how to go about answering the issues fully the responsibility of that pharmacist? While this position might ultimately be correct, it is too simplistic in this day and age of intensely busy and highly-technical pharmacy practices. Pharmacy technicians are interacting with patients more frequently and in much greater depth than even a few years ago. The scope of assistance that technicians provide to pharmacists is also increasing rapidly. This means that pharmacy technicians are more likely to encounter ethical questions and moral dilemmas on a first-hand basis. Pharmacy technicians may be of great assistance in gathering facts and clarifying issues so that those individuals who do have ultimate decision-making authority will be able to optimize the care of patients. Knowing the framework of ethical analysis and the kinds of issues that might be faced will help pharmacists, pharmacy technicians, patients, prescribers, caregivers and anyone else involved make the best decisions possible. Furthermore, a pharmacist might not always be present to decide how to act or what to say in a situation that requires an immediate decision by the pharmacy technician. In these rare but very realistic situations, the pharmacy technician might have to decide what to do without the availability of any authority figure. Even so, it is important to realize that many practice-based decisions are left up to professional discretion where there is no single right or wrong solution. These are sometimes called grey areas because there is no clear rule of behavior. In these situations, rather than relying solely on personal values to make judgment calls, pharmacists and pharmacy technicians may wonder what other pharmacy practitioners would do under the circumstances. These are the types of dilemmas that are the subject matter of professional ethics.

Codes of Ethics and Standards of Practice

One defining characteristic of a profession is the promulgation of a **code of ethics**. Codes of ethics predate organized government and the licensure laws that now regulate minimum behavioral requirements for health care practitioners. Today, codes supplement legal requirements and generally set higher standards of care than those required by law.

In pharmacy, the American Pharmacists Association (APhA) Code of Ethics has been widely followed by many state and even other national professional associations. The first APhA code was established in 1852 and was modeled after the 1848 Code of Ethics of the Philadelphia College of Pharmacy. The code has been revised several times to reflect changes in the pharmacy environment. The membership of APhA adopted a dramatic revision of its Code of Ethics for Pharmacists in 1994 (see Table 6). Some institutional organizations such as hospitals and nursing care facilities follow the Patient's Bill of Rights published by the American Health and Hospital Association. Other pharmacy organizations follow the National Association of Boards of Pharmacy's (NABP®) Pharmacy Patient's Bill of Rights. Some state-based pharmacy technician groups have also adopted codes. Depending on the employment situation, pharmacy technicians must determine which, if any, of these various statements will govern their practice at particular locations.

The American Association of Pharmacy Technicians (AAPT) adopted a Code of Ethics for Pharmacy Technicians (AAPT Code) in 1996 that is nearly identical to the 1994 APhA Code of Ethics for Pharmacists (APhA Code) as to the values it contains (see Tables 5 and 6). Some modifications were made to make it specific to the tasks, obligations and duties of pharmacy technicians. Read and compare the two codes for similarities and differences.

Table 5

American Association of Pharmacy Technicians, Inc.
Code of Ethics for Pharmacy Technicians

Preamble	Pharmacy Technicians are health care professionals who assist pharmacists in providing the best possible care for patients. The principles of this code, which apply to pharmacy technicians working in any and all settings, are based on the application and support of the moral obligations that guide the pharmacy profession in relationships with patients, health care professionals and society.
Principles	
I.	A pharmacy technician's first consideration is to ensure the health and safety of the patient, and to use knowledge and skills to the best of his/her ability in serving others.
II.	A pharmacy technician supports and promotes honesty and integrity in the profession, which includes a duty to observe the law, maintain the highest moral and ethical conduct at all times and uphold the ethical principles of the profession.
III.	A pharmacy technician assists and supports the pharmacist in the safe, efficacious and cost effective distribution of health services and health care resources.
IV.	A pharmacy technician respects and values the abilities of pharmacists, colleagues and other health care professionals.
V.	A pharmacy technician maintains competency in his/her practice, and continually enhances his/her professional knowledge and expertise.
VI.	A pharmacy technician respects and supports the patient's individuality, dignity and confidentiality.
VII.	A pharmacy technician respects the confidentiality of a patient's records and discloses pertinent information only with proper authorization.
VIII.	A pharmacy technician never assists in the dispensing, promoting or distribution of medications or medical devices that are not of good quality or do not meet the standards required by law.
IX.	A pharmacy technician does not engage in any activity that will discredit the profession, and will expose, without fear or favor, illegal or unethical conduct in the profession.
X.	A pharmacy technician associates with and engages in the support of organizations which promote the profession of pharmacy through the utilization and enhancement of pharmacy technicians.

Approved by the AAPT Board of Directors Jan. 7, 1996. All rights reserved.

Table 6
American Pharmacists Association Code of Ethics for Pharmacists

Preamble	Pharmacists are health professionals who assist individuals in making the best use of medications. This Code, prepared and supported by pharmacists, is intended to state publicly the principles that form the fundamental basis of the roles and responsibilities of pharmacists. These principles, based on moral obligations and virtues, are established to guide pharmacists in relationships with patients, health professionals and society.
Principles	
I.	A pharmacist respects the covenantal relationship between the patient and pharmacist. Considering the patient-pharmacist relationship as a covenant means that a pharmacist has moral obligations in response to the gift of trust received from society. In return for this gift, a pharmacist promises to help individuals achieve optimum benefit from their medications, to be committed to their welfare, and to maintain their trust.
II.	A pharmacist promotes the good of every patient in a caring, compassionate, and confidential manner. A pharmacist places concern for the well-being of the patient at the center of professional practice. In doing so, a pharmacist considers needs stated by the patient as well as those defined by health science. A pharmacist is dedicated to protecting the dignity of the patient. With a caring attitude and a compassionate spirit, a pharmacist focuses on serving the patient in a private and confidential manner.
III.	A pharmacist respects the autonomy and dignity of each patient. A pharmacist promotes the right of self-determination and recognizes individual self-worth by encouraging patients to participate in decisions about their health. A pharmacist communicates with patients in terms that are understandable. In all cases, a pharmacist respects personal and cultural differences among patients.
IV.	A pharmacist acts with honesty and integrity in professional relationships. A pharmacist has a duty to tell the truth and to act with conviction of conscience. A pharmacist avoids discriminatory practices, behavior or work conditions that impair professional judgment, and actions that compromise dedication to the best interests of patients.
V.	A pharmacist maintains professional competence. A pharmacist has a duty to maintain knowledge and abilities as new medications, devices, and technologies become available and as health information advances.
VI.	A pharmacist respects the values and abilities of colleagues and other health professionals. When appropriate, a pharmacist asks for the consultation of colleagues or other health professionals or refers the patient. A pharmacist acknowledges that colleagues and other health professionals may differ in the beliefs and values they apply to the care of the patient.

Table 6 *cont.*

American Pharmacists Association Code of Ethics for Pharmacists

Principles	
VII.	A pharmacist serves individual, community and societal needs. The primary obligation of a pharmacist is to individual patients. However, the obligations of a pharmacist may at times extend beyond the individual to the community and society. In these situations, the pharmacist recognizes the responsibilities that accompany these obligations and acts accordingly.
VIII.	A pharmacist seeks justice in the distribution of health resources. When health resources are allocated, a pharmacist is fair and equitable, balancing the needs of patients and society.

Adopted by the membership of the American Pharmaceutical Association, Oct. 27, 1994.

Conclusion

It is important that all pharmacy technicians know and understand the ethical standards, laws and regulations governing pharmacies, pharmacy personnel and pharmaceuticals in order to ensure that patient safety and confidentiality are not compromised. Pharmacy technicians play important roles when dealing with the ordering and filling of prescriptions for controlled substances. Pharmacy technicians have the responsibility of acting within the scope of their practice as outlined by state laws and their pharmacy's policies. Professional ethics in pharmacy practice creates rights and responsibilities for practitioners. The best interest of each patient forms the cornerstones of ethical health care behavior.

Bibliography

- Abood, R.R., Brushwood, D.B., Pharmacy Practice and the Law, 2nd edition, Gaithersburg, MD, 1996.
- Brushwood, D.B., Vivian, J.C., Ethical Perspectives: Guidelines for Dealing with Ethics in Pharmacy Practice, Kalamazoo, MI, 1988.
- Buerki, R.A., Vottero, L.D., Ethical Responsibility in Pharmacy Practice, American Institute of the History of Pharmacy, Madison, WI, 1994, pp. 40-43.
- Buerki, R.A., Teaching and Learning Strategies in Pharmacy Ethics, 2nd edition, Special Issue of Journal of Pharmacy Teaching, Vol. 6, No. 1/2, 1997.
- Department of Health and Human Services Office of Civil Rights, HIPAA Privacy Regulation Text, October 2002.
- Department of Health and Human Services Office of Civil Rights Guidance on Final Privacy Rule, Dec. 3, 2002.
- Fink, J.L., Vivian, J.C., Bernstein, I., Pharmacy Law Digest, Facts and Comparisons, St. Louis, MO, 40th edition, 2006.
- Haddad, A.M., Buerki, R.A., Ethical Dimensions of Pharmaceutical Care, Binghamton, NY, 1996.
- Haddad, A.M., Teaching and Learning Strategies in Pharmacy Ethics, 2nd edition, Binghamton, NY, 1997.
- Health Insurance and Accountability Act of 1996, PA, Title II, Part C, Sec. 1172, 42 USC §1320a-1327 et seq, pp. 104-191.
- Lawrence, J., Argument for Action: Ethics and Professional Conduct, Ashgate Publishing, Brookfield, VT, 1999, p. 5.
- Mintz, Levin, Cohn, et. al., HIPAA Privacy Standards: A Compliance Manual for Pharmacists, 2nd edition, National Association of Chain Drug Stores, 2002.
- Mongagle, J.F., Thomasma, D.C., Health Care Ethics. Critical Issues for the 21st Century, Gaithersberg, MD, 1998.
- Pharmacist's Letter, "HIPAA Made Simple: Pharmacist's Survival Guide," Vol. 2002.
- Purtilo, R., Ethical Dimensions in the Health Professions, 3rd edition, Philadelphia, PA, 1999.
- Smith, M., Strauss, S.B., John, H., Alberts, K., Pharmacy Ethics, Binghamton, NY, 1991.
- Weinstein, B., Ethical Issues in Pharmacy, Pharmacy Practice and the Law, Abood and Brushwood, Aspen, 1994, p. 311.
- Younger, P., Conner, C., Cartwright, K.K., Kole, S.M., Pharmacy Law Answer Book, Gaithersburg, MD, 1996.

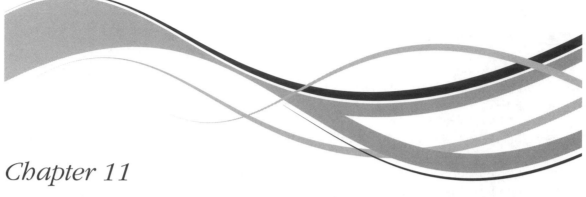

Chapter 11

REVIEW QUESTIONS

1. Which of the following is not a permitted use or disclosure of PHI?
   a. A use or disclosure of PHI for purposes of providing treatment, obtaining payment and performing the pharmacy's health care operations
   b. The pharmacist, using professional judgment and determining that it is in the patient's best interest, allowing a friend or family member to pick up a filled prescription for the patient
   c. The pharmacy discloses patient prescription records to a Board of Pharmacy
   d. Inspector investigating a possible violation of state pharmacy laws by the pharmacy
   e. The pharmacy sells a list of the names of its diabetic patients to a company that sells blood glucose monitors who will then use that information to send the pharmacy's patients brochures on the benefits of purchasing and using the monitors without first obtaining an authorization from the patients.

2. Which of the following best describes the minimum necessary requirement for using PHI?
   a. The pharmacy must limit the amount of PHI it uses or discloses to the "minimum necessary" to carry out treatment, payment and health care operations or other use or disclosure permitted by the Privacy Rule.
   b. The pharmacy must limit the amount of PHI it uses or discloses to the "minimum necessary" to carry out treatment, payment and health care operations or other use or disclosure permitted by the Privacy Rule, except for communications with the patient, communications between the pharmacy and other health care providers for treatment purposes and disclosures made pursuant to an authorization.
   c. The pharmacy must limit the amount of PHI it uses or discloses to the "minimum necessary" for communications with the patient, communications between the pharmacy and other health care providers for treatment purposes and disclosures made pursuant to an authorization.
   d. The pharmacy must limit the amount of PHI it uses or discloses to the "minimum necessary" to carry out treatment, payment and health care operations.

3. Which of the following statements is true regarding federal and state laws affecting pharmacy practice?
   a. When there is a conflict, federal law always prevails over state law.
   b. A state law cannot be stricter than a federal law.
   c. Licensure of professionals is regulated by federal law.
   d. Pharmacy technicians are licensed under federal law.

4. Which of the following is the regulation that prohibits the sale, purchase or trading of drug samples?
   a. Nonprofit Institutions Act
   b. Prescription Drug Marketing Act
   c. Controlled Substances Act
   d. OBRA '90

5. Which regulation requires pharmacists to perform drug use reviews for all Medicaid patients?
   a. Nonprofit Institutions Act
   b. Prescription Drug Marketing Act
   c. Federal Hazardous Substances Act
   d. OBRA '90

6. Under the requirements of OBRA '90, which of the following may a pharmacy technician do?
   a. Counsel a patient regarding drug therapy
   b. Screen patient profiles for drug-disease contraindications
   c. Call a prescriber and recommend a different drug dosage
   d. Make the offer to have the pharmacist counsel a patient, if permitted by state law

7. Federal law and DEA regulations provide a legal way for properly licensed and registered pharmacies to accept Schedule 2 prescriptions transmitted to the pharmacy electronically by a properly licensed and registered physician.
   a. True
   b. False

8. Which of the following is true regarding the principles found in a typical code of ethics?
   a. They are ironclad laws mandating prescribed behavior.
   b. They provide clear right and wrong decisions for each situation.
   c. They are only guidelines for behavioral standards.
   d. They eliminate personal discretion in deciding how to resolve ethical conflicts.

9. The AAPT Code compels pharmacy technicians to not do which of the following?
   a. Practice as a pharmacist when a pharmacist is unavailable
   b. Respect the diversity that exists in the pharmacy technician's patient population
   c. Refrain from knowingly using, dispensing or preparing for dispensing any medical or drug product that is substandard
   d. Promote and advance the profession of pharmacy through professional organizations

10. Which of the following is the law that protects the privacy rights of the patient?
    a. FRA
    b. ETA
    c. OBRA
    d. HIPAA

Chapter 12

PHARMACY OPERATIONS AND ADMINISTRATION

By Paul W. Bush, Pharm.D., MBA
Dianne E. Miller, R.Ph.
Kuldip R. Patel, Pharm.D.

Learning Objectives

This chapter seeks to prepare a pharmacy technician to:

- explain the concept of a pharmacy formulary (formulary system).
- explain the medication purchasing process.
- list concepts of inventory management.
- identify medication storage requirements for pharmaceuticals.
- list the common elements of the unit dose distribution system.
- define the terms "policy" and "procedure."
- explain why policies and procedures are needed and important.
- explain how a policy and procedure manual is organized.

Introduction

Pharmacy technicians are often involved in doing those things that keep the pharmacy running in a smooth and legal manner. Beyond helping to prepare prescriptions for a pharmacist to dispense, pharmacy technicians will be involved with (or may coordinate for the pharmacy) activities, such as managing inventory, drugs purchasing, preparing administrative reports and assisting nonpharmacists in their pharmacy-related duties. Formularies, while less common in community pharmacies, are traditionally found in institutional pharmacies, and they specify which medications a pharmacy will stock and dispense. Inventory policies and procedures allow the pharmacy to properly account for its inventory and appropriately manage medications that require special attention. To ensure that these special requirements are part of the normal operations of the pharmacy, they must be established in a procedure based on a policy, both documented for all to be trained on and follow.

Formulary System

The **formulary system** is a method for evaluating and selecting suitable drug products for an organized health setting (e.g., hospital, managed care plan). A **formulary** consists of those medications that are considered by the professional staff of that setting to be the most appropriate for the greatest number of patients. Hospital pharmacies, clinics and health maintenance organizations (HMOs) utilize this list of approved medications for stocking medications and dispensing them to patients. The professional staff who design the formulary will generally choose one agent from each class of commonly-prescribed medications to be put on the formulary. For instance, of the fluoroquinolone antibiotics (i.e., ciprofloxacin, levofloxacin, gatifloxacin, moxifloxacin, gemifloxacin, norfloxacin and ofloxacin), the hospital will choose to only carry and dispense levofloxacin rather than stock some quantity of each of these. By doing so, the pharmacy can control its costs by not having inventory sitting on the shelf not being used very often. Further, the pharmacy may now be able to purchase levofloxacin in bulk and buy it at a better price to increase the savings. The only way that this system will be effective is if the professional staff agree to enforce the exclusive nature of the formulary; that is, physicians must agree to use those agents found on the formulary and the pharmacy must agree not to stock formulary exceptions on a regular basis. To ensure that this process happens smoothly, most institutions establish guidelines for pharmacists to approve **therapeutic substitutions**. Unlike making a generic substitution, where the active ingredients are exactly the same between two manufacturers, a therapeutic substitution is where a different active ingredient, from the same class and with similar effects, is selected from a formulary. Using the example above, if a physician in this hospital writes a prescription for moxifloxacin, the pharmacist on duty will have the authority to translate that prescription into an order for levofloxacin (a therapeutic substitution) without having to call the physician and verify that this substitution is acceptable (since the therapeutic substitution agreement of the hospital permits this to be done). There will always be times when the formulary needs to be violated and a specific agent must be dispensed; there is a procedure that the physician may follow if she or he feels it absolutely necessary to not use the formulary agent. Generally, that physician will collaborate with a pharmacist, who will evaluate the request and determine whether or not the pharmacy can fulfill the request.

Although individual community pharmacies generally have no reasonable way to benefit from having a formulary, and therefore do not have one, there are formularies encountered in this setting as well. Most pharmacy benefit managers (PBMs) and health insurance companies have a formulary of covered medications. This formulary does not allow a pharmacist to make a therapeutic substitution without consulting with the prescriber; however, the substitution is generally required before the PBM will pay for the drug. Again, using the same example, if the PBM formulary says that levofloxacin is the preferred fluoroquinolone, and a prescription arrives at the pharmacy requesting that moxifloxacin be dispensed, the PBM may reject the claim for moxifloxacin entirely or may ask the patient to pay a substantially higher copayment (copay) than if levofloxacin were prescribed. In either case, the PBM will communicate the formulary alternative to the pharmacy, and the pharmacy will contact the prescriber to request that the agent be switched to the covered item. The patient may also elect to bypass their insurance and pay out-of-pocket for the originally-prescribed drug. Further, if the prescriber insists that the originally-prescribed agent is the better choice for the patient, they may contact that patient's PBM to request approval (called a **prior authorization**) for the drug to be covered (or be covered at a lower copayment). The PBM will evaluate this request and either stand by its formulary or grant the exception; generally, a PBM will employ a team of professionals (pharmacists, physicians and nurses) who make these decisions based on clinical guidelines and the clinical judgement of those health professionals.

Medication Purchasing and Inventory Control

A pharmacy will often receive medications from multiple sources and receive drugs every business day. Most pharmacies have a primary wholesaler from which they order the large majority of their drug supplies, and a secondary wholesaler from which they obtain those items that their primary wholesaler cannot get or cannot get at a reasonable price. Further, there are some rare instances where medications are still obtained directly from the manufacturer. Institutional settings may also receive medications from patients staying in the institution; these are maintenance medications that the patient will be continuing while in the hospital that are brought from home. These medications are stored in the pharmacy, dispensed by the pharmacy on the required schedule and then returned to the patient upon discharge. Generally the medications that this will be done with are those that are not on the formulary, those that are particularly expensive and those that are not expected to change while the patient is in the hospital or when they return home. Throughout all of these processes of ordering and receiving drugs, pharmacy technicians are integral in making this happen smoothly. Pharmacy technicians are often responsible for preparing and/or placing orders with wholesalers to replace depleted stock. Further, pharmacy technicians are often responsible for processing all of the paperwork associated with receiving these drugs. Finally, pharmacy technicians are usually responsible for storing these received medications for later dispensing.

With all of the drugs coming in and going out of a pharmacy each day, it is absolutely essential to keep accurate account of exactly which drugs remain in the pharmacy at any given moment. Pharmacy technicians are usually responsible for maintaining an inventory management system in place at the pharmacy and are sometimes called upon to design and implement an inventory management program. Inventory management involves many tasks that are within the scope of practice for a pharmacy technician, including monitoring the usage of each drug in the inventory and ensuring that unused drugs are sent back to the wholesaler (when appropriate); helping establish minimum stock levels for each drug in the inventory; reducing the number of look-alike or sound-alike medications that are stored in close proximity; verifying that current inventory accounts match the true on-hand inventory present in the pharmacy; selecting specific package sizes to order from a wholesaler to ensure that the inventory is continuously being used and that bulk savings are being captured; and preparing orders for items that need replenishing. Pharmacy technicians, through their daily duties, are most often in a position to identify fluctuations in a medication's use before a pharmacist. A pharmacy technician who can identify usage trends and, thus, avoid potential out-of-stock situations is a highly-valued member of the pharmacy team. One of the most frustrating situations in a pharmacy is when a medication is out of stock because someone neglected to reorder it or neglected to order enough to meet the patient needs. Every pharmacy employee is responsible for proactively identifying these situations in order to avoid patient harm and inconvenience.

Some pharmacy dispensing software track medication use to assist with ordering. A minimum level of stock is established for each medication so that the computer will trigger an automatic reorder of the product when stock levels go below that minimum level. Several other approaches to inventory management exist, including **just-in-time**, **Pareto's Law (80/20 analysis)** and **ABC inventory**.

Table 1
Approaches to Inventory Management

Approach	Description
Just-in-Time	With this system of inventory management, the pharmacy seeks to predict exactly when a medication will be needed and order just enough of that medication to have exactly enough to fulfill all of the day's orders, without having any significant stock of the medication left in the inventory.
Pareto's Law or 80/20 Analysis	This system examines the frequency of ordering and tries to maximize inventory turnover of high usage items. The numbers "80" and "20" refer to the goal of having 80 percent of the pharmacy's sales come from 20 percent of the pharmacy's inventory.
ABC Inventory	In this system, "A" is very important (20 percent of items representing 65 percent of the inventory's total value), "B" is moderately important (30 percent of items representing 25 percent of the inventory's total value), and "C" is the least important (50 percent of items representing 10 percent of the inventory's total value). After assigning a letter to each drug, replenishment is ordered accordingly.

In a just-in-time inventory management system, it becomes essential to evaluate exactly how much of a drug is being used on a daily basis so that the right number of packages can be ordered for the upcoming day (generally, pharmacies receive a delivery each business day). To do this, generally one would take the average quantity dispensed for the prescriptions that the pharmacy fills, multiply this by the typical number of prescriptions the pharmacy fills for that drug in a day, and then divide this by the quantity in each package (see example below). To calculate the number of packages of medication to order, the following formula may be used:

$$\frac{(\text{Average Quantity Dispensed } \times \text{ Average \# Prescriptions / Day}) - \text{\# Units Remaining at Day's End}}{\text{Quantity in Each Package}}$$

= Number of Packages to Order for Single-Day Supply

Wholesalers resell pharmaceuticals that have been purchased directly from pharmaceutical manufacturers in large quantities. **Wholesalers** do not manufacture pharmaceuticals; they are an intermediary in the distribution process. Drug wholesalers may enter into a **prime vendor agreement** with a pharmacy. Under a prime vendor agreement, the wholesaler agrees to provide pharmaceuticals to a pharmacy at their best price in exchange for the pharmacy's commitment to buy most, or all, of its drugs through that wholesaler. This is an advantage for the wholesaler because they can count on a certain volume of business, and the pharmacy benefits by getting the wholesaler's best price. Wholesalers will also enter into prime vendor agreements with generic manufacturers. These agreements allow the wholesaler to get the best price for generic drugs and stock their preferred vendor rather than having to stock some of each manufacturer's product. The advantage for pharmacies in

Example
Determining the Number of Packages of Medication to Order

A pharmacy typically dispenses 40 mg furosemide tablets in quantities of 34 tablets. The pharmacy orders 100-count bottles of 40 mg furosemide tablets from their wholesaler. If the pharmacy typically dispenses 12 prescriptions for 40 mg furosemide tablets each day, and there are no bottles of 40 mg furosemide tablets on the shelf, how many packages of furosemide must the pharmacy order to supply the next day's need?

Step 1: Fill in the equation.

$$\frac{(\text{Average Quantity Dispensed} \ \times \ \text{Average \# Prescriptions / Day}) - \text{\# Units Remaining at Day's End}}{\text{Quantity in Each Package}}$$

= Number of Packages to Order for Single-Day Supply

$$\frac{(34 \times 12) - 0}{100} = \text{Number of Packages to Order for Single-Day Supply}$$

Step 2: Solve the problem by multiplying the average quantity dispensed by the average number of prescriptions per day, subtracting the number of units remaining at day's end, and then dividing by the quantity in each package.

$$\frac{(34 \times 12) - 0}{100} = \frac{408 - 0}{100} = \frac{408}{100} = 4.08 \text{ rounded to } 5$$

Therefore, five bottles must be ordered to fulfill the next day's need. If four bottles are ordered, the pharmacy will be eight tablets short of its expected need and thus a fifth bottle must be ordered to ensure that the pharmacy has at least the expected need.

using a large wholesaler is that the bulk discounts received by wholesalers for having prime vendor agreements with manufacturers, coupled with the prime vendor agreements between wholesalers and pharmacies, mean that the price the pharmacy pays for most of its drugs is far less than if the pharmacy ordered directly from a manufacturer (not that this is realistic any longer as most manufacturers will not deal directly with a pharmacy as they once did).

Pharmacies may form a **group purchasing organization** (GPO), or be part of an organization that combines the purchasing power of the individual members (a **cooperative buying group**), in order to realize the volume discounts that can come from being a large pharmacy network ordering as one entity. The advantage for a pharmacy to be involved in a GPO or cooperative buying group is twofold: first, the pharmacy does not have to negotiate directly with the wholesaler as the group's representatives will take the time to do that on behalf of the group, and two, the buying group represents substantially more volume for a wholesaler than a single independent pharmacy and thus is more willing to provide price breaks for a large buying group than a lone pharmacy. Pharmacies and pharmacists that are involved with a GPO or cooperative buying group must take care not to violate any of the anti-trust (anti-monopoly) laws; however, there are very few downsides to joining a GPO or cooperative buying group.

Most wholesalers use a computer-based ordering system. In some cases, a perpetual inventory system automatically orders drugs for the pharmacy and there is not a human involved in this process unless an error occurs (where a drug is not ordered correctly). No matter how the orders are placed, orders generally arrive on the next business day and must be checked in, often by a pharmacy technician. A pharmacy technician must compare the items actually received to the invoice provided by the wholesaler of what drugs were shipped. The wholesaler must be contacted if any items are missing, received in error, are damaged or unusable, or are expired and accidentally sent to the pharmacy. Since pharmacists are ultimately responsible for the proper receiving of these drugs, most pharmacies have a process for a pharmacist to certify that the work done by the pharmacy technician who checked in the drugs was done correctly. Then the received drugs are integrated into the pharmacy's inventory. In addition to making sure that each drug is put away in the correct place on the shelf, it is important to ensure that the stock is being properly rotated. What is meant by **rotating the stock** is that newly received products must be placed behind products that are already on the shelf unless the newly received product will expire sooner than the product already on the shelf. This is also an opportunity for a pharmacy technician to note any change from what is currently on the shelf to what has been received (such as the same drug now coming from a different manufacturer) and take the appropriate action. This is also a chance for the pharmacy technician to see if this new package will cause confusion being where it is (e.g., if the drug on the shelf immediately below this new product looks nearly identical, then an alert flag can be placed on the shelf to alert others to the higher potential for taking the wrong drug from the shelf). After all of the newly-received medications are integrated into the pharmacy's inventory, the invoices (and other related paperwork, according to the pharmacy's procedure for receiving inventory) are filed according to the pharmacy's procedure, in compliance with the laws, both state and federal, governing record maintenance. This procedure may include providing a copy of the invoices to an accounting department responsible for paying the wholesaler for the received deliveries. Each pharmacy's procedure may be unique.

Borrowing Pharmaceuticals

The U.S. Food and Drug Administration (FDA) publishes a list of all of the approved drugs and all of the equivalent products approved for sale in the U.S. This book, called the **Orange Book**, is available on the FDA Web site. The Orange Book for 2011 is 1,252 pages; there is absolutely no way for any pharmacy to carry a sufficient supply of each and every one of these drugs. Occasionally, a pharmacy will receive a prescription for a drug, medical device, medical supply or other product that is not stocked by the pharmacy. If it is urgent, or if the patient simply is unwilling to wait to initiate the therapy after the pharmacy places an order for the drug from their wholesaler, the drug may be borrowed or purchased from another pharmacy. The regulations on such transactions will be different depending on the state or states involved in the transfer. Some states do not allow pharmacy-to-pharmacy sales, so borrowing (that is, Pharmacy A borrows drugs from Pharmacy B, Pharmacy A orders a new supply of the drug and then Pharmacy A replaces the drugs taken from Pharmacy B's inventory) may be the only option. In either case, borrowing or buying, detailed records must be kept by both pharmacies; the lot number, expiration date, national drug code (NDC), name, strength, dosage form and quantity being exchanged must be recorded by both pharmacies. Further, the pharmacists at each pharmacy who are authorizing the transaction must be noted. In the event of a recall on a product that has been borrowed or sold to another pharmacy, it is the obligation of each pharmacy to communicate knowledge of the recall to the other pharmacy to prevent the recalled medication from being dispensed to patients. Generally, there are more stringent requirements for borrowing or buying controlled substances from another pharmacy; however, unless barred by state law, Schedule 2 controlled substances can be purchased from another pharmacy by executing the proper order form **(DEA-222)**.

Managing Expired Medication

Each drug has an expiration date established by its manufacturer. Once a pharmaceutical product has reached its expiration date, it must be removed from active stock and placed in a designated area in the pharmacy for disposal processing. Each pharmacy will have a different policy for handling the examination of the pharmacy's inventory for expired items; however, most pharmacies will examine each item in their inventory monthly to remove those items that expire during the upcoming month. Due to the varying rules between manufacturers and the number of manufacturers, pharmacies generally do not return expired products directly to manufacturers. Most pharmacies have a relationship with a reverse distributor that will take expired medications from the pharmacy and attempt to obtain credit for the pharmacy from the manufacturers of the expired products. In appreciation for stocking and attempting to dispense their product, many manufacturers will give the pharmacy some level of credit when one of their products expires. A **reverse distributor** will also take responsibility for destroying medications in an environmentally-conscious and legal way if the manufacturer will not take the product back for destruction. Although the pharmacy will pay a modest fee to the reverse distributor for these services, a reverse distributor is generally better able to obtain credits for the pharmacy than the pharmacy would be able to get on their own; if a reasonable contract can be negotiated with a reverse distributor, the relationship is generally beneficial to the pharmacy. What the pharmacy must never do is simply discard expired medications into regular waste disposal systems. Beyond having a responsibility to the environment that is not met by this action, the release of these chemicals into the trash-handling system by a pharmacy may be illegal and may facilitate these drugs falling into the wrong hands.

Inventory Turnover

One measure of the success of an inventory management system is the inventory turnover rate, or turns. Generally, a pharmacy does not want to order a drug only to have it sit on the shelf for a long period of time. In most situations, a pharmacy will have to pay for a drug within two weeks of having ordered it; however, the drug might not be paid for until 30 days after it is dispensed. Therefore, most pharmacies seek to have the gap of time between paying for the drug and being paid for the drug to be as small as possible. One way to measure this is to figure out, on average, how many times a product is reordered and dispensed over a given period of time. In other words, finding out what percentage of the average inventory, at any given moment, is newly-purchased items will tell the pharmacy how much their inventory is turning over and being replaced with new bottles. To calculate an inventory's turns, the following formula may be used:

$$\text{Inventory Turnover Rate} = \frac{\text{Total Purchases During Period}}{\text{Average Inventory During Period}}$$

The period of time being measured is generally not less than one month and not more than one year. Further, each pharmacy will set its own goals for turns; however, most pharmacies seek to average one turn for each business day that the pharmacy is open. There are 20 business days in the average month, so many pharmacies target 20 turns as their goal for inventory management.

Example
Calculating Inventory Turnover Rate

A pharmacist examines her inventory and believes there are a lot of items that are simply not moving. She wants to verify her suspicions and begins to collect the necessary data to calculate her inventory's turns. She finds that for the previous month that she purchased $3,100,000 in drugs. Further, her dispensing system tells her that her average inventory for this same period was $650,000. The pharmacist wants to determine if the pharmacy is meeting the goal of 20 turns per month.

Step 1: Fill in the equation.

$$\text{Inventory Turnover Rate} = \frac{\text{Total Purchases During Period}}{\text{Average Inventory During Period}}$$

$$\text{Inventory Turnover Rate} = \frac{\$3,100,000.00}{\$650,000.00}$$

Step 2: Solve the equation by dividing the total purchases by the average inventory.

$$\text{Inventory Turnover Rate} = \frac{\$3,100,000.00}{\$650,000.00} = 4.769 = 4.8 \text{ turns}$$

The pharmacist's suspicions have been confirmed. The pharmacy's goal of 20 turns is a long way off and some adjustment must be made to the pharmacy's inventory management system.

Pharmacy technicians can help a pharmacy reach its inventory management goal by assisting in identifying products that are in the inventory but not turning over. If these products are unopened packages, they may be able to be returned to the pharmacy's wholesaler (depending on the wholesaler's terms for returning such products), or they may be able to sell the product to another pharmacy in the area that is using that product more regularly (depending on the regulations and laws of the state where the pharmacy operates). Further, pharmacy technicians are instrumental in selecting products to order from wholesalers and can help adjust ordering habits to prevent unneeded medication from being ordered.

Recalled Medications

Although the FDA has the authority, in some situations, to force a manufacturer to recall a product, the pharmaceutical and medical device industry have an established history of voluntarily recalling products when problems arise. Recalls are classified into one of three categories by the FDA:

■ **Class I**
These recalls are for dangerous or defective products that are highly likely to cause harm to consumers. Drugs used to treat a life-threatening condition, or that have a very narrow dosage range before being toxic, are recalled as Class I recalls. Examples include a specific lot number of a drug has been found to have sharp metal shavings

sticking out of a tablet, a nebulizer has been found to catch fire when plugged in or a specific lot number of a drug contains a lethal dose of the active ingredient rather than the dose printed on the label.

- **Class II**

    These recalls are for products that are outside of their standard specifications but the deviation is not likely to cause serious harm. Generally, drugs recalled under a Class II recall are not used to treat life-threatening conditions. Examples include three lot numbers of a cholesterol-lowering drug are found to have twice the labeled dose of active ingredient as is stated on the product's label and a cream containing a mild steroid used to treat simple rashes is found to be turning a brown color (rather than being white) after being packaged.

- **Class III**

    These recalls are for products that do not pose any likely danger to patients but that are in violation of FDA regulations on labeling, packaging or documentation requirements. An example: a manufacturer uses good manufacturing practices and produces what appears to be an acceptable product, but the FDA finds that, upon inspection, the quality assurance logs for that lot of product are not on file (as required), so that lot of the product must be recalled.

Pharmacy technicians are often charged with receiving notifications of recalls and examining a pharmacy's inventory for the presence of a recalled product. Further, pharmacy technicians may be employed to notify patients who may be in possession of a recalled product if that is part of the direction of the manufacturer or the FDA as part of the recall process for that drug. Most recalls involve removing the drug from a pharmacy's inventory and returning it to the manufacturer but do not involve recalling the product from patients.

Medication Storage

Being generally charged with maintaining a pharmacy's inventory, pharmacy technicians must become experts on drug storage requirements. Most drugs are stored at room temperature, however, some drugs require refrigeration or must be stored in a freezer. Deviations from these temperature requirements can be disastrous for the stability and efficacy of a drug product. Further, some drugs must be stored in refrigerated conditions by the pharmacy but are dispensed to a patient for storage at room temperature; these products often require the pharmacy to label the product with an expiration date during the dispensing of the product that is based on the date when the product is removed from refrigerated conditions. Another environmental factor that may affect a drug's stability is the drug's exposure to light. Some drugs are degraded by UV light and some by full-spectrum white light; these drugs must be stored in containers that are resistant to penetration by light. The standard for light protection is amber-colored glass containers; however, some plastic containers have been tested to provide an acceptable level of light-penetration resistance for storing sensitive medications. Further, some products are flammable, some are toxic (like cancer chemotherapy), some will evaporate if left in an open container and some will absorb water from the air and be unusable. There are many chemical requirements for the environment that drugs are stored in, and these requirements must be taken into consideration when any drug is received by the pharmacy. Beyond the stability issues associated with drugs, some drugs have the potential for theft (also called diversion) due to their potential street value or abuse potential. These drugs must be stored in a manner that minimizes the chance for diversion, without being inappropriately burdensome when they must be accessed for legitimate purposes, and in such a way that these medications can be more carefully monitored and tracked while in the pharmacy's inventory. Although pharmacists are usually a good resource for directing this aspect of inventory management, experienced pharmacy technicians are generally relied upon as the pharmacy's experts in drug storage.

Controlled Substances

It may seem odd to call some drugs controlled substances when all of the drugs that a pharmacy dispenses are substances that are controlled by laws and regulations; however, these drugs have more requirements and regulations and are, therefore, further controlled than other drugs. Although every state may have specific requirements for storing controlled substances in a pharmacy, generally one of two methods are employed. Either the controlled substances are dispersed throughout the pharmacy's inventory in such a way that they are virtually indistinguishable from all of the other drugs to the untrained eye, or the controlled substances are stored in a room, cabinet or safe that is accessible only by those with legitimate need to access those drugs. If the pharmacy's controlled substances are sequestered in a cabinet, the cabinet must be anchored to the building in such a way that the entire cabinet cannot be stolen or removed with significant destruction to the structure of the building. Some pharmacies employ a mixture of these two strategies and sequester their Schedule 2 controlled substances in a locked cabinet and then the Schedule 3-5 controlled substances are dispersed throughout the inventory. Controlled substances also have more record-keeping requirements than other drugs. Pharmacy technicians, especially those newly hired by a pharmacy, must take extra care to ensure that they are compliant with the pharmacy's procedures for handling controlled substances as well as being compliant with all applicable laws for the state in which they are working as a pharmacy technician.

Investigational Medications

Investigational medications used in a hospital are medications undergoing studies to prove their safety and effectiveness for the treatment of a particular disease. Investigational medications may only be used for those patients enrolled in a controlled study and may not be used on other patients. All investigative studies have a protocol that must be followed very closely to ensure that the results are accurate and without bias. Procedures for handling investigational drugs resemble those of dispensing controlled substances. Dispensing records and dose accountability are required for investigational medications. A specially-trained pharmacy technician may be involved in the inventory control, protocol management and distribution of these medications. Further, some investigational drugs require some amount of extemporaneous compounding before they may be dispensed, and a pharmacy technician is often involved in this preparation. Borrowing or loaning investigational medications is not permitted. Investigational drugs are supplied directly from the manufacturer in a tightly-controlled direct distribution channel to prevent these drugs from being integrated into a pharmacy's regular inventory. Restocking of investigational drugs may involve extensive procedures that include personnel from outside the pharmacy being involved in authorizing orders for these drugs. A procedure must be established to prevent the pharmacy from running out of an investigational drug, as this may significantly affect the outcome of the study results.

Packaging

Packaging pharmaceuticals for patient use is an important aspect of any pharmacy service. Medication packages are more than simply a holding vessel for drugs. There are not only legal requirements for packaging drugs, but the useability of a package may determine whether or not a patient can use a medication as prescribed. Functions of the package include the following:
- Identifying the medication completely and precisely. This must include, at minimum:

- the name of the medication.
- the strength of the medication.
- the dose form of the medication (e.g., tablet, c
- the intended route of administration for the medic
- any identifying numbers, such as an NDC, unique to
- the expiration or discard date of the medication.
- the quantity of medication dispensed in the container.

■ Preventing deterioration of the medication by:
- protecting the medication from light exposure.
- protecting the medication from excess air exposure.
- protecting the medication from liquid exposure (including moisture from t air).
- facilitating storage at the necessary temperature.
- protecting the medication from breakage, leakage, contamination or other damage.

■ Allowing safe and ready access to the medication while preventing unwanted access to the medication (such as by a child)

For medications that are not readily available as **unit-of-use** or **unit-dose** (see Figure 1) packages, pharmacy technicians are generally responsible for dividing bulk packages into customized packages for dispensing. This may involve taking a 500-count bottle of tablets and counting out the 34 tablets required to fill a prescription. It may also involved packaging several different drugs into unit-dose blister packs to assist a patient with remembering to take their medications. Some of the commonly-encountered types of repackaging are listed in Table 2. Regardless of the type of repackaging, there must be rigorous controls built into the system to ensure that this error-prone process is kept as error-free as is possible. Improper packaging errors can be fairly harmless, such as having the name misspelled on the package's label, or fairly serious, such as having the wrong drug in the package. Although pharmacists are continuing to take on more clinical roles and less dispensing roles, one aspect of dispensing that still attracts the full attention of pharmacists is collaborating with pharmacy technician to develop and implement error-prevention strategies for this repackaging processes. Whether it is preparing the label, selecting the correct drug to be repackaged or counting the correct number of doses into the new package, there must be specific procedures in place to ensure that each order is filled accurately.

Figure 1
Unit-Dose Package

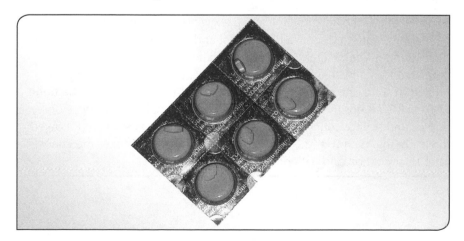

...erting an entire bulk package into unit-
... Generally, this is not done to directly fill a
... prepare for future orders. An example of this is
... pharmacies buy large packages of bisacodyl tablets
...00-count bottles) and divide the entire bottle into
... or four tablets since these small quantities are generally
... be taken during the preparation for a colonoscopy. The
... commercially-available package is 10 tablets, and so it is often
... expensive and more convenient for patients to buy this small supply
... from the pharmacy.

Table 2.

Bulk Package	A bulk package is a large container of medication (e.g., 1,000-count bottle of tablets). Generally, these packages are not intended for direct dispensing to a patient (they must be repackaged into smaller quantities to be dispensed). Further, these packages are often priced at a better rate (per tablet) than smaller packages and may allow the pharmacy to realize a significant savings on those drugs that are most often used.
Dispensing Package (Unit-of-Use)	A dispensing package is a package that comes from a manufacturer with the intention of being dispensed directly to the patient after being labeled by the pharmacy. Many examples of this type of packaging exist, for instance: a Medrol® dosepak, a Zithromax® Z-pak™, a 100 mL bottle of amoxicillin 400 mg/5 mL powder for reconstitution, most oral contraceptive products, and nearly all eye and ear drops.
Extemporaneous Repackaging	Extemporaneous repackaging is the same as batch repackaging; however, it refers to repackaging only a portion of the bulk package, rather than the entire package, in one sitting. This may be done in response to a specific prescription or may be done in preparation for future prescriptions.
don't need Prepackaging	Prepackaged products are those that are sold to a pharmacy in bulk cases of unit-dose packages. An example of this is lansoprazole orally-disintegrating tablets that come in a box of 100 tablets but each tablet is individually wrapped in a unit-dose package.
Repackaging	Repackaging is the act of taking any package of medication that would be inappropriate to dispense to a patient and putting some, or all, of that medication into a different container (usually with a new label of the container's contents) for dispensing to a patient. This process is not limited to solid oral dosage forms (tablets and capsules) and may be done with nearly all dosage forms (including creams, ointments, suspensions, liquids and suppositories) as long as appropriate procedures are followed to ensure that the process is done in a manner that minimizes the chance for contamination and patient harm.

Term	Definition
Unit-Dose Package	A unit-dose package, formally c⌐ package containing medication(s) v. dose of the medication(s) contained th⌐ packages may be linked together (such as _____ packages with each unit separated by a per⌐ackage, is a separable and dispensed individually), each do⌐ins only one package and not the entire card of packages. An e⌐unit-dose packages (linked together in a single card) is shown i⌐dose

Policies and Procedures

Before a policy can be written, first a standard must be established. Standards may be a⌐ by a society, a profession or an organization tasked with developing standards. Standards are ⌐ ally broad statements that categorize behaviors as being acceptable or unacceptable. An example o⌐ standard is in the United States only qualified individuals are permitted to operate a car on the public roadways. Society at large has set this standard that those individuals who are not qualified to drive, for whatever reasons, should not be allowed to drive. Standards often contain language of "should" or "should not" because standards inherently make a value judgment that one behavior is considered acceptable and another behavior is considered unacceptable. Notice that the standard does not tell anyone how to enforce the standard and that it does not establish any mechanism for deciding who meets the standard and who doesn't.

Once a standard has been established, then an organization tasked with enforcing that standard can create a policy that outlines how, generally, the organization will separate those behaviors that are considered unacceptable from those behaviors that are considered acceptable. Most laws enacted by state and federal legislatures are policies. Continuing the driving example, based upon the standard that unqualified drivers should not be allowed to drive on the roadways, the state legislature enacts a policy stating that only those individuals who are at least 15 years of age, and possess a license to operate a motor vehicle issued by the Secretary of State, will be permitted to drive. Further, the law then grants the Secretary of State the authority to determine the procedure for issuing and revoking such licenses. Notice that policies often include language of "will" and "shall" but don't themselves make a value judgment about an action or set of actions.

A procedure is a detailed set of instructions that outline exactly how a policy, based on a standard, will be carried out. These prescriptive recipes are the exact steps to be carried out each time the policy is enforced. So, if the standard is that only qualified drivers may drive, and the policy is that only those who have reached the correct age and have completed a training course may be considered qualified, then the procedure would be that the Secretary of State's office must receive proof of age and proof of training course completion before issuing a driver's license. Notice that the procedure must address each aspect of the policy in order to be complete. A properly written procedure will address all reasonable (and sometimes some unlikely) scenarios that may be encountered when executing a policy.

In the medical professions, accrediting agencies, such as The Joint Commission or the Healthcare Quality Association on Accreditation (HQAA), and professional boards, like the State Board of Pharmacy or the State Board of Medicine, are tasked with writing standards for professional practice. These standards are usually written to express the profession's understanding of its best practices. Then, each

at meet those standards
...el are tasked with devel-
... to be followed to fulfill the

pharmacy or health care organization is task...
and govern the actions of the organizatio...
oping, implementing, maintaining and ...plementation Process
policies. See Table 3 for an example...

Table 3
Standards, Policies...

...cal Equipment, Prosthetics, Orthotics and Sup-

(Based on th... ...al
plies (DM... ...armacy) provides appropriate education, training and safety instruc-
...patients), or their caregivers, as required by their payers (the patient's
Stan... ...mpany) on all equipment, devices, products (including enteral products) or
■ ...rovided. This process clearly identifies the client (patient), or caregiver, training
...ations. On admission to services provided in the client's (patient's) residence, the
...ganization (pharmacy) educates each client (patient), and caregiver, when applicable,
regarding the following:

- The client's (patient's) rights and responsibilities
- The client's (patient's) role in participation in the plan of care
- Options for rental and purchase of all equipment/devices provided
- The proper setup and use of the equipment or device that complies with the physician's order
- Infection control issues
- Residence safety and other appropriate safety considerations
- Handling emergencies and emergency preparedness
- Equipment or device maintenance/cleaning/troubleshooting/potential hazards
- A process for reporting injuries while using the equipment or device

■ The organization provides clear and concise printed teaching materials for all equipment or devices, related to the setup (including preparation of formulas), features, routine use, troubleshooting, cleaning and maintenance of the items provided to clients (patients). These materials include drawings or illustrations as needed. All materials disclose any known potential hazards or contraindications for use. Educational materials include troubleshooting instructions when available. If individualized instructions are created for a client (patient) based on the client's (patient's) need, language, etc., they are retained in the client's (patient's) record.

Policy Developed by the Manager of the Pharmacy

■ The pharmacy utilizes pharmacists to provide appropriate education, training and safety instruction to patients/caregivers on all drugs, equipment, devices, products and services provided. This process clearly identifies the patient/caregiver training expectations. On admission to services provided in the patient's residence, a pharmacist educates each patient/caregiver on the following:

- The patient's rights and responsibilities
- The patient's role in participating in the plan of care
- Options for rental and purchase of all equipment/devices provided

- Proper setup and use of the equipment or device that complies with the physician's order
- Infection control issues
- Safety considerations with the device
- Handling emergencies and emergency preparedness
- Equipment or device maintenance/cleaning/troubleshooting/potential hazards
- The pharmacy's process for reporting injuries while using the equipment or device

■ The pharmacy provides clear and concise printed teaching materials for all equipment or devices related to the setup (including preparation of formulas), features, routine use, troubleshooting, cleaning and maintenance of the items provided to patients. These materials include drawings or illustrations as needed. All materials disclose any known potential hazards or contraindications for use. Educational materials include troubleshooting instructions when available. If individualized instructions are created for a patient based on their unique needs, such materials are retained in the patient's record. The pharmacy also provides appropriate material, in a written form, to each patient for each drug, dispensed by a pharmacist pursuant to a prescription.

Procedure Developed by the Licensed Pharmacists Practicing at the Pharmacy

■ Each patient receiving a DMEPOS product will receive a patient information packet with the initial dispensing/billing of that device and each time a new prescription for that device is presented (generally, once annually). If multiple devices are received during the same calendar week, only one packet will be given unless the patient requests another copy. The packet shall include the following (not necessarily in this order):
- The pharmacy's policy on the release of medical records and information
- The pharmacy's billing procedures
- FDA prescription and over-the-counter drug return policy
- A set of frequently asked questions, with answers, written by the pharmacists practicing at the pharmacy
- The pharmacy's notice of privacy practices (HIPAA documentation)
- The Patient Bill of Rights (rights and responsibilities) established by the pharmacy
- Instructions for patients to follow in case of an emergency
- The pharmacy's procedures for lodging a complaint
- A document outlining the scope of services provided by the pharmacy
- For Medicare patients only (may be included in the packet for all patients but not addressed with non-Medicare patients):
  - Capped Rental and Inexpensive Item Notice (Medicare-designed form)
  - Medicare Supplier Standards (Abbreviated) (Medicare-designed form)
  - Warranty Information (Medicare-designed form)

■ New patient packets will be available on the pharmacy's Web site. Staff must print new patient packets from the Web site when needed. Copies will not be pre-printed; however, a master copy may be obtained from the pharmacy manager if the Web site is down or not working properly.

Table 3 cont.
Standards, Policies, Procedures and Implementation Process

- Pharmacists will provide education to patients/caregivers per the requirements set forth by Standard PS2-3 (elsewhere in the HQAA Manual). This shall include the patient's role in the plan of care, the proper setup of equipment, the proper cleaning of equipment, the proper use of equipment, infection control issues and safety issues.
- The pharmacy manager shall create and maintain a library of patient handouts that can be photocopied or referenced by any pharmacist that will facilitate the training on any DME provided by the pharmacy.
  - Prescription and OTC drugs, dispensed pursuant to a prescription, must be dispensed with the monograph on file with the pharmacy manager or an FDA-approved Medication Guide (or both). A pharmacist may highlight the relevant risks of using the medication before providing the monograph or Medication Guide to a patient or caregiver.
  - Pharmacists shall make an electronic progress note in the patient's chart whenever counseling services are provided (which are required on initial dispensing of any prescription product). The progress note shall have the following headings/sub-paragraphs and include details on the specific training provided by the pharmacist:
    - Patient Role
      - To include training on how to use the medication/device
      - To include nonpharmacological therapies recommended
      - To include nonprescription therapies recommended
      - To include an assessment of the patient's understanding of counseling and if additional education is appropriate
      - To include any other notes regarding the use of the medication/DMEPOS
    - Device/Medication Management
      - To include training on setup, cleaning, infection control and safety with the DMEPOS
      - To include proper storage instructions if specific to the product or otherwise unusual
      - Process for reporting injuries
    - Educational Materials
      - To include which handouts were provided (including drug monographs, device manuals/instructions, etc.)
      - To include any other counseling points stressed to the patient

This example makes it clear that these policies and procedures can be lengthy and can cover a wide variety of scenarios. This is only one standard from the HQAA manual that includes 11 chapters of standards (approximately 50 standards). HQAA is only one of more than a dozen accrediting agencies in the United States; each accrediting agency has its own manual of standards. The standards are generally the same, as they are the consensus of best practices throughout the profession. As mentioned, accrediting agencies are not the only groups with published standards; professional boards, professional organizations and patient advocacy groups will publish standards of practice. It is up to each individual pharmacy to create policies and procedures that meet the relevant standards for their organization. Some standards and the associated policies are actually laws (or have the full force of a law) and must be complied with and others are only enforced by the good conscience of the pharmacists and pharmacy technicians practicing at a pharmacy. Either way, pharmacy technicians are often an integral part of crafting these policies and procedures and are certainly integral to executing them. A wise pharmacy technician will become familiar with a pharmacy's policies and procedures upon starting to work for that pharmacy.

Conclusion

As more pharmacists spend their time counseling patients and assisting health care personnel in the appropriate use of medications, pharmacy technicians are being relied upon to handle the roles of managing the pharmacy's inventory, including receipt and storage. Pharmacy technicians, in assisting a pharmacist, must be aware of and follow not only the applicable laws, but also the policies and procedures established by each pharmacy. Following established policies and procedures is the first step to ensure that patients are kept safe from errors and that products dispensed by the pharmacy are consistent from one dispensing to the next. This standardization leads to improved patient and employee safety and reduced legal liability. By attending to the details of all actions relating to the processes of inventory management, pharmacy technicians help to enable pharmacists to provide patients with the highest level of care.

Bibliography

- American Society of Health-System Pharmacists, ASHP Guidelines, www.ashp.org/Import/ PRACTICFANDPOLICY/PolicyPositionsGuidelinesBestPractices/BrowsebyDocumentType/ GuidelinesMain.aspx, Feb. 2, 2011.
- Drug Enforcement Administration, Pharmacist's Manual, "An Informational Outline of the Controlled Substances Act Revised 2010," www.deadiversion.usdoj.gov/pubs/manuals/ pharm2/index.html, Feb. 2, 2011.
- FDA 101: Product Recalls, www.fda.gov/ForConsumers/ConsumerUpdates/ucm049070. htm, Feb. 8, 2011.
- Neubrecht, F., Pharmacy Technician Policy and Procedure Manual, 1st edition, Lansing, Mich., 1999.
- Webster's Eleventh New Collegiate Dictionary, Merriam-Webster, Springfield, M.A., 2003.

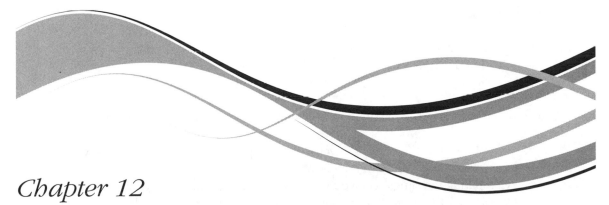

Chapter 12
REVIEW QUESTIONS

1. Which of the following best describes Pareto's law?
   a. Based on a "want book," orders are placed with wholesalers
   b. An inventory management system whereby drugs are categorized, based on importance, into one of three categories, designated A, B or C
   c. An inventory management system that tries to maximize inventory turnover of high usage items by having 20 percent of a pharmacy's inventory generate 80 percent of its revenue
   d. An inventory management system where little inventory is kept on hand

2. Which of the following does not describe a drug formulary?
   a. A formulary is a list of drugs that are considered by the professional staff of an institution to be the most useful in caring for the greatest number of patients
   b. A formulary is a list of medications approved for prescribing to patients within a given institution
   c. A formulary is a list of medications utilized in hospitals, clinics or health mainte nance organizations
   d. A formulary is a list of the therapies most recently approved by the FDA for every disease state or condition

3. Which entity acts as an intermediary between the manufacturer and the pharmacy in the drug distribution process?
   a. Cooperative buying group
   b. Wholesaler
   c. Pharmaceutical representative
   d. Pharmacist

4. In a typical prime vendor agreement, the pharmacy is under no obligation to order most of its drugs through the particular wholesaler with which the prime vendor agreement is signed.
   a. True
   b. False

5. What type of packaging is also called a dispensing package?
   a. Unit-of-use package
   b. Bulk package
   c. Batch repackage
   d. Repackage

6. Which of the following is generally a pharmacy technician's role in the ordering and inventory process?
   a. Examining the pharmacy's inventory for expired drugs and then removing the found expired drugs from the inventory
   b. Comparing the drugs received from a wholesaler to the invoices provided by the wholesaler to ensure that the invoices accurately represent the drugs actually received
   c. Ensuring that stock is rotated such that newly-received packages are placed behind packages already in the pharmacy's inventory unless the newly-received items will expire before the items already in the pharmacy's inventory
   d. All of the above

7. A pharmacy typically dispenses 500 mg cephalexin capsules in quantities of 40. The pharmacy purchases cephalexin in a 100-count package. If the pharmacy typically dispenses eight prescriptions for 500 mg cephalexin capsules each day, and at the end of the day there is a single bottle containing 17 capsules left on the shelf, how many 100-count packages of 500 mg cephalexin capsules must be ordered to be ready for the next day's anticipated need?

8. A pharmacy typically dispenses 600 mg ibuprofen tablets in quantities of 60. Packages of 600 mg ibuprofen tablets are purchased by the pharmacy in 1,000-count bottles. If the pharmacy typically dispenses 17 prescriptions for 600 mg ibuprofen tablets each day and there is a partial bottle of 25 tablets on the shelf at the end of the day, how many packages of 600 mg ibuprofen tablets must a pharmacy technician order to be ready for the next day's anticipated need?

9. Determine the annual inventory turnover rate if a pharmacy spent $2,715,000 on inventory and the average inventory value during the past year was $637,000 (round your answer to the nearest whole turn).

10. Determine the inventory turnover rate if a pharmacy spent $1,970,000 on inventory and the average inventory value during the past year was $786,000 (round your answer to the nearest tenth of a turn).

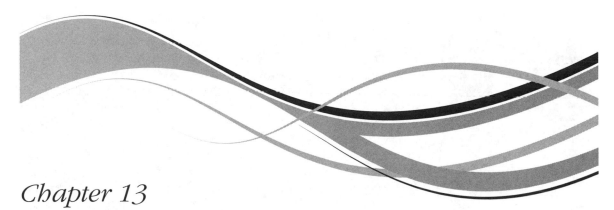

Chapter 13

EMERGENCY PREPAREDNESS

By Greg A. Pratt, R.Ph.

Learning Objectives

This chapter seeks to prepare a pharmacy technician to:

- identify recent disaster scenarios that have occurred in the United States that have underscored the importance of preparedness for pharmacists and pharmacy technicians.
- investigate the disastrous impact when a community is exposed to an intentional dissemination of either of the Category A biologic agents, a chemical agent or a radiologic agent.
- summarize the possible role the pharmacy technician should be prepared to play in anticipation of a terrorist or natural disaster event.

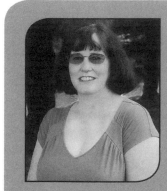

What role would a technician play in preparing for an emergency, such as a bioterrorism event, natural disaster or infectious disease outbreak?

"My pharmacy houses a 'CHEMPACK' that is set up and maintained by the Centers for Disease Control & Prevention (CDC). This pack contains antidotes that would be needed immediately in case of a biological incident. The technician along with the pharmacist would be directly involved in the deployment of this pack. It is important to know the proper deployment procedures to help the process flow smoothly if it's needed to save lives.

We also maintain medication stockpiles of antibiotics that may be used in any situation with a large number of patients. Maintenance includes keeping supplies stocked and up-to-date.

Practice for a mass vaccination clinic in the case of an infectious disease outbreak is performed annually at our hospital. We perform a practice drill each fall by providing a flu vaccination clinic for employees. In a four-hour time period, we have vaccinated nearly 500 people without any wait. We could also vaccinate more if needed. This clinic is staffed by nurses, nursing students, student pharmacists, pharmacy technicians and other staff members. Each year, we become more efficient and now use this as our main event for employee flu vaccinations."

Joan Williams, CPhT
Carilion Clinic
New River Valley,
Radford, Va.

Introduction

The United States has faced several national emergency events during the last 10 plus years, making emergency preparedness planning critical to future response.

■ **Sept. 11 Terrorist Attack**

On Tuesday, Sept. 11, 2001, operatives from the terrorist group known as Al-Qaeda initiated a long-planned attack on the United States by hijacking four airplanes. Two were intentionally flown into the World Trade Center buildings in New York City, one into the Pentagon in Virginia, and one was thwarted from flying into the White House by the passengers and crew who attempted to take back the airplane. The World Trade Center buildings each burned upon impact. Within two hours, both had collapsed, causing 2,605 deaths. The total death toll from this event is estimated to be more than 6,000 persons. This group is expected to continue its efforts to attack Americans on American soil using tools of terror to achieve its goals.

■ **Hurricane Katrina**

On Aug. 28, 2005, a Category 5 hurricane hit New Orleans and the surrounding region with long-term devastating effect. It is estimated that more than 1,800 people lost their lives, and countless people were left homeless. The widespread destruction from this storm left hospitals without power and left hospital patients and employees struggling to evacuate to areas of safety. The coordination of medical resources was made difficult by the breakdown in communication services and difficulties experienced by different aid agencies as they attempted to deliver and distribute key supplies. Natural disaster relief planning and response efforts have changed forever in the United States due to the perception that the effort made during this event did not rise to the occasion.

■ 2009 H1N1 Influenza Pandemic

Influenza pandemic planning has been in place for several years as experts anticipated the spread of the Avian H5N1 influenza virus. Caches of antivirals and protective equipment were in place and plans to deploy them were written and exercised. Unfortunately, the expectation that the next influenza pandemic would begin in Southeast Asia did not occur as anticipated. Instead, in April of 2009, reports began to circulate from California and Texas of a novel influenza virus, which seemed to be of swine origin, with the ability to circulate in humans.

A year later, the Centers for Disease Control & Prevention (CDC) estimated that 61 million people in the United States were infected with this virus, and approximately 12,400 people died as a result of this pandemic. The CDC reported the number of pediatric deaths (0-17 years of age), as of May 22, 2010, at 341.[1]

Local health departments and pharmacies worked together to coordinate the distribution of the federal supply of antiviral medications and the available vaccine. Along with this distribution process was a requirement that all of these assets be tracked to the ultimate user, and pharmacies were very helpful in assisting local health departments with this monumental task.

All crisis events are local. If the local response is absent, or inadequate, outside resources have no framework to build upon in support of that local community. Therefore, it is the responsibility of pharmacy professionals, as highly accessible health care workers, to be knowledgeable of the possible crisis events that may impact our communities. Daily, face-to-face contact with community members and the high level of trust placed in the profession of pharmacy puts both pharmacists and pharmacy technicians into key roles when an event does occur. Affected people will look to pharmacies for direction and guidance regarding medications, medication billing assistance for displaced friends and family, and general health care information.

Pharmacy professionals need to take an "All Hazards" approach to planning and be prepared for either a natural event, intentional (terrorist) event or pandemic event because the response to any, and all, of these can be safer, more effective and more efficient if pharmacy professionals take an active role in that response.

This chapter covers potential disaster scenarios, resources available to aid in response and recommendations as to how pharmacy professionals can play a role in planning, preparing and responding as a trusted health care provider to play a positive role in assuring a safe and efficient response to one of these events.

Chemical, Biological, Radiological, Nuclear and Explosive Events

CBRNE is a common acronym for the five types of crisis events that need response plans in anticipation of their eventuality; those include **C**hemical, **B**iological, **R**adiological, **N**uclear and **E**xplosive events. The following is a synopsis of each of these possible events and suggestions for how pharmacy technicians can assist in the response to exposure in one of these events.

Chemical

There are several different possible chemical agents that might be either intentionally or accidentally released into a community (see Table 1).

Table 1
Chemical Event

Class of Chemical Agent	Chemical Agents	Toxic Effects
Blood Agents	Cyanogen Chloride, Hydrogen Cyanide	Relatively nonspecific. May see shortness of breath, hypertension and increased heart rate among other symptoms
Incapacitating Agents	3-Quinuclidinyl benzilate (BZ)	Dry skin and mucus membranes, increased heart rate, facial flushing, elevated temperature
Irritant Agents	Ammonia, Chlorine, Mace, Pepper Spray, Phosgene	Immediate damage to pulmonary tissue with resultant airway obstruction
Nerve Agents	Sarin, Soman, Tabun, VX (Nerve Agent)	Overproduction of fluids by most organ systems of the body with seizures and respiratory depression
Vesicants	Lewisite, Mustard, Phosgene Oxime	Blistering of the patient's skin

The toxic effects of these agents are extensive and can be life threatening if exposure levels are high enough. These toxic effects, manifested by exposure to chemical agents, will probably be swift and cause large numbers of patients to self-report to hospitals and quickly overwhelm them and their capacity to respond. Hopefully, quick assessment of symptoms by clinicians will identify the offending agent and recommended countermeasures; but, until that point, command and control of the situation will require leadership and cooperation by all staff in every facility.

A pharmacy technician's ability to then assist with the compounding of antidotes and requesting them from alternate sources will be a crucial role in the response to this type of event.

Biological

A biological event will present much differently than a chemical one, but with its own complement of danger. The effects from an intentional release of one of these agents will not be apparent right away, which makes a biological event different from a chemical event. It may be days to weeks before the commonality of complaints being reported by patients are recognized by health care personnel and true disease investigation begins.

Bioterrorism is defined by the Model Emergency Health Powers Act as, "the intentional use of a pathogen or biological product to cause harm to a human, animal, plant or other living organism to influence the conduct of government and to intimidate or coerce a civilian population."

The CDC has designated the following biological agents listed in Table 2 to be of greatest risk because of their availability, stability and/or mortality rate.

Table 2
CDC's Category A Biological Agents

Agent	Agent Type	Key Identifier	Recommended Countermeasure
Anthrax	Bacterial	Widening of the mediastinum (membranous partition between two body cavities or two parts of an organ) on x-ray	Antibiotics
Botulism	Toxin	Skeletal muscle paralysis	Antitoxin and Long-term Respiratory Support
Hemorrhagic Fever Viruses	Virus	Hemorrhage (bleeding) from multiple sites	Supportive Care
Plague	Bacterial	Classic swelling of lymph nodes known as "bubo"	Antibiotics
Smallpox	Virus	Rash	Supportive Care
Tularemia	Bacterial	Ulcerations and sores in and around mucus membranes (such as the mouth and gums)	Antibiotics

Three of these agents will require mass dispensing of antibiotics to the exposed or possibly exposed population. Hospitals and public health departments have a plan in place to accomplish this and exercise these plans on a scheduled basis. A pharmacy technician's ability to assist with this dispensing process, as well as the management of these possibly affected patients, will be critical functions to ensure that this process is accomplished safely and effectively. If given the opportunity by either a hospital or health department to participate in a drill or exercise, pharmacy technicians are encouraged to take the opportunity to learn about the important role that they will play in the event of a real disaster.

Radiological/Nuclear Event

It is anticipated by response planners at all levels that the next terrorist event most likely to occur on American soil is that of an improvised explosive device, possibly containing a radioactive agent. A radioactive element is dangerous because it gives off energy in the form of particles (known as alpha or beta particles) or in the form of electromagnetic waves (known as gamma waves). Exposure to these high energy electromagnetic waves, or contamination by these high energy particles, can have very serious health consequences to the patient, depending upon the level and duration of exposure.

In preparation for an event involving radiation, it is important to know and understand these two key terms: **exposure** and **contamination**.

■ **Exposure**
If a person is exposed to a radiologic source, it can have very negative biologic effects. Those effects may manifest themselves very quickly or may develop slowly over time, even causing negative biologic effects throughout the rest of a person's life. If, however, one is only exposed (and not contaminated), then one does not carry any radioactive source and is therefore not at risk of exposing others to radiation. An example of this type of radiation would be from gamma radiation, which is energy in the form of electromagnetic waves that pass through the body. If the dose and duration are high and long enough, there will be damage to cells of the

body, but one does not retain the gamma rays in the system. Health care personnel are not at risk of radiation exposure when treating these patients.

■ **Contamination**

Contamination by a radioactive source indicates that one is carrying radioactive elements on, or within, one's body that is continuing to release energy as radioactivity, causing damage to all cells that it encounters and, therefore, to any other person in contact with the one contaminated. An example of this type of radiation would be from either alpha particles or beta particles. Health care personnel can protect themselves from the radioactive contaminated patient by using universal precautions.

Knowledge of these simple facts regarding exposure to the contaminated or exposed patient and of available radiation countermeasures within the community or region will allow a pharmacy technician to assist with planning of the deployment of these assets. Clear thinking, and knowledge of available assets, will be critical to the successful response to this type of event.

Explosive Event

On May 1, 2010, in Times Square, terrorist Faisal Shazad built and lit a bomb in a parked vehicle and waited for it to erupt. Luckily for a city that has already seen much suffering and tragedy due to the terrorist attacks of 9/11, this one did not ignite. An alert bystander, noticing white smoke coming from the vehicle, notified police who immediately began evacuation of the area. When pressed by Judge Cedarbaum during his trial in U.S. District Court, questioning why he would target civilians, Shazad replied, "Well the people select the government; we consider them all the same."[2]

Explosive events, like the near-miss described above, have become a mainstay for many areas of the world, and for the front pages of newspapers. When a terrorist group is successful in detonating an explosion on United States soil, the closest health care facilities will probably be overwhelmed with trauma casualties.

If a pharmacy technician is present at, or nearby, the actual event, it is critical for him or her to follow some long-established recommendations in order to initiate a response that is likely to bring order to the chaos and save as many people as possible. The Disaster Paradigm Triage/Treatment protocol that follows in Table 3 will help provide guidelines for efficient response. M.A.S.S. triage is a disaster triage model that utilizes military triage categories with a proven means of handling large numbers of casualties in a mass casualty incident (MCI). M.A.S.S. stands for **M**ove, **A**ssess, **S**ort, **S**end.

Also utilized in the M.A.S.S. triage model is the "ID-me" categories, which include **I**mmediate, **D**elayed, **M**inimal, **E**xpectant. This is an easy to remember phrase that incorporates a mnemonic for sorting patients during MCI triage.

Table 3
Disaster Paradigm Triage/Treatment Model[3]

M.A.S.S. Triage Model	
MOVE	Anyone who can walk is told to MOVE to a collection area Remaining victims are told to MOVE an arm or leg
ASSESS	Assist remaining patients who didn't move (assist these victims first)
SORT	Categorize patients by "ID-me" triage categories (see below)
SEND	Transport patients with immediate needs to hospitals Others may go to secondary treatment facilities
"ID-me" Triage Categories	
IMMEDIATE	Obvious threat to life or limb. Most often this will be patients who have some alteration in their ABC (Airway, Breathing, Circulation)
DELAYED	In need of definitive medical care but should not decompensate rapidly if care is initially delayed
MINIMAL	"Walking wounded" (those with abrasions, contusions, minor lacerations, etc., and stable vital signs)
EXPECTANT	Little or no chance of survival; resources are not utilized initially to care for them unless additional resources become available

Strategic National Stockpile

The **Strategic National Stockpile (SNS)** is a federal cache of pharmaceuticals that is intended to supply, or resupply, a community that is overwhelmed by an event and in need of critical medical supplies. The SNS is not a "fixed" asset. Rather, it is an asset that is intended to be somewhat flexible, depending upon the nature of the crisis event that requires its deployment. Some of those caches include the following:

- **SNS Pushpack**
  The **SNS Pushpack** is a cache of pharmaceuticals that is intended to be the first response of medical assets to resupply a community with a wide variety of medical supplies. It consists of approximately seven semi-truckloads full of supplies weighing around 50 tons and costing approximately three million dollars. There are 12 Pushpack sites around the United States, and they are guaranteed to arrive in a state within 12 hours of the approval of the request by the CDC SNS team.

- **Managed Inventory**
  In order to provide some flexibility to the system, the SNS has reached agreements with various wholesalers and manufacturers around the U.S. to expand their inventories of key pharmaceuticals and supplies that can be requested by the SNS if/when the need arises. Since these assets are not pre-staged, like the Pushpacks, they will take longer to reach the state and community in need.

- **Vaccines**
  The SNS purchases several vaccines that would be in great need as countermeasures to outbreaks of anthrax, smallpox, H5N1 and others. They are cached in large quantities and are ready to be deployed upon request.

■ **Federal Medical Stations**

These are mobile units with enough supplies and equipment to provide non-acute and special needs care for up to 250 persons for three days. These modular units would require a large facility to set up in, and will need staffing assistance to meet the needs of the affected persons.

■ **CHEMPACK**

The **CHEMPACK** program, though not a true "SNS" asset, is still a CDC managed and monitored asset. The CHEMPACK is a cache of pharmaceuticals placed geographically around a state that are filled with countermeasures for a nerve agent exposure. When an incident involving a nerve agent occurs, access to this asset will have to be well coordinated and efficiently managed so that these life-saving medications can be brought to the area of greatest need. A facility may have a CHEMPACK on site, and, if so, a pharmacy technician should be aware of the facility CHEMPACK contacts who will help ensure that this asset is accessed as quickly as possible when requested.

Mass Dispensing

As mentioned in the CBRNE section, intentional dissemination of anthrax, tularemia or plague would require mass dispensing of life-saving antibiotics as soon as possible. This mass dispensing of medications will have to be accomplished by hospitals to employees, and by local health departments to all possibly affected persons.

Hospitals and local health departments must write and exercise a plan to screen patients for key clinical information, make prescribing and dispensing decisions, and do so efficiently, effectively and safely. Management of potentially thousands of anxious persons within a very tense environment will require medical personnel to be comfortable and confident in their plan and in their ability to make the right decisions under this unique type of pressure.

In either setting, having pharmacy technicians assisting will be of great value. Pharmacy technicians are uniquely qualified to assist with an endeavor such as this due to their experience with order processing, no matter what their practice setting. This dispensing must be done in an organized and controlled manner, and pharmacy technicians have the experience of filling and processing orders while under pressure to ensure that accuracy and organization are not ignored.

Pharmacy technicians' experience in dealing with patients in multiple clinical situations becomes valuable when managing the flow of patients in the mass dispensing process.

Pandemic Flu

Each year, seasonal flu is responsible for approximately 36,000 deaths and 226,000 hospitalizations. While this is always of great concern to health care decision makers, it is the threat of pandemic flu that causes even greater concern.

A **pandemic** is an epidemic that is geographically widespread, occurring throughout a region or even throughout the world. An influenza pandemic is of great public health concern due to a lack of human immunity to such a novel virus. Infants, the elderly and those with underlying disease states will be at highest risk.

With the 2009 H1N1 pandemic, the impact was widespread. That pandemic was particularly virulent toward those 18 years of age and younger and pregnant women. Even those without underlying disease states were at high risk of contracting this infection and suffering severe consequences. As a result, even a somewhat prepared society was not prepared for the unpredictable effect upon worker absenteeism, school closures and organizing vaccine programs around pre-defined priority groups.

Based on the 2009 H1N1 pandemic, there are several best practices learned to help guide future decision making and planning:

■ **Morbidity and Mortality**

As in epidemics past, the greatest risk of infection will be to those who are most susceptible to its consequences. This is most often infants, the elderly and those with underlying disease states such as diabetes and asthma. Planning for influenza pandemics must always consider prioritizing care for these groups.

■ **Health Care System**

With cutbacks in hospital beds and staffing over the last several years, it is likely that emergency rooms and health care systems will soon be overwhelmed in an influenza pandemic with a low attack rate. This was exemplified in some areas of the United States during the 2009 H1N1 pandemic.

■ **Workforce**

It is assumed that during a pandemic, up to 40 percent of the workforce may become ill and up to 10 percent will be absent from work at one time. Adding to this is the burden of school closure, which requires that some healthy adults stay at home to deal with unanticipated day care issues.

■ **Critical Infrastructure**

The impact upon suppliers, utility companies, emergency service and other critical daily service functions is unpredictable. Employers may have to be flexible in their expectations of supplier service levels.

■ **Vaccine Production Capacity**

The influenza vaccine manufacturers did prove during the 2009 H1N1 pandemic that they were capable of making a safe and effective vaccine in a somewhat timely fashion. But, until the manufacturing process is shifted from its present reliance upon poultry eggs for production of each dose to a more efficient system, the time frame will be at least three months.

Pharmacy technicians, as well as all health care personnel, are in an ideal position to communicate to patients key messages regarding seasonal and pandemic flu. During the 2009 H1N1 pandemic, new information became available quite often and sometimes seemed contradictory to the previous message(s). It is the responsibility of pharmacy professionals to sift through this information and be a source of accurate, timely and practical information that aids patients in their preparation and response to the pandemic.

Pharmacy Billing Assistance During a Disaster Event

During large catastrophic events, such as Hurricane Katrina, one of the results that requires the assistance of the pharmacy profession is the medication management of potentially thousands of displaced persons. It is a reasonable assumption that during events of this magnitude, a great majority of displaced persons will not have their medications with them. And even if they have the foresight to bring their medications with them, they may quickly run out.

Due to experience with this dilemma in the past, there are now some tools in place to assist pharmacy professionals in their attempt to access these patients' medication records and provide billing assistance. With the pharmacy technician's expertise in prescription processing and navigation of billing programs, no one is better poised to assist these patients and ensure that their medication needs are met, no matter where they are displaced. Below are a few programs that pharmacy technicians need to be familiar with, in anticipation of future response efforts:

■ **Rx Response**

Rx Response is an information sharing and problem-solving forum for the pharmaceutical supply system. It works to ensure that information regarding pharmaceutical supplies is communicated to decision makers during a disaster event so that important pharmaceutical assets are sent to areas of greatest need.

Rx Response is also able to track the re-opening of pharmacies within a declared disaster area as recovery begins. This will aid not only patients in need of pharmacy services but also all pharmacies looking to support each other's efforts during a disaster event. Registered pharmacies can also use their site to access pharmacy-specific information during the event as Rx Response tracks supplies and other key information.

The Rx Response Web site is located at www.rxresponse.org.

■ **Emergency Prescription Assistance Program**

The Emergency Prescription Assistance Program (EPAP) is a program managed by the Department of Health and Human Services. When activated during a disaster, it can be utilized to assist displaced persons by providing financial assistance for their medication needs. Pharmacies can sign up to be a part of this network at any time, in order to learn about the program and be ready to implement it when needed.

To enroll, call (866) 561-5933.

It is advisable for pharmacy technicians to make an attempt to access these sites and learn to navigate them before an event occurs. Knowledge of passwords and how to use these resources so that the response is timely and accurate will help to ensure that the best care is provided to the people in need. During the actual event is not the time to attempt to sign up and become oriented to these sites.

Response Liability Protections

Of concern to all volunteer personnel who respond to a request for volunteers during an event is liability. It is human nature to want to assist people in need during these events; but, unfortunately, it is also sometimes human nature for some to assign blame and seek financial gain as a result of the event. Fortunately, there are state and federal regulations in place to provide liability protection to those who respond to the call and assist response agencies in their efforts. Federal programs (e.g., the Emergency Medical Assistance Compact, the Federal Volunteer Protection Act) and state laws that are implemented when that state's governor declares a state of emergency are intended to provide the assurance that liability protection is in place at multiple levels.

To assist response planners in ensuring that you are covered under these laws, it is helpful if you take the opportunity to pre-register on your state's volunteer registry. This allows them to verify licensure and certifications so that all volunteers are placed in areas of response that best fits their expertise. This also gives access to trainings and key information about the events as they develop.

Conclusion

Initial response to any event must begin at the local level. Health care professionals who have knowledge of cached pharmaceutical assets and key communication pathways, as well as have established relationships with other local response planners, can be a part of a successful response to a crisis event.

Pharmacy technicians who have learned about billing assistance and medication history assistance Web sites will be of great value during the event. Several Web sites of interest to reference can be found in Table 4. Displaced individuals will be facing a myriad of health care issues as a result of this displacement; and, to be able to assist with the replacement and dispensing of their medications will be extremely important.

Basic knowledge of potential terrorist agents and natural disaster events for a community will help pharmacy technicians to assist decision makers in their initial response to these events. A well-prepared pharmacy technician will be aware of the following in anticipation of their emergency preparedness role:

The Pharmacy Technician Response Plan "Need to Know" List

1. Who is the "lead" pharmacist or administrator when an emergency is declared within the pharmacy, department or facility?
2. What is my initial role and responsibility when an emergency is declared?
3. How can I participate in drills and exercises to help increase my knowledge and expertise regarding my department's disaster response plan?
4. Do I have multiple options for notifying family members of the possibility of my detainment at work for an extended period of time?
5. What is the departmental plan to maintain functional capacity of the department during the event?
6. How will the department return to "business as usual" after the event?

Table 4
Emergency Preparedness Web sites of Interest

Billing Assistance Web site	Pharmaceutical Research and Manufacturers of America (PhRMA): www.rxresponse.org
General Bioterrorism Web sites	CDC: www.bt.cdc.gov Federal Emergency Management Agency (FEMA): www.ready.gov
Pandemic Flu Websites	Centers for Disease Control and Prevention (CDC): www.cdc.gov/flu Immunization Action Coalition (IAC): www.immunize.org. U.S. Department of Health and Human Services (HHS): www.pandemicflu.gov
Radiation Response Web site	Radiation Emergency Medical Management: www.remm.nlm.gov

References

1. Centers for Disease Control and Prevention, www.cdc.gov/flu/weekly, June 29, 2010.
2. www.military.com, "Times Square Bomber Details Plot," June 22, 2010.
3. Dallas, Cham E Ph.D., et al, *Basic Disaster Life Support Provider Manual Version 2.6*, 2007, pp. 1-26.

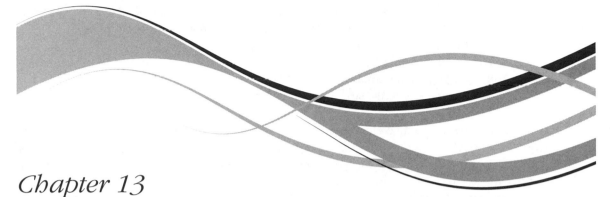

Chapter 13
REVIEW QUESTIONS

1. To build a successful response plan, a community must begin with the assumption that all crisis events are local.
    a. True
    b. False

2. What does CBRNE represent?
    a. A federal agency
    b. Five steps in a response plan
    c. Five crisis events as part of an "all hazards" response
    d. Five medical countermeasures

3. Which of the following is not a chemical agent that causes an event to which emergency responders must respond?
    a. Nerve agents
    b. Vesicants
    c. Blood agents
    d. Smallpox

4. A key difference between release of a biologic agent and a chemical one is that the effects of a chemical release will be noticed immediately; whereas, the effects of a biologic agent may take days to weeks.
    a. True
    b. False

5. Match the Category A Biologic agent with its key identifier:

    a. Anthrax   _____skeletal muscle paralysis
    b. Plague   _____widening of the mediastinum
    c. Tularemia   _____hemorrhage from multiple sites
    d. Smallpox   _____rash
    e. Botulinum Toxin   _____swelling of lymph nodes, or bubos
    f. Hemorrhagic Fever   _____ulcerations in and around mucus membranes

6. Intentional release of which of the following agents will require mass dispensing of life-saving antibiotics by hospitals and health departments to protect or treat the affected population?
   a. Botulinum toxin, plague, anthrax
   b. Smallpox, tularemia, plague
   c. Anthrax, plague, tularemia
   d. Hemorrhagic fever virus, smallpox, nerve agent

7. If you are carrying radioactive elements on, or within, your body that are continuing to release energy as radioactivity and causing damage to all cells that it encounters, as well as any other person that comes into contact with you, then you are considered to be_____ radiation.
   a. exposed to
   b. contaminated with

8. Which of the following make up the flexible response strategy of the SNS?
   a. Pushpack
   b. Vaccines and vaccine purchasing ability
   c. Managed inventory
   d. All of the above

9. Pharmacy technicians who have participated in mass dispensing exercises and have contributed to writing and developing these plans will be counted on to play a key role in any response.
   a. True
   b. False

10. Pandemic flu differs from seasonal flu, in that:
    a. a vaccine is available quickly.
    b. it is easily contained and treated.
    c. it is not expected it to have an impact upon school closures.
    d. even outbreaks with low attack rates will quickly overwhelm our current health care system.

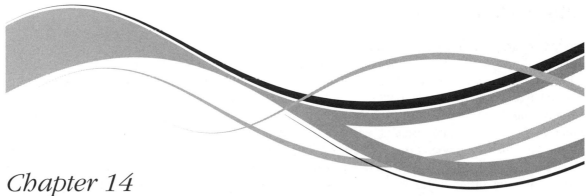

Chapter 14

IMMUNIZATIONS

By Jacqueline A. Morse, Pharm.D., BCPS

Learning Objectives

This chapter seeks to prepare a pharmacy technician to:

- explain the importance of vaccines and the role that pharmacy teams can play in increasing vaccination rates.
- describe each vaccine-preventable disease and the vaccine used to prevent it.
- discuss how to properly store and manage vaccines.
- explain the pharmacy technician's role in pharmacy-based immunization programs.

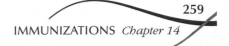

Introduction

Vaccines prevent many transmissible diseases that were once common causes of illness and death in the United States and around the world. Approximately 500,000 Americans were infected with measles each year before 1963.[1] Since a vaccine to prevent measles was introduced in 1963, rates have dropped by more than 98 percent.[1] Though once common, polio has been eradicated in the United States because of successful vaccination efforts. However, if vaccinations end, these and many other vaccine-preventable diseases, which were once common and often deadly, could and would return. **Vaccines** are preparations of dead or living (but weakened, or **attenuated**) organisms that are given to a patient to stimulate the body's production of antibodies that work to protect a person from disease. **Immunization** is the act, or process, of administering a vaccine to a person to stimulate an immune response.

Though there have been many successes with vaccines in the United States, vaccine-preventable diseases, and their complications, still claim the lives of approximately 50,000 American adults each year.[2] More than 36,000 people die from influenza-related complications each year, the vast majority of patients who die from influenza-related complications being over the age of 65.[2] Also, there have been outbreaks of pertussis (commonly known as whooping cough) in recent years; this increase in pertussis cases is due to the need for "booster" doses of pertussis-containing vaccines not being administered to adults, which has led to people contracting pertussis even though they were immunized as children.

It is cases such as the recent increase in pertussis infections that highlight the need to not only continue the nationwide vaccination efforts already in place but also expand those efforts to ensure that vaccine-preventable diseases do not surge now that they are under control. Pharmacists are becoming key players in vaccine delivery. Since 2009, pharmacists in all 50 states are legally able to administer vaccines. Each state has specific guidelines that may be different from those regulations in other states.

Pharmacists are among the most trusted health care professionals, and community pharmacists, in particular, are easily accessible and convenient for patients. Accessibility and society's understanding that vaccination is within the scope of a pharmacist's practice make pharmacy perfectly positioned to help increase immunization rates. Certified pharmacy technicians can play an important role in increasing immunization rates in their communities by being vaccine advocates and can help ensure safe and efficient delivery of vaccines by assisting with pharmacy-based vaccination programs.

Overview of Vaccines

Vaccines are made from the viruses or bacteria they are designed to protect against. Vaccines are considered medications, and, like other medications, they contain an active ingredient. The active ingredient in a vaccine is called the **antigen**. An antigen is any foreign substance that can stimulate the body's immune response. Many vaccines are made from small pieces of the offending bacteria or virus that contain only the antigen; these types of vaccines, called inactivated or dead vaccines, are designed to eliminate any unnecessary viral or bacterial material from being delivered to the patient, that may be linked to adverse effects from receiving the vaccination. The immune response, following vaccination, results in the production of antibodies, that destroy the antigen, and the production of "memory" immune cells that provide protection from future infection by the offending bacteria or virus. It takes approximately two weeks for the body to develop a protective level of antibodies after vaccination.

Most vaccines consist of dead organisms, and, therefore, vaccines cannot cause the disease they are designed to prevent. Some vaccines, however, contain live organisms that have been altered so that they do not cause disease. The antigen in live vaccines must replicate, or make copies of itself, in the body in order to produce the immune response (e.g., the live influenza vaccine is given intranasally and is "cold-adapted," which means that it must replicate in the cooler nasal passages in order to work but cannot withstand the warmer parts of the body where it could cause disease). Live vaccines typically result in a greater immune response than inactivated vaccines. Live vaccines come with more precautions and cannot be given to certain populations, including pregnant women and those with a weakened immune system. These groups may be more susceptible to adverse effects and/or a reduced effect from the vaccine.

Vaccines come in a variety of dosage forms. From multiple-dose vials to single-use prefilled syringes to capsules for oral dosing, vaccines present a challenge to anyone, such as a pharmacy technician seeking to become familiar with the availability of these products. Likewise, vaccines are administered by various routes depending on the type of vaccine. Intramuscular vaccines are given in the thigh in infants and young children or in the deltoid (large muscle of the upper arm) for older children and adults. Some vaccines are given subcutaneously, into the fatty layer under the skin on the back of the upper arm. Though most vaccines are given either intramuscularly or subcutaneously, there are a few vaccines delivered orally, intranasally and by other routes.

Because there does not exist a vaccine that will always produce full immunity in all patients, sometimes multiple doses of a vaccine must be given to patients who do not respond to their first dose of the vaccine (e.g., it is recommended to dose varicella vaccine again if immunity is not achieved from the first dose). With other vaccines, multiple doses spread out over time are given to boost antibody levels that naturally decrease over time. This natural decrease in antibody levels is why tetanus and diphtheria (Td) booster doses must be given every 10 years for a patient to retain immunity to these two diseases.

Since most vaccines are injected, reactions (side effects) occurring around the site of the injection are common (e.g., warmth, redness, muscle pain with intramuscular vaccines and bruising). Systemic reactions (those side effects occurring away from the injection site) are far less common (e.g., fainting, slight fever and, very rarely, **anaphylaxis**, which is a severe allergic reaction that may lead to shock and can be fatal if left untreated). There are many misconceptions about vaccine safety. The Food and Drug Administration (FDA) and Centers for Disease Control and Prevention (CDC) have done extensive research into trying to identify a link between vaccines and problems (e.g., autism, mercury toxicity, sudden infant death syndrome (SIDS) and fainting). The FDA and CDC have found no credible evidence that a link exists between these ailments and vaccines.

Vaccine-Preventable Diseases: Viral

■ **Influenza**

Influenza is a viral illness that is easily spread by a cough or sneeze. Classic symptoms of influenza include fever, chills, body aches, tiredness, an occasional cough and sore throat (it should be noted that "stomach flu" (gastroenteritis) is not caused by the influenza virus.) Influenza resolves without intervention for most people, but it can lead to pneumonia and other complications in some people and is a significant cause of hospitalizations and death in older patients. More than 90 percent of deaths due to influenza and its complications occur in people 65 years of age and older.[3] Influenza activity is usually highest from December through March of each year, with peak influenza activity usually occurring in January or February.[3] In any given season, though, multiple waves of influenza activity can occur, and each wave often affects a different group (e.g., children in the first wave, elderly in the next and health care workers in the third).

Part of the reason for the wave-action observed in some influenza infection seasons is because influenza viruses, in an effort to avoid destruction by our immune system, change the chemicals presented on the outside, or surface, of their "bodies." These chemicals are the antigens that cause irritation to our immune system, leading to the symptoms we call "the flu."

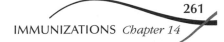

Because these surface antigens change so rapidly, and because the seasonal influenza vaccine can only contain a limited number of surface antigens each season, a new vaccine is created every year based on the combinations of surface antigens expected to be most common during the flu season for which the vaccine is designed. Each year, the seasonal influenza vaccine contains antigens from three strains, or types, of influenza virus that experts from the CDC and elsewhere, predict will be the most commonly circulating strains causing disease for the upcoming flu season. Severe outbreaks, like the 2009 H1N1 influenza pandemic, occur when the surface antigens seen in common influenza viruses change drastically and unpredictably from season to season; the experts use the best available data and science to predict which strains to cover each season, but there will always be unaccountable surprises.

There are two available dosage forms of influenza vaccine. The first is a dead, inactivated vaccine given intramuscularly, and the second is a live, attenuated vaccine given intranasally. The inactivated vaccine is approved for individuals six months of age and older. A new, high-dose, inactivated vaccine became available in 2009 for people 65 years of age and older since those over 65 do not produce as many antibodies compared to younger adults when given the traditional influenza vaccine; it has been shown that a higher dose is better at protecting a person over 65 years of age from contracting influenza. The live attenuated influenza vaccine (LAIV) is approved for healthy people from two to 49 years of age. Since LAIV is given intranasally, the most common reactions involve the nose and the surrounding tissues (e.g., runny nose, sore throat, congestion and cough).[3] See Table 1 for more information on influenza vaccines and on the other vaccines presented in this section.

Though it is recommended to vaccinate all eligible patients six months of age or older, there are certain target groups who are more likely to suffer from influenza complications and, therefore, must be prioritized for vaccination during vaccine shortages. These high-risk groups include pregnant women, those with certain chronic health conditions, like diabetes or heart disease, and the elderly. Immunizers should start giving the influenza vaccine as soon it becomes available (usually late August or early September) and continue until the season's supply is gone, as influenza can circulate throughout the year and has more than one peak.

■ Varicella

Varicella is a virus that first presents as **chicken pox** (widespread, itchy lesions on a person's body). Varicella is highly contagious to those who have not previously been infected or vaccinated, and it is spread by contact with contaminated respiratory droplets with the lesions of an infected person. Usually mild in children, chicken pox is typically worse in adults and can occasionally lead to bacterial infections, pneumonia and other complications.

A live vaccine, Varivax®, is recommended for the prevention of varicella infection in children ages 12-15 months, followed by a second dose at four to six years of age. Older individuals who do not have evidence of varicella immunity may also receive the vaccine.

Following chicken pox, the varicella virus remains in the body in an inactive state. Sometimes, the virus can resurface later in life; this resurgence is usually due to advancing age, a weakened immune system or another trigger. This secondary infection is called **zoster** (shingles); a zoster infection appears as a localized rash that can be very painful and can result in long-term nerve pain once the rash has resolved. A live vaccine to prevent shingles, Zostavax®, is available and approved for adults 60 years of age and older. Zostavax® contains the same antigen as Varivax® but at a much higher dose. This higher dose is necessary to stimulate immunity in older adults who tend to have an increasingly weakened immune response.

■ **Hepatitis A and B**

Although **hepatitis**, which generally refers to inflammation of the liver, can be caused by noninfectious sources, infectious hepatitis is caused by a group of viruses. These viruses are grouped based on the accompanying symptoms, severity and duration of hepatitis that they cause. Many cases of hepatitis A reported in the United States are due to contaminated food or international travel. **Hepatitis A** begins suddenly with symptoms such as jaundice (yellowing of the skin and/or eyes), fever, upset stomach and/or vomiting. These symptoms do not usually last longer than two months.[4] **Hepatitis B** is typically a sexually-transmitted infection in the United States, but it can also be transmitted through sharing infected needles (especially during drug injection). It is usually slower in onset, compared to hepatitis A, and often presents with jaundice, fever and influenza-like symptoms. Though a hepatitis B infection is cleared naturally and without intervention by the immune system in most adults, approximately 10 percent of adults (and 90 percent of infants) will later develop chronic hepatitis B that can lead to cirrhosis, liver cancer and death.

It is recommended for all children one year of age and older, as well as adults traveling to countries with high rates of hepatitis A or who have other risk factors, to be vaccinated with a two-dose series of the inactivated hepatitis A vaccine. The inactivated hepatitis B vaccine is given routinely to infants as a three-dose series; the first dose is given shortly after birth and then the other two are part of the usual pediatric immunization schedule. People with HIV, those who abuse injectable drugs, those with liver disease and other high-risk adults must also be vaccinated against hepatitis B if they were not vaccinated as an infant. This high-risk group also includes certain health care workers (e.g., immunizing pharmacists and pharmacy technicians) who must be vaccinated against hepatitis B to protect against contracting it from a patient if a needle-stick or other exposure occurs.

■ **Human Papillomavirus**

Human papillomavirus (HPV) is a very common sexually transmitted infection causing genital warts. It is the most common cause of cervical cancer. There are currently two inactivated vaccines approved to prevent HPV. Gardasil® and Cervarix® protect against cervical cancer, with Gardasil® having additional protection against genital warts. Both vaccines are recommended routinely as three doses for girls aged nine through 26. Additionally, Gardasil® may be used in boys and men of the same age range for the prevention of genital warts.[5] There is also a growing interest in using Gardasil® for the prevention of anal and rectal cancers in men who have sex with men, due to such cancers being linked to HPV, but evidence does not yet exist for the FDA to approve its use for this purpose.

■ **Measles, Mumps and Rubella**

Though measles, mumps and rubella are three viral illnesses no longer commonly seen in the United States, routine vaccination is still recommended. **Measles** often presents as a body rash (with or without fever), common cold-like symptoms and blue-white spots on the mucus membranes. Signs and symptoms of **mumps** include rash, swollen salivary glands, headache, fever and (possible) testicular inflammation in males. **Rubella** appears as a full body rash, with or without fever, and is usually mild compared to measles; however, if it occurs during pregnancy, rubella can cause significant problems, including miscarriage or serious birth defects. Vaccination of all children with a two-dose series of the live, attenuated measles, mumps and rubella (MMR) vaccine is currently recommended. Additionally, certain at-risk adults (health care workers, international travelers, nonpregnant women of childbearing age, etc.) are recommended for vaccination if they do not have evidence of immunity (generally confirmed by a simple blood test).

- **Poliomyelitis**

Though most infections with polio are not symptomatic, **paralytic poliomyelitis** can cause lasting paralysis of the limb muscles (most often involving the leg). Polio was once common throughout the northern hemisphere; but, it has been eliminated in the United States since 1979 due to successful vaccination efforts.[6] Because polio is still present in, and therefore can be brought in from, other countries, routine vaccination of all infants and travelers to areas of the world where polio is present is still recommended. Vaccination consists of a four-dose series with an inactivated vaccine, IPOL®.

- **Rotavirus**

Almost all children by age five have been infected with **rotavirus**, a major cause of diarrhea worldwide. Severe or prolonged diarrhea due to rotavirus may result in dehydration and possible hospitalization. There are currently two rotavirus vaccines on the market, RotaTeq® and Rotarix®, given as a two-dose or three-dose series depending on the brand. Rotavirus is one of the few oral vaccines on the market. To give the vaccine, a sweetened suspension containing live, weakened rotavirus virus is squeezed into the infant's or child's mouth to be swallowed.

Vaccine-Preventable Diseases: Bacterial

- **Pneumococcal Disease**

Pneumococcal disease is caused by the *Streptococcus pneumoniae* bacteria and can cause **pneumonia** (an infection of the lung that causes fluid to accumulate in the lungs), **meningitis** (an infection of the spinal column) or **sepsis** (an infection of the blood). Any of these infections, especially meningitis and sepsis, may be fatal if left untreated. In children under the age of five, *S. pneumoniae* is the leading cause of bacterial meningitis and can also cause ear infections.[7] Symptoms of pneumococcal disease vary depending on which type of *S. pneumoniae* infection is present. Pneumococcal disease can occur at any time of the year and is a common bacterial complication following infection with the influenza virus. Resistance to antibiotics is common with *S. pneumoniae*; with treatment becoming increasingly difficult, prevention through vaccination is becoming even more important.

To prevent *S. pneumoniae* infections, an inactivated vaccine is given as a four-dose series to all infants and children. The pneumococcal conjugate vaccine, known as PCV-13 or Prevnar-13®, protects against 13 different strains of the pneumococcal bacteria known to cause disease. Prevnar-13® was approved in early 2010 and replaces the previous vaccine (PCV-7) that covered only seven strains of *S. pneumoniae*. In addition, there is another type of pneumococcal vaccine; the pneumococcal polysaccharide vaccine (PPSV) is marketed under the brand name Pneumovax 23®. PPSV is 23-valent (i.e., protecting against 23 strains of the bacteria) and is recommended for all adults 65 years of age (and older) and those two through 64 years of age with certain chronic health problems. Unlike the seasonal influenza vaccine, PPSV is administered once; select patients are eligible for a second dose five or more years after the first dose for a maximum of two lifetime doses.

It is important to realize that the pneumococcal vaccine cannot be called the "pneumonia vaccine" since *S. pneumoniae* is not the only cause of pneumonia; other bacteria, and some viruses, can cause pneumonia. To further complicate matters, although the vaccine has been shown to reduce infections from *S. pneumoniae*, it has not been show to reduce the rate of pneumococcal pneumonia presentation in adults.[7]

■ **Tetanus, Diphtheria and Pertussis**

Tetanus results from spores of the bacteria *Clostridium tetani* (found in soil, dust and elsewhere) entering a skin lesion or wound. The spores produce a toxin that causes severe muscle spasms, muscle rigidity, lockjaw and sometimes death. **Diphtheria** is caused by *Corynebacterium diphtheria*. *C. diphtheria* can infect many body sites but most commonly appears as a thick, bluish-white membrane on the back of the throat that can lead to obstruction of breathing, other complications and sometimes death. Though rarely seen anymore in the United States, other countries have had diphtheria outbreaks as recently as the 1990s.[8] Nearly all cases of tetanus and diphtheria occur in people who are not vaccinated (or up-to-date with their vaccines). **Pertussis**, or whooping cough, is caused by the *Bordatella pertussis* bacteria and is characterized by severe and frequent coughing fits; sometimes, these coughing fits can be severe enough to make it difficult for a person to breathe. Pertussis is most severe in young children and can lead to pneumonia, seizures and sometimes death. In recent years, there have been several outbreaks of pertussis in the United States.

There are a number of inactivated vaccines available to protect against tetanus, diphtheria and/or pertussis. DtaP is a vaccine recommended for infants and children to protect against all three diseases. Td is the tetanus and diphtheria booster vaccine typically given every 10 years and sometimes after a deep wound occurs. Tdap is a vaccine for adolescents and adults designed to replace a one-time Td booster dose. Tdap was approved in 2005 when it was found that adolescents and adults were losing immunity to pertussis and serving as carriers of the virus.[9] Although these adults rarely presented with symptoms, young children who came into contact with them were contracting full-blown cases of whooping cough. Notice that the names of these vaccines correspond to the component diseases covered by the vaccines; capital letters are used to denote the parts of the vaccine that will provoke the greatest immune response after giving that particular vaccine. An "a" before a "P/p" means that the pertussis portion is acellular (meaning that the whole cell of the bacteria is not used in the vaccine).

■ **Meningococcal Disease**

Meningococcal disease is transmitted through contact with infected respiratory droplets and can cause symptoms such as headache, neck stiffness and sensitivity to light. The disease is commonly called **meningitis**; however, meningitis refers specifically to an inflammation of the meninges, membranes that are a part of the central nervous system, caused by the *Neisseria meningitidis* bacterium. Meningococcal disease may also lead to sepsis and death if the bacteria infect the blood. There are currently three meningococcal vaccines on the market: one polysaccharide vaccine (Menomune®) and two conjugated vaccines (Menactra® and Menveo®). The conjugate vaccines are preferred in those under 56 years of age. Target groups for vaccination include all adolescents, travelers to certain countries, certain individuals living in close quarters (like college students living in dorms and military basic training personnel) and others at risk.

■ **Haemophilus Influenzae Type B**

Prior to vaccine approval, *Haemophilus influenzae* type B (Hib) was the leading cause of bacterial meningitis in children under the age of five.[10] Invasive Hib can lead to hearing impairment and other serious long-term effects. All infants and young children are recommended to receive the inactivated Hib vaccine. Though Hib is rarely seen in those over five years of age, vaccination may be considered for older children and adults with certain risk factors.

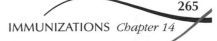

Other Vaccines

There are vaccines, such as the rabies vaccine and several vaccines used primarily in travel medicine, which are less likely to be encountered in the pharmacy setting. These vaccines are not covered here. Some pharmacies, however, do offer travel medicine services to help prepare international travelers by protecting them against infectious diseases they may encounter. Vaccines are an important part of these programs. Several vaccines commonly used in travel medicine include hepatitis A, typhoid fever, Japanese encephalitis and yellow fever. Some vaccines require special authorization, such as yellow fever vaccination, before they can be administered or provided. It is very important to work closely with the traveling patient's physician, the local health department and CDC to determine precisely what is needed.

Many vaccines are combinations (e.g., Twinrix® consists of both hepatitis A and hepatitis B antigens) that mean fewer injections and improved patient acceptance, particularly with young children. However, this can lead to errors in records and dosing, so it is always important to document each individual vaccine a patient is given and not just the name of the combination.

As their role in providing vaccines continues to expand, pharmacists and pharmacy technicians can help prepare to administer immunizations during a bioterrorism event. More information on this topic is available in Chapter 13, Emergency Preparedness. Bioterrorism, which involves the intentional release of a virus, bacteria or other agent, is a threat to which the medical community must be prepared to respond. Though not discussed here, vaccines against smallpox, anthrax and others are available, on a restricted basis, through the federal government and may be mobilized during a terrorist attack or outbreak.

Table 1
Vaccine Characteristics[11,12]

Vaccine	Brand Name(s)**	Type	Dose	Route	Doses / Frequency	Pharmacy Storage
Diphtheria, Tetanus, Pertussis (DTaP, DT, Tdap, Td)	Adacel (Tdap), Daptacel (TDaP), Decavac (Td)	Inactivated	0.5 mL	IM[a]	4-dose primary series with DTaP, followed by 1-time Tdap and Td every 10 years	Refrigerated[b]
Haemophilus Influenza Type B (Hib)	ActHIB, Hiberix, PedvaxHIB	Inactivated	0.5 mL	IM	2-3 dose primary series	Refrigerated
Hepatitis A (HepA)	Havrix, Vaqta	Inactivated	≤ 18 yrs: 0.5 mL ≥ 19 yrs: 1.0 mL	IM	2-dose primary series	Refrigerated

Vaccine	Brand Name(s)**	Type	Dose	Route	Doses / Frequency	Pharmacy Storage
Hepatitis B (HepB)	Engerix-B, Recombivax HB	Inactivated	≤ 19 yrs: 0.5 ml *; ≥ 20 yrs: 1.0 mL *Recombivax can be given as a 1.0 mL 2-dose series in persons 11-15 yrs	IM	2-3 dose primary series	Refrigerated
Human Papillomavirus (HPV)	Cervarix, Gardasil	Inactivated	0.5 mL	IM	3-dose primary series	Refrigerated
Influenza, Live Attentuated (LAIV)	FluMist	Live	0.2 mL	Nasal Spray	1 dose annually (2 doses 4 weeks apart for children 2-8 yrs receiving for first time)	Refrigerated
Influenza, Trivalent Inactivated (TIV)	Afluria, Fluvirin, Fluzone, FluLaval	Inactivated	6-35 mos: 0.25 mL ≥ 3 yrs: 0.5 mL	IM	1 dose annually (2 doses 4 weeks apart for children 6 mo-8 yrs receiving for first time)	Refrigerated
Measles, Mumps and Rubella (MMR)	M-M-R II	Live	0.5 mL	SQ^c	2-dose primary series	Refrigerated or Frozen^d (Diluent. Refrigerated or at RT^e)
Meningo-ccocal Conjugate (MCV)	Menactra, Menveo	Inactivated	0.5 mL	IM	1 dose (2nd dose considered 5 years after 1st for highest risk groups)	Refrigerated

Table 1 *cont.*
Vaccine Characteristics[11,12]

Vaccine	Brand Name(s)**	Type	Dose	Route	Doses / Frequency	Pharmacy Storage
Meningo-coccal Polysaccha-ride (MPSV)	Menomune	Inactivated	0.5 mL	SQ	1 dose (2nd dose considered 5 years after 1st for highest risk groups)	Refrigerated (Diluent: Refrigerated or at RT)
Pneumococc-al Conjugate (PCV13)	Prevnar-13	Inactivated	0.5 mL	IM	4-dose primary series	Refrigerated
Pneumococc-al Polysacc-haride (PPSV23)	Pneumovax 23	Inactivated	0.5 mL	IM or SQ	1 dose (1-time revaccination indicated for some)	Refrigerated
Polio, Inactivated (IPV)	IPOL	Inactivated	0.5 mL	IM or SQ	4-dose primary series	Refrigerated
Rotavirus (RV)	Rotarix, RotaTeq	Live	2.0 mL (RotaTeq), 1.0 mL (Rotarix)	Oral	2-3 dose primary series	Refrigerated
Varicella (Var)	Varivax	Live	0.5 mL	SQ	2-dose primary series	Frozen
Zoster (Zos)	Zostavax	Live	0.65 mL	SQ	1 dose	Frozen

**All rights to all brand names and trademarks are held by their respective owners. There may be additional brand names for some of the products listed.*

a *IM: intramuscular*
b *Refrigeration: 35-46°F (2-8°C)*
c *SQ: subcutaneous*
d *Frozen: 5°F (-15°C) or below*
e *RT: room temperature*

Immunization Programs in a Pharmacy Setting

- **Workflow**

There are several ways to incorporate immunizations into a pharmacy, and a pharmacy technician may be asked to assist in managing workflow when doing so. Vaccines can be given during clinics (e.g., a three-hour pre-scheduled event where patients can come in any time). Clinics tend to work well for vaccines in high demand (e.g., influenza in the fall). Scheduled appointments, on the other hand, may work well for vaccines that you may need to order or for travel-related vaccination services. Finally, immunizations can be processed like a regular prescription, and a patient requesting a vaccination would have to wait to be vaccinated just as they would for a medication to be dispensed. A pharmacy technician may be responsible for scheduling appointments, advertising for a clinic, preparing patients (helping them fill out paperwork) prior to an immunization, preparing supplies needed during the vaccination (e.g., cotton swab, band aid, gloves), preparing the vaccination space or countless other tasks essential to executing a successful immunization program.

- **The Vaccine Prescription**

Vaccines can be prescribed by a patient's personal physician, by the pharmacist working under a physician-authorized standing order and, in some states, independently by a pharmacist. Further, each state varies on who may administer a vaccination once it is prescribed. Some states allow pharmacy technicians to administer vaccinations, after receiving proper training, while working under a pharmacist who has been given authority to administer vaccinations. It is important that pharmacy technicians know what is allowed in their state. In addition, states vary on what pharmacists are allowed to do when administering vaccines; some states have limitations on types of vaccines a pharmacist may give and some allow pharmacists to vaccinate only certain patients (such as those 18 years of age and older). Prescriptions for vaccinations generally are required to have the same elements as prescriptions for other drugs. The prescription must clearly specify the patient for whom the vaccination is being selected, the date that the order is written, the vaccination to be given (preferably the exact combination of vaccinations and not a brand name), the route of administration and the identity of the prescriber.

- **Screening a Patient**

Pharmacy technicians may be asked to assist the pharmacist in screening patients prior to vaccination. The purpose of screening is to determine if a patient is an appropriate candidate for a vaccine. Screening helps to rule out patients with contraindications or characteristics that will likely lead to harm if the vaccine is given (e.g., prior severe allergic reaction to an influenza vaccine, HIV status, pregnancy status). Screening also allows the pharmacist to determine if any precautions exist. Precautions are characteristics that may lead to patient harm or may make the vaccine less effective if given. The Immunization Action Coalition (IAC) has a standard screening questionnaire for all vaccines that can be found online at www.immunize.org.

- **Documentation and Paperwork**

Maintaining proper documentation is extremely important when any medical service is provided to a patient; immunization records are no less important than other health records for a patient. Many pharmacies and institutions require patients, or caregivers, to sign a consent form prior to being vaccinated. Also, all patients need to be screened prior to receiving a vaccine and must be given a copy of the most recent **Vaccine Information Statement (VIS)** that explains the risks and benefits of a particular vaccine. The person administering the vaccine is required to record certain details about each vaccine given (e.g., manufacturer, lot number, dose given). It is also a good practice to update each patient's immunization record card or to provide them with one if they do not have one. All immunization records must be maintained for a patient's lifetime; so, all records need to be stored in a secure area where they will not be disposed. It is also a good idea to share, with a patient's expressed permission, that an immunization has been given with the patient's other health care providers; in some instances, pharmacists are required to provide a copy of the patient's immunization record to the patient's primary care physician. Further, some states and municipalities require reporting of immunization events to a centralized database; assisting with any step of the record-keeping process is definitely within the scope of practice for a pharmacy technician.

■ Payment

Some insurance companies will reimburse pharmacies for both the cost of certain vaccines and the cost of administering the vaccine. Medicare Part B (medical benefit through the federal government) covers influenza, pneumococcal and (sometimes) the hepatitis B vaccine for beneficiaries. Medicare Part D plans typically cover Zostavax® and will likely cover additional vaccines for adults approved in the future. Commercial insurance plans (i.e., insurance plans not administered by the government) are covering pharmacist-provided immunizations more and more. An important thing to keep in mind is whether billing an insurance company or charging a patient directly, vaccine reimbursement must always include both the cost of the vaccine and the cost of administering the vaccine. Some plans will only cover the vaccine itself and, in these cases, pharmacies must charge the patient directly for the administration (often around $10-20). Patients must always be given a payment receipt that clearly shows all of the services/products that were administered/rendered and the cost associated with each service/product. In some cases, patients must submit such a receipt for reimbursement to an employer, insurer or health savings account administrator.

■ Emergency Situations

Pharmacy technicians must always be prepared for an emergency situation following any vaccination. A pharmacist will not be able to perform all of the functions necessary to assist a patient experiencing a severe reaction following a vaccination. As part of the vaccination program administered by pharmacists, all pharmacy technicians must be trained on their responsibilities during any medical emergency. After a vaccine is administered, fainting may occur; appropriate safeguards must be in place to avoid injury to both the patient and the pharmacy team. Though extremely rare, anaphylaxis may also occur following a vaccine dose. The following are several things a pharmacy technician can do to help avoid emergency situations:

- Appropriately screen all patients, and have patients seated securely in a chair (with arms) during vaccination
- Have injectable epinephrine and diphenhydramine readily available in the case of a severe allergic reaction (or whatever drugs and supplies are specified in your pharmacy's emergency protocol)
- Have a manual blood pressure monitor and stethoscope available
- Have a clipboard with a pre-set checklist of what to do in an emergency with space to record the events and times of events that occur during the emergency.

Also, it is generally recommended that patients remain in the vaccination area for approximately 15-20 minutes following vaccination to monitor for any adverse events. If a patient reports an adverse reaction or problem following a vaccine, the individual who gave the vaccine must be informed immediately, as it is vaccinator's responsibility to report significant events to the Vaccine Adverse Event Reporting System (VAERS).

Vaccine Storage and Handling

Vaccines, like many pharmaceutical products, can be very expensive and often have strict storage requirements. Vaccines that are not stored appropriately may become contaminated or lose potency. All vaccines on the U.S. market today are either refrigerated or frozen. Appropriate refrigeration temperatures range from 35°F to 46°F (2-8°C) with a target of 40°F. In general, vaccines must be stored in the middle of the refrigerator unit (not in vegetable bins, against sides, etc.). Frozen vaccines must be maintained at 5°F (-15°C) or colder. Dormitory-style units, with a freezer box in the same compartment as the refrigerator, are not appropriate for vaccine storage. If storing frozen vaccine, the freezer must be separate and sealable from the refrigerator compartment. The public health standard is to check and log temperatures of every unit vaccine is stored in, twice daily.

All pharmacy personnel, including pharmacy technicians, must be trained on how to receive vaccines and maintain the **cold chain**. A properly executed cold chain means that the vaccine's storage conditions meet the manufacturer's specifications from the time the vaccine is manufactured to the time the vaccine is administered. Upon delivery, vaccine shipments must be opened immediately. Temperature indicator cards, if included, must be viewed to determine if the vaccine has fallen out of the acceptable temperature range. If no indicator card is present, ice packs must be checked to ensure they are still frozen or cold.[13] Whenever vaccine is transported from one site to another, it must always be done in an insulated cooler with a thermometer. If, at any time, the cold chain appears to be broken (e.g., due to inappropriate transport or refrigerator power failure) the vaccine must be separated and labeled "do not use." Every cold chain problem must be documented. Local health departments, or the vaccine manufacturer, must be contacted for information on what action to take for storage problems.

In addition to the cold chain, there may be other vaccine storage requirements pharmacy teams will need to consider. Many vaccines must be protected from light and stored in the original packaging. Also, some vaccines must be given within a specified period of time following reconstitution. As with all drugs, vaccines also have an expiration date – even if they have been stored properly. Vaccines must be examined, along with all drugs in the pharmacy, on a regular basis to ensure that expired products are removed from stock (to prevent them from being dispensed to a patient) and processed using the pharmacy's protocol for expired medications.

Vaccine stock must be rotated as is done with other medications (i.e., vaccines with the earliest expiration date are placed in front of those with expiration dates farther out). There cannot be any food or beverages stored in areas that vaccines are located. This does not mean that vaccines may be stored on one shelf of a refrigerator that also contains food; drugs and food must be maintained in totally separate refrigerators. Refrigerators can be lined with water bottles and freezer units can be lined with ice packs to help ensure a consistent temperature. Pharmacy teams must review vaccine package inserts to determine storage requirements.

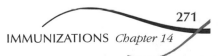

The Pharmacy Technician's Role

Depending on the situation in which a pharmacy technician is practicing, his or her responsibilities relating to vaccine administration may be as light as stocking the cotton balls or as rigorous as walking patients through the entire process. Pharmacy technicians are frequently called upon to do the following:

- Process the vaccine prescription
- Appropriately bill for both the cost of the vaccine and its administration
- Provide and assist patients with forms
- Maintain order during a vaccine clinic
- Ensure patient privacy
- Maintain overall workflow of the pharmacy during vaccine administration
- Process patient payment for vaccines administered
- Assist with documentation, faxing physicians and filling
- Assist in emergency situations (e.g., call 911, record activities of the pharmacist for future record and access and emergency kit)
- Ensure proper vaccine receipt and storage

An important role of pharmacy technicians that is often overlooked is that of an immunization advocate. Pharmacy technicians who understand the importance of vaccination, and begin asking patients about their vaccination status when interacting with them, can do a great public service by increasing the vaccinated population.

Immunization Resources

There are useful immunization resources that pharmacy technicians can access. The CDC is the authority on immunization practices in the United States and always has the most accurate and up-to-date information. They provide current immunization schedules, vaccine information sheets, vaccine storage guidelines and training, information on current controversies surrounding vaccines and much more. The CDC's immunization Web site is available at www.cdc.gov/vaccines. The IAC is an organization supported by the CDC that has many resources (e.g., screening questionnaires, sample standing orders and a supplies checklist) designed for vaccine providers. IAC's resources can be accessed at www.immunize.org. In addition to these national resources, many state health departments have immunization resources and information geared toward issues in a particular state.

Conclusion

Understanding the importance of vaccines, as well as the role that a pharmacy technician can play in immunization services, can help make any pharmacy-based vaccination program a success. In addition to this, it is important that pharmacy technicians have a basic understanding of vaccine-preventable disease and their vaccines. Finally, knowing how to appropriately store and manage vaccines is essential to protecting this fragile, and often expensive, pharmaceutical product. Pharmacy-based immunization programs are designed to increase vaccination rates in communities and function as an additional source of revenue for the pharmacy. Certified pharmacy technicians can help make both of these goals a reality.

References

1. Centers for Disease Control and Prevention, *Measles*, Epidemiology and Prevention of Vaccine-Preventable Diseases, Atkinson, W., Wolfe, S., Hamborsky, J., McIntyre, L., 11th edition, Public Health Foundation, Washington, D.C., 2009, pp. 157-176.

2. National Foundation for Infectious Diseases, Facts about adult immunization, www.nfid.org/pdf/factsheets/adultfact.pdf, July 9, 2010.

3. Centers for Disease Control and Prevention, *Influenza*, Epidemiology and Prevention of Vaccine-Preventable Diseases, Atkinson, W., Wolfe, S., Hamborsky, J., McIntyre, L., 11th edition Public Health Foundation, Washington, D.C., 2009, pp. 135-156.

4. Centers for Disease Control and Prevention, *Hepatitis A*, Epidemiology and Prevention of Vaccine-Preventable Diseases, Atkinson, W., Wolfe, S., Hamborsky, J., McIntyre, L., 11th edition, Public Health Foundation, Washington, D.C., 2009, pp. 85-98.

5. Centers for Disease Control and Prevention, *FDA Licensure of Quadrivalent Human Papillomavirus Vaccine (HPV4, Gardasil) for Use in Males and Guidance from the Advisory Committee on Immunization Practices (ACIP)*, MMWR, 2010, 59(20), pp. 630-632.

6. Centers for Disease Control and Prevention, *Poliomyelitis*, Epidemiology and Prevention of Vaccine-Preventable Diseases, Atkinson, W., Wolfe, S., Hamborsky, J., McIntyre, L., 11th edition, Public Health Foundation, Washington, D.C., 2009, pp. 231-244.

7. Centers for Disease Control and Prevention, *Pneumococcal Disease*, Epidemiology and Prevention of Vaccine-Preventable Diseases, Atkinson, W., Wolfe, S., Hamborsky, J., McIntyre, L., 11th edition, Public Health Foundation, Washington, D.C., 2009, pp. 217-230.

8. Centers for Disease Control and Prevention, *Diphtheria*, Epidemiology and Prevention of Vaccine-Preventable Diseases, Atkinson, W., Wolfe, S., Hamborsky, J., McIntyre, L., 11th edition, Public Health Foundation, Washington, D.C., 2009, pp. 59-70.

9. Centers for Disease Control and Prevention, *Pertussis*, Epidemiology and Prevention of Vaccine-Preventable Diseases, Atkinson, W., Wolfe, S., Hamborsky, J., McIntyre, L., 11th edition, Public Health Foundation, Washington, D.C., 2009, pp. 199-216.

10. Centers for Disease Control and Prevention, *Haemophilus influenzae type b*, Epidemiology and Prevention of Vaccine-Preventable Diseases, Atkinson, W., Wolfe, S., Hamborsky, J., McIntyre, L., 11th edition, Public Health Foundation, Washington, D.C., 2009, pp. 71-84.

11. Immunization Action Coalition, "Administering Vaccines: Dose, Route, Site and Needle Size," www.immunize.org/catg.d/p3085.pdf, July 7, 2010.

12. Centers for Disease Control and Prevention, Vaccine Management, www.cdc.gov/vaccines/pubs/pinkbook/downloads/appendices/C/storage-handling.pdf, July 9, 2010.

13. Centers for Disease Control and Prevention, *Importance of Maintaining the Cold Chain*, www.cdc.gov/vaccines/ed/shtoolkit/pages/cold_chain.pdf, July 9, 2010.

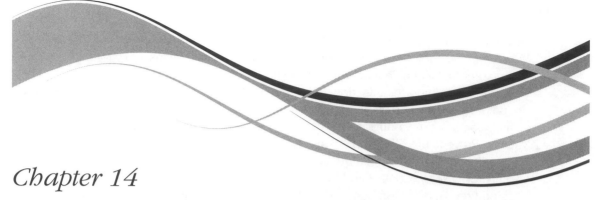

Chapter 14

REVIEW QUESTIONS

1. Which of the following is true?
    a. There are no longer outbreaks of vaccine-preventable diseases in the U.S.
    b. Vaccine-preventable diseases and their complications kill about 50,000 U.S. adults every year.
    c. There is no need to continue worldwide vaccination efforts.
    d. Some states still do not allow pharmacists to vaccinate.

2. Which of the following is not true about vaccines?
    a. Vaccines are considered medications.
    b. The active ingredient in a vaccine is called the antigen.
    c. Live vaccines must replicate in order to work.
    d. Many vaccines are 100 percent effective.

3. Local reactions following an intramuscular vaccine can include all of the following except:
    a. redness.
    b. swelling.
    c. anaphylaxis.
    d. muscle pain.

4. Which of the following are common symptoms of influenza?
    a. Severe cough and difficulty breathing
    b. Fever and body aches
    c. Vomiting and diarrhea
    d. Rigid muscles and sensitivity to light

5. Which of the following is not true about influenza vaccines?
    a. Because influenza viruses alter their surface antigens regularly, a new vaccine is necessary each year.
    b. Side effects of LAIV can include runny nose, congestion and cough.
    c. Influenza vaccination should begin as soon as the vaccine becomes available each year.
    d. Influenza vaccines should not be given to children under two years of age.

6. For which of the following vaccines is a booster dose recommended every 10 years?
   a. Pneumococcal polysaccharide (PPSV23)
   b. Tetanus and diphtheria (Td)
   c. Tetanus, diphtheria and pertussis (Tdap)
   d. Hepatitis B (HepB)

7. Which of the following is an inactivated vaccine?
   a. Human papillomavirus (HPV)
   b. Measles, mumps and rubella (MMR)
   c. Rotavirus (RV)
   d. Varicella (VAR)

8. Which of following must pharmacies always do when seeking vaccine reimbursement?
   a. Ensure they are reimbursed for both the cost of dispensing the vaccine and the cost of administering the vaccine
   b. Bill Medicare Part B for all vaccines administered to Medicare patients
   c. Provide a payment receipt only to those patients who paid an insurance copayment for their vaccine
   d. Charge all patients directly for vaccination services so that patients can seek reimbursement on their own

9. How often must the temperature on vaccine storage units be checked and recorded?
   a. Twice daily
   b. Twice daily for one month, then once weekly
   c. Once daily
   d. Once weekly

10. While participating in an immunization program, pharmacy technicians can do all of the following, except:
   a. assist patients with completing forms.
   b. process the vaccine prescription and collect payment.
   c. prescribe the vaccine to the patient.
   d. maintain refrigerator temperature logs.

Chapter 15

POISONINGS AND EMERGENCY MEDICINE

By Justin K. Rak, Pharm.D.
    Cherry Kwong, Pharm.D.

Learning Objectives

This chapter seeks to prepare a pharmacy technician to:
- explain the general supportive measures utilized in medication overdoses and poisonings.
- describe the different approaches used for gastrointestinal decontamination after a medication overdose or poisoning.
- recognize the signs and symptoms of medication overdoses covered in this chapter.
- identify antidotes available for the management of specific overdoses covered in this chapter.

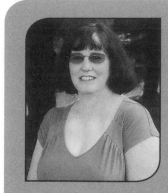

Introduction

A **poison** is any substance that when ingested, inhaled, injected or diffused through the skin causes harmful effects to the body in the amount (dose) that is absorbed into the body. Even a prescription or over-the-counter medication can act as a poison if taken or given in sufficient amount.[1,2] American Poison Control Centers reported approximately 2.5 million cases of human toxic substance exposures in 2009. This represented an increasing trend compared to previous years. Poisoning is one of the top 20 causes of death in the U.S., accounting for 36,204 deaths in 2007. Nearly 80 percent of fatal exposures were ingested orally, followed by inhalation and then parental (intravenous) injection. More than 80 percent of all the exposures were unintentional and related to medication misuse, such as accidental double-dosing, taking the wrong medication, taking an incorrect dosage, taking doses too frequently or using medications prescribed for another individual. Although most exposures can be managed at home, more serious cases may require medical attention and hospitalization.[1-3]

Analgesics rank as the No. 1 cause of poisoning deaths.[3,4] The majority of these cases originate from the misuse of acetaminophen and acetaminophen-based combination products, methadone and oxycodone. Following analgesics for causing poisoning deaths are cardiovascular medications, antidepressants, stimulants and street drugs. Table 1 shows the substances most frequently involved in adult exposures in 2009.[3]

Table 1

Substances Most Frequently Involved in Adult Overexposures in 2009[3]

Incidence	Substances
148,780	Analgesics
127,708	Sedative/Hypnotics/Antipsychotics
70,294	Antidepressants
69,924	Cleaning Substances (Household)
60,507	Cardiovascular Drugs
54,237	Alcohols
46,322	Bites and Envenomations
41,301	Pesticides
32,313	Anticonvulsants
31,571	Cosmetics/Personal Care Products

Supportive Care

Stabilization of the patient's airway, breathing and circulation, known as the "ABC," are the main components of initial supportive measures.[1,2,4] Maintaining breathing is essential for oxygenation and to prevent stomach contents from being inhaled into the lungs (aspiration). In some cases, intubation and mechanical ventilation may be required, especially in patients who are unresponsive or who have an altered mental status. Supplemental oxygen may also be necessary to provide an adequate level of oxygen saturation throughout the body, and IV fluids may be necessary to provide an adequate volume of circulating.[1,2] Unconscious patients are often given a combination of IV thiamine, dextrose and naloxone, referred to as the "coma cocktail." Each component in this recipe serves a unique purpose. Thiamine (Vitamin B_1) provides nutrients to the brain to prevent neurological complications resulting from being unconscious, especially in the case of alcohol overdose. Dextrose is given to reverse the effects of low blood glucose, while naloxone is used to reverse reduction in consciousness, breathing and blood pressure commonly seen in opioid overdose.[2,4] In the event of a seizure, anticonvulsants, such as lorazepam or diazepam, may be required while cardiopulmonary resuscitation (CPR) must be started immediately if vital signs are absent.[2]

Decontamination

Decontamination is the removal of a toxic substance from the body to prevent further exposure and damage.[1,2,4] As mentioned earlier, toxic substances can enter the body through the skin, eyes, mouth, lungs or injection into a vein. Skin decontamination includes the removal of contaminated clothing and cleaning of the exposed area with gentle soap and water. For eye exposures, the eye must be flushed with water, or use of an eye wash solution must be started immediately.[1,2] The majority of the toxic exposures occur orally; therefore, this section will focus on decontamination of the gastro-intestinal (GI) tract.[3]

■ Reducing Absorption

Syrup of ipecac irritates the GI lining and stimulates the nausea center in the brain to induce vomiting (**emesis**). It was once a widely used agent after toxic ingestion; however, with the risk of serious side effects, including esophageal tearing and aspiration, it is no longer recommended by most guidelines. It is considered if the patient is fully alert, able to maintain breathing and if it can be used within one hour of oral exposure. It is contraindicated in patients exposed to corrosives and petroleum products because emesis of these substances can lead to serious damage of the GI tract and lungs via aspiration. Ipecac is avoided in patients receiving antiemetic agents.[1,2,4] **Activated charcoal** is used most commonly for GI decontamination. It works by binding toxins to its surface; this prevents further absorption and allows removal of the toxins through the GI tract.[1,2,4] It is usually administered as a single dose. Repeated use of activated charcoal will further remove some toxic substances even after being absorbed, a method called multiple-dosed activated charcoal. Use of this method can cause charcoal aspiration, which may lead to pneumonia and other respiratory complications, especially in unconscious patients.[1,2] Although activated charcoal is well-tolerated and effective, substances such as potassium, iron, lithium and alcohols cannot be bound and thus cannot be removed with this method.[1,2,4]

Gastric lavage is a procedure that utilizes a large tube and pump system to flush out and remove the contents of a patient's stomach.[1,2,4] Water is poured continuously into the stomach through a tube that is inserted through the mouth. At the same time, the water is suctioned out until all stomach contents are removed.[1,2] It is best used within one hour of ingestion but may sometimes be used up to 12 hours after ingestion of a toxin.[1,2,4] Gastric lavage is commonly used for ferrous sulfate and lithium overdoses that cannot be removed by activated charcoal.[1,2]

Catharsis is a way to force bowel evacuation with the use of laxatives, such as magnesium citrate or sorbitol, to increase GI elimination of toxic substances.[1,2,4] It is often used with activated charcoal to speed up the removal of charcoal-bound toxins. Sorbitol is the preferred agent for catharsis because it has fewer side effects than other agents. A single dose is used with the first dose of activated charcoal to minimize adverse side effects such as diarrhea.[1,2]

Whole bowel irrigation is the complete cleansing of the bowel to push tablets or packages through the GI tract.[1,2,4] Osmotic laxatives, such as polyethylene glycol (Miralax®) and electrolyte solutions (Colyte®, Golytely®), are products available for this method.[1,2] Whole bowel irrigation can be a good option when patients have ingested extended-release products that cannot be removed by catharsis or activated charcoal.[1,2,4] This method may cause bowel inflammation and is not recommended in patients who have certain GI problems such as GI bleeding.[1,2]

■ Enhance Elimination

Few pharmacological methods are available to enhance elimination of toxins from the body. The fluid-loading method (forced diuresis) may be used to increase the patient's urine output, and hence eliminate toxins that are cleared by the kidneys. Alteration of the urine pH with sodium bicarbonate can also increase the removal of salicylates and phenobarbital. Hemodialysis, hemoperfusion or hemofiltration are methods that can be considered to remove toxins directly from the blood but are beyond the scope of this text.[1,2]

Common Medication Overdoses

Some of the common medication overdoses and their antidotes are matched in Table 2.[1,4,5] An **antidote** is a substance used to neutralize, or counteract, the damage caused by a specific toxin or favorably alter the toxic effects of the poison. Not all poisons have antidotes. In such cases, symptomatic management is employed.[1]

■ **Acetaminophen**

Acetaminophen (Tylenol®) is one of the most widely available and utilized drugs.[1,4,5] It is also the most common agent that leads to toxicity requiring hospitalization in the United States.[1,3-5] Many prescription and over-the-counter pain relievers and cough and cold products contain acetaminophen. Hence, it is easy for consumers to reach or exceed the maximum daily dose of 4,000 mg if they do not pay attention to the active ingredients in the products they are taking.[1,4] It is important for all patients, particularly those buying a medication for a child, to check the acetaminophen content. Normally, acetaminophen is metabolized to nontoxic metabolites through enzymes in the liver.[1,3] Acute overdose of acetaminophen can overwhelm these pathways; un-detoxified, reactive metabolites of acetaminophen can lead to severe and life-threatening liver injury. Chronic use of alcohol and/or seizure medications, malnutrition and HIV/AIDS patients are at a higher risk for acetaminophen toxic overdose due to a depletion of these liver enzymes.[1,4] Initial symptoms of overdose are usually delayed and include nausea, vomiting and abdominal pain. If untreated, it may progress to liver failure in three to 10 days.[1,4,5] When a patient presents within four hours of overdose, a single dose of activated charcoal is recommended.[1,5] N-acetylcysteine is the antidote for acetaminophen overdoses. It replenishes liver enzymes, which allows the proper metabolism of acetaminophen, and is effective when used up to 36 hours after the exposure. There are two formulations for N-acetylcysteine; it can be given orally in divided doses over 72 hours as Mucomyst® or IV over 21 hours as Acetadote®. It is dosed based on a patient's weight. The major side effects of using the oral formulation are nausea and/or vomiting that may require the use of an antiemetic. Oral administration is, therefore, avoided in patients with a GI bleed or a decreased level of consciousness. The IV formulation has a higher risk of allergic/anaphylactic reactions (hypotension, rash, wheezing and shortness of breath) and is typically reserved for patients unable to take or tolerate the oral formulation.[1,4,5]

■ **Opioids/Narcotics**

Narcotic analgesics act within the central nervous system (CNS) and have the potential for both dependence and abuse.[1] Mild to moderate overdoses can lead to low blood pressures, constipation, drowsiness and constricted (a.k.a. pinpoint) pupils. The patient may experience respiratory depression and coma if exposed to higher doses, and, in some cases, seizures may result from a narcotic overdose. Naloxone (Narcan®) injection is a short-acting antidote used to reverse narcotic toxicity.[1,4,5] It can be administered via IV push or as a continuous infusion. Naloxone generally begins to work in two minutes and then it lasts for a short period of time. Repeat doses may be necessary in overdoses with longer-acting narcotics or narcotics formulated as extended-release products.[1,5] When administering this antidote, close monitoring is needed due to the risk of precipitating withdrawal effects such as hypertension, sweating, agitation and irritability.[1,4,5]

■ **Benzodiazepines**

Benzodiazepines are used widely in the community, as well as the health-system, pharmacy setting. They have multiple therapeutic uses, such as sedation, insomnia, muscle relaxation, seizure control and anxiety but can cause significant central nervous system depression particularly at high doses. Symptoms of overdose may include extreme tiredness, slurred speech, muscle in-coordination, respiratory depression and coma induction. Flumazenil (Romazicon®) directly blocks benzodiazepine activity to prevent these actions.[1,4,5] Therefore, it is often used after surgery and overdose to reverse the sedative effects of benzodiazepines.[1,5] It has a very short duration of action, thus repeat dosing may be required.[1,4,5] Flumazenil is contraindicated in patients with a history of seizures, chronic benzodiazepine use and possible tricyclic antidepressant overdose as it may precipitate seizure activity in these patients. Side effects include precipitation of withdrawal effects, dizziness, sweating, headache and blurred vision.[1,4,5]

■ Digoxin

Digoxin (Lanoxin®) is used in heart failure and to regulate certain heart rhythms.[1,4,5] Patients who have reduced kidney function, who are elderly or have low blood potassium and magnesium levels have a greater risk for digoxin toxicity.[1,5] Symptoms of toxicity include confusion, fatigue, abdominal pain, color distortion, blurred vision, low heart rate, abnormal heart rhythm and high potassium levels. Laboratory digoxin levels can also support diagnosis. Digoxin Immune Fab (Digibind® or DigiFab®) are molecules used to bind digoxin.[1,4,5] Dosing is calculated either using the dose of digoxin ingested or using the digoxin level found in the blood.[1,5] Reversal of toxicity may lead to low blood potassium and the reappearance of the abnormal heart rhythm that was being controlled by digoxin.[1,4,5]

■ Iron

Most iron tablets are green or red in color and look very much like candy. This potential confusion for children may explain why it is the most common unintentional overdose in children.[4] Acute overdose of 10-20 mg/kg elemental iron mostly results in GI irritation.[1,4,5] More than 40 mg/kg may require hospitalization due to severe toxicity.[1,5] Symptoms of toxicity appear in stages. Victims will experience transient vomiting and diarrhea, followed by CNS and cardiovascular problems, bloody vomit and diarrhea. After a few days, progression to liver failure may occur; after a few weeks, progression to GI obstruction, or scarring, may occur.[1,4,5] Deferoxamine (Desferal®) binds to iron forming a stable compound.[1,5] Patients may experience a change in the color of their urine if deferoxamine is ever necessary for them. This reddish-orange color is a sign that the drug has bound to iron in the system and is helping to eliminate it from the body through the kidneys.[1,4] Reddish-orange urine color could also result while the stable complex is excreted through the kidney.[1,4] It is given through a slow infusion due to potential serious cardiac and skin side effects. Due to the possible development of acute respiratory distress syndrome (ARDS), deferoxamine is not used for more than 24 hours.[1,4,5]

Table 2
Common Medication Overdoses and Their Antidotes[1,4,5]

Overdoses**	Antidotes**
Acetaminophen (Tylenol)	N-acetylcysteine (Mucomyst, Acetadote)
Benzodiazepines	Flumazenil (Romazicon)
Digoxin (Lanoxin)	Digoxin Immune Fab (Digibind or DigiFab)
Iron salts (Feosol)	Deferoxamine (Desferal)
Opioid / Narcotics	Naloxone (Narcan)

**All rights to all brand names and trademarks are held by their respective owners.

Prevention

Since the incidence of toxic substance exposures is rising each year, it is more important than ever to prevent such events from occurring. Proper medication usage and limiting the access of children to medications and household poisons using child-proof containers and locks on cabinets containing household chemicals is incredibly important.

Conclusion

Since not all poisons and overdoses have an antidote, symptomatic management and rapid assessment by a poison control specialist, or medical personnel, are crucial in such cases.[1,2,4] If a poisoning is suspected, the local regional poison control center can be reached with the national toll-free number (800) 222-1222. These centers are staffed by trained nurses, pharmacists, physicians and pharmacologists, 24 hours each day, providing technical information to guide callers in the assessment and management of any poisoning or toxic ingestion.[1,2,4] It is recommended that everyone have this number programmed into their mobile phone and have it available at each pharmacy to direct patients to the proper help during an emergency.

Acknowledgement

The authors wish to acknowledge Susan C. Smolinske, Pharm.D., for her extensive contributions to this chapter in a previous edition of this Manual.

References

1. Chyka, P.A., Pharmacotherapy: A Pathophysiologic Approach, Clinical Toxicology, 6th edition. McGraw Hill, Chicago, IL, 2005, pp. 125-148.

2. Mokhlesi, B., Leiken, J.B., Murray, P., Corbridge, T.C., "Adult Toxicology in Critical Care: Part I: General Approach to the Intoxicated Patient," *Chest*, Northbrook, IN, Vol. 123, No. 2, pp. 577-592, February 2003.

3. Bronstein, A.C., et al., "2009 Annual Report of the American Association of Poison Control Centers, National Poison Data System (NPDS): 27th Annual Report," *Clinical Toxicology*, Vol. 48, No. 10, pp. 979-1178, December 2010.

4. Michigan Pharmacists Association, Pharmacy Certified Technician Training Manual, 11th edition, Lansing, MI, pp. 607-614, 2008.

5. Mokhlesi, B., Leiken, J.B., Murray, P., Corbridge, T.C., "Adult Toxicology in Critical Care: Part II: Specific Poisonings," *Chest*, Northbrook, IN, Vol. 123, No. 3, pp. 897-922, March 2003.

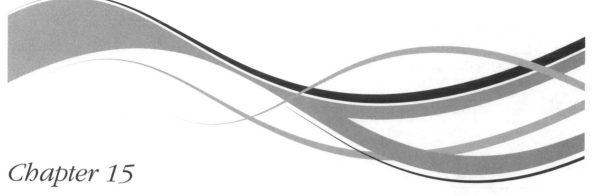

Chapter 15

REVIEW QUESTIONS

1. Which of the following is utilized as a supportive measure for a medication overdose or poisoning?
   a. Whole Bowel Irrigation
   b. Ipecac Syrup
   c. Stabilize airway, breathing and circulation
   d. N-acetylcysteine

2. Which of the following, though rarely used due to the risk of side effects, causes emesis and can be given for GI decontamination?
   a. Activated Charcoal
   b. Ipecac Syrup
   c. Whole Bowel Irrigation
   d. Laxative

3. What method is commonly used for GI decontamination in iron toxicity?
   a. Ipecac Syrup
   b. Whole Bowel Irrigation
   c. Activated Charcoal
   d. Gastric Lavage

4. Which of these decontamination methods enhances elimination?
   a. Hemodialysis
   b. Activated Charcoal
   c. Gastric Lavage
   d. Digibind®

5. Which of the following toxicities occurs most commonly in children?
   a. Acetaminophen
   b. Narcotics
   c. Iron
   d. Benzodiazepines

6. Liver damage can occur in later stages of toxicity with which of the following medications?
   a. Warfarin
   b. Benzodiazepines
   c. Digoxin
   d. Acetaminophen

7. Flumazenil is an antidote for which of the following medication overdoses?
   a. Benzodiazepines
   b. Narcotics
   c. Heparin
   d. Salicylates

8. Which of the following antidotes is used for narcotic toxicity?
   a. Digibind®
   b. Narcan®
   c. N-acetylcysteine
   d. Flumazenil

9. Why should deferoxamine be discontinued after 24 hours during treatment for iron poisoning?
   a. It is expensive
   b. It has a reduced effectiveness over time
   c. Acute respiratory distress syndrome may develop
   d. Another agent is better

10. What is the national, toll-free number for poison control centers?
    a. (800) 888-2888
    b. (800) 222-1222
    c. (800) 222-2222
    d. (800) 522-5225

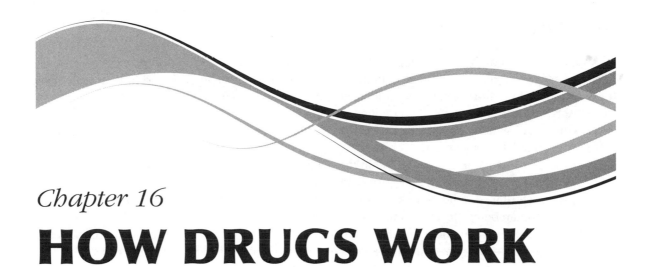

Chapter 16

HOW DRUGS WORK

By Tracey A. Okabe-Yamamura, Pharm.D.

Learning Objectives

This chapter seeks to prepare a pharmacy technician to:

- ■ describe the processes of absorption, distribution, metabolism and elimination of medications.
- ■ explain the differences between pharmacokinetics and pharmacodynamics.
- ■ describe age-related changes that affect drug action.

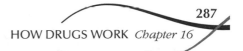

Introduction

One definition of the term "**drug**" is "a chemical substance used in the treatment, cure, prevention or diagnosis of disease."[1] Other definitions for the term "drug" can be found in pharmacy laws and regulations from the federal government and each state. For example, the Michigan Public Health Code (Act 368 of 1978, §333.17703) defines a drug as:

(a) a substance recognized or for which the standards or specifications are prescribed in the official compendium.

(b) a substance intended for use in the diagnosis, cure, mitigation, treatment, or prevention of disease in human beings or other animals.

(c) a substance, other than food, intended to affect the structure or a function of the body of human beings or other animals.

(d) a substance intended for use as a component of a substance specified in subdivision (a), (b), or (c), but not including a device or its components, parts, or accessories.[2]

Pharmacists are integrally involved in the appropriate use of drugs; thus, a thorough understanding of a drug's activity in the body is essential. This chapter will review the basic concepts of pharmacokinetics, pharmacodynamics and age-related changes that can affect drug therapy.

Overview

Drugs can be classified as prescription or nonprescription (e.g., over-the-counter or OTC). Nonprescription drugs can be sold directly to the consumer without a valid prescription written by a licensed provider such as a physician or dentist.

Each drug is generally described by three different names. The first is the **structural name** that describes the drug's molecular structure. The structural name is usually too technical and cumbersome for general use. The second name of a drug is its **generic name**, the official, chemical name of the drug that is not protected by patent or trademark. The third name is the **brand name** that identifies a specific product and is registered to a manufacturer holding the trademark on that name. Some popular drugs may even have a nickname used in advertising as a fourth name. Let's look at an example:

> **Brand name:** Prilosec®
> **Generic (chemical) name:** omeprazole
> **Structural name:** 5-methoxy-2-((4-methoxy-3,5-dimethylpyridin-2-yl)[3] methylsulfinyl)-1H benzo[d]imidazole

While a drug can have several brand names if it is manufactured by different manufacturers, a drug will have only one structural name and one generic name. A drug patent typically lasts 17 to 20 years, and during this time period, the original manufacturer has exclusive rights to produce the drug. Once this period expires, other manufacturers may apply to the Food and Drug Administration (FDA) to produce the drug.

Many generic and brand names of drugs can either look similar in spelling or sound similar when spoken. These drugs are called **"Look-Alike, Sound-Alike" drugs** or **LASA drugs**. An example is the pair of chemotherapy drugs, vincristine and vinblastine. There have been mix-ups between the two medications, and because the dosing differs between them, serious medication errors have resulted. Organizations such as the Institute for Safe Medication Practices (ISMP) have developed strategies to avoid such errors. Strategies include the following:

1. Using "tall man" lettering to distinguish the differences in the spelling of the two drugs (e.g., "vinCRIStine" and "vinBLAStine")
2. Physically separating the two drugs where they are stocked in the pharmacy or in other locations such as a nursing unit floor-stock in an automated dispensing cabinet
3. Using auxiliary labels or special stickers to identify the drugs more clearly
4. Educating all health care professionals and patients of the potential for errors in order to heighten awareness[4]

Pharmacokinetics and Pharmacodynamics

Clinical **pharmacokinetics** describes the processes of absorption, distribution, metabolism and elimination of drugs in the body.[5,6] It is the study of what the body does to the drug. In contrast, **pharmacodynamics** is the study of the relationship between the concentration of the drug in the body and the response, to the drug, from the body. It is the study of what the drug does to the body.[7] Refer to Figure 1.

Figure 1
Pharmacokinetics & Pharmacodynamics

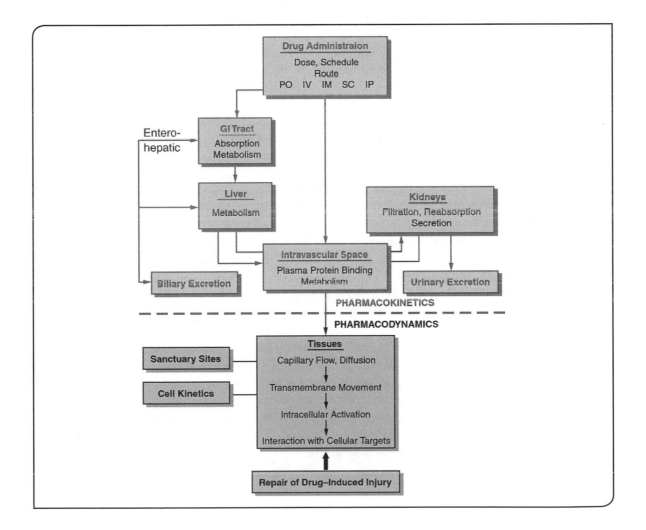

Pharmacokinetics

The four key processes of clinical pharmacokinetics are absorption, distribution, metabolism and elimination. In order for a drug to have its therapeutic effect, the drug must be moved from outside of the body into the body and then to the site of action. Pharmacokinetics is how the processes occurring to accomplish this biological feat are expressed. After a drug completes its action, it must be processed for removal (metabolized) and then eliminated from the body to complete the cycle.

■ Absorption

Absorption is the process that brings the drug from the site of administration into the body. There are several different ways to get a drug into the body (also called routes of administration). The most common routes of administration include the following (with common pharmacy abbreviations):

1. Oral (by mouth) – PO
2. Intravenous (through the vein) – IV
3. Intramuscular (through the muscle) – IM
4. Subcutaneous (under the skin) – SC or SQ
5. Sublingual (under the tongue) – SL
6. Rectal (through the rectum) – PR
7. Buccal (through the buccal cavity between the cheek and gum)
8. Transdermal (through the skin)
9. Inhalation (through the lungs)

Drugs are formulated into different entities (e.g., tablets, capsules, injections, patches) that are then administered using one or more of these routes of administration. **Parenteral solutions** of drugs can often be given IV, IM or SC. There may be situations where an oral drug can be given sublingually; if the patient cannot swallow tablets or capsules and an oral liquid preparation is not available, or if faster absorption than what is achieved by swallowing a tablet is required, a sublingual tablet may be used.

Except for IV administration, all other routes require that the drug is first absorbed into the systemic (blood) circulation. Oral drugs must be swallowed, dissolved and then absorbed through the gastrointestinal (GI) system (or GI tract). The absorption of drugs is almost always faster from the small intestine than from in the stomach. Like most things absorbed from the intestines, orally-administered drugs go straight to the liver in a process called the **first-pass effect**.[8] Due to the first-pass effect, some metabolism of the drug may occur before it ever reaches the systemic circulation or where it must go to exert its effect. **Bioavailability** is the term used to describe the amount of the drug that reaches the systemic circulation unchanged. Assessment of bioavailability from concentration-time data usually involves determining the maximum (peak) drug concentration, the time at which maximum drug concentration occurs (peak time) and the area under the concentration-time curve (AUC), as indicated in Figure 2. Ideally, 100 percent of a drug would reach the systemic circulation; however, there are many factors that can reduce a drug's bioavailability. Drugs that are not **water soluble** (do not dissolve in water) will be less likely to be absorbed from the GI tract. Further, as previously mentioned, the first-pass effect may lower the amount of drug that reaches the systemic circulation.[8] Other factors that affect bioavailability include age, sex, regularity of physical activity, other drugs and genetics (see Figure 2).[9]

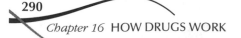

Figure 2
Drug Bioavailability Concentration-Time Curve

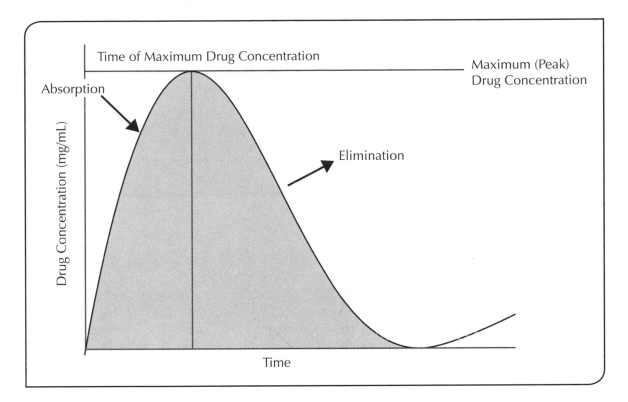

■ Distribution

The process of drug **distribution** moves the drug from the systemic circulation to the area where it will exert its pharmacologic effect.[10] Drugs, generally, do not distribute evenly throughout the body. Factors that can affect the distribution of drugs include: blood flow to an area (i.e., **perfusion**), **pH** of an area, permeability of the cell membranes in an area, and the affinity of a drug to bind to a specific tissue.

Distribution from the blood to other tissues occurs more easily when a tissue is highly vascular (has a high perfusion) because more blood circulating to a particular tissues will more quickly deliver more drug to the area. Some drugs will stay in the watery tissues of the blood or muscles, while other drugs may accumulate in specific organs such as the liver. The volume of distribution is a value used to describe how well a drug distributes throughout the body; using how much drug is administered and how much of the drug is found in the plasma (a part of blood), the volume of distribution can be calculated. Some drugs will bind to proteins in the blood, e.g. albumin, to varying degrees; the level of protein binding affects the amount of drug that is available to be distributed to tissues other than the blood and therefore exert a pharmacologic effect. Bound drug is kept in the systemic circulation, while unbound drug is available for distribution. For example, if the protein binding of a drug is 90 percent, then only 10 percent of the drug is free to exert its effect.

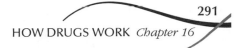

■ Metabolism

Metabolism is the process that prepares the drug for elimination. The liver is the primary organ responsible for metabolism. There are several enzyme systems within the body that change a drug into molecules, called **metabolites**, better suited for elimination. These enzyme systems use processes such as **oxidation**, **conjugation**, **hydrolysis** and **reduction**, to accomplish this event. Metabolites can be active or inactive; active metabolites are those metabolites that exert their own pharmacologic effect. This pharmacologic effect may be the same or completely different from the effects of the original drug (e.g., the opioid meperidine is given for pain relief and is metabolized into the active metabolite normeperidine, which has less analgesic effect. Normeperidine can be toxic to the central nervous system (brain), causing hyper-excitability and seizures.

One of the most important enzyme systems in Phase I metabolism is the cytochrome-P (CYP) 450 system. The primary role of the CYP-450 system is the oxidative metabolism of many drugs. There is a high concentration of CYP-450 enzymes in the liver and small intestine. There are more than 30 human CYP-450 isoenzyme systems that have been identified. The major isoenzymes used in drug metabolism are CYP3A4-7, CYP1A2, CYP2A6, CYP2B6, CYP2C8-9, CYP2C18-19, CYP2D6 and CYP2E1. The CYP-450 system, especially while working on a drug, can either induce or inhibit the metabolism of other drugs. These changes to normal drug metabolism can result in significant drug interactions; the identification of these interactions is essential to proper use of the involved drugs. Many times, for such interactions, a pharmacist is called upon to modify the administered dose of one or both of the drugs in the interaction in order to achieve the blood-level and effect required for each drug, while minimizing the harmful effects of the interaction.

In Phase II metabolism, glucuronidation is the most common pathway; glucuronidation occurs only in the liver. Glucuronides are excreted into the bile. They break down drugs into water-soluble metabolites that can then be excreted by the kidneys in the urine. Glucuronidation is not directly affected by age; however, this process can be immature in a newborn (therefore, some drugs that require glucuronidation may not be usable in newborns).

■ Elimination

Elimination is the final step of the process that takes the drug out of the body. Most elimination occurs through the kidneys and into the urine. Renal (kidney) function is an important monitoring element when dosing medications; changes in renal function can affect how quickly a drug will be eliminated from the body. Renal function is monitored by measuring or estimating **glomerular filtration rate (GFR)** or **creatinine clearance (CrCl)**. The **Cockcroft-Gault equation** is one commonly-used method by pharmacists for estimating CrCl:

$$\text{CrCl (mL/min)} = \frac{(140 - \text{age}) \times \text{Weight} (\times\, 0.85 \text{ if female})}{(72 \times \text{SCr})}$$

CrCl = Creatinine clearance (estimated) in milliliters/minute (mL/min)
Age = The patient's age in whole years
Weight = The patient's weight in kilograms (kg)
SCr = The patient's blood level of creatinine (in mg/dL)

Some drugs may be eliminated via the **biliary system**. Changes in a patient's liver function can alter drugs eliminated by this route. Liver function may be measured in a variety of ways; most commonly a blood test is done to measure a patient's alanine transaminase (ALT) and aspartate transaminase (AST) levels, which are indicators of liver function.

Pharmacodynamics

Pharmacodynamics is the study of what a drug does to the body. In the majority of cases, the pharmacologic effect of the drug will depend on its binding to target receptor. The concentration of drug at the target site will influence how much of a response the body will have to the drug. There are, however, examples of drugs that participate in a chemical reaction that affect the body without binding to a target receptor. An example of such a chemical reaction is when an acid and a base cancel each other out to produce a neutral solution; specifically, this is seen when antacids (bases) are given to neutralize stomach acids.

■ Effects of Aging

As people age, there is a natural physiologic deterioration of the body's functions.[11] Nearly all organ systems will be slower in an elderly patient when compared to a younger adult patient.

Metabolism and elimination are generally slower in the elderly. A pharmacist can use this knowledge to properly adjust a drug's dose, frequency of dosing or both to minimize unwanted side effects. There is a progressive reduction in blood flow through the liver as we age;[11] this reduction in blood flow contributes to a reduction in first-pass metabolism. Renal function also declines as a person ages.

In terms of pharmacodynamics, changes in drug sensitivity can occur as a patient ages, but the effect is not always consistent from drug to drug. There can also be changes in drug-receptor interactions that occur over time. Elderly patients tend to be more sensitive than their younger adult counterparts to particular drug classes (e.g., drugs with anticholinergic effects). This class of medications includes tricyclic antidepressants, nonselective antihistamines and some antipsychotic drugs. Anticholinergic effects can include constipation, urinary retention, blurred vision, orthostatic hypotension and dry mouth. The elderly are also more sensitive to drugs that affect the central nervous system, such as opiate analgesics that may cause more drowsiness and confusion.

Drug-related problems in the elderly can be the result of:
- an inappropriate drug due to dose, route or frequency of administration
- duplicate medications (multiple drugs used for the same indication).
- a lack of recognition of drug-drug interactions.
- a lack of appropriate monitoring.
- under-treatment or over-treatment of a particular disease.[9]

■ Adverse Events and Toxicities

Adverse events can be defined as unintended effects that occur when a drug is given.[10] The term "adverse event" encompasses both side effects and toxicities. A **side effect** occurs as an unavoidable condition of the drug. An example of a side effect is sedation (drowsiness) from an opioid analgesic or dry mouth caused by an anticholinergic drug. **Toxicities** occur when a drug's plasma concentration is higher than the recommended level. Toxicities are often more troublesome than side effects because they are often harmful to the body rather than annoying like most side effects. An example of a toxicity is the renal damage that can be caused by the aminoglycoside antibiotics (e.g., gentamicin and tobramycin) if the blood level of such a drug is allowed to remain too high.

Many drugs are monitored by measuring the drug's plasma concentration (e.g., aminoglycoside antibiotics, vancomycin, digoxin, theophylline and lithium). To realize the therapeutic benefits of a drug, while avoiding its toxicities, requires the plasma concentration of the drug to remain within the drug's therapeutic window, or therapeutic index. The **therapeutic window** gives the range of plasma concentrations that will generally provide therapeutic benefit and avoid toxicity. It should be noted that some patients may experience toxicity while their plasma concentration for a drug is still within the therapeutic window. Pharmacists, and the pharmacy technicians assisting them, must remember to treat patients based on their symptoms and appearance rather than solely based on their lab value (see Figure 3.)

Figure 3
Therapeutic Window Range

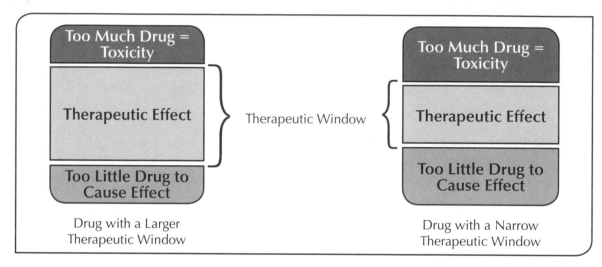

Too Much Drug = Toxicity

Therapeutic Effect

Too Little Drug to Cause Effect

Drug with a Larger Therapeutic Window

Therapeutic Window

Too Much Drug = Toxicity

Therapeutic Effect

Too Little Drug to Cause Effect

Drug with a Narrow Therapeutic Window

■ **Drug Interactions**

When two or more drugs are administered at the same time, there is always the potential that an interaction may occur between the drugs. If two drugs have the same effect, the actions can be additive or synergistic. An **additive effect** occurs when two or more drugs interact to produce a combined effect that is the sum of the individual drugs alone. A **synergistic effect** is when the combined effect of the two drugs together is greater than the sum of the individual drugs alone. Drug interactions can also be antagonistic where the interaction reduces the effectiveness of one or more of the interacting drugs. For example, one drug can stimulate the CYP-450 system and, in doing so, increase the metabolism of a second drug. Since the metabolism of the second drug is increased, there will be less drug available to exert a therapeutic effect.

Additive 1+1=2
Synergism 1+1 >2

Conclusion

Medication therapy is affected by both a drug's pharmacokinetic and pharmacodynamic properties. Understanding how both a patient's body will likely affect each of their drugs and how each of those drugs could affect the patient, a pharmacist, assisted by a pharmacy technician, can help design a drug therapy regimen that can be therapeutic and minimize the patient's experience of side effects and toxicities.

References

1. Dictionary.com, www.dictionary.com, July 23, 2010.
2. Michigan Legislature, www.legislature.mi.gov, July 24, 2010.
3. Drug Bank, www.drugbank.ca/drugs, July 31, 2010.
4. Institute for Safe Medication Practices, www.ismp.org, Aug. 2, 2010.
5. Diasio, R.B., Principles of Drug Therapy, and Goldman, L. and Ausiello, D., Cecil Medicine, Saunders Elsevier, Philadelphia, PA, 2007, www.mdconsult.com, July 23, 2010.
6. Neely, M.N. and Reed, M.D., Pharmacokinetic-Pharmacodynamic Basis of Optimal Antibiotic Therapy, and Long, S.S., Principles and Practice of Pediatric Infectious Diseases, Churchill Livingston, 2008, www.mdconsult.com, July 24, 2010.
7. Shriner, L.B. and Steimer, J.L., "Pharmacokinetic/Pharmacodynamic Modeling in Drug Development," *Annual Review of Pharmacology and Toxicology*, Vol. 40, pp. 67-95, 2000.
8. Kwan, K.C., "Oral Bioavailability and First Pass Effects," *Drug Metabolism and Disposition*, Vol. 25, pp. 1329-1336, December 1997.
9. The Joint Commission, www.jointcommission.org, Aug. 3, 2010.
10. The Merck Manual for Healthcare Professionals, www.merck.comm/mmpe, Aug. 1, 2010.
11. Mangoni, A.A. and Jackson, S.H.D., "Age-related Changes in Pharmacokinetics and Pharmacodynamics: Basic Principles and Practical Applications," *British Journal of Clinical Pharmacology*, London, Vol. 57, pp. 6-14, 2003.

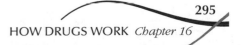

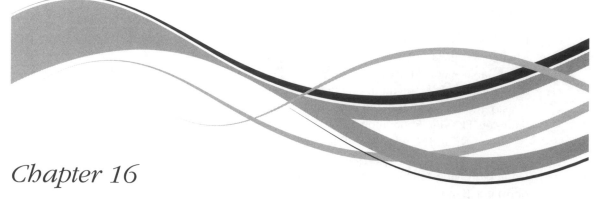

Chapter 16

REVIEW QUESTIONS

1. The processes of absorption, distribution, metabolism and elimination describe which of the following?
    a. Pharmacodynamics
    b. Elimination
    c. Pharmacokinetics
    d. Pharmacogenomics

2. Pharmacodynamics is:
    a. the quantitative aspects of elements of drug disposition: absorption, distribution, metabolism and elimination.
    b. not only what the drug does to the body but also where the drug works and how the drug works.
    c. when the drug dose exceeds the recommended range, when therapy exceeds the recommended duration or if a drug is not monitored properly.
    d. when a drug lacking effect of its own increases the effect of a second, active drug.

3. The amount of drug that reaches the systemic circulation unchanged is its:
    a. first-pass effect.
    b. maximum concentration.
    c. bioavailability.
    d. elimination rate.

4. Which drug will not undergo the first-pass effect when administered as specified?
    a. Acetaminophen 650 mg oral tablets
    b. Omeprazole 20 mg capsule
    c. Ceftriaxone 250 mg IV piggyback
    d. None of the above

5. The process that takes the drug out of the body is which of the following?
    a. Absorption
    b. Distribution
    c. Metabolism
    d. Elimination

6. The Cytochrome P-450 enzyme system is:
    a. an oxidative system of Phase I metabolism.
    b. an oxidative system of Phase II metabolism.
    c. a glucuronidation system of Phase I metabolism.
    d. a conjugation system of Phase II metabolism.

7. What is the major organ for elimination?
    a. Liver
    b. Kidneys
    c. Small intestine
    d. Lungs

8. Which of the following is an example of a side effect?
    a. Renal failure from tobramycin overdose
    b. Seizures from meperidine overdose
    c. Sedation from morphine
    d. Liver failure from acetaminophen overdose

9. When two or more drugs combine to provide a response that is greater than the sum of the individual drugs, it is called:
    a. an additive effect.
    b. synergism.
    c. antagonism.
    d. absorption.

10. Drugs that are not water soluble:
    a. do not dissolve in water.
    b. cannot be taken with water.
    c. are more likely to be absorbed from the GI tract.
    d. have a greater likelihood of being absorbed if formulated as a tablet.

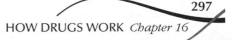

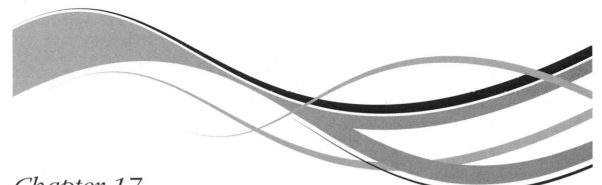

Chapter 17

DRUGS AND DRUG NAMES

By   Derek J. Quinn, Pharm.D.

Learning Objectives

This chapter seeks to prepare a pharmacy technician to:

- discuss the three different names for a drug and when the use of each name is appropriate.
- identify the parts of a National Drug Code (NDC).
- discuss the anatomy of the label used on commercially-prepared prescription medication stock bottles.
- be familiar with the brand name, generic name and common use for roughly 200 drugs.

Introduction

Throughout the world, different names are given to the same drug. Further, within each country, most drugs have at least three names—its structural name, brand (or trade) name and generic (or chemical) name. Since all three names describe the same chemical, they are generally interchangeable; however, there are circumstances where one of the three names is most appropriate to use. Since the choice of a name, specifically the brand name, falls to the pharmaceutical companies, this chapter will also discuss the requirements of a pharmaceutical company on labeling a drug being brought to market.

Structural Name

Every drug has a name that describes the chemical structure of the drug. Generally, this name is used only by researchers and chemists who are interested in the exact structure of the molecule. There are very few, if any, uses for this name in everyday practice. This name can always be found in the full prescribing information provided by the manufacturer if the need ever arises to reference this name. The **structural name** can generally be identified as the very long descriptive name listed directly above or below the drawing of the chemical structure in the full prescribing information provided by the manufacturer. For instance, the structural name of atorvastatin (Lipitor®) is: [R-(R*, R*)]-7-[2-(4-Fluorophenyl)-5-(1-methylethyl)-3-phenyl-4-(phenylaminocarbonyl)-1H-pyrrol-1-yl]-3,5-dihydroxyheptanoic acid calcium salt.[1] Based on that one structural name, it is easy to see why this name is generally not used in practice and is rarely included on lists of drug names.

Chemical (Generic) Name

Each drug is assigned a **chemical name** that describes the function (or class) that the drug fits into. This is the name that the drug will generally be known as, and this name is generally universal throughout the world. This name is often called the **generic name** because that is the name that the drug will go by when generic equivalents are released into the market. Each drug is assigned its chemical name before the original brand makes it to market and can be found on every drug product's packaging. An example of a chemical name is atorvastatin (the chemical name for Lipitor®). Although not every drug that ends in "statin" is used to lower cholesterol, there is a common theme that drugs in the class known as "HMG-CoA Reductase Inhibitors" are given a chemical name that ends in "statin." Thus, the class bears the nickname "the statins." This happens commonly with drug names to assist in keeping the drugs separated into their classes.

Brand (Trade) Name

The manufacturer who discovers and markets a drug is permitted to give that chemical a marketing name—something catchy that will help the company market that drug to health care providers and patients. This is known as the **brand or trade name,** as it is the brand identity for a drug. Because drugs, upon first release, are only available as a brand name drug, providers and patients become familiar with the brand name and will often continue to call the drug by its brand name forever (even after generic equivalents of the drug become available). Further, the brand name can be different in every country of the world if the manufacturer believes that it can be better marketed under a different name. An example of a brand name is Lipitor®.

In some cases, multiple companies seek to market a drug as the first manufacturer and present their applications to the Food and Drug Administration (FDA) at the same time. In these instances, there sometimes is cause for the FDA to allow both manufacturers to bring the drug to market at the same time with both being considered a brand name. One such example is the blood pressure lowering drug lisinopril. Lisinopril, though generically available from many manufacturers, is marketed under both the brand name Prinivil® and the brand name Zestril®. Patients who request to use "the original brand" must specify which original brand they wish to use if the drug is lisinopril. Also, the drug company that discovers a drug may not be the company that ultimately markets and sells the drug. Further, the original manufacturer of a brand name drug may sell the rights to that brand name to another company that may produce the drug in exactly the same way or may reformulate the inactive ingredients. Either way, the new company may use the brand name in its marketing of the product.

Anatomy of a National Drug Code

The FDA requires that each drug licensed for use in the United States be assigned a unique NDC. The NDC constitutes three important pieces of information: the manufacturer, the drug and strength, and the package size. For example, Lipitor® 10 mg tablets packaged in a 90-count bottle have the NDC: 00071-0155-23.[1] The first set of digits identify the manufacturer; in this case, 00071 corresponds to Pfizer. The 0155 identifies that "drug #155" at Pfizer is 10 mg Lipitor®. Finally, the 23 is the code that Pfizer has chosen to identify the 90-count package; note that Lipitor® 10 mg tablets also come in a 5,000-count bottle and has the NDC: 00071-0155-34.[1] The NDC for the 5,000-count bottle differs from the 90-count bottle only in the final two digits, which represent the package size. Although common NDC for packages used in a pharmacy may become familiar to a pharmacy technician, it is important to verify that the NDC on the package matches the NDC requested on the prescription label for every fill in order to minimize the chance for a dispensing error.

Anatomy of a Manufacturer's Drug Package Label[2]

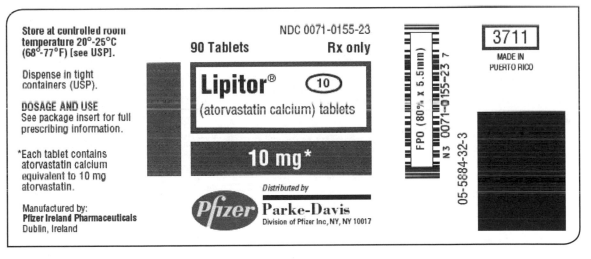

Although every label is different, there are some commonalities, including the following:[2]

1. **Storage Information**
   Lipitor® must be stored between 20-25° C.

2. **Location of Manufacturer**
   This package of Lipitor® was made in Dublin, Ireland.

3. **Manufacturer**
   Lipitor® is made by Pfizer.

4. **NDC**
   0071-0155-23. The NDC is not required to be on the package.

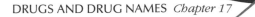

5. **Rx Only**

   This is generally required for prescription drugs marketed in the United States.

6. **Package Size**

   90

7. **Generic / Chemical and Brand / Trade Names**

   Lipitor® (atorvastatin calcium)

8. **Dosage Form**

   Tablets

9. **Strength**

   10 mg

10. **Barcode**

    This barcode corresponds to the NDC.

11. **Lot Number and Expiration Date**

    Where the black box in the right-hand bottom corner is in the example above, the lot number (or control number) and expiration date would be stamped or printed.

Top 200 Generic Drugs

Every year, *Drug Topics* magazine publishes a series of "Top 200" lists that examine the top brand name drugs and generic drugs either based on dollar value dispensed or in units dispensed. The following list uses the *Drug Topics* top 200 generic drugs of 2010, based on units dispensed, and also provides at least one brand name (some drugs are marketed under multiple brand names) and at least one common **indication** (though there may be many more reasons to use each of these drugs). When many brand names exist, an "et al." will end the list of brand names to indicate that there are others not listed here. This list is not intended to be memorized; however, since it is expected that a pharmacy technician can freely convert between brand and generic names for drugs (as well as list at least one use for each drug), this list will hopefully serve as an initial exposure to these commonly used drugs.

Table 1
Top 200 Generic Drugs

Rank[3]	Generic Name[3]	Brand Name(s)[4**]	Indication
1	Hydrocodone / APAP	Vicodin, Lortab, Norco	Pain
2	Metoprolol Succinate	Toprol XL	High Blood Pressure
3	Oxycodone	OxyIIR	Pain
4	Pantoprazole	Protonix	Acid Reflux
5	Omeprazole	Prilosec	Acid Reflux
6	Simvastatin	Zocor	High Cholesterol
7	Amphetamine Salt Combo SR	Adderall XR	Attention Deficit Disorder
8	Fentanyl Transdermal	Duragesic	Pain
9	Azithromycin	Zithromax	Bacterial Infections
10	Valacyclovir HCl	Valtrex	Viral Infections
11	Venlafaxine ER	Effexor	Depression
12	Fexofenadine	Allegra	Allergies
13	Gabapentin	Neurontin	Nerve Pain
14	Oxycodone / APAP	Percocet	Pain
15	Lisinopril	Zestril, Prinivil	High Blood Pressure
16	Amlodipine Besylate / Benazepril	Lotrel	High Blood Pressure
17	Lansoprazole	Prevacid	Acid Reflux
18	Levothyroxine	Synthroid	Thyroid Disorder
19	Amoxicillin / Potassium Clavulanate	Augmentin	Bacterial Infections
20	Amlodipine Besylate	Norvasc	High Blood Pressure
21	Fluticasone (Nasal Spray)	Flonase	Allergies
22	Alprazolam	Xanax	Anxiety
23	Tamsulosin HCl	Flomax	Benign Prostatic Hyperplasia
24	Budesonide	Bumex	Fluid Retention
25	Metformin	Glucophage	Diabetes
26	Sertraline	Zoloft	Depression
27	Bupropion XL	Wellbutrin XL	Depression
28	Cefdinir	Omnicef	Bacterial Infections
29	Losartan Potassium	Cozaar	Hypertension
30	Risperidone	Risperal	Psychosis

Table 1 *cont.*

Top 200 Generic Drugs

Rank[3]	Generic Name[3]	Brand Name(s)[4**]	Indication
31	Pravastatin	Pravachol	High Cholesterol
32	Amoxicillin	Amoxil	Bacterial Infections
33	Divalproex Sodium	Depakote	Seizures
34	Claravis	Accutane	Severe Acne
35	Fluoxetine	Prozac	Depression
36	Zolpidem Tartrate	Ambien	Sleep
37	Lamotrigine	Lamictal	Seizures
38	Topiramate	Topamax	Seizures
39	Lovastatin	Mevacor	High Cholesterol
40	Diltiazem CD	Cardizem, Diltzac, Tiazac	High Blood Pressure
41	Tramadol	Ultram	Pain
42	Levetiracetam	Keppra	Seizures
43	Lisinopril / Hydrochlorothiazide	Prinzide, Zestoretic	High Blood Pressure
44	Citalopram HBr	Celexa	Depression
45	Lorazepam	Ativan	Anxiety
46	Warfarin	Coumadin	Blood Clots
47	Losartan Potassium / Hydrochlorothiazide	Hyzaar	High Blood Pressure
48	Ocella	Yasmin	Birth Control (Oral)
49	Clonazepam	Klonopin	Anxiety, Muscle Spasms
50	Alendronate	Fosamax	Low Bone Density
51	Hydrochlorothiazide	HydroDiuril	High Blood Pressure
52	Sumatriptan (Tablets)	Imitrex	Migraines
53	Pramipexole Dihydroc	Mirapex	Parkinson's Disease
54	Carvedilol	Coreg	High Blood Pressure
55	Fentanyl Citrate	Actiq	Pain
56	Amphetamine Salt Combo	Adderall	Attention Deficit Disorder
57	Budeprion XL	Wellbutrin XL	Depression
58	Metoprolol Tartrate	Lopressor	High Blood Pressure
59	Atenolol	Tenormin	High Blood Pressure
60	Enoxaparin Sodium	Lovenox	Deep Vein Thrombosis
61	Fenofibrate	Lofibra	High Triglycerides
62	Paroxetine	Paxil	Depression
63	Cephalexin	Keflex	Bacterial Infections

Rank[3]	Generic Name[3]	Brand Name(s)[4]**	Indication
64	Finasteride	Proscar, Propecia	Enlarging Prostate / Hair Loss
65	Metaxalone	Skelaxin	Muscle Spams
66	Imiquimod	Aldara	Actinic Keratosis, Warts
67	Tacrolimus	Prograf	Organ Transplant Rejection
68	Cyclobenzaprine	Flexeril	Muscle Spasms
69	Oxcarbazepine	Trileptal	Seizures
70	Furosemide Oral	Lasix	Fluid Retention
71	Endocet	Percocet	Pain
72	Buproprion SR	Wellbutrin SR	Depression
73	Ondansetron	Zofran	Nausea
74	Nifedipine ER	Procardia XL, Adalat CC	High Blood Pressure
75	Ibuprofen	Motrin	Inflammation
76	Albuterol (Nebulizer Solution)	Proventil	Trouble Breathing
77	Carisoprodol	Soma	Muscle Spasms
78	Oxycodone HCl CR	Oxycontin	Pain
79	Fexodenadine / Pseudo	Allegra	Allergies
80	Oxybutynin Chloride ER	Ditropan XL	Over-Active Bladder
81	Ranitidine HCl	Zantac	Acid Reflux
82	Famciclovir	Famvir	Cold Sores
83	Ciprofloxacin HCl	Cipro	Bacterial Infections
84	Morphine Sulfate ER	MSContin	Pain
85	Clonidine	Catapres	High Blood Pressure
86	Potassium Chloride ER	K-Dur, Klor-Con	Low Potassium
87	Propoxyphene-N / Acetaminophen	Darvocet N	Pain
88	Meloxicam	Mobic	Inflammation
89	Klor-Con	Klor Con	Low Potassium
90	Ramipril	Altace	High Blood Pressure
91	Phentermine	Ionamin, Pro-Fast HS, Adipex P	Attention Deficit Disorder, Obesity
92	Venlafaxine	Effexor	Depression
93	Trimethoprim / Sulfametoxazole	Bactrim, Sulfatrim, Septra	Bacterial Infections
94	Gianvi	Yaz	Birth Control
95	Spironolactone	Aldactone	Fluid Retention
96	Temazepam	Restoril	Insomnia
97	Trazodone HCl	Desyrel	Insomnia

Table 1 *cont.*
Top 200 Generic Drugs

Rank[3]	Generic Name[3]	Brand Name(s)[4**]	Indication
98	Dorzolamide HCl / Timolol	Cosopt	Glaucoma
99	Potassium Chloride	Not Available	Low Potassium
100	Mycophenolate Mofetil	Cellept, Myfortic	Organ Transplant Rejection
101	Diclofenac Sodium SR	Voltaren	Inflammation
102	Prednisone Oral	Deltasone	Inflammation
103	Triamterene / Hydrochlorothiazide	Dayzide, Maxzide	High Blood Pressure
104	Buproprion ER	Wellbutrin SR or XL	Depression
105	Naproxen	Naprosyn	Inflammation
106	Verapamil SR	Calan SR	High Blood Pressure
107	Polyethylene Glycol	Miralax	Constipation
108	Hydroxyzine	Atarax, Vistaril	Itching
109	Diazepam	Valium	Anxiety
110	Clindamycin (Capsules)	Cleocin	Bacterial Infections
111	Isosorbide Mononitrate	ISMO, ImDur, Monoket	Chest Pain
112	Ropinirole HCl	Requip	Parkinson's Disease
113	Acetaminophen / Codeine	Tylenol with Codeine	Pain
114	Paroxetine SR	Paxil CR	Depression
115	Felodipine ER	Plendil ER	High Blood Pressure
116	Fluconazole	Diflucan	Fungal Infections
117	Clobetasol	Temovate	Skin Inflammation
118	Enalapril	Vasotec	High Blood Pressure
119	Metformin HCl ER	Glucophage	Diabetes
120	Promethazine Tablets	Phenergan	Nausea
121	Gemfibrozil	Lopid	High Triglycerides
122	Glyburide	Glucovance	Diabetes
123	Tri-Sprintec	Tri-Sprintec, Ortho-Cyclen	Birth Control
124	Clozapine	Clozaril	Psychosis
125	Nabumetone	Relafen	Inflammation
126	Dronabinol	Marinol	Loss of Appetite
127	Glimepiride	Amaryl	Diabetes
128	Morphine Sulfate CR	MSContin	Pain
129	Mirtazapine	Remeron	Depression
130	Mupirocin	Bactroban	Bacterial Infections

Rank[3]	Generic Name[3]	Brand Name(s)[4]**	Indication
131	Doxycycline	Vibramycin, Adoxa, Vibra-Tabs, Periostat	Bacterial Infections
132	Methadone HCl	Dolophine	Pain
133	Minocycline	Minocin	Bacterial Infections
134	Desoximetasone	Topicort	Skin Inflammation
135	Methylprednislone	Medrol	Inflammation
136	Albuterol Sulfate / Ipratropium	DuoNeb	Trouble Breathing
137	Allopurinol	Zyloprim	Gout
138	Busipirone HCl	Buspar	Anxiety
139	Desmopressin Acetate	DDAVP	Bedwetting
140	Tobramycin / Dexamethasone	Tobradex	Bacterial Eye Infections
141	Tretinoin	Retin-A	Acne
142	Tramadol HCl / Acetaminophen	Ultracet	Pain
143	Phenytoin Sodium ER	Dilantin	Seizures
144	Tizanidine HCl	Zanaflex	Muscle Spasms
145	Acyclovir	Zovirax	Viral Infections
146	Clarithromycin	Biaxin	Bacterial Infections
147	Amitriptyline	Elavil	Insomnia
148	Nitrofmtoin Monohydrate Macrocrystals	Macrobid	Bacterial Infection
149	Glyburide / Metformin HCl	Glucovance	Diabetes
150	Carbidopa / Levodopa	Sinemet	Parkinson's Disease
151	Hydralazine	Apresoline	High Blood Pressure
152	Sumatripta (Stat Refill)	Imitrex	Migraines
153	Benazepril	Lotensin	High Blood Pressure
154	Calcium Acetate	PhosLo	Kidney Failure
155	Hydromorphone HCl	Dilaudid	Pain
156	Aviane	Aviane-28	Birth Control
157	Triamcinolone Acetonide	Kenalog	Skin Inflammation
158	Clotrimazole / Betamethasone	Lotrisone	Bacterial Skin Infections
159	Dextroamphetamine Sulfate	DextroStat	Attention Deficit Disorder
160	Calcitriol	Rocaltrol	Low Bone Density
161	Nitroglycerin	Nitro-Stat	Chest Pain
162	Methotrexate	Trexall	Rheumatoid Arthritis
163	Meclizine HCl	Antivert, Dramamine	Vertigo

Table 1 *cont.*
Top 200 Generic Drugs

Rank[3]	Generic Name[3]	Brand Name(s)[4**]	Indication
164	Diltiazem	Cardizem	High Blood Pressure
165	Quinapril	Accupril	High Blood Pressure
166	Ursodiol	Actigall, Urso	Gall Stones
167	Ketoconazole (Topical)	Nizoral	Fungal Infections
168	Fluorouracil	Carac, Efudex	Cancer
169	Trinessa	Ortho-Tri-Cyclen	Birth Control
170	Nystatin Systemic	Mycostatin	Fungal Infections
171	Nifedical XL	Procardia XL, Adalat CC	High Blood Pressure
172	Glipizide ER	Glucotrol XL	Diabetes
173	Terbinafine HCl	Lamisil	Fungal Infections
174	Cefprozil	Cefzil	Bacterial Infections
175	Benzonatate	Tessalon	Cough
176	Clindamycin / Benzoyl Peroxide	Cleosin	Bacterial Skin Infections, Acne
177	Ondansetron ODT	Zofran ODT	Nausea
178	Propranolol HCl	Inderal	High Blood Pressure
179	Famotidine	Pepcid	Acid Reflux
180	Nifedipine	Procardia	High Blood Pressure
181	Medroxyprogesterone	Depo-Provera	Birth Control
182	Colchicine	Colcrys	Gout
183	Penicillin VK	Veetids	Bacterial Infections
184	Digoxin	Lanoxin	Congestive Heart Failure
185	Hydrocodone / Ibuprofen	Vicoprofen	Pain and Inflammation
186	Promethazine / Codeine	Phenergan with Codeine	Cough
187	Anastrozole	Arimidex	Breast Cancer
188	Folic Acid	Not Available	Low Folic Acid Anemia
189	Butalbital / Acetaminophen / Caffeine	Fioricet	Migraines
190	Hydroxychloroquine	Plaquenil	Rheumatoid Arthritis
191	Galantamine HBr	Razadyne	Alzheimer's Disease
192	Terazosin	Hytrin	High Blood Pressure
193	Labetalol	Normodyne, Trandate	High Blood Pressure
194	Glipizide	Glucotrol	Diabetes
195	Clindamycin (Topical)	Cleocin	Bacterial Skin Infections
196	Baclofen	Lioresal	Muscle Spasms
197	Tramadol HCl ER	Ultram ER	Pain
198	Etodolac	Lodine	Inflammation
199	Donepezil	Aricept	Dementia
200	Testosterone Cypionate	Depo-Testosterone	Low Testosterone

***All rights to all brand names and trademarks are held by their respective owners.*

Conclusion

Drugs have multiple names. Pharmacy technicians are expected to convert freely between the brand and generic names of medications (at least the commonly used ones) without effort. Books, software and many other tools are available to assist in learning both the brand and generic names for drugs; however, the best teacher is time spent working with the medications. It is also imperative that a pharmacy technician be familiar with the labeling requirements for prescription drugs so as to easily separate prescription from over-the-counter medications.

References

1. Pfizer, www.pfizer.com/files/products/uspi_lipitor.pdf, Aug. 15, 2010.
2. Label Data Plus, www.labeldataplus.com/detail.php?c=13095, Aug. 15, 2010.
3. Drug Topics Magazine, www.drugtopics.modernmedicine.com/Pharmacy+Facts+&+Figures.htm, June 14, 2011.
4. Wolters Kluwer Health, www.factsandcomparisons.com, Aug. 15, 2010.

Chapter 17

REVIEW QUESTIONS

1. The structural name for a drug is rarely used in practice for which of the following reasons?
   a. It's too short to reasonably use
   b. It doesn't use enough Greek letters to be appropriate for pharmacy use
   c. It is too long to reasonably use
   d. It uses too many Greek letters to be appropriate for pharmacy use

2. The generic (chemical) name can sometimes indicate the class that the drug belongs to.
   a. True
   b. False

3. The FDA determines what the brand name for a drug will be.
   a. True
   b. False

4. The manufacturer's label must include all of the following except:
   a. the name of the manufacturer.
   b. the quantity of product contained in the package.
   c. the address of the manufacturer's headquarters.
   d. the lot (or control) number for that package.

5. Which of the following is the brand name for metoprolol succinate?
   a. Toprol XL®
   b. Lopressor®
   c. Topamax®
   d. Medrol®

6. Which of the following is the generic name for Ceftin®?
   a. Cefpodoxime
   b. Cephalexin
   c. Ceftriaxone
   d. Cefuroxime Axetil

7. Sporanox® is used to treat which of the following conditions?
   a. Bacterial infections
   b. High blood pressure
   c. Fungal infections
   d. High cholesterol

8. Allopurinol has the brand name of _____ and is used for _____.
   a. Methotrexate, rheumatoid arthritis
   b. Coreg®, high blood pressure
   c. Zyloprim®, gout
   d. Zantac®, acid reflux

9. Are Pepcid® and ranitidine used for the same condition?
   a. Yes
   b. No

10. When _____ was first released, it was a miracle drug for those who suffer with _____.
   a. Imitrex®, migraines
   b. Indocin®, inflammation
   c. Topamax®, eye infections
   d. Altace®, high cholesterol

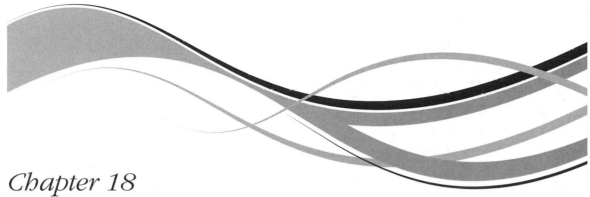

Chapter 18

VITAMINS AND MINERALS

By Andrea D. Goodrich, Pharm.D., BCPS

Learning Objectives

This chapter seeks to prepare a pharmacy technician to:

- define a nutrient.
- explain the importance of maintaining proper nutrition and health.
- discuss the updated guideline recommendations by the Dietary Advisory Committee.
- identify interactions with prescription medications and nutrients.

Introduction

Many Americans do not meet the government-approved dietary recommendations for optimal health. The groups who often fall short of these recommendations include the elderly, the chronically ill, vegetarians, patients with gastrointestinal (GI) malabsorption (which includes those who have had gastric bypass surgery), alcohol-dependent individuals, infants, adolescents, pregnant women and select ethnic populations.[1]

The number of Americans who take supplements continues to rise. The Third National Health and Nutrition Examination Survey (NHANES II) estimates that approximately 50 percent of Americans use vitamins regularly. From 1988 to 1994, it was found that the prevalence of supplement use ranged from 24 to 55 percent. Supplement users tend to be healthy people with positive attitudes about their diets and their health. The use rates for vitamins were highest among females, the well-educated and health professionals (including physicians, dietitians and pharmacists). The study pointed out that using supplementation is strongly associated with increased knowledge about nutrition and health. The reason for taking vitamins is to protect a patient from disease and supplement an inadequate diet.[1] Maintaining proper nutrition is key to optimal health in order to reduce the risk of chronic disease. Choosing a well-balanced, healthy diet is the best way to reduce this risk. Obtaining additional nutrients from multivitamins and/or supplements can also help in meeting required nutritional needs. Consumers may not always be well-informed about the type and amount of supplementation that they may need to make the best selection when purchasing a product.

Even though many Americans are using dietary supplements, it doesn't necessarily mean that Americans are knowledgeable about what products they are taking. A report published in 2009 from the U.S. Government Accountability Office states that consumers do not have the proper information to make good decisions about purchasing dietary supplements and may have difficulty understanding product labels.[2] The Government Accountability Office stated that this may place consumers' health at risk. Consumers need to receive more education on and assistance with nutritional supplements in order to make safe and appropriate choices.

The Dietary Guidelines

Every five years, the dietary guidelines for Americans are developed by the U.S. Department of Agriculture (USDA) and the U.S. Department of Health and Human Services (HHS) to ensure that all Americans are able to have the most current and nutritionally sound advice available. These guidelines are evidence-based and "designed to prevent and reduce diet-related chronic disease while promoting good and healthy weight gain among Americans ages two and older."[3] The most recent set of guidelines were finalized in December 2010 and consumer products and promotional materials were released in 2011.

In the 2010 report, the USDA and HHS decided that obesity is the largest problem facing the public's health today and that this is especially true for children (whose incidence of obesity has tripled in the past 30 years). The importance of eating behaviors and weight control is also discussed. The four nutrients that Americans are lacking, according to the report, are: fiber, potassium, Vitamin D and calcium. The foods, or ingredients, that the committee identified as being over-consumed by Americans include sodium, saturated fats and trans-fats.[3]

The 2010 report recommendations included:

- **Sodium** – the previous goal was less than 2,300 mg/day. This goal is now reduced to less than 1,500 mg/day.
- **Saturated fats** – the previous goal was less than 10 percent of daily calories to come from saturated fats. The goal is now reduced to less than 7 percent of daily calories.
- **Omega-3 fatty acids** – now, eight ounces of seafood per week is recommended. This will provide 250 mg of omega-3 fatty acids/day.[3]

Dietary Definitions

The following are key to understanding labeling and explaining labels to patients.

- **Recommended Dietary Allowance (RDA)** is the average dietary intake of the nutrient that prevents deficiency in approximately 98 percent of the population.
- **Adequate Intake (AI)** is the goal for each person for those nutrients that do not have a RDA.
- **Tolerable Upper Intake Level (UL)** is the highest level of the nutrient that is likely to pose no risk of adverse health effects in 98 percent of the population.
- **Dietary Reference Intakes (DRI)** are quantitative estimates of nutrient intakes to be used for planning and assessing diets for healthy people. The DRI include both RDA and UL.[3]

Nutrients

A **nutrient** is a chemical that humans need for the body to grow and survive. Nutrients build and repair tissues, give energy and provide sustenance. Organic nutrients are carbohydrates, fats, proteins and vitamins. Inorganic nutrients are minerals, water and oxygen.[3]

Proteins are produced from amino acids that are needed for tissue growth and repair. After water, protein is the most abundant substance in the body. After the age of two, a person needs about two to three servings of protein-rich food daily. Examples of a protein serving include one ounce of meat, poultry or fish; one-fourth cup cooked dry beans, one egg, one tablespoon of peanut butter or one-half ounce of nuts or seeds. Foods that are high in protein are meat, fish, eggs, milk and poultry. Plant sources that have proteins include beans, peas, nuts, bread and cereal.[3]

Carbohydrates, which include starch and sugars, are the body's main energy source. It is recommended to obtain 45 to 65 percent of one's daily calories from carbohydrates; the best source of carbohydrates are those sources that are rich in fiber, whole grains and have little added sugar. Most Americans consume about half of their calories in carbohydrates, but in countries such as Asia and Africa, carbohydrates are about four-fifths of their calories. Foods that are high in carbohydrates include vegetables, rice, wheat, corn and fiber rich fruit.[3] Refined sugars are considered nonessential foods, or "empty calories," because they provide only calories and no nutritional value. These should be eaten in moderation.[3]

Fats and oils are a concentrated form of energy; they provide nine calories/gram. This is more than twice the calories from a carbohydrate that supplies four calories/gram. For those two years and older, total fat intake is recommended to be between 20 and 35 percent of total calories; further, of the consumed fats, less than 10 percent is to come from saturated fats (e.g., fatty meat, dairy product, tropical oils such as coconut oil), less than 300 mg/day is to be in the form of cholesterol, and trans fats (e.g., cakes, cookies, crackers, pies) consumption is to be as low as possible. Fats are used to ensure that vitamins are absorbed into the body, to protect vital organs and to help maintain the body's core temperature. Fats are found in all cells within the body. **Saturated fats** are fats that come from animal products and can raise cholesterol, increasing the risk for heart disease. Therefore, it is recommended that dietary fat come from monounsaturated and polyunsaturated fat, which comes from plant, olive and peanut oils, and omega-3 unsaturated fats found in fatty fish such as salmon, sardines and shellfish.[3]

Vitamins

Vitamins are a group of organic nutrients that are required in small amounts for a body's survival. As the body cannot make them on its own, they must be supplied by the body's diet. Vitamins perform essential metabolic reactions in the body. Vitamins are often separated into two categories: fat soluble and water soluble. **Fat-soluble vitamins** include A, D, E and K; these vitamins can be stored in the body for long periods of time and have the potential to cause toxicity when they build up in the body. Vitamin C, the B vitamins, folate and biotin are all **water-soluble vitamins**. These vitamins are not stored in the body; excessive amounts of these chemicals are excreted in the urine. Laboratory tests are useful to confirm the suspicion of a vitamin deficiency. The first sign of a deficiency is usually a decrease in the amount of the vitamin found in the blood. Toxicity can be observed the same way (especially with fat-soluble vitamins). Patients must be warned against starting any high-dose vitamin supplementation without proper medical supervision. Table 1 lists the recommended daily allowances and adequate intake by the USDA for common vitamins.[3]

Fat-Soluble Vitamins

Vitamin A (**Retinol** or **Beta Carotene**) is essential for the development of bones, skin and eyesight. It strengthens the immune system and therefore creates resistance to infection and disease. It also regulates growth by regulating the expression of the growth hormone gene.

- ■ **Deficiency:** blindness (night blindness), dermatitis, itchy skin, hair changes and poor growth
- ■ **Toxicity:** birth defects, liver toxicity, hyperlipidemia, dry skin, scaly skin, fatigue, nausea, loss of appetite, bone pains, joint pains and headaches
- ■ **Sources:** oily fish, dairy, liver, kidneys, eggs and most fruits/vegetables that are the following colors when eaten: yellow, orange and dark green (e.g., oranges, carrots, broccoli, spinach and watercress)[4,5,6]

Vitamin D (Calciferol) has gained much publicity over the past few years because taking vitamin D, along with calcium, can significantly increase bone mass in growing children, and taking these supplements as adults could decrease bone loss and prevent fractures. Vitamin D is naturally present in very few foods; therefore, it must either be fortified into food or be taken as supplements. Vitamin D is produced when ultraviolet (UV) rays from the sun are absorbed through the skin and trigger vitamin D synthesis from vitamin D precursors already present in certain skin cells. Unfortunately, using sunscreen, with a UV protection above the sun protection factor (SPF) of eight, blocks the synthesis of vitamin D from UV rays. Although the main chemical that is vitamin D is calciferol, there are slight chemical variations of calciferol that occur in the body and have vitamin D activity. Vitamin D_3 (cholecalciferol) is considered to be three times as effective as vitamin D_2 (ergocalciferol) in raising serum (blood) vitamin D levels and maintaining those levels for a longer period of time; thus, the preferred form of vitamin D in supplements is D_3. The entire cycle of vitamin D, from precursors and UV light being converted into to both vitamin D_2 and D_3, is beyond the scope of this chapter. Forty units of vitamin D corresponds to 1 mcg of cholecalciferol.

Vitamin D, needed for calcium absorption and proper bone growth, also plays a role in the prevention of cancers, specifically colon cancer, prostate cancer and breast cancer. New research is also emerging that vitamin D may assist in the prevention and treatment of diabetes (both type I and II) and hypertension. In 2008, the American Academy of Pediatrics (AAP) increased its recommendation for the amount of vitamin D that all children need each day to twice the previously recommended amount. The USDA has not yet increased its recommendation for the amount of vitamin D that children need daily; therefore, a consensus has not been reached on the proper amount of vitamin D needed by children to maintain healthy growth.[7] For adults, the American Academy of Family Physicians (AAFP) recommends increased amounts of vitamin D that are twice the current USDA recommendations; AAFP states that sufficient evidence exists to support this higher dose of vitamin D because it reduces the risk of fractures and maintains bone health better than the lower dose.[8] Taking vitamin D, along with calcium, has been shown to decrease falls, fractures and bone loss in elderly patients.

- **Deficiency:** thin bones, brittle bones, misshapen bones, rickets, osteomalacia and osteoporosis
- **Toxicity:** nausea, vomiting, poor appetite, weight loss, weakness, constipation, changes in mental status, heart rhythm abnormalities and increased calcium levels[9]
- **Sources:** cod liver oil, salmon, tuna and fortified products (such as milk, yogurt and orange juice)[4,5,6] and from vitamin D precursors activated by UV light

Vitamin E (alpha-Tocopherol) is an antioxidant that intercepts free radicals. Vitamin E, which is an essential part of the immune system, is also important for the function of sex organs and the protection of cells from inflammation. This protection from inflammation has led to vitamin E supplements being used for a variety of conditions involving increased inflammation. Further, it has effects on the body's system for forming blood clots; therefore, patients taking anti-clotting drugs (e.g., warfarin) may be at a greater risk for bleeding if vitamin E is taken without supervision from a pharmacist or physician. Also, patients using insulin may find that the dose of insulin needed to control blood sugar levels may change if vitamin E supplementation is initiated or terminated.

- **Deficiency:** nerve damage, muscle damage, membrane damage, impaired balance, impaired coordination and hemolysis
- **Toxicity:** bleeding
- **Sources:** vegetable oils, nuts, seeds, beans, avocados, margarine, egg yolks, flour, whole grains and green leafy vegetables.[4,5,6]

Vitamin K$_1$ (Phytonadione) plays a vital role in blood clotting. Vitamin K$_1$ also plays a vital role in binding calcium to the bones. Vitamin K$_1$ is used to reverse the anticoagulation actions of the drug warfarin. There are several forms of vitamin K$_1$, one produced by plants, one produced by animals (including humans) and a large range of types that are synthesized by bacteria in the small intestine of humans. Humans are able to use the vitamin K$_1$ that is produced by the bacteria in the small intestines; therefore, vitamin K$_1$ deficiency is rare in adults with a functioning GI tract. In some rare cases, vitamin K$_1$ deficiency is seen in patients taking warfarin and those with severe liver abnormalities.

- **Deficiency:** bleeding
- **Toxicity:** no significant toxicities
- **Sources:** Vitamin K is found in dark green vegetables (e.g., spinach, romaine lettuce, broccoli, brussels sprouts, soy beans and olives) and oils[4,5,6]

Water-Soluble Vitamins

Vitamin B$_1$ (Thiamine) plays an important role in the production of energy. Thiamine is essential for the metabolism of carbohydrates into energy that cells need to function. It is particularly essential for the nervous system, the heart, the brain, the gastrointestinal system and the muscles. Patients on dialysis, those with diseases that affect absorption of nutrients and those with alcoholism tend to be deficient in vitamin B$_1$.

- **Deficiency:** anorexia, fatigue, depression, impaired memory/concentration, paresthesia, lactic acidosis, congestive heart failure, Wernicke-Korsakoff's syndrome (alcoholic brain injury), peripheral nerve damage and beriberi
- **Toxicity:** lactic-acidosis
- **Sources:** unrefined rice cereals, legumes (beans and lentils), flour, yeast, dried fruit, potatoes, pork, fortified white rice and fortified white flour[4,5,6]

Vitamin B$_2$ (Riboflavin) maintains healthy eyes, healthy skin and a healthy nervous system. Children under the age of 12 and people experiencing kidney failure are not recommended to receive supplementation with vitamin B$_2$ beyond what is obtained from their diet. Diuretics may increase riboflavin requirements. Alcoholics have a higher risk of riboflavin deficiency as a result of decreased intake and decreased absorption.

- ■ **Deficiency:** dry skin, red skin, flaky skin, cracked lips, sore throat, sore tongue, irritated eyes, light sensitivity, poor concentration, memory loss, a burning sensation in the feet and decreased red blood cell levels
- ■ **Toxicity:** No significant toxicities
- ■ **Sources:** Vitamin B_2 is found in milk (dairy products), enriched white flour and enriched white bread[4,5,6]

Vitamin B_3 (Niacin) assists functions of the nervous system, digestive system, food metabolism, forming red blood cells and forming skin cells. Niacin is used to treat **pellagra**; pellagra is a condition that nearly always is attributed to a niacin deficiency and is characterized by "the four Ds": dermatitis, diarrhea, dementia and death. Niacin is also recommended for dizziness, premenstrual syndrome (PMS) and arthritis. Niacin can also be useful for those with high cholesterol, mental illness and severe stress problems. Flushing and gastrointestinal distress can be seen with vitamin B_3 administration. Patients taking niacin, especially in high doses for cholesterol reduction, are often recommended a single 325 mg aspirin approximately 30 minutes before taking niacin to reduce the flushing seen with niacin administration.

- ■ **Deficiency:** pellagra, **glossitis** (inflammation or infection of the tongue) and headaches
- ■ **Toxicity:** facial flushing and liver disease
- ■ **Sources:** meat, fish, bread, yeast, nuts, seeds, soy beans, potatoes, dried fruit, tomatoes and peas[4,5,6]

Vitamin B_5 (Pantothenic Acid) is responsible for turning fats, proteins and carbohydrates into energy and brain activity. It is also responsible for the production of blood as well as the metabolism of toxins by the liver. Vitamin B_5 is used to prevent stress, relieve headache, treat insomnia, treat arthritis, reduce food intolerance, correct hair problems and stop teeth grinding.

- ■ **Deficiency:** fatigue, malaise, headache, insomnia, vomiting and abdominal cramps
- ■ **Toxicity:** doses greater than 1,200 mg may cause nausea and heartburn
- ■ **Sources:** peanuts, liver, kidneys, avocado, mushrooms, seeds, nuts, pumpkin, avocados, sweet potatoes, egg yolks, broccoli, dairy products, fish, chicken, whole grain cereals, bread and bananas [4,5,6]

Vitamin B_6 (Pyridoxine) gives red blood cells the ability to carry oxygen throughout the human body. Vitamin B_6 regulates metabolism, digestion and fluid balance. Neurotransmitters in the nervous system are synthesized using enzymes that need vitamin B_6. Vitamin B_6 supplementation is recommended for those who suffer from cardiovascular disease, morning sickness, insomnia, anxiety and PMS.

- ■ **Deficiency:** nervousness, irritation, confusion, dry flaky skin, tongue inflammation and ulcers in the mouth
- ■ **Toxicity:** sensory neuropathy (damage to the nerves leading to pain, numbness and tingling)
- ■ **Sources:** cereals, brown rice, brown bread, wheat germ, yeast, nuts, seeds, lentils, potatoes, baked beans, soy beans, bananas, white fish and meat[4,5,6]

Folic Acid (Folate) is essential to women during pregnancy, and while breastfeeding, to promote cell growth, cell development and nervous system functioning in their growing children (folic acid decreases the risk of a growing child developing neural tube defects). Alcoholics, people who suffer from depression, people with a variety of mental illnesses and patients with Alzheimer's disease may benefit from folate supplementation. A folate-rich diet is associated with a decreased risk of developing cardiovascular disease.

- ■ **Deficiency:** anemia, diarrhea, glossitis, **angular stomatitis** (inflammation at the corners of the mouth), fatigue, difficulty concentrating, irritability, headache, palpitations, shortness of breath, heart failure, tachycardia, postural hypotension, lactic acidosis and neural tube defects (an opening in the spinal cord/brain that can occur very early in human development)
- ■ **Toxicity:** doses greater than 400 mcg may cause anemia and may mask symptoms of a vitamin B_{12} deficiency
- ■ **Sources:** spinach, brussel sprouts, broccoli, yeast, fortified cereals, citrus fruit juices, legumes, liver, kidneys and oranges[4,5,6]

Vitamin B_{12} (Cobalamin, Cyanocobalamin) plays a role in the formation of red blood cells, the formation of bone marrow, the metabolism of carbohydrates, the metabolism of fats, the metabolism of proteins and the production of genetic materials. Supplementation may be required either for deficiency in the diet or from an inability to absorb vitamin B_{12} into the body. Some individuals develop an inability to absorb vitamin B_{12} and must receive supplementation through injecting cyanocobalamin either subcutaneously or intramuscularly. The risk of this occurring goes up with age; those over the age of 60 years are at the greatest risk of developing absorption-related vitamin B_{12} deficiency. Because 10-30 percent of older people may not absorb food-bound B_{12} well, it is advisable for individuals older than 50 years of age to meet their RDA mainly by consuming foods fortified with B_{12} (or from a supplement containing vitamin B_{12}). Two other groups are at higher risk for developing vitamin B_{12} deficiency: vegetarians and alcoholics.

- ■ **Deficiency:** anemia, exhaustion, irritation, depression, shortness of breath, difficulty walking, memory loss, mood swings, disorientation, dementia and constipation
- ■ **Toxicity:** doses greater than 3,000 mcg may cause eye conditions
- ■ **Sources:** meat, poultry, fish, eggs, seaweed, fortified cereals and (to a lesser extent) dairy products[4,5,6]

Biotin is generally classified as part of the vitamin B family (known as a B-complex vitamin) that is responsible for turning fats, proteins and carbohydrates into energy. This means that biotin plays a role in DNA replication and transcription. Biotin supplements are used to promote skin, nail and hair growth.

- ■ **Deficiency:** skin loss, nail loss, hair loss, weakness, depression, hallucination, numbness, fatigue, irritation, rashes and loss of appetite
- ■ **Toxicity:** no significant toxicities
- ■ **Sources:** bread, brown rice, bran cereals, egg yolk, yeast, nuts, beans, milk, liver, kidneys and fish[4,5,6]

Vitamin C (Ascorbic Acid) is needed for the synthesis of collagen, tendons, bones, teeth, blood vessels and muscles. Vitamin C is an antioxidant that assists in fighting viral and bacterial infections and helps to heal damage induced by free radicals. It is used in skin products to enhance skin vitality and it plays a role in wound healing. Vitamin C supplements are also used to reduce the severity and duration of symptoms of infections. People who smoke, drink alcohol or use oral hormones may benefit from vitamin C supplementation. Severe deficiency is known as **scurvy**.

- ■ **Deficiency:** bruising, bleeding, skin loss and hair loss
- ■ **Toxicity:** GI disturbances, kidney stones and excess iron absorption
- ■ **Sources:** fresh fruit, fresh vegetables and fruit juice[4,5,6]

Table 1
Vitamins:
Recommended Dietary Intakes for Individuals

Lifestage Group	Vitamin					Thiamine mg/d	Riboflavin mg/d
	A µg/d[a]	C mg/d	D µg/d[b]	E mg/d[c]	K µg/d		
Infants							
0–6 mo	400	40	5	4	2.0	0.2	0.3
7–12 mo	500	50	5	5	2.5	0.3	0.4
Children							
1–3 y	**300**	**15**	5	**6**	30	**0.5**	**0.5**
4–8 y	**400**	**25**	5	**7**	55	**0.6**	**0.6**
Males							
9–13 y	**600**	**45**	5	**11**	60	**0.9**	**0.9**
14–18 y	**900**	**75**	5	**15**	75	**1.2**	**1.3**
19–50 y	**900**	**90**	5	**15**	120	**1.2**	**1.3**
51–70 y	**900**	**90**	10	**15**	120	**1.2**	**1.3**
> 70 y	**900**	**90**	15	**15**	120	**1.2**	**1.3**
Females							
9–13 y	**600**	**45**	5	**11**	60	**0.9**	**0.9**
14–18 y	**700**	**65**	5	**15**	75	**1.0**	**1.0**
19–50 y	**700**	**75**	5	**15**	90	**1.1**	**1.1**
51–70 y	**700**	**75**	10	**15**	90	**1.1**	**1.1**
> 70 y	**700**	**75**	15	**15**	90	**1.1**	**1.1**
Pregnancy							
18 y	**750**	**80**	5	**15**	75	**1.4**	**1.4**
19–50 y	**770**	**85**	5	**15**	90	**1.4**	**1.4**
Lactation							
18 y	**1200**	**115**	5	**19**	75	**1.4**	**1.6**
19–50 y	**1300**	**120**	5	**19**	90	**1.4**	**1.6**

Source: Food and Nutrition Board, Institute of Medicine—National Academy of Sciences Dietary Reference Intakes, 2004.

Bold type *is the Recommended Daily Allowances (RDA). Plain type is the Adequate Intake (AI)*

[a] *Retinol activity equivalents (RAEs). 1 RAE = retinol 1 mcg, beta-carotene 12 mcg, alpha-carotene 24 mcg, or beta-cryptoxanthin 24 mcg. The RAE for dietary provitamin A carotenoids is 2-fold greater than retinol equivalents (RE), whereas the RAE for preformed vitamin A is the same as RE.*

[b] *Cholecalciferol. 1 mcg = vitamin D 40 units. These values based on the absence of adequate exposure to sunlight.*

[c] *As alpha-tocopherol.*

Niacin mg/d	Vitamin B_6 mg/d	Folate µg/d[d]	Vitamin B_{12} µg/d	Pantothenic Acid mg/d	Biotin µg/d	Choline mg/d[f]	Lifestage Group
							Infants
2	0.1	65	0.4	1.7	5	125	0–6 mo
4	0.3	80	0.5	1.8	6	150	7–12 mo
							Children
6	**0.5**	**150**	**0.9**	2	8	200	1–3 y
8	**0.6**	**200**	**1.2**	3	12	250	4–8 y
							Males
12	**1.0**	**300**	**1.8**	4	20	375	9–13 y
16	**1.3**	**400**	**2.4**	5	25	550	14–18 y
16	**1.3**	**400**	**2.4**	5	30	550	19–50 y
16	**1.7**	**400**	**2.4**[e]	5	30	550	51–70 y
16	**1.7**	**400**	**2.4**[e]	5	30	550	> 70 y
							Females
12	**1.0**	**300**	**1.8**	4	20	375	9–13 y
14	**1.2**	**400**	**2.4**	5	25	400	14–18 y
14	**1.2**	**400**	**2.4**	5	30	425	19–50 y
14	**1.5**	**400**	**2.4**[e]	5	30	425	51–70 y
14	**1.5**	**400**	**2.4**[e]	5	30	425	> 70 y
							Pregnancy
18	1.6	600	2.6	6	30	450	18 y
18	1.9	600	2.6	6	30	450	19–50 y
							Lactation
17	2.0	500	2.8	7	35	550	18 y
17	2.0	500	2.8	7	35	550	19–50 y

[d] *Dietary folate equivalents (DFE). One DFE = food folate 1 mcg = folic acid 0.6 mcg from fortified food or as a supplement consumed with food = 0.5 mcg of a supplement taken on an empty stomach.*

[e] *Because 10 to 30 percent of older people may not absorb food-bound B_{12} well it is advisable for individuals older than 50 years of age to meet their RDA mainly by consuming foods fortified with B_{12} or a supplement containing B_{12}.*

[f] *Although AIs have been set for choline, there are few data to assess whether a dietary supply of choline is needed at all stages of the life cycle, and it may be that the choline requirement can be met by endogenous synthesis at some of these stages.*

Minerals

Minerals make up approximately four percent of a person's body weight. Minerals are found everywhere in the body, cannot be made by the body and need to be obtained from the diet. The body uses minerals for many different activities, such as water balance, bone development and nerve conduction. There are two types of minerals. **Macro minerals** include calcium, chloride, magnesium, phosphorus, potassium and sodium. These minerals are needed in larger quantities, on a daily basis, than trace minerals. **Trace minerals** include boron, chromium, cobalt, copper, fluoride, iodine, iron, manganese, molybdenum, nickel, selenium and zinc. Table 2 lists the RDA and adequate intake for the minerals recommended by the USDA.[3,6,10]

Calcium is essential for the preservation of the human skeleton and human teeth. It also assists the functions of nerves and muscles and is involved in many steps in activating blood clotting. There have also been studies showing that calcium may be beneficial in preventing symptoms of PMS. Calcium is best absorbed when it is taken in smaller doses more frequently (i.e., 500 mg taken three times a day is better absorbed than 1,500 mg taken once daily). Many reasons, beyond low dietary intake, exist for low blood calcium including parathyroid dysfunction, kidney failure and alcoholism.

- **Deficiency:** osteoporosis, bone deformity, behavior and personality disorders, muscle spasms, cramps, and mental and growth impairment
- **Toxicity:** doses greater than 2 g/day can cause kidney stones, anorexia, nausea, vomiting and constipation
- **Sources:** milk, milk products, sardines, clams, oysters, vegetables, nuts and beans[5,6,10]

Chloride (Chlorine) is used to maintain water balance, as a carrier to bring nutrients through the body, and to aid in absorption.

- **Deficiency:** no deficiency found
- **Toxicity:** coughing, chest pain, water retention in the lungs, skin irritation, eye irritation and respiratory system irritation.
- **Sources:** table salt[5,6,10]

Chromium is an essential nutrient to enhance the action of **insulin** (a hormone critical to the metabolism and storage of carbohydrate, fat and protein in the body). Chromium appears to be directly involved in carbohydrate, fat and protein metabolism. Chromium has been sold as a weight loss product; however, it has not been proven to be beneficial in reducing weight. Levels of chromium decrease with age.

- **Deficiency:** glucose intolerance, peripheral neuropathy, increased total cholesterol and triglycerides, weight loss, glucosuria (sugar in the urine) and impaired protein use
- **Toxicity:** concentration problems and fainting
- **Sources:** fish, liver, meats, milk, corn oil and grains[5,6,10]

Copper is found everywhere in the body; however, copper levels are highest in the liver, brain, heart and kidneys. Copper is needed for the appropriate functioning of the CNS, as well as helping to regulate blood pressure and heart rate. It is also needed to help absorb iron from the stomach.

- **Deficiency:** decrease in white blood cells, anemia, osteoporosis, hair/skin depigmentation, dermatitis, anorexia, diarrhea, mental decline and high cholesterol
- **Toxicity:** excess of 250 mg/day causes vomiting; **Wilson's disease**, the inability to eliminate copper, leads to: liver cirrhosis, diarrhea, vomiting and metal taste.
- **Sources:** tap water, seafood, liver, cherries, whole grains, wheat bran, lentils and chocolate[5,6,10]

Fluoride is found in tooth enamel and in bones. Fluoride is important for preventing cavities by making the tooth enamel stronger. Doses greater than 2 g in adults and 0.5 g in children are toxic and may lead to death.

- **Deficiency:** dental cavities and osteoporosis
- **Toxicity:** chalky-white, irregular, patches on the surface of the teeth, brown and yellow stained teeth, death, tremors, seizures, respiratory and heart failure
- **Sources:** fluoridated drinking water[5,6,10]

Iodine is involved primarily in the production of thyroid hormones. Thyroid hormones are important for determining how your body grows and uses nutrients.

- **Deficiency: hypothyroid goiter** (swelling in the thyroid gland), postnatal mortality, mental impairment, impaired fertility and, in severe cases, **cretinism** (stunted physical and mental growth)
- **Toxicity:** sore teeth and gums, burning in the mouth, unpleasant taste and hypothyroidism
- **Sources:** fortified table salts[5,6,10]

Iron is involved in oxygen transport throughout the body. It is also essential for the regulation of cell growth. Iron supplements can cause GI discomfort and constipation. This can be reduced by taking iron with food, though doing this reduces absorption of iron by approximately 50 percent.

- **Deficiency:** anemia, weakness, fatigue, feeling cold, headache, difficulty swallowing, nail changes, tingling of the skin and decreased mental function
- **Toxicity:** vomiting, diarrhea, electrolyte imbalance, shock and death
- **Sources:** red meats, fish, poultry, egg yolks, enriched grains and dark green vegetables[5,6,10]

Magnesium is important for muscle function, nerve function, bone development, immune system maintenance and heart rhythm maintenance. It helps maintain blood pressure levels and assists in regulating blood sugar. There is new interest in magnesium's role in hypertension, cardiovascular disease and diabetes. Severe magnesium deficiency can result in low blood levels of calcium and potassium. Magnesium is cleared from the body by the kidneys; therefore, kidney disease increases the risk of toxicity.

- **Deficiency:** numbness, tingling, muscle contractions, muscle cramps, seizures, personality changes, abnormal heart rhythms and coronary spasms
- **Toxicity:** diarrhea and abdominal cramping
- **Sources:** green vegetables, beans, nuts, seeds and whole grains.[5,6,10] People on long-term parenteral nutrition are at a higher risk of developing molybdenum deficiency.

Manganese is found in the body's liver, pancreas, kidney, muscle and bone. Manganese is needed for processing glucose and affects the body's ability to use steroids, cholesterol and fatty acids.

- **Deficiency:** nausea, vomiting, dermatitis, hair color changes, hypercholesterolemia, growth delay, defective carbohydrate metabolism and defective protein metabolism
- **Toxicity:** Parkinson-like symptoms, hyper-irritability, hallucinations and libido disturbances
- **Sources:** whole grains, nuts, vegetables and fruits[5,6,10]

Table 2

Minerals:

Recommended Dietary Intakes for Individuals

Lifestage Group	Calcium mg/d	Chromium µg /d	Copper µg/d	Fluoride mg/d	Iodine µg/d	Iron mg/d	Magnesium mg/d
Infants							
0–6 mo	210	0.2	200	0.01	110	0.27	30
7–12mo	270	5.5	220	0.5	130	**11**	75
Children							
1–3 y	500	11	**340**	0.7	90	**7**	**80**
4–8 y	800	15	**440**	1	90	**10**	**130**
Males							
9–13 y	1,300	25	**700**	2	**120**	**8**	**240**
14–18y	1,300	35	**890**	3	**150**	**11**	**410**
19–30y	1,000	35	**900**	4	**150**	**8**	**400**
31–50y	1,000	35	**900**	4	**150**	**8**	**420**
51–70 y	1,200	30	**900**	4	**150**	**8**	**420**
> 70 y	1,200	30	**900**	4	**150**	**8**	**420**
Females							
9–13 y	1,300	21	**700**	2	**120**	**8**	**240**
14–18 y	1,300	24	**890**	3	**150**	**15**	**360**
19–30 y	1,000	25	**900**	3	**150**	**18**	**310**
31–50 y	1,000	25	**900**	3	**150**	**18**	**320**
51–70 y	1,200	20	**900**	3	**150**	**8**	**320**
> 70 y	1,200	20	**900**	3	**150**	**8**	**320**
Pregnancy							
18 y	1,300	29	**1,000**	3	**220**	**27**	**400**
19–50 y	1,000	30	**1,000**	3	**220**	**27**	**350**
Lactation							
18 y	1,300	44	**1,300**	3	**290**	**10**	**360**
19–50 y	1,000	45	**1,300**	3	**290**	**9**	**310**

Source: Food and Nutrition Board, Institute of Medicine—National Academy of Sciences Dietary Reference Intakes, 2004.

Bold type *is the Recommended Daily Allowances (RDA). Plain type is the Adequate Intake (AI)*

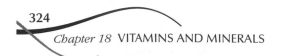

Man-ganese mg/d	Molyb-denum µg/d	Phos-phorus mg/d	Sele-nium µg/d	Zinc mg/d	Potas-sium g/d	Sodium g/d	Chlo-ride g/d	Lifestage Group
								Infants
0.003	2	100	15	2	0.4	0.12	0.18	0–6 mo
0.6	3	275	20	3	0.7	0.37	0.57	7–12 mo
								Children
1.2	17	460	20	3	3	1	1.5	1–3 y
1.5	22	500	30	5	3.8	1.2	1.9	4–8 y
								Males
1.9	34	1,250	40	8	4.5	1.5	2.3	9–13 y
2.2	43	1,250	55	11	4.7	1.5	2.3	14–18 y
2.3	45	700	55	11	4.7	1.5	2.3	19–30 y
2.3	45	700	55	11	4.7	1.5	2.3	31–50 y
2.3	45	700	55	11	4.7	1.3	2	51–70 y
2.3	45	700	55	11	4.7	1.2	1.8	> 70 y
								Females
1.6	34	1,250	40	8	4.5	1.5	2.3	9–13 y
1.6	43	1,250	55	9	4.7	1.5	2.3	14–18 y
1.8	45	700	55	8	4.7	1.5	2.3	19–30 y
1.8	45	700	55	8	4.7	1.5	2.3	31–50 y
1.8	45	700	55	8	4.7	1.3	2	51–70 y
1.8	45	700	55	8	4.7	1.2	1.8	> 70 y
								Pregnancy
2.0	50	1,250	60	12	4.7	1.5	2.3	18 y
2.0	50	700	60	11	4.7	1.5	2.3	19–50 y
								Lactation
2.6	50	1,250	70	13	5.1	1.5	2.3	18 y
2.6	50	700	70	12	5.1	1.5	2.3	19–50 y

Molybdenum is involved in many biological processes, including development of the nervous system, removing waste in the kidneys and producing energy in the cells.

- ■ **Deficiency:** rapid heart rate, rapid breathing, altered mental status, visual changes, headache, nausea and vomiting
- ■ **Toxicity:** gout-like symptoms (painful joints) and increased urinary copper
- ■ **Sources:** beans, peas, lentils, grains, dark green leafy vegetables, liver and nuts[5,6,10]

Phosphorus is found throughout the body and is stored in the bones. Phosphorus is needed for strong bones, all cell functions, cell membranes and parathyroid hormone regulation.

- ■ **Deficiency:** weakness, anorexia, pain and bone loss
- ■ **Toxicity:** diarrhea and stomach pain
- ■ **Sources:** dairy products, fish, meats, poultry, nuts and eggs[5,6,10]

Potassium is involved in many major biologic processes (e.g., muscle contractions, nerve impulses, nucleic acid synthesis, protein synthesis and energy production). Deficiency is usually caused by severe vomiting, severe diarrhea, using (certain) diuretics, kidney disease or the overuse of laxatives. Toxicity is usually caused by using (certain) diuretics and kidney disease.

- ■ **Deficiency:** muscle paralysis or abnormal heart beats that can be fatal
- ■ **Toxicity:** stomach upset, muscle weakness, intestinal problems and abnormal heart rhythms
- ■ **Sources:** fresh fruits and vegetables [5,6,10]

Selenium is found everywhere in the body; however, its highest concentration is found in both the kidneys and liver. Selenium has antioxidant properties; it helps prevent cellular damage from free radicals. **Free radicals** are natural by-products of oxygen metabolism that may contribute to the development of chronic diseases such as cancer and heart disease.

- ■ **Deficiency:** muscle weakness/pain and heart disease
- ■ **Toxicity:** nausea, vomiting, hair/nail loss, tooth decay, skin lesions, irritability, fatigue and peripheral neuropathy
- ■ **Sources:** meats, grains, onions and milk[5,6,10]

Sodium helps maintain normal fluid balance and blood pressure. Sodium plays a key role in normal nerve and muscle function. The body receives sodium through foods and loses it through urine and sweat. Most Americans get much more sodium than the body needs. Excess body sodium can lead to an increase in blood pressure for some individuals. The most common causes of toxic sodium are dehydration, diarrhea, kidney disease and using (certain) diuretics.

- ■ **Deficiency:** confusion, muscle twitches, seizures, coma and death
- ■ **Toxicity:** confusion, muscle twitches, coma and death
- ■ **Sources:** table salt and processed foods

Zinc plays a role in immune function, protein synthesis, wound healing and DNA synthesis. The body cannot store zinc; therefore, a daily intake is required to maintain a steady state.

- ■ **Deficiency:** dermatitis, **alopecia** (hair loss), diarrhea, depression, growth retardation, impaired wound healing and an impaired immune system
- ■ **Toxicity:** gastric distress, nausea, dizziness and death
- ■ **Sources:** oysters, shellfish, red meats, poultry, beans, nuts, whole grains, fortified breakfast cereals and dairy products[5,6,10]

Drug Interactions with Vitamins and Minerals

Most people, when listing the medications that they take, do not include over-the-counter medications unless they are specifically asked to list over-the-counter medications. Medications taken with vitamins/minerals have the potential to cause serious drug interactions; Table 3 lists examples of some of these interactions. Taking a thorough medication history from each patient, including all nonprescription drugs, will help enhance a pharmacist's ability to ensure the proper use of all drugs being used by the patient, including the vitamins and minerals being taken.

Table 3
Medication Interactions with Vitamins and Minerals[11]

Vitamin / Mineral Supplementation	Medication**	Effect of Interaction	How to Manage Interaction
Aluminum and Magnesium	Fluoroquinolones, Tetracyclines, Bisphosphonates, Levothyroxine	Decreased effectiveness of the medication	Separate doses by at least two hours
Calcium	Fluoroquinolones, Tetracyclines	Decreased effectiveness of the antibiotic	Avoid calcium supplementation while taking the antibiotic
	Bisphosphonates, Levothyroxine	Decreased effectiveness of the medication	Separate by at least four hours
Folic Acid	Methotrexate	Prevents adverse events from methotrexate; almost always used in combination	Recommend that patients take folic acid with methotrexate for rheumatoid arthritis or psoriasis
Iron	Digoxin, Fluoroquinoles, Levothyroxine, Tetracyclines	Decreased effectiveness of the medication	Separate doses by at least two hours
	Methyldopa	Worsening of hypertension	Avoid using the two medications together
Niacin	HMG-CoA Reductase Inhibitors (a.k.a. Statins)	Decreased effectiveness / Risk of myopathy or rhabdomyolysis	Use a carbidopa / Avoid self treatment with niacin and monitor physician-guided treatment closely
Potassium	ACE Inhibitors, ARBs, Digoxin, Indomethacin, Potassium-sparing Diuretics[6]	Hyperkalemia (high-blood potassium)	Avoid potassium supplementation and salt substitutes (containing KI) without physician/pharmacist supervision

Table 3 *cont.*
Medication Interactions with Vitamins and Minerals

Vitamin / Mineral Supplementation	Medication**	Effect of Interaction	How to Manage Interaction
Vitamin A	Accutane (Isotretinoin) and Soriatane (Acitretin)	Risk of toxicity: nausea, vomiting, dizziness, blurred vision, poor muscle coordination	Avoid using in combination
Vitamin B$_6$	Levodopa	Decreased effectiveness of levodopa, leading to Parkinson symptoms	Use a carbidpoa / levodopa combination
	Dilantin (Phenytoin)	Decreased phenytoin effectiveness: risk of seizures	Discontinue vitamin B$_6$ supplementation or increase phenytoin dose
Vitamin E	Coumadin (Warfarin)	Increased risk of bleeding	Avoid doses > 800 IU / day of vitamin E
Vitamin K	Coumadin (Warfarin)	Decreased effectiveness of warfarin: risk of clotting (vitamin K is the antidote for warfarin overdose)	Maintain consistent vitamin K intake and adjust warfarin dose as needed

**All rights to all brand names and trademarks are held by their respective owners.

Conclusion

Vitamin and mineral supplementation may be needed based on a patient's dietary intake, metabolic needs, how well their body is able to absorb vitamins/minerals and potential drug interactions. A pharmacy technician trained in dietary supplementation basics may help identify patients in need of assistance with vitamins and minerals to a pharmacist. Further, pharmacy technicians trained in the use of these products may be better-equipped to assist in marketing and displaying such products most effectively. Finally, a pharmacy technician who has successfully completed this chapter will be less surprised to see prescriptions from physicians for the drugs called vitamins and minerals that are required for the health and well-being of every body.

References

1. Millen, A.E., Dodd, K.W., Subar, A.F., "Use of vitamin, mineral, nonvitamin, and nonmineral supplements in the United States: The 1987, 1992, and 2000 National Health Interview Survey Results," *Journal of the American Dietetic Association*, Vol. 104, pp. 942-950, 2004.

2. Government Accountability Office, www.gao.gov/new.items/d09250.pdf, July 2010.

3. United States Department of Agriculture, www.cnpp.usda.gov, July 2010.

4. Bender, D.A., Mayes, P.A., "Chapter 44, Micronutrients: Vitamins & Minerals," in Murray, R.K., Bender, D.A., Botham, K.M., Kennelly, P.J., Rodwell, V.W., Weil, P.A., Harper's Illustrated Biochemistry, 28e: www.accesspharmacy.com/content.aspx?aID=5229785, Aug. 20, 2010.

5. Lenntech, www.lenntech.com, August 2010.

6. Berdari, R.R., Handbook of Nonprescription Drugs: An Interactive Approach to Self-care, Washington, D.C., 2006, pp. 441-474.

7. Wagner, C.L., Greer, F.L., Section on Breastfeeding and Committee on Nutrition, "Prevention of Rickets and Vitamin D Deficiency in Infants, Children and Adolescents," *American Academy of Pediatrics*, Vol. 122, No. 5, pp. 1145-1152, November 2008.

8. Langan, R.C., Bordelon, P., Ghetu, M.V., "Recognition and Management of Vitamin D," *American Family Physician*, Vol. 80, No. 8, pp. 841-846, October 2009.

9. Office of Dietary Supplements, http://ods.od.nih.gov, July 2010.

10. Chessman, K.H., Kumpf, V.J., "Chapter 143, Assessment of Nutrition Status and Nutrition Requirements," In: DiPiro, J.T., Talbert, R.L, Yee, G.C., Matzke, G.R., Wells, B.G., Posey, L.M., Pharmacotherapy: A Pathophysiologic Approach, 7th edition, www.accesspharmacy.com/content.aspx?aID=3222376, Aug. 20, 2010.

11. Ezzo, D.C., Marzella Sulli, M., "Drug Interactions with Vitamins and Minerals Drug Interactions with Vitamins and Minerals," *US Pharmacist*, Vol. 1, pp. 42-55, 2007.

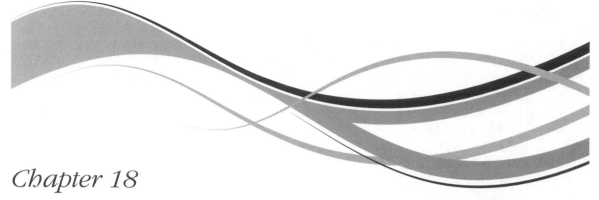

Chapter 18

REVIEW QUESTIONS

1. Which of the following is a nutrient?
    a. Protein
    b. Vitamin
    c. Mineral
    d. Carbohydrate
    e. All of the above

2. Which of these is a fat-soluble vitamin?
    a. Vitamin B
    b. Vitamin C
    c. Vitamin D
    d. Niacin
    e. All of the above

3. Using sunscreens with a UV protection above a SPF of ____ blocks the synthesis of vitamin D from UV rays.
    a. 4
    b. 8
    c. 10
    d. 15
    e. 30

4. What vitamin or mineral counteracts the blood-thinning action of warfarin?
    a. Vitamin A
    b. Vitamin C
    c. Vitamin D
    d. Vitamin K
    e. All of the above

5. Which vitamin or mineral is fortified into tap water to prevent dental cavities?
    a. Copper
    b. Thiamine
    c. Fluoride
    d. Vitamin A
    e. All of the above

6. What vitamin or mineral is needed for bone health?
    a. Phosphorus
    b. Calcium
    c. Vitamin D
    d. Vitamin K
    e. All of the above

7. What vitamin or mineral is responsible for thyroid function?
    a. Chloride
    b. Iodine
    c. Vitamin E
    d. Pyridoxine
    e. All of the above

8. Pregnant/lactating women do not need an increased amount of this vitamin or mineral (compared to women who are not pregnant/lactating).
    a. Folate
    b. Vitamin A
    c. Copper
    d. Calcium
    e. All of the above

9. Which vitamin or mineral below interacts with levothyroxine?
    a. Iron
    b. Calcium
    c. Magnesium
    d. Aluminum
    e. All of the above

10. The 2005 USDA guidelines and the 2008 American Academy of Pediatrics disagree on the proper dose for children of which of the following vitamins or minerals?
    a. Vitamin D
    b. Selenium
    c. Pantothenic acid
    d. Molybdenum
    e. All of the above

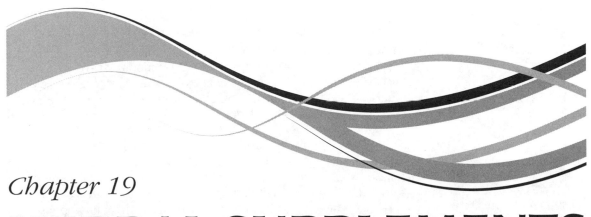

Chapter 19

HERBAL SUPPLEMENTS

By Jean C. Lee, Pharm.D., BCPS, AAHIVE

Learning Objectives

This chapter seeks to prepare a pharmacy technician to:

- distinguish between a "dietary supplement" and an "herbal supplement."
- describe the regulatory requirements and oversight for herbal supplements in the United States.
- discuss current concerns with the safety and efficacy of herbal supplements.
- explain the importance of collecting a complete medication history from patients taking herbal supplements.
- identify situations, involving herbal supplements and dietary supplements, when patient counseling by a pharmacist is required.

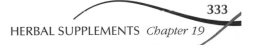

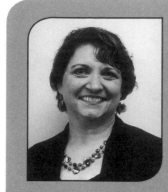

In relation to vitamins, supplements and herbals, what kinds of questions do you receive?

"Working in a small, independent community pharmacy, we consistently receive inquiries about vitamins, supplements and herbals. As a CPhT, it's important to be knowledgeable of the uses, benefits and risks of these products.

Though I have seen many vitamins, supplements and herbals gain and lose popularity through the years, there are a few that remain constant. Some of the more common products we regularly get asked about include zinc or vitamin C for colds; Lutein for eyes; glucosamine/chrondroitin/MSM for joints; calcium/vitamin D_3 for bones; Saw Palmetto for prostate; and Black Cohosh for menopause.

The most popular question asked would have to be, 'does this really help?' And, I'll leave it up to you to learn and determine how best to answer."

Doreen Kern, CPhT,
The Prescription Shop,
Glen Arbor, Mich.

Introduction

The use of alternative medicine, including herbal supplements, has increased over time. The annual use of herbal supplements has increased from 2.5 percent of Americans in 1990, to 12.1 percent in 1997,[1] to 14.2 percent in 1999, to 18.8 percent in 2002,[2] and finally 17.7 percent in 2007.[3] The amount of money spent by consumers has also steadily increased from $5.1 billion in 1997[1] to $14.8 billion in 2007.[4] With the increasing popularity of herbal supplements, likely due to ease of access and perceived efficacy, it continues to be important for all health care professionals, and paraprofessionals, to become familiar with this area of medicine.

Complementary and alternative medicine (CAM) is the label given to the varied health care systems, practices and products that are not considered part of conventional Western medicine. Being a different branch of medicine, the traditional regulatory agencies do not have jurisdiction over CAM. So, the National Center for Complementary and Alternative Medicine (NCCAM) was established to help oversee CAM in the United States; NCCAM is the lead government agency within the National Institute of Health (NIH) responsible for overseeing CAM. NIH supports and funds clinical scientific research and distributes authoritative information to the public and health care professionals.[5] As there are thousands of products, and many different CAM treatments, being used by people in the United States, health care professionals, particularly pharmacists and pharmacy technicians, need to be familiar with these treatment options.

In December 2008, NCCAM and the National Center for Health Statistics of the Center for Disease Control and Prevention (CDC) released new information from the 2007 National Health Interview Survey. The results indicated that the use of CAM by adults in the United States had increased from 36 percent of the U.S. population in 2002 to 38.3 percent in 2007. For 2007, in children, the use of CAM was 11.8 percent[3] (see Figure 1). Further, the use of CAM was greater in women and those with higher levels of education and economic status. CAM use was highest in the American Indian/Alaska native group, at 50.3 percent of that population, followed by Caucasian-Americans (43.1 percent) and then Asian-Americans (39.9 percent). The age group with the highest use was those between 50 and 59 years of age (44.1 percent).[3]

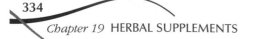

Figure 1
Complementary Alternative Medicine Use by U.S. Adults and Children[3]

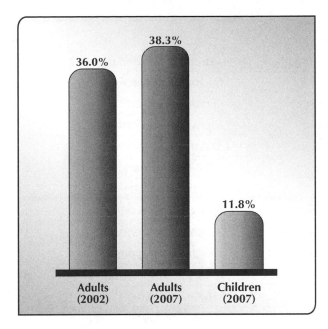

The differences in CAM utilization between ethnic groups within the United States may be attributable to cultural differences in acceptance of such therapies. Herbal supplements play a large role in the traditional practices of some cultures. Herbal products (e.g., Astragalus and gingko) are still being used to treat a variety of conditions in Traditional Chinese Medicine (TCM). Originating in India, Ayurvedic medicine uses naturally occurring substances such as plants, oils and common spices (e.g., ginger, turmeric) for both treatment of disease and for health maintenance. The Native Americans also continue to use herbs as part of their healing traditions (e.g., dandelion, goldenseal).[6] These are only a few examples; many cultures throughout history have used herbals in the prevention and treatment of ailments and some continue to do so. Some herbal products have been so effective and well-tolerated that they have been approved as over-the-counter (OTC) or prescription medications; some examples are included in Table 1.[7]

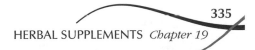

Table 1
Medications Originating from Plants[7]

Medication	Plant	Use / Indication
Atropine (prescription)	*Atropa belladonna*	Pupil Dilation
Capsaicin (OTC)	*Capsicum frutescens*	Pain
Cocaine (prescription)	*Erythroxylon coca*	Pain
Codeine (prescription)	*Papaver somniferum*	Pain
Colchine (prescription)	*Colchicum autumnale*	Gout
Digoxin (prescription)	*Digitalis purpurea*	Congestive Heart Failure
Ephedrine (OTC)	*Ephedra sinica*	Asthma
Ipecac (OTC)	*Cephaelis ipecacuanha*	To Induce Vomiting
Physostigmine (prescription)	*Physostigma venenosum*	Alzheimer's Disease
Quinine (prescription and OTC)	*Cinchona officinalis*	Malaria
Reserpine (prescription)	*Rauvolfia serpentina*	High Blood Pressure
Senna (OTC)	*Cassia acutifolia*	Constipation
Salicylin (OTC)	*Salix purpurea*	Pain / Inflammation
Scopolamine (prescription)	*Datura fatuosa*	Nausea (Motion Sickness)
Taxol (prescription)	*Taxus brevifolia*	Cancer
Vincristine (prescription)	*Catharanthus roseus*	Cancer

Regulation of Herbal Supplements

A **dietary supplement** is defined by the U.S. Food and Drug Administration (FDA) as "a product containing a vitamin, a mineral, an herb or other botanical, an amino acid, a dietary substance for use by man to supplement the diet by increasing the total dietary intake (e.g., enzymes or tissues from organs or glands), or a concentrate, metabolite, constituent or extract."[8] In 1994, dietary supplements, which include herbal supplements, were defined by the Dietary Supplement Health and Education Act (DSHEA), which gives regulatory authority to FDA. As per DSHEA, manufacturers of herbal supplements may claim the product will benefit by supporting "the structure or function in humans or describing general well-being from consumption" of the herbal product. The manufacturer may not, however, claim that the product treats, cures, prevents or may be used to diagnose any known disease of the human body. Manufacturers are required to indicate on the product label, in boldface, that any such claim "...has not been evaluated by the Food and Drug Administration. This product is not intended to diagnose, treat, cure or prevent any disease."[8] Each herbal product must be labeled as a "dietary supplement"[9] and follow all labeling requirements for dietary supplements required by the FDA.

An **herbal supplement** is "any form of a plant or plant product, including leaves, stems, flowers, roots and seeds."[10] Herbal supplements are considered a type of dietary supplement that contain a sole herb or a mixture of products.[6] An herbal, being an unstandardized, naturally-occurring product, may contain chemicals at varying levels; so manufacturers wishing to provide a quality product with the predictable results must develop a standardized process of manufacturing to ensure consistency in the final product. However, manufacturers may develop different processes to produce their herbal products, which may result in significant differences between similar products. Further, this variation may not only occur between manufacturers but also within different lots from the same manufacturer.[7,10]

In 2007, Congress required manufacturers to register, by passage of the Bioterrorism Act, with FDA prior to the manufacture or marketing of any supplements in the U.S. Currently, companies that manufacture, package or hold dietary supplements are required to establish and follow current Good Manufacturing Practices (cGMP) to ensure the correct identity, purity and quality of their products.[9]

Some argue that DSHEA did not go far enough when it defined herbal products as dietary supplements, because dietary supplements do not undergo the level of scrutiny by the FDA that OTC drugs must undergo. Both OTC and prescription medications must show, through scientific study, that they are both safe for human consumption and efficacious as treatments for a specific condition to be approved for marketing in the U.S. by the FDA. DSHEA requires that manufacturers are responsible for ensuring the safety and accurate labeling of their products and that they have some evidence that their claims are valid; however, there is neither a requirement to have manufacturers submit this evidence to the FDA, nor a standard to have the FDA evaluate these claims. The FDA is, however, responsible for ensuring the safety of the public by restricting the sale of products known to be harmful to the public. Thus, the burden of proof is on the FDA to prove that an herbal supplement is not safe before action, such as removing it from the market, is taken against an unsafe product. To assist the FDA in its responsibility to ensure the public's safety, manufacturers are required to submit any reported adverse reactions to the FDA for evaluation.[8,9] Because of this regulatory structure, it is important for patients and health care professionals to conduct their own review of a product's safety record prior to taking or recommending a particular herbal product.

Considerations of Efficacy

It has been estimated that there are more than 20,000 herbal products available in the United States,[7] and the list is growing. Generally, there is limited data to show the efficacy of each of these products. Although information is available for the commonly used herbs, there is considerably less information on the remaining thousands of products. Further, the available information generally applies to the herbal in general and not to a specific manufacturer's product. Having little or no information does not necessarily mean there is no benefit from using a particular product; however, it simply means that there is a deficiency in conclusive studies, either positive or negative, regarding the efficacy of the product.

Properly-designed, well-executed, rigorous scientific studies are the best way to determine the efficacy of any therapy; however, this standard, which is generally always required for OTC and prescription medications, is not typically required for herbal products to make it to market. The herbal industry argues that to conduct properly-designed clinical trials would be too costly, with estimates for the research being around $350 million to determine both safety and efficacy of a product.[7] The industry also states that it would cost much less to patent the drug than to conduct these studies.[7] Most of the studies currently done on herbal products are now conducted and funded by independent researchers from universities, companies and the NIH.[5,11,12] Further, many of these herbal efficacy studies are conducted outside the U.S., where herbal products are often more strictly regulated.[7]

Although not technically an herbal supplement, omega-3 fatty acids (fish oil) are available not only as a dietary supplement but also as a prescription drug, Lovaza™; omega-3 fatty-acids are used to lower high triglycerides (a component of cholesterol). Multiple clinical trials using Lovaza™ have established it as an effective agent to treat high triglycerides. When some OTC products were reviewed for quality in one study, investigators found that some products did not meet their own label statements, including finding that some products did not contain the amount of omega-3 fatty-acids claimed on the label.[13]

Safety of Herbal Supplements

As herbal products are directly derived from plants, they are often perceived as "natural" and therefore safe to take; however, many herbal products, as well as conventional medications derived from plants, may be toxic. Unlike with conventional drugs, clinical studies to determine the most appropriate dose, common side effects and drug interactions are typically not conducted on herbal supplements. As some supplements may be a mixture of a variety of herbs or, compared to their labeled contents, may be adulterated, contaminated or misidentified, this may lead to a product having adverse effects. These side effects are likely under-recognized and under-reported to the manufacturer and therefore to the FDA. Also, since safety studies are not required, herbal products do not have to be tested for safety to growing fetuses, for cancer-causing potential or for potential harm to those with serious medical conditions. Since less than 1 percent of all adverse effects from dietary supplements are believed to be reported to the FDA,[14] consumers should inform their health care professionals about their use of these products in order to receive careful monitoring while taking these supplements. Common side effects for popular herbal products are shown in Table 2.

Ephedra Example

Ephedra, also known as Ma Huang, is a natural source of ephedrine alkaloids commonly found as nonprescription bronchodilators (drugs that make it easier to breathe), decongestants and appetite suppressants (e.g., ephedrine, pseudoephedrine and norephedrine). In combination with natural sources of caffeine (e.g., guarana, green tea and kola nut) and other extracts, such products were marketed as diet aides, exercise enhancers and energy boosters.[15] Reported adverse events, including nervousness, anxiety, tachycardia (fast heart rate), hypertension (high blood pressure), insomnia, appetite suppression, kidney stones, psychosis, seizures, heart attack, stroke and death, led investigators to determine that ephedra was a likely cause for these adverse events.[16]

Gurley, et al., studied the content of 20 ephedra-containing supplements. It was determined that the total ephedra-alkaloid content ranged from 0 mg to 18.5 mg per dose. Significant variation was observed even between lots from the same product; further, one alkaloid, (+) norpseudoephedrine, a Schedule IV controlled substance, was often found when it would be illegal for such products to contain that alkaloid. Authors found that, of the 20 ephedra-containing dietary supplements that they studied, the alkaloid content differed from that claimed on the label and was inconsistent between lots for some of the products.[15] A systematic review of ephedra studies shows a modest, short-term weight loss compared to placebo; however, it also shows that there is a two- to three-fold increase in the chance of experiencing adverse events (e.g., nausea, vomiting, heart palpitations and psychiatric symptoms) over placebo.[17]

In 2001, the mounting evidence on ephedra's potential to harm took center stage in the American media. A woman in Alaska who suffered a stroke after taking an ephedra-containing product manufactured by E'Ola Inc. was awarded $13.3 million in punitive and compensatory damages. Companies settled nearly three dozen personal injury or wrongful death lawsuits between 1994 and 1999; this case in Alaska was the first case to go to trial.[18] In February 2004, the FDA ruled that ephedra-containing supplements posed an unreasonable risk of illness or injury to the public. This ruling went into effect in April 2004 and prohibited the sale of ephedra-containing products in the U.S.[19,20] This issue with ephedra prompted many health care professionals, especially those practicing conventional Western medicine, to view herbal products in a negative light.

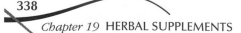

Drug-Herbal Interactions

Herbals that may be safe to take alone may be dangerous when combined with certain conventional medications and other herbals. A telephone survey of more than 2,500 adults showed that 14 percent of participants took at least one herbal supplement.[21] Among the 81 percent of those surveyed who were prescription-drug users, 16 percent of them also took an herbal supplement in the preceding week.[21] The 2002 National Health Interview Survey showed that 21 percent of people who use prescription drugs also take at least one herbal product and, of these, 69 percent have not discussed their use of the herbal product(s) with their physician.[22] As many people take both prescription and herbal products, drug-herbal interactions may occur, including when both are metabolized by the liver through similar pathways. Some of these interactions are well-documented (Table 2), but others are not or are occurring without the scientific community being aware of the interaction. Extreme caution should be used by patients taking both herbal products and conventional medications.

A classic example of a drug-herbal interaction is the interaction between St. John's Wort, which is commonly used for depression, anxiety and nervousness, and many other medicatons.[23] Reviews of published studies suggest that St. John's Wort is well tolerated and more efficacious than placebo in short-term treatment of mild to moderate depression. Research conducted in the early 2000s showed that St. John's Wort was a potent inducer of a variety of cytochrome P450 liver enzymes (specifically CYP3A4).[24-27] Cytochrome P450 enzymes are pathways in the liver that play a part in the metabolism of many chemicals, including some medications and some herbal products. Chemicals of any sort, if metabolized by the same pathway, may compete for that metabolism (as only one substance can go down a particularly pathway at once), which can result in a higher concentration of the losing product. That can lead to toxicity or over-effectiveness. A serious interaction between St. John's Wort and traditional drugs has been shown with organ-transplant anti-rejection drugs. Studies using both drugs at the same time showed a decreased cyclosporine blood concentration that, in many cases, resulted in either normalization of cyclosporine level when St. John's Wort was stopped, a required increase in cyclosporine dose, or rejection of the transplanted organ.[28]

With thousands of herbal products available and hundreds of new products introduced each year, herbal-drug interactions need to be routinely examined to protect those patients who take cocktails of prescriptions, over-the-counters and herbal products; often without the knowledge of their health care professionals.

Special Populations

Pharmacy technicians are expected to use the same decision-making process in referring patients inquiring about OTC medications as those inquiring about herbals. In light of the safety concerns and drug interactions that are possible with herbals, a pharmacy technician is expected to recognize those patients who are in need of a consultation with a pharmacist. Patients who are especially in need of a pharmacist's expertise before using herbals include the following:

- Pregnant or breast-feeding women
- Patients with a history of allergies
- Children
- Those scheduled for surgery
- Those using more than one herbal product
- Those self-treating a serious or chronic condition
- Patients experiencing a side effect related to a herbal supplement
- Those inquiring about a herbal product with significant side effect potential
- Anyone taking prescription medications
- Anyone with a history of high blood pressure or diabetes

Now, more than ever, it is essential for patients to share their entire medication use history, including herbals, with all of their health care professionals. Pharmacy technicians are expected to assist pharmacists in collecting medication histories and lists of currently used medications from patients. This task is made more difficult every day by the increasing diversity of herbals and the number of supplements containing multiple herbal ingredients. Also, many multi-herbal products may change ingredients without changing their product name. A chronological history may be required for a pharmacist to determine all of the drug/herbal-related side effects or interactions a patient may be experiencing. Obtaining the dose and frequency is also an important part of the record. Many pharmacists and physicians request that patients bring in their supplement bottles to ensure that accurate lists of ingredients can be obtained when recording a complete medication list.

Resources

There are a number of Web sites that provide information regarding herbal supplements. Many, however, do not provide adequate information for a patient to make an informed decision about the safety or efficacy of a particular product. Among 338 retail Web sites evaluated, 81 percent made one or more health claims and 55 percent claimed to treat, prevent, diagnose or cure specific diseases even though this is not legal in the U.S.[29] Of the sites with an health claim, 52 percent omitted the standard, and required, FDA disclaimer that must appear on the product packaging if the product is sold in the U.S.[29] Only 12 percent of 443 sites provided referenced information without a link to a distributor.[29]

Patients should be informed of potential misinformation on retail Web sites promoting herbal supplements. In addition to the expertise provided by a pharmacist, a patient may be referred to any of the following sites to find information based on available scientific evidence:

- FDA Dietary Supplement regulation: www.fda.gov/Food/DietarySupplements
- National Council for Complementary and Alternative Medicine: http://nccam.nih.gov
- National Institute of Health, Office of Dietary Supplements: http://ods.od.nih.gov
- Clinical trials (completed/ongoing) studying herbal products: www.clinicaltrials.gov

Conclusion

For a pharmacy technician, knowledge of the increasing utilization of CAM, which includes herbal supplements, is paramount to effectively assisting today's pharmacists. These products are widely advertised in stores and online; herbals are also being added to beverages, snack foods and other consumables. A pharmacy technician, knowledgeable of current regulatory structure, requirements to test for the efficacy and safety of herbal supplements, and populations who are particularly at risk for problem associated with using herbals, is an absolutely essential resource for a pharmacist wishing to obtain a complete medication history or assist a patient in making informed health care decisions.

Table 2

Commonly Used Herbal Products and Potential Drug-Herb Interactions [6,23,27-32]

Herbal	Commonly Uses	Common Adverse Effects	Sample Interacting Conventional Drug(s)	Known Potential Problem(s)
Echinacea	Treat or prevent colds, flu and infections. Stimulate the immune system and treat acne or boils	Allergic reactions (including anaphylaxis), rash, worsening asthma, stomach / intestinal upset	Anabolic steroids, methotrexate, amiodarone, ketoconazole	Liver toxicity
			Immunosuppressants	Reversing the desired effect
Evening Primrose Oil	Treat cancer, diabetes, eczema, rheumatoid arthritis, menstrual symptoms (i.e., breast pain or premenstrual syndrome)	Stomach / intestinal upset, headache	Anti-convulsants	Increased risk of seizures
Feverfew	Treat fever, headaches, stomach aches, toothaches, insect bites, infertility, menstrual problems, problems with labor during childbirth, migraine headaches, rheumatoid arthritis, psoriasis, allergies, asthma, tinnitus, dizziness, nausea / vomiting	Allergic reactions, canker sores, swelling / irritation of lips / tongue, loss of taste, nausea, digestive problems, bloating, headaches, nervousness, difficulty sleeping, stiff muscles and joint pain, and uterine contractions leading to miscarriage or premature delivery	Nonsteroidal anti-inflammatory drugs	
			Warfarin	Altered bleeding time
Garlic	Treat high cholesterol, heart disease, high blood pressure, stomach cancer, colon cancer	Breath / body odor, heartburn, upset stomach, allergic reactions, inappropriate bleeding	Warfarin	Increased bleeding
			Ritonavir	Increased stomach / intestinal problems
			Saquinavir	Decreased saquinavir blood levels
Ginger	Treat stomachache, diarrhea, nausea, rheumatoid arthritis, osteoarthritis, joint / muscle pain	Gas, bloating, heartburn, nausea (mostly with powdered ginger)	Warfarin	Altered bleeding time
Gingko	Treat asthma, bronchitis, fatigue, tinnitus, Alzheimer's disease, dementia, intermittent claudication, sexual dysfunction, multiple sclerosis	Headache, nausea, stomach upset, diarrhea, dizziness, allergic skin reactions, increased bleeding risk, seizures, death	Warfarin, trazodone and aspirin	Increased bleeding reactions

Table 2 cont.
Commonly Used Herbal Products and Potential Drug-Herb Interactions [6,23,27-32]

Herbal	Commonly Uses	Common Adverse Effects	Sample Interacting Conventional Drug(s)	Known Potential Problem(s)
Ginseng	Improve health of those recovering from illness, increase sense of well-being, increase stamina, increase mental and physical performance, treat erectile dysfunction, hepatitis C, symptoms of menopause, lower blood glucose, control blood pressure	Headaches, insomnia, stomach / intestinal problems, allergic reactions, menstrual irregularities, increased blood pressure	Phenelzine sulfate	Mania
			Estrogens, corticosteroids	Additive effects
			Digoxin	Interference with drug-level monitoring
			Insulin, sulfonylureas, metformin	Altered blood-sugar levels
Hawthorn	Treat heart disease, digestive problems, kidney problems, heart failure, angina	Upset stomach, headache, dizziness	Digoxin	Interference in drug level monitoring
Kava	Treat asthma, urinary tract infections, fatigue, insomnia, anxiety, menopausal symptoms	Liver damage (hepatitis and liver failure), dystonia, scaly / yellow skin, drowsiness		Additive sedative effects, coma, lethargy, disorientation
Saw Palmetto	Treat urinary symptoms from benign prostatic hyperplasia, chronic pelvic pain, bladder disorders, decreased sex drive, hair loss, hormone imbalance, prostrate cancer	Stomach discomfort	Benzodiazepines, cimetidine, terazosin	Reduced iron absorption

Herbal	Commonly Uses	Common Adverse Effects	Sample Interacting Conventional Drug(s)	Known Potential Problem(s)
St. John's Wort	Treat mental disorders, nerve pain, anxiety, depression, sleep disorders, malaria, wounds / burns, insect bites	Sensitivity to sunlight, anxiety, dry mouth, dizziness, stomach / intestinal upset, fatigue, headache, sexual dysfunction	Mono-amine oxidase inhibitors (MAOI), serotonin re-uptake inhibitors	Serotonin syndrome
			5-aminolevulinic acid, amitriptyline, cyclosporine, digoxin, indinavir, midazolam, nefazodone, nevirapine, oral contraceptives, simvastatin, tacrolimus, theophylline, warfarin, phenytoin, phenobarbital, irinotecan	Changed concentrations of drug listed
			Iron	Reduced iron absorption
Valerian	Treat sleep disorders, anxiety, headaches, depression, irregular heartbeat, trembling	Headaches, dizziness, upset stomach, tiredness (the morning after its use)	Barbiturates, any central nervous system depressant	Additive effects, excessive sedation

References

1. Elsenberg, D.M., Davis, R.B., Ettner, S.L. et al., "Trends in Alternative Medicine Use in the United States, 1990-1997: Results of a Follow up National Survey," *Journal of the American Medical Association*, Vol. 280, No. 18, pp. 1569-1575, 1998.

2. Kelly, J.P., Kaufman, D.W., Kelley, K. et al., "Recent Trends in Use of Herbal and Other Natural Products," *Archives of Internal Medicine*, Vol. 165, pp. 281-286, 2005.

3. Barnes, P.M., Bloom, B., Nahin, R., CDC, 2007 National Health Statistics Report #12, Complementary and Alternative Medicine Use Among Adults and Children: United States, Dec. 10, 2008.

4. Nahin, R.L., Barnes, P.M., Stussman, B.J., Bloom, B., Costs of Complementary and Alternative Medicine (CAM) and Frequency of Visits to CAM Practitioners: United States, 2007 National Health Statistics Reports, No. 18, U.S. Department of Health and Human Services, Hyattsville, MD, 2009.

5. National Center for Complementary and Alternative Medicine, NCCAM Facts at a Glance and Mission, National Institute of Health, http://nccam.nih.gov/about/ataglance, Aug. 2, 2010.

6. National Center for Complementary and Alternative Medicine, Herbs at a Glance: A Quick Guide to Herbal Supplements, National Institute of Health, U.S. Department of Health and Human Services, Publication No. 10-6248, June 2010.

7. Winslow, L.C., Kroll, D., "Herbs as Medicines," *Archives of Internal Medicine*, Vol. 158, pp. 2192-2199, 1998.

8. FDA Regulatory Information, Dietary Supplement Health and Education Act of 1994, www.fda.gov/RegulatoryInformation/Legislation/FederalFoodDrugandCosmeticActFDCAct/SignificantAmendmentstotheFDCAct/ucm148003.htm, Aug. 3, 2010.

9. FDA, Overview of Dietary Supplements, www.fda.gov/Food/DietarySupplements/ConsumerInformation/ucm110417.htm, Aug. 3, 2010.

10. Bent, S., "Herbal Medicine in the United States: Review of Efficacy, Safety and Regulation," *Journal of General Internal Medicine*, Vol. 23, No. 6, pp. 854-859, 2008.

11. National Institute of Health Clinical Trials, www.clinicaltrials.gov, Aug. 19, 2010.

12. Office of Cancer Complementary and Alternative Medicine, National Cancer Institute, www.cancer.gov/cam, Aug. 28, 2010.

13. Sadovsky, R., Collins, N., Tighe, A.P., Brunton, S.A., Safeer, R., "Patient use of dietary supplements: a clinician's perspective," *Current Medical Research and Opinion*, Vol. 24, pp. 1209-1216, 2008.

14. Woo, J.J., "Adverse event monitoring and multivitamin-multimineral dietary supplements," *American Journal of Clinical Nutrition*, Vol. 85, pp. 323S-324S, 2007.

15. Gurley, B.J., Gardner, S.F., Hubbard, M.A., "Content versus label claims in ephedra containing dietary supplements," *American Journal of Health-System Pharmacists*, Bethesda, MD, Vol. 57, pp. 963-969, 2000.

16. Haller, C.A., Benowitz, N.L., "Adverse Cardiovascular and Central Nervous System Events Associated with Dietary Supplements Containing Ephedra Alkaloids," *New England Journal Medicine*, Vol. 343, pp. 1833-1838, 2000.

17. Shekelle, P.G., Hardy, M.L., Morton, S.C., "Efficacy and Safety of Ephedra and Ephedrine for Weight Loss and Athletic Performance: A Meta-analysis," *Journal of the American Medical Association*, Vol. 289, No. 12, pp. 1537-1545, 2003.

18. Gugliotta, G., "Woman Wins $13.3 Million Against Dietary Company," www.crnusa.org/Mshellmedia020901wpcopy.html, Aug. 15, 2010.

19. FDA Register Final Rule – FR69 6787, Final Rule Declaring Dietary Supplements Containing Ephedrine Alkaloids Adulterated Because They Present an Unreasonable Risk, Feb. 11, 2004, www.fda.gov/Food/DietarySupplements/GuidanceComplianceRegulatoryInformation/ RegulationsLaws/ucm079733.htm, Aug. 15, 2010.

20. FDA Statement: FDA Announces Rule Prohibiting Sale of Dietary Supplements Containing Ephedrine Alkaloids Effective April 12, 2004, www.fda.gov/NewsEvents/Newsroom/PressAnnouncements/2004/ucm108281.htm, Aug. 15, 2010.

21. Kaufman, D.W., Kelly, J.P., Rosenberg, L., Anderson, T.E., Mitchell, A.A., "Recent Patterns of Medication Use in the Ambulatory Adult Population of the United States: The Slone Survey," *Journal of the American Medical Association*, Vol. 287, pp. 337-344, 2002.

22. Gardiner, P., Graham, R.E., Legedza, A.T., Eisenberg, D.M., Phillips, R.S., "Factors Associated With Dietary Supplement Use Among Prescription Medication Use," *Archives of Internal Medicine,* Vol. 166, pp. 1968-1974, 2006.

23. De Smiet, P., "Herbal Remedies," *New England Journal of Medicine*, Vol. 347, pp. 2046-2056, 2002.

24. Durr, D., Stieger, B., Kullak-Ublick, G.A. et al., "St. John's Wort induces intestinal P-glycoprotein/MDR1 and intestinal and hepatic CYP3A4," *Clinical Pharmacology & Therapeutics*, Vol. 68, pp. 598-604, 2000.

25. Roby, C.A., Anderson, G.D., Kantor, E., Dryer, D.A., Burstein, A.H., "St. John's Wort: Effect on CYP3A4 Activity," *Clinical Pharmacology & Therapeutics*, Vol. 67, pp. 451-457, 2000.

26. Wang, Z., Gorski, J.C., Hamman, M.A., Huang, S.M., Lesko, L.J., Hall, S.D., "The Effects of St. John's Wort (Hypericum perforatum) on Human Cytochrome P450 Activity," *Clinical Pharmacology & Therapeutics*, Vol. 70, pp. 317-326, 2001.

27. Mannel, M., "Drug Interactions With St. John's Wort: Mechanisms and Clinical Implications," *Drug Safety*, Vol. 27, No. 11, pp. 773-797, 2004.

28. Hu, Z., Yang, X., Ho, P.C.L. et al, "Herb-Drug Interactions: A Literature Review," *Drugs*, Vol. 65, No. 9, pp. 1239-1282, 2005.

29. Moris, C.A., Avorn, J., "Internet Marketing of Herbal Products," *Journal of the American Medical Association*, Vol. 290, pp. 1505-1509, 2003.

30. Vickers, A., Zollman, C., "ABCs of Complementary Medicine: Herbal Medicine," *British Medical Journal*, Vol. 319, pp. 1050-1053, 1999.

31. Miller, L.G., "Herbal Medicinals," *Archives of Internal Medicine*, Vol. 158, pp. 2200-2211, 1998.

32. Izzo, A.A., Ernst, E., "Interactions Between Herbal Medicines and Prescribed Drugs: An Updated Systematic Review," *Drugs*, Vol. 69, No. 13, pp. 1777-1798, 2009.

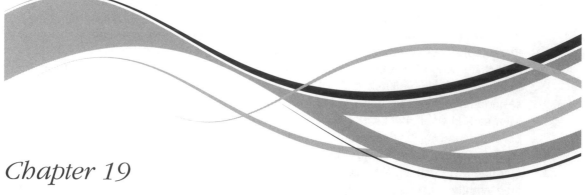

REVIEW QUESTIONS

1. Which of the following is not considered a dietary supplement?
    a. Feverfew
    b. Vitamin C
    c. Orange juice
    d. Omega-3 fatty-acids

2. The use of herbal products, as part of complementary/alternative medicine has increased since 1990.
    a. True
    b. False

3. The Dietary Supplement and Health Education Act regulates the use of dietary supplements in the United States.
    a. True
    b. False

4. Which of the following can be on the label of a dietary supplement?
    a. "Approved by the FDA"
    b. "… may treat osteoporosis"
    c. "… may be used to prevent infection from insects"
    d. "… may be used to support mental well-being"

5. It is the responsibility of the herbal manufacturer to inform the FDA of any adverse reactions reported to them by patients; but, it is up to the FDA to prove an herbal product unsafe.
    a. True
    b. False

6. Which of the following Internet sites could a pharmacy technician or pharmacist use to obtain evidence-based information about dietary supplements?
   a. Herbs at a Glance: A Quick Guide to Herbal Supplements from NCCAM
   b. National Council for Complementary and Alternative Medicine
   c. National Institute of Health, Office of Dietary Supplements
   d. All of the above

7. As herbal products are plants or derivatives from plants, they are often perceived as "natural" and therefore as safe to take even when their safety has not been well-studied and when certain patients should not use such products due to interactions with other medications.
   a. True
   b. False

8. Which of the following is an example of a harmful drug interaction?
   a. Saw palmetto causing hives in a patient with a history of allergies
   b. A woman having a stroke after taking more than what was on the label of an ephedra-containing product
   c. Bleeding in a 26-year-old woman taking only ginseng
   d. Rejection of an organ transplant in a patient taking St. John's wort and cyclosporine

9. Which herbal product was declared unsafe and taken off the market by the FDA?
   a. Echinacea
   b. Ma huang
   c. Green tea
   d. Gingko biloba

10. Which of the following patients should be referred to a pharmacist for counseling?
    a. A 30-year-old, pregnant women who is considering taking feverfew for psoriasis
    b. An 83-year-old man who is taking high blood pressure medications and would like to also take Hawthorn
    c. A 58-year-old woman who is being admitted next week for elective surgery. She would like to know where the garlic capsules are because she heard it can improve her cholesterol levels
    d. All of the above

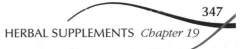

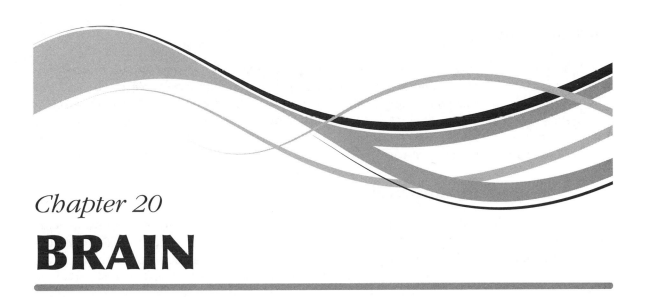

Chapter 20

BRAIN

By Sister Phyllis Klonowski, Pharm.D.

Learning Objectives

This chapter seeks to prepare a pharmacy technician to:

- explain brain and nerve structure and function.
- name the two cell families involved with central nervous system function and explain how they differ.
- describe the primary types of transmitters and receptors.
- define the primary families of glial cells and other specialty cells for transport and protection.

Introduction

It is important for pharmacy professionals to understand how disruptions, injuries or variations in normal functioning of the brain and nervous system can affect medication choices and regimens. This chapter seeks to review the anatomy (structure) and physiology (operation) of the brain and nervous system in relationship to other parts of the human body. Further, understanding the anatomy and physiology of the brain will give a pharmacy technician a better understanding of how psychiatric disorders, discussed in Chapter 21, can result from structural or functional abnormalities of the brain.

Views of the Body and Brain

For anatomical purposes, the body is viewed and defined from a standing erect, forward-facing view. Further, descriptions of direction (left/right) are always from the perspective of the body being described rather than from the perspective of the observer. Having a basic understanding of the anatomy will help in the understanding of diseases – especially those that originate in one part of the brain but ultimately affect somewhere other than that origin. Understanding the celluar anatomy is helpful to understand the complex relationship between the **neurotransmitters**, chemical messengers that brain cells use to communicate, and how their dysfunction can lead to visible signs of illness. This understanding also gives a framework for the types of drugs and other therapies that are available to those afflicted with abnormalities of the structure and function of the brain. The brain is one of the most difficult organs to see in action because it cannot be removed from the body or artificially supported with machines. Thus, advanced imaging techniques have been developed to look at the brain and other organs functioning inside a live patient. A **Computed Tomography (CT) Scan** and a **Magnetic Resonance Image (MRI)** are the most common brain scans used to visualize the functioning brain. The pictures generated by these scans are composites of many images taken throughout the scan. Generally, an image of a very thin slice of the brain is taken with each pass of the scan; once the many thousands of images are compiled into a single image, the picture becomes a three-dimensional image of the functioning brain. A modern clinician must use physical assessment, lab values and these valuable images when making a diagnosis or recommending a change in therapy.

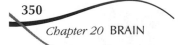

Figure 1
The Brain

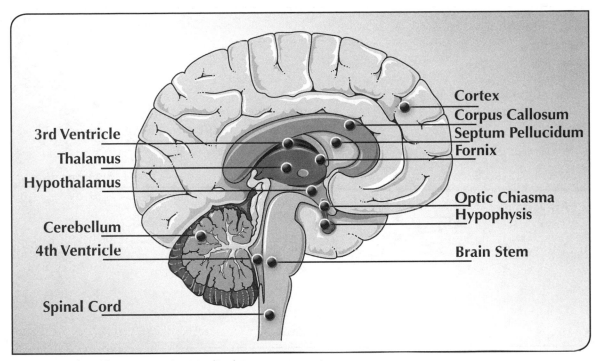

Figure produced using Servier Medical Art, www.servier.com

Brain Structure and Function

The brain has three major sections: the forebrain, midbrain and hindbrain (see Figure 1 for an overall picture of the brain). The front and top of the head is called the **forebrain**; the forebrain includes the **cortex/cerebrum** (also known as the **frontal lobe** and **upper parietal lobe**). The forebrain is associated with interpreting, understanding, organizing, directing and planning. Damage to this part of the brain means a potential loss in skills such as problem-solving, financial management, planning complex tasks and following complex directions. The cortex is connected to almost every other part of the body. There are recognized locations within the cortex associated with motor function, sensory perception and the functioning of other body organs. Nerves, or nerve-tracts, extend from the part of the cortex closest to the front and top of the brain to the tips of the fingers and the tips of the toes.

The **midbrain** has gained greater importance as the vital functions covered by the small distinct areas of this location have continued to be clarified. The midbrain is associated with emotional responses, especially anxiety, panic, worry and fear. The midbrain is also responsible for processing sensory signals from throughout the body (e.g., pain and temperature). Currently, these areas and their related functions, are believed to be as follows (see Figure 2):

- **Thalamus:** relays outside sensory information to the cortex
- **Amygdala:** screens for danger or threats to survival and sends alerts to the forebrain for direction
- **Hippocampus:** stores memory
- **Anterior Cingulate Gyros (ACG):** integrates signals and language from outside the CNS, concisely sends these messages to the cortex and then sends a return message from the cortex to the appropriate part of the body that needs to respond. Damage to this part of the brain appears to compromise flexibility.

Figure 2
Midbrain

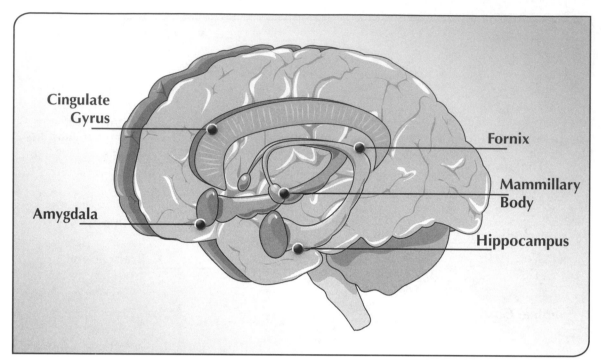

Figure produced using Servier Medical Art, www.servier.com

The **hindbrain** consists of the **pons**, **medulla oblongata** and **cerebellum**. The hindbrain is associated with basic functions, such as breathing and heart function, as well as voluntary or skeletal muscle coordination and alertness. This area is sometimes referred to as the reptilian brain because it is the part of the anatomy that humans have in common with nearly all animals, including reptiles, and is the part of the brain that reacts without thinking and keeps an animal alive in the face of danger. The amygdala may screen our surroundings for threats, but the hindbrain forces the action often referred to as the "fight or flight" response. Other functions controlled by the hindbrain are the subconscious actions that the body must do just to stay alive.

Spinal Cord

The **spinal cord** is a column of tissue that is surrounded by bone (called vertebrae) for the protection of the length of nerve fibers running between the brain and the body's trunk. Nearly all of the nerves that are responsible for controlling the body outside the brain originate in the brain and travel through the spinal cord to reach the area that they control. Further, any nerve that is responsible for sensing a body's environment and then relaying that sensory information to the brain must also travel through the spinal column. Damage to the spinal cord generally means that any nerves that connect further away from the brain than the injury are affected by that injury.

Cells and Structures for Communication

Neurons enable communication, via an electrical charge or current, between the brain and the other parts of the body or within the brain. Neurons that are connected to areas outside the brain often use the spinal cord to traverse the distance between the brain and the target end of the neuron.

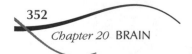

Neuron cells are like any other cells in the body, with the exception that neurons usually have dendrites and an axon (see Figure 3). **Dendrites** are neuron cell fibers that carry impulses to and from the cell body. Dendrites do not usually connect neurons to each other; dendrites usually carry sensory signals to the main body of the neuron for processing or for the message to be passed along to another neuron. Dendrites look like the roots (or branches) of a tree; they are named from the Greek word for tree: dendro. Another projection that usually comes from the main body of a neuron is called an **axon**; axons are single fibers that usually carry impulses from the main body of a neuron either to other neurons or to a muscle or a gland in order for that area to respond to the sensory stimulus that first came down a dendrite to the neuron's main body. Axons are often quite long; they can branch many times and may connect to hundreds of other neurons or nerve tracts. Bundled neuron fibers are called **nerves** or **nerve tracts**. **Glial cells** are the support cells that allow neurons to function normally; glial cells prevent inappropriate foreign substances (including bacteria and viruses) from entering the brain, protect neurons from exposure to toxic chemicals and facilitate the removal of waste from the brain.

Figure 3
Neuron

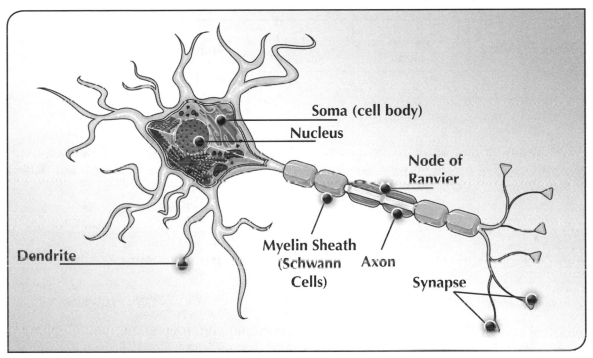

Figure produced using Servier Medical Art, www.servier.com

Neurons are responsible for communicating between one another and with other cells. Depending on the types of cells doing the communication and the type of connection between the neuron and the other cell, a different name exists for each type of connection. **Nodes** are compact areas where individual neurons in a nerve tract come close enough to each other to share information without having a direct physical connection. A **junction** is a connection between a nerve and a non-nerve tissue (such as a muscle cell). Finally, a **synapse** is a direct physical connection between two nerves. Communication that occurs at a node is passive, in that there is no control mechanisms in place to control how the communication is spread from neuron to neuron. At either a junction or a synapse, there is a complex pathway of receptors and chemicals that is used to control exactly how messages are sent from one neuron to another. The chemicals that neurons use to talk to one another, and to other cells, are called neurotransmitters. Generally, receptors exist on cells such that, when a neurotransmitter attaches to that receptor, a chemical change inside the cell occurs. This change generally starts or stops a cascade of chemical reactions that ultimately lead to some effect. For instance, one cell may use serotonin, a neurotransmitter, to send a signal to another cell that the stomach is full and that eating can stop. The second neuron, upon getting this message that a neuron attached to the stomach has received the full signal, instructs every other neuron around it to release serotonin in response to this stimulus. In this way, the nerve attached to the stomach has communicated, using neurotransmitters, to the entire brain that the stomach is full. This process is also part of feeling tired after eating a large meal, the extra serotonin that is released into the brain causes drowsiness, and the more one eats the more serotonin is released after becoming full. At a synapse, the neuron that is sending the signal is called the **pre-synaptic neuron** and the neuron that is receiving the signal is called the **post-synaptic neuron**.

See Table 1 for drugs often associated with the brain and its function. For a broader listing of drugs associated with psychiatric disorders, see Chapter 21.

Table 1
Drugs Often Associated with Brain Function

Drug Class(es)	Generic Name(s)**	Brand Name(s)**	Indication(s)	Available Dose Form(s)
Anticonvulsant	Carbamazepine	Carbatrol, Epitol, Equetro, Tegretol, Tegretol XR	Alcohol Withdrawal, Bipolar Disorder, Post-Traumatic Stress Disorder, Restless Leg Syndrome, Schizophrenia, Seizures	Capsule, Chewable Tablet, Suspension, Tablet
Anticonvulsant	Divalproex Sodium or Valproic Acid or Valproate Sodium	Depacon, Depakene, Depakote, Depakote ER, Depakote Sprinkle, Stavzor	Behavior Disorders in Alzheimer's Disease, Bipolar Disorder Mania, Migraine Prophylaxis, Seizures, Status Epilepticus	Capsule, Gel Cap, Injectable, Syrup, Tablet
Anticonvulsant	Gabapentin	Neurontin	Bipolar Disorder, Chronic Pain, Peripheral Neuropathy, Post-Herpetic Neuralgia, Seizures, Social Anxiety Disorder	Capsule, Solution, Tablet
Anticonvulsant	Lamotrigine	Lamictal, Lamictal ODT, Lamictal Starter Kit, Lamictal XR	Bipolar Disorder, Seizures	Extended-Release Tablet, Orally-Disintegrating Tablet, Tablet

Drug Class(es)	Generic Name(s)**	Brand Name(s)**	Indication(s)	Available Dose Form(s)
Anticonvulsant	Levetiracetam	Keppra, Keppra XR	Bipolar Disorder, Migraine Prevention, Seizures	Extended-Release Tablet, Injectable, Solution, Tablet
Anticonvulsant	Oxcarbazepine	Trileptal	Bipolar Disorder, Seizures	Suspension, Tablet
Anticonvulsant	Phenytoin	Dilantin, Dilantin Infatabs, Phenytek	Seizures	Capsule, Chewable Tablet, Injectable, Suspension
Anticonvulsant	Topiramate	Topamax, Topamax Sprinkle	Bipolar Disorder, Cluster Headache, Migraine Prophylaxis, Neuropathic Pain, Seizures	Capsule (Sprinkle), Tablet
Anti-Migraine	Acetaminophen / Butalbital / Caffeine with or without Codeine (some are Schedule 3)	Esgic-Plus, Fioricet, Fiorinal	Migraines	Capsule, Liquid, Tablet
Anti-Migraine	Sumatriptan	Alsuma, Dosepro, Imitrex, Imitrex Stat-Dose, Sumavel	Migraines	Injectable, Nasal Spray, Tablet
Anti-Parkinson's Disease	Carbidopa / Levodopa	Parcopa, Sinemet, Sinemet CR	Parkinson's Disease	Extended-Release Tablet, Orally-Disintegrating Tablet, Tablet
Anti-Parkinson's Disease	Ropinirole	Requip, Requip XL	Parkinson's Disease, Restless Leg Syndrome	Extended-Release Tablet, Tablet
Cholinesterase Inhibitor	Galantamine	Razadyne	Alzheimer's Disease	Extended-Release Capsule, Solution, Tablet
Dopamine Receptor Agonist (Long-Acting)	Cabergoline	Dostinex	Low Prolactin Levels	Tablet
Methylxanthines	Theophylline	Theo-24, Uniphyl	Asthma	Capsule, Liquid, Tablet

*All rights to all brand names and trademarks are held by their respective owners.

Transmitters and Receptors

The major neurotransmitters in the brain include **gamma-aminobutyric acid (GABA)**, **glutamate**, **norepinephrine (NE)**, **serotonin (5-hydroxytryptamine, 5-HT)**, **dopamine (DA)**, **acetylcholine** and **histamine**. Each plays a specific role in brain function. To add to the complexity and confusion associated with brain pathophysiology, each neurotransmitter can interact with different subtypes of receptors specific to that neurotransmitter. For example, there are at least 14 subtypes of receptors that bind serotonin. Each receptor subtype has different anatomical distribution throughout the brain and different functions.

GABA is the most important inhibitory neurotransmitter in the CNS. When GABA receptors are stimulated, the chemical processes that unfold will stop or slow down the action of the nerve. This becomes quite interesting when multiple neurons with GABA receptors are chained together along a nerve tract. If the action of the first neuron is to slow down the actions of the second neuron and then GABA is exposed to the first neuron, inhibiting its action, then the second neuron will act without restraint. The opposite may also be true: if the first neuron must fire for the second neuron to fire, then, in the presence of GABA, the second neuron will not fire because its trigger, the first neuron, is inhibited. Brain circuits with too little GABA activity may be responsible for seizures and anxiety disorders. Among the drugs that affect the GABA system, the most widely prescribed are the benzodiazepines, such as alprazolam, diazepam and lorazepam, used to treat anxiety. Many commonly used sleep aids also enhance GABA activity (e.g., temazepam, zolpidem). Side effects of drugs that increase the activity of GABA neurons include performance impairment and undesirable sedation.

Glutamate is the most important stimulatory neurotransmitter in the CNS. Glutamate-containing neurons are found throughout the forebrain. When glutamate-releasing neurons are stimulated, they have an excitatory effect on the next neuron in a circuit. Insufficient activity in the glutamate system may be responsible in part for the symptoms of schizophrenia (thought disorder). Excessive glutamate activity can lead to seizures. There are relatively few drugs that directly affect glutamate or glutamate receptors at the time of this publication, but there is great interest in this system for a number of psychiatric disorders.

NE neurons originate from small, discrete areas in the hindbrain, but the neurons diffuse throughout the brain to influence the actions of other neurons in many different areas. The functions of NE in the CNS include regulation of sleep-wake cycles, central blood pressure control, food and water intake, mood, anxiety, learning, memory and attention. With so many effects from NE, it is easy to predict that disrupting the normal activity of norepinephrine-containing neurons can have widespread desirable or adverse effects. Drugs that block the reuptake of norepinephrine are useful in treating depression and attention deficit hyperactivity disorder (ADHD), a problem with attention and motivation. They are also associated with peripheral side effects, such as tremor, tachycardia and hypertension.

Like NE, 5-HT neurons originate in a small, discrete area of the brain. From this small area in the hindbrain, 5-HT neurons spread across many areas of the brain to have regulatory roles over many functions. 5-HT actions include regulation of the release of other neurotransmitters and control of basic human behaviors, such as sleeping, eating and sexual activity. 5-HT also functions to regulate mood, anxiety, attention and alertness. For this reason, drugs that affect 5-HT have utility in many different disease states. Some side effects that follow directly from the physiological action of 5-HT include insomnia, changes in appetite, changes in weight and sexual disturbances.

Dopamine is confined to four neuron tracts that start in very small areas of the brain and spread to areas of influence smaller than those of NE and 5-HT. Consequently, dopamine is limited to effects on thought, emotion, certain muscle movements, reward and motivation, and release of prolactin (a hormone related to the formation and secretion of milk). Problems in the different dopamine tracts are believed to be responsible for such diverse conditions as schizophrenia (a thought disorder), Parkinson's Disease (a movement disorder), ADHD (a problem with attention and motivation) and, possibly, substance abuse (problems with reward and motivation). Each of these conditions is the result of changes in dopamine signals in one or more of the four dopamine tracts. Most of the drugs used to treat these conditions directly affect the dopamine system either by blocking dopamine receptors or by enhancing the action of dopamine.

Acetylcholine neurons start in discrete areas of the brain and, like NE and 5-HT neurons, spread across wide areas of the brain. This neurotransmitter has functions associated with learning, memory and arousal. One prominent disorder associated with disturbance of the brain-acetylcholine system is Alzheimer's disease. It is believed that this condition is caused by loss of acetylcholine-containing neurons, and the most effective drugs available to treat this disease reduce the enzymatic destruction of acetylcholine. Many drugs block acetylcholine receptors, leading to "anticholinergic" side effects. These effects include confusion, memory problems, blurred vision, exacerbation of angle closure glaucoma, tachycardia, constipation, urinary retention and dryness of the eyes, mouth, nasal passages and skin. Histamine is found in an area of the forebrain called the **hypothalamus**. From there, histamine-containing neurons spread throughout the brain to affect many brain activities. The normal functions of histamine-containing neurons include regulation of alertness, cognition, sensory information processing, regulation of the release of pituitary hormones and control of appetite. Many drugs have antihistaminic side effects, including increased appetite, weight gain, dryness and sedation.

The actions of neurotransmitters, released into a synapse, are terminated by three mechanisms. The most important mechanism by which neurotransmitter action is stopped is reuptake of the neurotransmitter back into the presynaptic nerve ending. Once transported back into the presynaptic neuron, the neurotransmitter is either destroyed by enzymes or recycled for future use. The second method by which the action of a neurotransmitter is stopped is through diffusion of the neurotransmitter out of the synapse away from the receptors sensitive to the neurotransmitter's influence. Finally, the neurotransmitter may be destroyed by enzymes found pre-synaptically or post-synaptically. Inhibition of neurotransmitter reuptake, and inhibition of enzymatic destruction of neurotransmitters, are two mechanisms by which drugs work to relieve depression. In addition to control by electrical signals traveling down neurons, release of neurotransmitters is also regulated through presynaptic autoreceptors. When activated, these receptors alter the release of the neurotransmitter from the presynaptic nerve terminal. Some autoreceptors increase the release of a neurotransmitter, while others decrease the release of a neurotransmitter. An autoreceptor may bind the same neurotransmitter released from the presynaptic nerve terminal, or it may bind a different neurotransmitter. A neurotransmitter found interacting with an autoreceptor may originate from the same presynaptic nerve ending on which the autoreceptor is located, or it may come from a separate neuron. In the latter case, a synapse between the second neuron and the autoreceptor on the first neuron must exist. A neurotransmitter can be released from a second neuron, diffuse across the synapse, bind to the autoreceptor on the first neuron and induce some change in the release of a neurotransmitter in the first neuron. For example, in parts of the cortex in the forebrain, 5-HT receptors are located on neurons that release dopamine. When the serotonin-binding autoreceptor is stimulated, it decreases the release of dopamine from the presynaptic neuron. Atypical antipsychotics may act, in part, by blocking these presynaptic serotonin autoreceptors, and that enhances the release of dopamine from the neurons.

Specialty Cells for Protection and Transport

Axons are covered by a fatty material called **myelin**. Myelin provides both protection and insulation to the axon. This insulation may allow for signals to travel faster down an axon. Membrane construction in the **peripheral nervous system (PNS)** uses specialized glial cells called **Schwann cells** that wrap around the axon in layers. **Neuroglia** or **glial cells**, as mentioned previously, are support cells that ensure that neurons continue to function properly. One way to distinguish between neurons and glial cells is that glial cells do not reproduce, whereas neurons do possess the ability to reproduce. There are six differentiated families of glial cells in the CNS. Each has a special function.

- **Astrocytes (astroglia)** have numerous projections that anchor these cells to the blood system. They regulate the external chemical environment of the neurons by removing excess ions and recycling neurotransmitters. They are also part of the blood-brain barrier (discussed in detail later). These cells are also believed to regulate calcium levels in neurons.
- **Oligodendrocytes** are the building blocks of the myelin of the CNS.
- **Ependymocytes** line the cavities of the CNS, make up the walls of the brain's ventricles and create **cerebrospinal fluid (CSF)**. These cells have **cilia** (small hairs that project from the cell membrane and beat in a sweeping motion) that circulate CSF.
- **Radial glial cells** generate neurons and a skeletal framework to hold new neurons when the CNS is developing. Once matured, two sites in the brain retain these cells. **Bergmann cells**, found in the cerebellum, regulate synaptic plasticity. **Muller cells**, found in the retina, are part of bidirectional communication with neurons.
- **Satellite cells**, found in the PNS, form a covering for neurons in sensory, sympathetic and parasympathetic ganglia. They are interconnected, like the astrocytes, to gap junctions, respond to ATP (adenosine triphosphate) and increase intracellular calcium. These cells are associated with chronic pain following injury and/or inflammation.
- **Enteric glial cells** are located in the intrinsic ganglia of the digestive tract. Ongoing investigation is clarifying the specific functions of these cells, but they could be related to muscle contractility and secretory regulation of digestion.

Another type of specialty cell that makes up the tissue barriers for the brain, and CNS, are the **Blood Brain Barrier (BBB)** and the **Blood-Cerebrospinal Fluid Barrier (BCSFB)**. The human BBB is a network of capillaries with an endothelial lining known to have a significant lack of openings between the cells and an energy-requiring transport system. The need for transport applies to both essential nutrients and cellular building block material into the brain and its nerves, and of waste/excess material being eliminated from the brain and neurons. An added exterior protection of glial astrocytes attach to the BBB capillaries, forming almost two extra layers of cell membrane, plus cell content, as protection.

Conclusion

A thorough understanding of the brain requires extensive study, and this chapter only offers a very basic understanding of this complex system. The brain is broadly made up of three areas: the hindbrain, midbrain and forebrain. These three areas are connected by neurons that communicate with both electrical and chemical signals. In order to maintain this system, many cells must coordinate to support the function of neurons. Further, many drugs seek to enhance or interrupt the functions of this system to achieve a therapeutic benefit. There are many potential targets for malfunction that can lead to disease; this has resulted in many different classes of drugs used to affect the function of the brain.

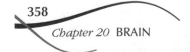

Bibliography

- Barrett, K.E., Barman, S.M., Boitano, S., Brooks, H., "Neurotransmitters and Neuromodulators," Chapter 7, Ganong's Review of Medical Physiology, 23rd edition, 2010, pp. 129-148.
- Barrett, K.E., Barman, S.M., Boitano, S., Brooks, H., "Overview of Cellular Physiology in Medical Physiology," Chapter 2, Ganong's Review of Medical Physiology, 23rd edition, 2010, pp. 31-62.
- Bloom, F.E., "Neurotransmitters and the Central Nervous System," Chapter 12, Part III, In: Goodman & Gilman's The Pharmacological Basis of Therapeutics, 11th edition, 2006, pp. 317-340.
- Bloom, F.E., Kupfer, D., Psychopharmacology: The Fourth Generation of Progress, New York, NY, 1995, pp. 397-405, 461-469.
- Chapter, M.C., White, C.M., DeRidder, A., Chadwick, W., Martin, B., Maudsley, S., "Chemical modification of Class II G protein-coupled receptor ligands: Frontiers in the development of peptide analogs as neuroendocrine pharmacological therapies," Pharmacology and Therapeutics, Vol. 125, 2010, pp. 39-54.
- Cogan, T.A., Thomas, A.O., Rees, L.E.N., Taylor, A.H., Jepson, M.A., Williams, P.H., Ketley, J., Humphrey, T.J., "Norepinephrine increases the pathogenic potential of Campylobacter jejuni," International Journal of Gastroenterology and Hepatology, Vol. 56, 2007, pp. 1060-1065.
- Cohen, B.J., Taylor, J.J., Memmler's The Structure and Function of the Human Body, 8th edition, Philadelphia, pp. 114-115, 139-144.
- Crimson, M.L., Buckley, P.F., "Schizophrenia," Pharmacotherapy: A Pathophysiologic Approach, 6th edition, New York, NY, 2005, pp. 1209-1233.
- Dalziel, S., Veryard, C., "Therapeutics for neurological indications American Chemical Society 234th National Meeting August 19-23, 2007," IDrugs, Vol. 10, 2007, pp. 676-677.
- Hardman, J.G., Limbird, L.E., Gilman, A., The Pharmacological Basis of Therapeutics, 10th edition, New York, NY, 2001, pp. 293-320.
- Hitchcock, S.A., Pennington, L.D., "Structure-Brain Exposure Relationships," Journal of Medicinal Chemistry, Vol. 49, No. 26, 2006, pp. 7559-7583.
- Hosie, A.M., Clarke, L., da Silva, H., Smart, T.G., "Conserved site for neurosteroid modulation of GABA$_A$ receptors," Neuropharmacology, Vol. 56, 2009, pp.149-154.
- Huang, G.T.J., Lee, H.W., Lee, H.S., Lee, G.H., Huh, S.Y., Choi, G.W., Park, S.H., "Localization of substance P-induced upregulated interleukin-8 expression in human dental pulp explants," International Endodontic Journal, Vol. 41, 2008, pp. 100-107.
- Kalant, H., Roschlau, W., Principles of Medical Pharmacology, 6th edition, Functional Organization of the Central Nervous System, New York, NY, 1998, pp. 217-240.
- Kalant, H., Roschlau, W., Principles of Medical Pharmacology, 6th edition, New York, NY, 1998, pp. 135-148.
- Konradi, C., Heckers, S., "Molecular Aspects of Glutamate Dysregulation: Implications for Schizophrenia and its Treatment," Pharmacology Therapeutics, Vol. 97, No. 2, 2003, pp. 153-179.
- Lidsky, T.I., Schneider, J.S., "Lead neurotoxicity in children: basic mechanisms and clinical correlates," Brain, Vol. 126, pp. 5-19, 2003.
- Lu, B., Su, Y., Das, S., Wang, H., Wang, Y., Liu, J., Ren, D., "Peptide neurotransmitters activate a cation channel complex of NALCN and UNC-80," Nature, Vol. 457, No. 5, 2009, pp. 741-745.
- MacDermott, A.B., Role, L.W., Siegelbaum, S.A., "Presynaptic Ionotropic Receptors and the Control of Transmitter Release," Annual Reviews of Neuroscience, Vol. 22, 1999, pp. 443-485.

- Nicholls, J., Martin, A., Wallace, B., Fuchs, P., From Neuron to Brain. 4th edition, Sunderland, MA, 2001.

- Parker, D., "Pharmacological Approaches to Functional Recovery After Spinal Injury," Current Drug Topics-CNS Neurological Disorders, Vol. 4, 2005, pp. 195-210.

- Reddy, D.S., "Mass spectrometric assay and physiological-pharmacological activity of androgenic neurosteroids," Neurochemistry International, Vol. 52, 2008, pp. 541-553.

- Ricardo, M., Trzaska, K. A., Rameshwar, P., "Neurokinin-A inhibits cell cycle activators inn K562 cells and activates Smad4 through a noncanonical pathway: a novel method in neural-hematopoietic axis," *Journal of Neuroimmunology*, Vol. 204, 2008, pp. 85-91.

- Richelson, E., "Interactions of Antidepressants with Neurotransmitter Transporters and Receptors and Their Clinical Relevance," *Journal of Clinical Psychiatry*, Vol. 64, No. 13, 2003, pp. 5-12.

- Waxman, S., "Signaling in the Nervous System," Chapter 3, Clinical Neuroanatomy, 26th edition, 2010, pp. 19-32.

- Wenzel, J., Grabinski, N., Cordula, A., Knopp, A.D., Manjunath, R., Randeva, H.S., Ehrhart-Bornstein, M., Dominiak, P., Johren, O., "Hypocretin/orexin increases the expression of steriodogenic enzmes in human adrenocortical NCI H295R cells," *American Journal Physiology – Regulatory Integrative and Comparative Physiology*, R1601-R1609, Sept. 30, 2009.

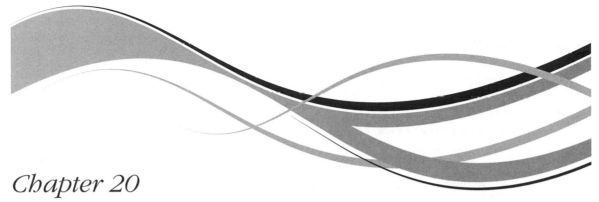

Chapter 20
REVIEW QUESTIONS

1. The brain is made up of three major sections, including the forebrain, midbrain and hindbrain.
    a. True
    b. False

2. The midbrain is associated with which kind of response?
    a. Pain
    b. Basal functioning
    c. Emotional
    d. A and C

3. The hindbrain includes which of the following?
    a. Amygdala
    b. Cortex
    c. Medulla oblongata
    d. Hippocampus

4. Which of the following is a fiber that carries impulses from sensory areas to the cell body?
    a. Dendrite
    b. Neuron
    c. Axon
    d. Node

5. Which of the following is a space between nerves and a tissue?
    a. Node
    b. Gap
    c. Synapse
    d. Junction

6. Which of the following transmitters is the most important stimulatory neurotransmitter in the CNS?
    a. GABA
    b. Glutamate
    c. Norepinephrine
    d. Dopamine

7. Schizophrenia is believed to be caused by a problem with which transmitter?
    a. Histamine
    b. Acetylcholine
    c. Dopamine
    d. GABA

8. Which prominent disorder is associated with the brain's acetylcholine system?
    a. Alcoholism
    b. Parkinson's disease
    c. Schizophrenia
    d. Alzheimer's disease

9. Which glial cells are the building block of the CNS myelin?
    a. Astrocytes
    b. Oligodendrocytes
    c. Ependymocytes
    d. Radial glial cells

10. Glial cells are distinguished from neurons by their ability to reproduce.
    a. True
    b. False

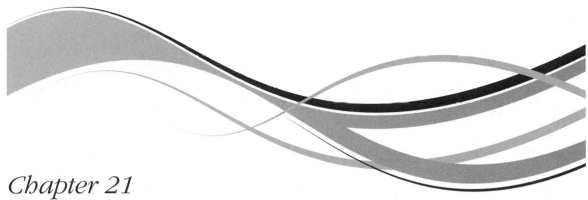

Chapter 21

PSYCHIATRIC DISORDERS

By   David W. Kaiser, Pharm.D.

Learning Objectives

This chapter seeks to prepare a pharmacy technician to:
- describe the signs, symptoms and characteristics of each discussed psychiatric disorder.
- describe how symptoms respond to effective medications.
- identify the neurotransmitter(s) involved in the pathophysiology of each psychiatric disease discussed.
- describe the role of each therapeutic alternative.
- describe the advantages and disadvantages for each therapeutic alternative.

Introduction

Health is defined by the World Health Organization as "a state of complete physical, mental and social well-being and not merely the absence of disease or infirmity."[1] Although there is no universally accepted definition for mental health, the term has largely been used to describe a level of cognitive or emotional well-being or an absence of a mental disorder.[2] A person who is mentally "healthy" is considered to be able to withstand many of life's adversities, and has achieved a certain degree of resilience to the normal day-to-day stressors of life.

The term "psychiatric disease" encompasses a number of mental disease states; each one is classified and distinguished by its predominant symptomotology and underlying neuropathophysiology. Regardless of the underlying cause, however, mental illness can be an incapacitating condition affecting numerous aspects of an individual's self esteem and interpersonal functioning in society.

There is a great deal of social stigma attached to mental illness. It is believed by uninformed people that patients with mental illness should be able to control the symptoms of their condition just by willing themselves well. Psychiatric conditions have physical causes, and it is no more possible for a person with a mental illness to will themselves well than it is possible for a person with diabetes to consciously control their blood glucose concentration. Mental illnesses are physical problems like most medical conditions, and, with proper treatment, the symptoms can be controlled.[3]

Depression

Depression is part of a group of disorders referred to as "affective" disorders. An **affective disorder** is a mental disorder characterized by a consistent, pervasive alteration in one's thoughts, emotions and behaviors. Depression is characterized by a mood of great sadness, despair and feelings of hopelessness. Depressed individuals often complain of lethargy, an inability to concentrate, sleep difficulties and a lack of interest in those activities that once brought them pleasure. Whatever the symptoms, depression is different from normal sadness in that it engulfs one's day-to-day life; it interferes with one's ability to work, study, eat, sleep and have fun. The feelings of helplessness, hopelessness and worthlessness are intense and unrelenting with little, if any, relief. These patients may begin to feel worthless, and guilty, and may dwell on thoughts of suicide, death or dying. Patients may also experience anxiety and physical symptoms, such as pain or muscle aches.

It is estimated that depressive disorders affect approximately one in six people. The true prevalence of depression is hard to determine because it is estimated that only one-third of sufferers seek treatment. Depression has a strong genetic component; it occurs in up to 20 percent of people who have a first-degree relative with depression and up to 40 percent in people with an identical twin with the disorder.[4] Depression may also be a side effect of a medication or the result of a medical condition.

Depression occurs two to three times more often in females than in males. Depression is also more prevalent in adults between the ages of 25 and 44 (more than any other age group).[4] Depressive episodes are often triggered by a psychosocial stressor, such as the death of a loved one, the loss of employment or financial problems. Suicide, which occurs in 15 percent of depressed patients, is the most serious outcome associated with depression.[4] Other problems that may develop if depression is inadequately treated include anxiety disorders, bipolar disorders, alcoholism or other substance abuse(s).

The symptoms of depression are believed to be caused by reductions in the effects of neurotransmitters responsible for controlling mood, primarily serotonin, norepinephrine and, possibly, dopamine. This may involve a decline in neurotransmitter concentration, a malfunction in regulation of these neurotransmitters or impairment in the sensitivity of neurotransmitter receptors. Most drugs effective for treating depression increase, or extend, the action of one or more of these neurotransmitters in the synapse.[3]

Treatment of depression generally focuses on alleviating the depressive symptoms in a patient and then preventing the occurrence of new depressive episodes. Treatment can be divided up between pharmacologic and nonpharmacologic therapies, with a combination of the two often providing the best outcomes for severely depressed patients.

Antidepressants are now required by the Food and Drug Administration (FDA) to contain a warning regarding the increased possibility of suicide associated with their use. While this might at first seem counterintuitive, the proposed rationale lies in the symptoms the patient is experiencing during a depressed period. Generally, depressed individuals exhibit low energy levels and a lack of motivation. These symptoms, however, are generally the first to respond to antidepressant therapy. An increase in energy levels typically precedes an elevation in mood; and thus, the patient who had suicidal thoughts and lacked the energy to carry out these thoughts now has the energy required to plan and carry out such acts before the medication has had a chance to improve his or her mood. Thus, patients starting antidepressant medications must be closely monitored for increases in suicidal thoughts in the first few weeks of beginning an antidepressant. Also, patients must be counseled about the time required to respond to a given medication and the possibility that they may initially feel worse before feeling better. Ensuring that the patient has adequate family and peer support during this initial period can also help to increase the odds of a successful treatment outcome.

The **selective serotonin reuptake inhibitors (SSRIs)** have been around for many years and continue to be the cornerstone of antidepressant therapy. These drugs have a proven record of efficacy, safety and tolerability and are largely considered to be "first-line" treatment for patients with signs and symptoms of depression. They are first-line because their side effect profile is generally mild and well-tolerated and because they are safer in overdose as compared with other antidepressants. Additionally, more family practice physicians are becoming comfortable writing prescriptions for these medications, which makes them more accessible to the general public. This, coupled with the fact that most of these agents are generically available, also adds to their popularity. Common adverse effects include nausea, vomiting, diarrhea, headache and sexual dysfunction. These agents may also cause insomnia or fatigue in some patients. It is important that pharmacy technicians understand these side effects and that tolerance usually develops to these side effects so they are not a reason to discontinue the drug.

Prior to the development of SSRIs, **tricyclic antidepressants (TCAs)** were the mainstay of antidepressant therapy. TCAs work in a similar fashion to SSRIs, but they act by blocking the reuptake of both serotonin and norepinephrine into the presynaptic nerve terminal. These agents also bind to a variety of other receptors as well, which accounts for the numerous side effects of these drugs that contributes to the potential deadly nature of these medications in overdose. Some of the side effects include dry mouth, urinary retention, constipation, blurred vision, tachycardia and other cardiac conduction problems.

Still, regardless of the side effect profile, these drugs are inexpensive and are as effective as the newer agents at relieving the signs and symptoms of depression. Their use as antidepressants is not as prevalent anymore, and many practitioners are using them to treat sleep disorders, chronic pain syndromes, fibromyalgia and to help augment the effects of other antidepressants.

Venlafaxine, desvenlafaxine and duloxetine are antidepressants that also act by blocking the reuptake of norepinephrine and serotonin. Since these agents act almost exclusively at these receptor sites, these agents are referred to as **serotonin/norepinephrine reuptake inhibitors (SNRIs)**. Some practitioners believe that the "dual mechanism" of these drugs allows them to work in some cases where other drugs might be ineffective, although this is still widely disputed in the medical community. Because these drugs increase the amount of norepinephrine available in the body, they would not be drugs of choice in a patient with elevated blood pressure or cardiac rhythm abnormalities. Some of the other common side effects shared by these drugs include nausea, constipation, sweating and sexual dysfunction. Like the TCAs, duloxetine (Cymbalta®) has established itself not only as an antidepressant, but also as being FDA-approved for the treatment of diabetic nerve pain (neuropathy) and fibromyalgia.

Trazodone is another antidepressant seen more as an adjunctive (add-on) treatment rather than as monotherapy for depression. Because this drug has very potent histamine binding properties, it is often used in depressed patients who have difficulty falling asleep. In fact, this agent is more often prescribed as a sleep aid than as an antidepressant. A rare, but serious, side effect of this medication for men that warrants immediate medical attention is priapism (a painful, sustained erection). Thus, all male patients must be counseled about this potential side effect. Another agent similar to trazodone is nefazodone. Brand name nefazodone (Serzone®) has been voluntarily withdrawn from the U.S. market due to an increase in liver damage associated with its use. Generic forms of the drug are still available, but this agent is rarely used anymore due to concerns over this potential side effect.

Bupropion is the only antidepressant that has a major effect on the reuptake of dopamine as well as norepinephrine. In addition to its antidepressant effects, it has been shown to decrease cravings for nicotine. It is marketed under the brand names Wellbutrin® and Aplenzin® (Wellbutrin® being bupropion hydrochloride and Aplenzin® being bupropion hydrobromide) as an antidepressant and as Zyban® for smoking cessation. It differs from the other antidepressants in that it causes fewer, if any, sexual side effects. It is, however, able to lower the seizure threshold in some individuals, making them more likely to sustain a seizure during therapy with this drug. Its use is contraindicated in patients with a history of an eating disorder or a previous seizure. Because this compound affects norepinephrine reuptake in the body, it can cause significant central nervous system (CNS) activation in some individuals, leading to such side effects as insomnia and, in some cases, tremor.

Mirtazapine is a tetracyclic antidepressant. It acts by blocking two types of serotonin receptors on the post-synaptic neuron, and increasing the release of norepinephrine and serotonin from presynaptic neurons.[5] Because, like trazodone, it has potent histamine receptor blockade, it is associated with both sedation and the potential for weight gain. Thus, those patients who experience weight loss and insomnia from their depression might well benefit from a trial of this agent. This compound has few drug interactions, and, like bupropion, causes few, if any, sexual side effects.

The **monoamine oxidase inhibitors (MAOIs)** act by blocking the enzymatic destruction of certain neurotransmitters in the brain, specifically serotonin and norepinephrine. These drugs are not used much anymore due to the potential for some very serious drug-drug and drug-food interactions. Still, for the right patient, these drugs can be highly effective. All patients on MAOIs must receive written information from a health care provider regarding the potential for food-drug interactions; specifically, they must limit their intake of foods containing the amino acid tyramine. A dietitian is usually involved in this initial consult with the patient, but a pharmacy technician must be able to recognize these medications on a patient's profile and refer any questions to a pharmacist.

Not all patients will respond to monotherapy for a major depressive disorder. Patients receiving antidepressant monotherapy may be partially, or totally, resistant to treatment in 10-30 percent of cases.[6,7] In patients who have experienced only partial treatment results, a clinician must first consider optimizing the patient's antidepressant dosage or lengthening therapy beyond the traditional trial period of six weeks. If this still does not elicit the desired response, the practitioner may opt to switch the patient to a different antidepressant or use a combination of antidepressants to achieve a different therapeutic response than that produced by the use of either drug alone. This practice is not without risks, however, and must be closely monitored by a health care professional to avoid the potential for drug-drug interactions.

Augmentation therapy can also involve the addition of other agents not traditionally thought of as having antidepressant activity. Lithium has been the most widely used, and extensively studied, augmentation agent. It's believed to enhance serotonin transmission by reducing the activity of post-synaptic serotonin (5-HT) receptors. This, in turn, reduces the negative feedback to serotonin-releasing cells and thereby increases serotonin levels in the **synaptic cleft**. Lithium may also have effects on other neurotransmitter systems and neuromodulators.[8] Other agents used in antidepressant augmentation include thyroid hormone and buspirone.

Antipsychotic agents are also now receiving FDA approval as adjunctive "add on" therapy to antidepressants. As of this writing, only two agents have this indication: aripiprazole and extended-release quetiapine. Although the exact mechanism of action by which these drugs help as adjunctive therapy in depression is not fully understood, it is postulated that aripiprazole acts more as a dopamine stabilizer, blocking its effects in some areas of the brain while enhancing its activity in others. There is also (in the case of quetiapine) a significant degree of norepinephrine reuptake inhibition exhibited by the active metabolite, which is assumed to be partially responsible for its efficacy with major depressive disorders.

Nonpharmacologic therapies include psychotherapy, cognitive or behavioral therapy (CBT), light therapy (commonly employed in individuals with seasonal affective disorder), and electro-convulsive therapy (ECT). Depending on the individual, some of these therapies can be combined with medications. It is important to keep in mind that the process of choosing the best regimen is largely a process of trial and error. Once a treatment regimen has been established, the patient and their family must be counseled that it takes time to see the full antidepressant effect of these medications and that compliance is essential to successful treatment.

Bipolar Disorder

Bipolar disorder (BD) is a disorder of mood like depressive disorders. Formerly known as "manic depression," the majority of patients with this disorder experience episodes of both mania and depression at various points in their lives. Thus, BD is distinguished from unipolar depression by the presence of intermittent manic episodes in which a patient's mood is unreasonably elevated and euphoric for a period of at least one week. In addition to an elevated mood, patients may also have inflated self-esteem, an increased need to speak, racing thoughts or increased distractibility. They may also become overly engaged in pleasurable activities that may have adverse consequences, such as excessive spending sprees or extreme participation in recreational activities. Bipolar patients often find that they are "more productive and creative" during these manic episodes, in part, due to a decreased need for sleep.

It is important to understand the classifications of bipolar disorder as well. Bipolar disorder is classified into two major categories: type I and type II. There are other categories, but for purposes of this review, we will focus on these two main categories. Type I is the designation for the classic variety of bipolar disorder characterized by full-blown manic attacks and deep, paralyzing depressions. Bipolar I is what physicians refer to as a "relapsing-remitting" illness; during the course of the illness, its symptoms come and go, making it difficult to diagnose and even more difficult to treat.[9]

In contrast, bipolar type II is characterized by fully-developed, debilitating, depressive episodes and transient episodes of hypomania. **Hypomania** is differentiated from mania in that these individuals do not suffer from impairment in their daily activities but would appear to be productive and driven during these periods. Classic symptoms of hypomania include mild euphoria, a flood of ideas, endless energy and a desire for success.[9] Often in those who have experienced their first episode of hypomania, there will have been a long or recent history of depression prior to the emergence of manic symptoms, and commonly this surfaces in the mid to late teens. Due to this being an emotionally charged time, it is not unusual for mood swings to be passed off as hormonal or teenage ups and downs and for a diagnosis of BD to be missed until there is evidence of an obvious manic/hypomanic phase.[10] Additionally, since BD type II patients seem to have more problems with depression, they might get misdiagnosed with major depressive disorder and subsequently do not receive treatment for BD at all.[9]

Bipolar disorder affects approximately 5.7 million American adults, or about 2.6 percent of the U.S. population 18 years of age and older, in a given year. The disorder seems to affect both men and women equally, with the median age of onset at about 21 years of age. There is a noticeable genetic trend in the disease; if one parent has been diagnosed with BD, then the risk of that parent's children getting the disorder is in the range of 15-30 percent. Further, if both parents have been diagnosed with BD, the risk to the child increases dramatically to between 50-75 percent.[11] There are numerous inconclusive theories regarding the neurochemistry of BD; however, no one theory is considered superior to another in this regard. As with depression, there are certain medical conditions and medications that may precipitate mania; however, in order for a patient to be clinically diagnosed with BD, neither the manic nor depressive episodes can be the result of such conditions or medications. Patients may be described as "mixed" if they experience both manic and depressive episodes within the same day, nearly every day for at least one week. Patients may be described as "rapid cyclers" if they have at least four episodes of mania and/or depression in one year.[11] And finally, some patients may develop psychotic symptoms as part of their bipolar disease. Medications are used to treat symptoms of BD but are not able to cure the disorder; thus long-term adherence to medication therapy is paramount in the management of this disease.

Bipolar disorder may be managed by either nonpharmacologic or pharmacologic means. Nonpharmacologic methods used in the treatment of the disorder include psychotherapy, CBT, light therapy and, in some refractory cases, ECT. Not surprisingly, the most effective treatment(s) involve a combination of both pharmacologic and nonpharmacologic modalities implemented and monitored jointly by a medical professional, the patient and the patient's family.[12]

Pharmacologic treatment options for BD include the mood stabilizers lithium, valproic acid, carbamazepine, lamotrigine, oxcarbazepine, gabapentin and topiramate. These drugs help to balance an individual's thoughts and behavioral patterns and, thus, help to minimize the number of extreme behaviors associated with BD. Occasionally, however, a patient may not respond to just one mood stabilizing agent. In these cases, the physician may prescribe another mood stabilizing agent; or, if the patient is exhibiting psychotic symptoms, then the practitioner may also decide to add an antipsychotic drug to the patient's medication regimen. Patients may also be put on an antidepressant if the practitioner believes that the patient is suffering more from depressive, rather than manic, episodes, or if the patient's family has a history of depression. Care must be taken, however, and the patient must be monitored closely as the addition of an antidepressant can precipitate a manic episode in certain subsets of patients with BD.

Lithium, carbamazepine and valproic acid have long been the first-line agents used in the treatment of bipolar disorder. The choice of which of these agents to use depends on the presentation and symptomotology of the patient, the side effect profile of the selected agent and lastly, patient and prescriber preference. It is important to note that these drugs require routine blood-level monitoring, so the patient must be willing to have these tests as often as is deemed necessary by the prescriber. All three of these drugs are teratogenic (capable of harming a developing fetus), so female patients of childbearing age must be counseled about appropriate contraceptive measures while on these medications.

Lithium is the drug of choice for BD patients with mania as their predominant symptom.[13] No other mood stabilizer has been shown to be more effective in this type of patient; however, lithium is less effective than valproic acid or carbamazepine for patients whose disease is "rapid cycling," "mixed" or characterized by psychotic symptoms. Although highly effective, its use is limited by several factors including gastrointestinal (GI) upset, tremor and kidney dysfunction. There are numerous drug interactions between lithium and other drugs both prescription and over-the-counter (OTC), including NSAIDs like ibuprofen and naproxen, diuretics and ACE inhibitors. Patients on lithium must be counseled about these potential drug interactions and the need to seek medical help if they develop any unusual side effects during therapy.

Valproic acid is another first-line alternative for BD. It is generally well-tolerated and is effective for certain subtypes of BD. It is a better choice in BD patients when the patient's disease is "rapid cycling" or "mixed."[13] Side effects of valproic acid include GI upset, sedation and weight gain. Serious, but rare, side effects of valproic acid include hematologic effects, liver toxicity and pancreatitis.

Valproic acid is also involved in many drug interactions, so the patient must be counseled not to start any new medications, including OTC, until speaking with a pharmacist or physician.

Carbamazepine is another effective therapy for BD; it is especially effective when a patient's disease is described as "rapid cycling" or "mixed," as with valproic acid.[3] It may also be considered when extreme anger or irritability is part of the patient's presenting symptomatology. It is used somewhat less frequently than lithium or valproic acid due to CNS side effects. Common side effects include sedation, dizziness, blurred vision and headache. Rare side effects include rashes and blood disorders. Like lithium and valproic acid, carbamazepine has many clinically significant drug interactions and is not used much for this reason.

Antipsychotic agents may be considered for patients who also have psychotic symptoms in addition to their bipolar disorder. Their use is becoming increasingly more popular in treating refractory patients or in those patients with a significant family history of psychosis or schizophrenia. Of these agents, the newer, atypical, agents (olanzapine, quetiapine, risperidone, ziprasidone, paliperidone, iloperidone and asenapine) generally have fewer side effects than some of the older agents on the market (haloperidol, chlorpromazine, fluphenazine), and may be preferred if the patient's insurance covers these medications.

The benzodiazepines clonazepam and lorazepam have been used for the treatment of acute mania, alone or in combination with mood stabilizers. Due to the risk of dependency with these controlled substances, they are almost never used as monotherapy. Instead, these agents are used mostly for agitation and insomnia during acute manic episodes or as part of maintenance therapy while the mood stabilizer is titrated. Benzodiazepines are used most frequently in bipolar patients as adjunctive therapy in combination with other more specific antimanic agents.

Lamotrigine is FDA-approved for use in treating BD. Many clinical trials indicate that, although it is not effective in acute mania or in the prevention of manic episodes, it is very helpful in the prophylaxis of depressive episodes and, as such, is a widely used agent in the treatment of BD.[14] Lamotrigine is also associated with a serious rash called Stevens-Johnson syndrome that seems to occur most often when the dose is titrated too fast. To minimize the risk of developing this, and other rashes, patients are started on a low dose for two weeks and gradually increased every two weeks until an effective dose is reached. While taking lamotrigine, patients must be encouraged to report any new rash, hives, fever, swollen glands, sores in the mouth and on the eyes, and swelling of the lips or tongue to a physician or pharmacist. Lamotrigine must also be tapered when the patient is going off the medication and switching to another agent.

Alternatives to the above drugs include anticonvulsants, such as topiramate, gabapentin and oxcarbazepine. These drugs are not FDA-approved for BD; however, clinicians use them in patients who fail, or are inappropriate candidates for more well-established alternatives.

Anxiety Disorders

Anxiety is an emotional state experienced by everyone, to a certain extent, when faced with a stressful event or a situation in which there is real or perceived danger. It is also a frequent symptom of other medical and psychiatric conditions. Common symptoms of anxiety include irritability, worry, restlessness, muscle tension and sleep disturbances.[15] Anxiety disorders are chronic, disabling, cause a significant loss of productivity at work and cause difficulty relaxing at home. The common symptom of anxiety disorders is the fear of the unknown and is often accompanied by increases in heart rate, difficulty breathing, choking sensations, hyperventilation and other autonomic responses. It should also be noted that there exists a strong association between anxiety and depression, and, most often, those patients suffering from anxiety disorders also suffer from some degree of depression.[16]

An anxiety disorder occurs when an individual experiences a disproportionate, or excessive, amount of stress secondary to a particular event or when anxiety causes a significant impairment in the individual's normal functioning ability. Anxiety disorders must also be distinguished from medical disorders in which anxiety is either a component of that disease, a response to knowing that one has the disease or the result of using medications or illicit drugs. The remainder of this section will focus on three specific anxiety disorders rather than anxiety as a symptom of other conditions. Anxiety disorders discussed in this chapter include generalized anxiety disorder (GAD), panic disorder (PD) and obsessive-compulsive disorder (OCD).

Anxiety disorders are some of the most common in the practice of medicine. They are experienced by one quarter of the population, but only one quarter of those people will receive treatment. As with mood disorders, anxiety disorders are often precipitated by a life stressor. The annual cost of anxiety to the U.S. economy is estimated at $100 billion. Anxiety disorders typically develop before age 30 and are more common in women and individuals whose families have a history of depression or anxiety. Those with anxiety disorders often develop other mental illnesses (e.g., depression, another anxiety disorder or a substance abuse disorder).[17]

The true cause of anxiety, as with other psychiatric illnesses, is unknown. Models, or theories, proposed to explain anxiety include alterations in the functioning of different brain structures and alterations in the amount of, or response to, different neurotransmitters. The anatomical structures involved in the conscious perception of anxiety are located in the forebrain. Neurotransmitters implicated in anxiety include norepinephrine, gamma aminobutyric acid (GABA) and serotonin. Therefore, medications used to treat anxiety disorders primarily alter the function or quantity of these neurotransmitters or their receptors.[3]

Management of anxiety depends on the individual disorder. Formal anxiety disorders are typically chronic diseases, with symptoms that come and go, and few patients ever are completely free of symptoms. Treatment of anxiety disorders is aimed at reducing the frequency, severity and duration of the patient's symptoms of anxiety; improving the patient's overall functioning and quality of life; and preventing future anxiety symptoms.[3]

Generalized Anxiety Disorder

Generalized anxiety disorder (GAD) is diagnosed when a person worries excessively about a variety of everyday problems for at least six months.[15] People with GAD can't seem to get rid of their concerns, even though they usually realize that their anxiety is more intense than the situation warrants. They can't relax, startle easily and have difficulty concentrating. Often they have trouble falling asleep or staying asleep. Physical symptoms that often accompany GAD include fatigue, headaches, muscle tension, muscle aches, difficulty swallowing, trembling, twitching, irritability, sweating, nausea, lightheadedness, having to go to the bathroom frequently, feeling out of breath and hot flashes. GAD affects about 6.8 million American adults, including twice as many women as men.[17] The disorder develops gradually and can begin at any point in the life cycle, although the years of highest risk are between childhood and middle age.[17] There is also evidence that genes play a modest role in GAD. The pathophysiology of GAD most likely involves excessive activity of serotonin or norepinephrine neurons.

Therapy for GAD usually involves nonpharmacologic interventions, psychotherapy and/or medications. Nonpharmacologic therapies include stress management training. CBT can help to support patients in forming effective coping strategies and overcoming their fears. Drugs that are generally avoided in patients with GAD include caffeine, "diet pills" and stimulants (both prescription and OTC). Drugs effective for GAD include antidepressants, benzodiazepines, buspirone, hydroxyzine, gabapentin and propranolol.[3]

The drugs of first choice for treating GAD are SSRI antidepressants. This is because SSRIs are safe, effective for a broad range of anxiety disorders and have less abuse potential than many other alternative drugs. They are believed to work in GAD by blocking presynaptic reuptake of serotonin. This leads to an increase of serotonin in the synapse and prolonged exposure of post-synaptic serotonin receptors to this neurotransmitter. Paroxetine and escitalopram are FDA-approved for GAD; but, all available SSRIs are probably effective for this condition. One limitation of using antidepressants to treat anxiety disorders is that response to these agents is delayed compared to benzodiazepines that act very quickly to improve anxiety symptoms. SSRIs must be taken regularly to be effective in GAD. Intermittent, "prn" (as needed), use is ineffective.[3]

Other antidepressants used to treat GAD include venlafaxine and mirtazapine. As with the SSRIs, response to these drugs is delayed for several weeks, and side effects are the same as those seen in depression. Extended-release venlafaxine is FDA-approved for the treatment of GAD.

The benzodiazepines are very effective for reducing anxiety; however, their role in the management of this disorder has fallen to second-tier therapy due to concerns of abuse, addiction and dependence. Consequently, these medications are controlled substances. They work by enhancing the effects of GABA, which reduces the activity of both norepinephrine and serotonin.[3] These drugs are superior to other medications in their ability to reduce the physical symptoms of anxiety and agitation (especially muscle tension and sleep abnormalities). The advantage to these agents is that they can be taken on an "as needed" basis for patients with transient anxiety symptoms. All benzodiazepines possess anxiolytic (anti-anxiety) properties (primarily due to their sedative qualities); but, to date, only seven are FDA-approved as anxiolytics, including alprazolam, chlordiazepoxide, clonazepam, clorazepate, diazepam, lorazepam and oxazepam. The adverse effect profile of benzodiazepines includes confusion, memory impairment and stumbling gait upon arousal. As such, benzodiazepines are not generally recommended for elderly patients, as they greatly increase an elderly patient's risk of fractures secondary to falls. Although generally well-tolerated, the sedative effect of these drugs, when combined with alcohol, is greatly increased and can potentially lead to respiratory arrest and death. Anyone taking these agents continuously for more than eight weeks must avoid abrupt discontinuation of these agents because of the risk of withdrawal.

Buspirone acts to reduce the activity of serotonin-containing neurons, which leads to improvement in anxiety symptoms. Advantages with this drug include little CNS depression (sedation, confusion, etc.), safety in overdose and low abuse potential. Studies have demonstrated that buspirone is as effective as any benzodiazepine after four weeks of therapy, but conflicting data exist regarding buspirone's onset of action. Some authors report that the onset of action of buspirone is delayed for several weeks. Buspirone must be taken regularly to be effective. It is not effective when taken on an "as needed" basis. Patients who have recently taken benzodiazepines for anxiety may not perceive much benefit from buspirone. Common side effects include headache, dizziness and nausea.[17]

Propranolol, a beta-adrenergic blocking agent (beta-blocker) often used to treat hypertension, is a second-line agent to treat anxiety. Because it acts to slow a patient's heart rate, it may be especially useful in patients with physical symptoms of anxiety (such as tremor, sweating, chest pain, palpitations or increased heart rate).[17] It is not as effective as a benzodiazepine for relieving other anxiety symptoms.[17] As with benzodiazepines, propranolol must not be discontinued abruptly or without the knowledge and advice of a physician. Side effects include fatigue and low blood pressure.

Hydroxyzine is an antihistamine that has anxiolytic properties. It is a second-line agent due to having only limited studies conducted on its use in patients with anxiety disorders. While its mechanism of action as an anxiolytic is not fully understood, it is thought that it relieves anxiety by the general sedating properties associated with antihistamines. It is especially useful in patients with substance abuse problems who must avoid benzodiazepines and patients who have not responded to, or don't want to take, antidepressants. One advantage of hydroxyzine is that it can also be taken on an "as needed" basis like the benzodiazepines. Side effects include those common to all anticholinergic agents, such as dry mucus membranes, constipation, tachycardia, blurred vision and others.

Gabapentin, FDA-approved for seizures and neuropathic pain, is occasionally used for anxiety as well. The mechanism by which it helps anxiety is unknown. Gabapentin has low abuse potential and is usually well-tolerated by patients. It is not approved for GAD, and studies supporting its use for this condition have not been conducted.

With appropriate therapy, patients with anxiety disorders can regain normal levels of functioning and improve the quality of their lives. By decreasing the financial burden associated with anxiety disorders, additional benefit will be realized in the health care system and society at large. Patients, their families and their employers will benefit from increased productivity and fewer missed days of work.

Panic Disorder

Panic disorder (PD) is characterized by the occurrence of episodic panic attacks. **Panic attacks** are brief, intense periods of extreme anxiety or fear that cause significant discomfort for the patient.[17] Panic attacks usually last less than 30 minutes and do not have an identifiable source of the fear. Symptoms present during panic attacks include increased heart rate, sweating and shortness of breath. Many of the symptoms of a panic attack resemble the symptoms of serious physical problems (such as a heart attack). For this reason, panic disorder is frequently misdiagnosed or worked up as a purely physical problem rather than one with a psychiatric component.

Panic disorder affects about six million American adults and is twice as common in women as men.[18,19] Panic attacks often begin in late adolescence or early adulthood, but not everyone who experiences panic attacks will develop panic disorder.[19] Many people have just one attack and never have another. The tendency to develop panic attacks appears to be inherited.[20] While the exact cause of panic attacks is unknown, it is believed that excessive activity of norepinephrine-containing and/or serotonin-containing neurons is the suspected precipitant of panic attacks. It is also thought that there may be a greater influence from norepinephrine neurons in PD than that seen in GAD.[20] Some people's lives become so restricted because of panic attacks that they avoid normal activities (such as grocery shopping or driving). About one-third of patients with panic attacks become housebound or are able to confront a feared situation only when accompanied by a spouse or other trusted person.[19] When the condition progresses this far, it is called agoraphobia, or fear of open spaces. People with PD are more receptive to treatment if they understand that the disorder involves both physical and psychologic processes and that treatment must address both. Drug therapy and behavior therapy can generally control the symptoms.[21]

Antidepressants and benzodiazepines are the drugs of choice to treat PD. SSRIs, TCAs and MAOIs have all been shown to be effective in reducing the occurrence of panic attacks. With medication, 60-80 percent of patients may experience remission of symptoms. This effect is typically delayed for three to five weeks and may take up to 12 weeks in some patients.[22] All medications for panic disorder, including benzodiazepines, need to be taken on a regular basis in order to prevent the occurrence of panic attacks. It is important to note that patients with PD are extremely sensitive to side effects from medications. For this reason, anti-panic medications must be started at lower than usual doses, and the doses must be increased very slowly to effective levels. Effective doses in panic disorder are often higher than the doses needed to treat other psychiatric conditions for which anti-panic medications are used. Consequently, it may take a considerable amount of time before a patient is at an effective dose of medication.

The SSRIs are the drugs of choice for PD due to their safety, efficacy and lack of abuse potential. Although paroxetine, fluoxetine and sertraline are the only SSRIs approved for PD, all agents in this class are effective. Side effects, mechanism of action and other limitations of SSRIs are the same as those seen when SSRIs are used to treat GAD. As previously stated, maximum benefit from SSRIs may be delayed for several weeks after an effective dose is found, so patients must be encouraged to be compliant through this waiting period.

Benzodiazepines are good second-line agents for PD. They are rapidly effective and are used first-line if the patient needs immediate relief from a panic attack (e.g., if the discomfort is unbearable or the patient is at risk of losing a job). Alprazolam and clonazepam are FDA-approved for the treatment of panic disorder, but all agents in the class are effective if given in equivalent doses. Side effects, mechanisms of action and other limitations of benzodiazepines are the same as those seen when benzodiazepines are used to treat GAD.

TCAs and MAOIs are both effective classes of drugs to treat panic disorder; however, due to the problem of drug and food interactions and side effects, their use is limited to patients in whom SSRIs and benzodiazepines are contraindicated, not tolerated or fail. TCAs are potentially fatal in overdose, and their side effects are often not tolerated; whereas, MAOIs have many significant food and drug interactions. These issues relegate these medications to a second-tier, or even third-tier, status in the treatment of PD.

Obsessive-Compulsive Disorder

Obsessive-compulsive disorder (OCD) is an anxiety disorder characterized by the presence of both obsessions and compulsions. **Obsessions** are recurrent and persistent thoughts, ideas, images or impulses that are intrusive, inappropriate and produce significant anxiety. Obsessions commonly concern contamination; the patient requires that things be in a certain order or be repeated to check that something was done (see Table 1). **Compulsions** are behaviors or actions that are intentional, purposeful and repetitive and commonly done in response to an obsession (see Table 2). It is important to note that performing such compulsive rituals is not pleasurable. At best, it produces temporary relief from the anxiety created by obsessive thoughts.[21] Contrary to schizophrenic patients who do not recognize their behaviors and thoughts as abnormal, patients with OCD usually recognize the irrational nature of their thoughts and behaviors. To get a diagnosis of OCD, the obsessions or compulsions must consume a significant amount of time each day (hours), cause significant distress or impair normal functioning.[15]

Table 1
Common Obsessions

Concern about becoming ill
Concern over dirt / germs
Disgust concerning bodily waste
Fear of embarrassing acts
Fear of harm to self/others
Fear of losing things
"Forbidden" sexual thoughts
Need for symmetry or exactness
Need to count or check things
Need to know or remember
Need to say or apologize
Somatic obsessions

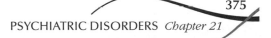

Table 2
Common Compulsions

Arranging rituals
Avoiding public settings
Checking health status
Cleaning/washing rituals
Counting or checking rituals
Hoarding rituals
Seeking reassurance about health

OCD affects about 2.2 million American adults, and the problem can be accompanied by eating disorders, other anxiety disorders or depression.[18,19,23,24] It strikes men and women in roughly equal numbers and usually appears in childhood, adolescence or early adulthood.[19] One-third of adults with OCD develop symptoms as children, and research indicates that OCD might run in families.[25]

A specific cause for OCD has not been pinpointed, but serotonin plays a key role. Evidence supporting this belief comes from the observation that the most effective drugs for OCD are serotonin reuptake inhibitors.[26] Recently, dopamine has been suggested to play a role in the manifestation of OCD, but dopamine-blocking agents (antipsychotics) are used only as adjunctive therapy to SSRIs in OCD. Serotonin and dopamine are intimately related in parts of the forebrain, so the additive benefit of these combination therapies isn't entirely unexpected.[27] Current treatments for OCD are inadequate, so much so that high doses of medications are often required in return for small reductions in the frequency of compulsive behaviors. Patients are often willing to put up with medication side effects in order to get even small improvements in their symptoms. Even with adequate treatment, many studies reveal only 40 percent improvement in "responders."[26] While OCD is incurable, and it is unrealistic to expect elimination of symptoms, therapy is directed at achieving as great a reduction in symptoms as can be accomplished.

As noted above, drugs with serotonin-reuptake blocking properties are the drugs of choice for the treatment of OCD. Practically, these include all the SSRI antidepressants and clomipramine, a TCA with greater reuptake inhibition of serotonin than norepinephrine.[28] Patients are frequently treated with the highest doses of these drugs that can be tolerated. Even with high doses, response to treatment is modest in most cases. Medications for OCD must be taken on a regular basis for prolonged periods to be effective.[29]

SSRIs are the drugs of choice for OCD due to their efficacy and safety. Fluvoxamine, fluoxetine and paroxetine are currently approved for OCD. An adequate trial of any drug for OCD is at least 10 weeks at the maximum recommended or maximally tolerated dose.

Although SSRIs are the drugs of choice for OCD, clomipramine, a TCA, is arguably the most effective medication for this condition.[30] A number of systematic reviews have shown it to be consistently more effective than SSRIs; however, it has the same adverse effect profile as other agents in the TCA class.[31-33] For this reason, as well as its increased risk of seizure induction, it may be withheld as a second-line agent in the treatment of OCD.

As in depression, antipsychotics have been used to augment SSRI treatment in OCD as well. Although antipsychotics are not FDA-approved for OCD, there is substantial evidence that probably all antipsychotics can benefit at least a subset of OCD patients. Due to the side effects associated with antipsychotics, these agents are reserved for severely ill patients and those refractory to monotherapy with SSRIs and clomipramine.[29]

Moderate symptom improvement can be expected in approximately 80 percent of patients taking either an SSRI or clomipramine.[26] Although achieving only modest improvement is not ideal, patients typically prefer this to their pretreatment level of functioning and are willing to take high doses of medications and tolerate adverse effects in order to obtain this response. Occasionally, OCD patients may take medications for only a few years; but, the majority of these patients require lifelong treatment. Taking medication for longer periods of time helps to avoid relapse and can enable the patient to continually experience the modest benefit of appropriate therapy for this disabling condition.

Schizophrenia

Schizophrenia is a disorder of thought characterized by misperceptions of sensory stimuli (hallucinations) or false beliefs (delusions). For example, schizophrenic patients frequently hear voices when no one is talking to them or believe that they have special powers. Symptoms of schizophrenia are classified as positive or negative. The positive symptoms can be thought of as enhancements to the normal life experience. Examples of positive symptoms include delusions, hallucinations and bizarre behavior. Negative symptoms can be thought of as restrictions to normal life experience. Examples of negative symptoms include social withdrawal, lack of motivation, inability to experience pleasure and reduced communication.

Schizophrenia has an average worldwide incidence of approximately one percent; the prevalence of which seems to be similar among all cultures.[34] The disease seems to affect both men and women equally; however, the age of onset differs somewhat significantly between the sexes. Schizophrenia often first appears in men in their late teens or early 20s. In contrast, women are generally affected in their 20s and early 30s.[34]

Schizophrenia is believed to be caused by a disturbance in dopaminergic signal transduction in certain areas of the forebrain. The negative symptoms are believed to be from too little dopamine activity in one area of the brain (specifically, the mesocortical area); whereas, the positive symptoms are believed to be from too much dopamine activity in another area of the brain (specifically, the mesolimbic area). Recent evidence implicates abnormal glutamate activity as another possible cause of schizophrenia; however, glutamate and dopamine are intimately connected in the brain, and it is difficult to separate the activity of the two neurotransmitters.[35] All drugs that have been shown to benefit patients with schizophrenia act, at least in part, as post-synaptic dopamine receptor blockers.[35]

The medications used to treat schizophrenia and other types of psychoses are referred to as antipsychotics or neuroleptics. The term "neuroleptic" refers to the slowness of thought and movement usually associated with the earlier (first-generation) drugs used to treat psychiatric disorders. Although there is a theoretical distinction between the two terms, clinicians will often use the terms interchangeably. Many times, the term "neuroleptic" is preferred due to the many indications (both FDA-approved and off-label) for these drugs; a person taking one of these agents is not necessarily delusional or psychotic and may find the term anti-psychotic to be disgraceful. As previously stated, these drugs can be divided up into traditional, first-generation agents (e.g., haloperidol, chlorpromazine and fluphenazine) and atypical agents (second-generation antipsychotics) like clozapine, olanzapine, quetiapine, risperidone, ziprasidone, paliperidone, iloperidone and asenapine. Clozapine is unique in that it is not a new compound. Due to its distinctive pharmacology, it is more closely related to the atypical agents and is generally considered part of this class.

All of the antipsychotics are FDA-approved for the treatment of schizophrenia. Other than clozapine, which is used for severely ill schizophrenic patients, all of the antipsychotics (regardless of generation) are classically considered equally effective for the treatment of positive symptoms. The atypical antipsychotics, however, appear to be more effective than first-generation antipsychotics for treating negative symptoms. In order to be effective in schizophrenia, these drugs are usually taken on a routine basis. Occasionally however, a prescriber may write for these medications to be taken on an "as needed" basis for "breakthrough" episodes of anxiety or agitation. Until recently, these compounds were used to treat the psychosis that sometimes accompanies dementia in elderly patients. While effective, studies showed that these patients had almost twice the risk of death when taking these agents as compared to those who did not take these medications. As a result of this, these agents are no longer recommended for use in this patient population and bear a black-box warning as such.

As a class, antipsychotics are associated with a group of adverse effects known as **extrapyramidal side effects (EPSEs)**. These are four different problems caused by their effects on dopamine and how the body handles dopamine. See Table 3 for a list of the EPSEs and their common symptoms. **Tardive dyskinesia** is a significant problem because there is no treatment for it, and it may become permanent if allowed to persist for a prolonged period of time. The first-generation antipsychotics have a greater risk of causing EPSEs than the atypical antipsychotics; but, the atypical antipsychotics can cause these side effects, too.[36-38]

Table 3
Extrapyramidal Side Effects of Antipsychotics

Side Effect	Common Presentation
Akathisia	Restlessness, need to be in constant motion, pacing, mental unease or discomfort
Drug-induced Parkinsonism	Tremor, stiffness, muscle rigidity, shuffling gait, slowness of thought
Dystonia	Frequently painful muscle contractions that may affect almost any muscle group but usually affecting muscles of the jaw, tongue, neck, back or eyes
Tardive Dyskinesia	Usually painless irregular muscle movements; may affect almost any muscle group of the body, but usually affects muscles of the tongue, small muscles of the face (tics and grimaces) or hands

The first-generation antipsychotics have been available since the late 1950s. They are classified as high potency (e.g., haloperidol) and low potency (e.g., chlorpromazine). Both potency classes are equally effective in the treatment of schizophrenia, although a patient may respond to one agent and not another similar drug. These agents are very effective for positive symptoms of schizophrenia, but they are frequently ineffective for negative symptoms to the point where negative symptoms may become worse when a patient is using one of these agents. The potency classes are different in the side effects they are most likely to cause. The high-potency neuroleptics are more likely to cause EPSEs than are the low-potency neuroleptics. The low-potency agents have slightly less risk of EPSEs than the high-potency neuroleptics; but, they are more likely to cause anticholinergic side effects (dry mouth, blurred vision, constipation, etc.), dizziness when the patient stands up and sedation. Compared to the atypical antipsychotics, the first-generation agents are very inexpensive. Atypical antipsychotics are the drugs of choice to treat schizophrenia and other psychotic disorders due to a reduced risk of EPSEs compared to first-generation antipsychotics, and perhaps are better at calming negative symptoms. These drugs block post-synaptic dopamine receptors like the first-generation antipsychotics, but they also block presynaptic serotonin receptors; this action seems to convey a reduced risk of EPSEs with these drugs. They are as effective as the first-generation antipsychotics against positive symptoms; but, they are more effective than first-generation antipsychotics against negative symptoms of schizophrenia.[34] As a class, the atypical antipsychotics seem to have a greater risk than first-generation antipsychotics for causing problems in patients with, or at risk of developing, diabetes, weight gain or problems with blood lipids (collectively called metabolic problems).[39]

Clozapine is the most effective antipsychotic in patients with treatment-refractory schizophrenia. It also has the lowest risk of causing EPSEs. Unfortunately, it has a 1-2 percent risk of a potentially fatal blood condition called agranulocytosis. This is a reduction in the white blood cells in the body which normally act to fight infection. When their numbers are reduced, patients are at risk of developing serious infections. Patients on this medication must consent to routine blood draws, the results of which are sent to the pharmacy and the patient's physician. These lab values are analyzed by the pharmacist and, if satisfactory, the drug is dispensed. If the results are not satisfactory, the pharmacist must contact the prescribing physician about whether or not the medication is to be continued. Clozapine can also induce seizures, has many drug interactions and has many other less serious, but bothersome, side effects. For these reasons, clozapine is usually reserved for only the most severely ill schizophrenic patients.[34]

As of this writing, risperidone is currently the only drug in this very expensive group of medications that is available generically. It is FDA-approved for the treatment of bipolar disorder as well as schizophrenia. It is one of only a few agents available as a long-acting injection (Risperdal® Consta®). It is also one of the most likely antipsychotics to cause increases in the hormone prolactin, which is an action that is usually antagonized by dopamine.[35] Thus, by inhibiting dopamine, prolactin levels rise, causing menstrual irregularities and milk formation in females, development of female-type breasts in men and sexual problems in both men and women. Risperidone has an intermediate risk of causing metabolic problems. Still, as indicated previously, due to its lower cost, most insurances prefer that a patient has at least tried and failed this agent before paying for a more expensive medication in this class.

Olanzapine has a modest, dose-dependent risk of EPSEs. It is often well-tolerated by patients. It is available in oral dosage forms as well as an immediate release and long-acting (Zyprexa® Relprevv™) intramuscular injection. Unfortunately, as of this printing, it is the most expensive medication in this class and has the greatest risk of metabolic problems (including weight gain and unmasking of diabetes).[39] Olanzapine is approved for both bipolar disorder and schizophrenia. A combination product is also available (Symbyax®), containing both olanzapine and fluoxetine. This product is FDA-approved for the treatment of both bipolar disorder and in treatment-resistant depression.

Other than clozapine, quetiapine has the lowest risk of causing EPSEs among the antipsychotics. It is generally well-tolerated with sedation being the most common side effect. Consequently, it is usually dosed at bedtime. It is moderately priced, depending on the dose used, and is only available in oral dosage forms. Quetiapine is available in both immediate-release and extended-release tablets; the latter dosage form allows the practitioner to get to a therapeutic dose faster while avoiding the dose-dependent side effects sometimes seen with titrating the immediate-release formulation up to a therapeutic dose. Quetiapine is approved as an adjunctive medication in the treatment of major depressive disorder as well as a primary treatment option in both bipolar disorder and schizophrenia.

Ziprasidone was the first atypical antipsychotic to be available in an injectable form. It has relatively little, if any, effect on weight and other metabolic effects, and, with one exception, its side effect profile is reasonable. The exception to the side effect profile is that ziprasidone is the most likely among the atypical antipsychotics to cause heart conduction problems. For this reason, prescribers must be sure that a patient isn't taking any interacting medication and doesn't have any other medical condition that could lead to heart problems. In such patients, ziprasidone must be avoided. This agent is approved for the treatment of both bipolar disorder and schizophrenia.

The pharmacology of aripiprazole is slightly different than other atypical antipsychotics. Aripiprazole is classified as a dopamine *partial* agonist. When aripiprazole binds to dopamine receptors in the CNS, it can enhance or reduce the effects of naturally-occurring dopamine depending on the amount of dopamine present at the site of action. The clinical advantage of this difference in mechanism of action is not clear, but it is postulated that it contributes to fewer EPSEs. Like ziprasidone, aripiprazole has few adverse effects on weight and metabolic problems. Aripiprazole is available in oral dosage forms as well as an immediate-release injectable formulation. Like quetiapine, it is FDA-approved for bipolar disorder, schizophrenia and as adjunctive therapy in the treatment of major depressive disorder.

Paliperidone is the active metabolite of risperidone. It is FDA-approved for the acute and maintenance treatment of schizophrenia. The tablet is formulated with a technology that releases the medication over time and, as such, is dosed once daily. Risperidone is often dosed twice daily to achieve symptom remission in schizophrenia. Due in part to the long half-life of the compound, it attains lower peak plasma (blood) levels and, therefore, is purported to have a lower incidence of EPSE and sedation compared to risperidone. Paliperidone is also available as a long-acting injection and is the third in the arsenal of long-acting injectable depot formulations. In this form, it is marketed under the brand name of Invega Sustenna®.

Asenapine is a newer atypical antipsychotic that claims to have minimal metabolic disturbances as well as minimal weight gain associated with its use. It is FDA-approved for both bipolar disorder and schizophrenia. It is a sublingual tablet and must be allowed to dissolve under the tongue in order to be effective. The most common side effects seen during therapy so far have been oral hypoesthesia (numbing sensation in the mouth and tongue) and taste disturbances.

Iloperidone is also a new atypical agent indicated for schizophrenia. Like ziprasidone, it can alter myocardial conduction, so it is generally avoided in patients with a history of cardiac problems. It is also associated with significant drops in blood pressure if not titrated appropriately. Unfortunately, this titration requires several days; this prolonged titration limits its utility in the acute treatment of schizophrenia.

Within this discussion of medications that may treat certain psychiatric diseases, the point is illustrated that many psychiatric medications are no longer used only for the conditions for which they were originally approved. Examples of this are the many anticonvulsants described previously to treat BD or the role of using antipsychotics as mood stabilizers and adjunctive therapy in depression. This also demonstrates that a suitably qualified clinician's judgment is paramount when deciding which medication to initiate in a particular patient. Patients may also be prescribed combinations of agents to best manage their illness. With the aid of these medications, patients can see improvement in their level of functioning and have an improved quality of life.[3]

Attention Deficit Hyperactivity Disorder

Attention deficit hyperactivity disorder (ADHD) is classified as a neurobehavioral developmental disorder. It is primarily characterized by the coexistence of attention problems, hyperactivity and symptoms starting before seven years of age.[41] The childhood beginning sets this condition apart from the other disorders in this chapter. All of the previously mentioned diseases usually start in late adolescence or adulthood. The three hallmark behavioral symptoms of ADHD are hyperactivity, impulsivity and inattention inappropriate for an individual child at a given age and stage of development. Hyperactivity is seen as excessive running or "horsing around," difficulty remaining seated or still, and excessive activity during sleep. Impulsivity is often seen as acting before thinking, changing activities frequently, disorganization, talking in class when not called upon, difficulty waiting for one's turn at an activity and increased need for supervision. Inattention is seen as difficulty listening or concentrating, distractibility and failure to finish an activity. All of these do not need to be present for a diagnosis of ADHD, but according to the American Academy of Child and Adolescent Psychiatry, the symptoms must create a "real handicap" in at least two of the following areas of a child's life in order to qualify as ADHD:

- In the classroom
- On the playground
- At home
- In the community
- In social settings

It is estimated that 3-5 percent of children have ADHD.[37] Genetics play a significant role in ADHD diagnoses as shown by the observations that 50 percent of children of parents with a history of ADHD, and up to 92 percent of identical twins whose twin has the disorder, will develop ADHD. Increased incidence of ADHD is also seen as a result of meningitis, lead poisoning and fetal alcohol syndrome. According to the National Institutes of Health, ADHD must occur by the age of seven and typically occurs around the age of three.[37] Girls develop ADHD three times less often than boys and exhibit more inattention than hyperactivity or impulsivity. Children may "outgrow" ADHD over time, or it may extend into adulthood as attention deficit disorder (ADD).

It is suspected that ADHD is caused by anatomic abnormalities or neurotransmitter regulation problems in dopamine-containing and/or norepinephrine-containing parts of the forebrain. Deficiency of dopamine leads to an inability to maintain one's attention on a given target. Norepinephrine is involved in levels of arousal and activity. The connections between these two neurotransmitters and the symptoms of ADHD are reinforced by the observation that drugs effective in ADHD block the reuptake of dopamine and/or norepinephrine.[3]

Medications are highly effective at managing the symptoms and associated behaviors of ADHD, although improved outcomes are generally seen when a combination of medication and behavioral therapy is employed.[37]

Stimulants, such as methylphenidate and mixed amphetamine salts, are generally considered first-line therapy. These medications increase dopamine and norepinephrine activity, although their exact mechanism of symptom alleviation is uncertain. Common side effects include stomachache, nausea, insomnia, headache, anorexia and weight loss. Side effects are a common reason for noncompliance in the younger population. Atomoxetine is also indicated for ADHD and is not a stimulant but rather a norepinephrine reuptake inhibitor (NERI). Bupropion and TCAs, such as imipramine, desipramine and nortriptyline, are considered second-line therapy, but are sometimes prescribed in addition to a stimulant to achieve a greater effect. Bupropion is associated with less anorexia than stimulants, fewer adverse effects than TCAs, and lower toxicity than TCAs. Compared to stimulants, TCAs have less insomnia, nausea and abuse potential, but have an increased frequency of other adverse effects and a higher risk of fatal overdose. TCAs also have a longer duration of action compared to the stimulants. Clonidine and guanfacine, which are more commonly used for hypertension, are third-line choices and act by modifying norepinephrine activity in the brain. These can be added to other therapies to help control aggression and improve sleep. They are less effective than stimulants when used alone. Lithium, valproic acid and carbamazepine are sometimes used to control aggressive and explosive behavior. Some antipsychotics are also being used to control hyperactivity, impulsivity and aggression. Adverse effects, as mentioned in the schizophrenia section, limit their use in ADHD since more effective agents are available.[37]

A careful diagnosis by a qualified professional is necessary because a response to these medications does not mean that a patient has ADHD. This is because all persons, regardless of whether or not they have ADHD, will exhibit increased attention, improved task completion and decreased arousal when given a stimulant.[3] While the effects of stimulants in individuals who do not suffer from ADHD lend to its abuse potential, these medications can be critical for those who need them. Recognition of this fact has led to increased prescribing rates of medications for ADHD. Between 1991 and 1995, the rate of stimulant use tripled, and the rate of clonidine use increased 28-fold.[37] Many children are inadequately treated despite this. While some parents might hesitate to initiate pharmacotherapy in their child, the consequences of untreated ADHD, such as low self-esteem or impaired social or academic abilities, must be considered in the decision of which therapies to use.

Sleep Disorders

Insomnia is defined as difficulty initiating, or maintaining, sleep or getting nonrestful sleep. This is the most common sleep disturbance in the U.S., affecting up to one-third of the population, with one in two insomniacs complaining of serious symptoms. Despite this, only one in 20 patients with insomnia seeks treatment, and one out of every 10 to one out of every 20 self-medicate with OTC products or alcohol.[38] Insomnia is actually a risk factor for the development of disorders, such as depression, anxiety disorders and certain cardiovascular complications. In fact, epidemiological studies have demonstrated an association of short sleep duration with increased cardiovascular morbidity. **Hypersomnia** is excessive sleepiness that lasts at least one month and can include **narcolepsy** (a condition of irresistible sleep attacks). **Parasomnias** are abnormal behavioral or physiological events occurring during, or immediately before or after sleep. Examples include nightmares, sleep terror disorders and sleepwalking.[38]

Insomnia and hypersomnia are common symptoms of depression, anxiety disorders, BD and schizophrenia. Patients are often misdiagnosed with a psychiatric illness because of how a sleep disturbance can affect mental functioning. Anergia (or lack of energy), impaired concentration and impaired memory can occur in patients with sleep apnea. **Sleep apnea**, a type of insomnia, may also lead to the development of depression because of its disruption to a patient's life. Patients with narcolepsy may be misdiagnosed as psychotic because of the hallucinations that may occur at the onset or end of their sleep. Patients with parasomnias may behave in such a way during sleep that they also are misdiagnosed with a psychiatric illness.[38]

Treatment of sleep disorders may include pharmacotherapy, behavioral modification, psychotherapy, and treatments such as continuous, or bilevel, positive airway pressure (CPAP or BiPAP) for sleep apnea. Sleep disorders related to a mental or medical condition will hopefully resolve if the other condition is adequately treated. Otherwise, a hypnotic (sleep-inducing agent) or stimulant may be needed. If a medication, or other substance, is found liable for the sleep disturbance, its use must be discontinued or modified if possible.

Medications used to treat insomnia include benzodiazepines and benzodiazepine-receptor agonists that act like benzodiazepines. Some antidepressants, antihistamines, barbiturates, alcohol and quetiapine are also effective. The agents approved for insomnia are indicated in patients with parasomnias, and they may also be given these medications with the hope that they will improve sleep maintenance.

Benzodiazepines approved for their hypnotic effects include estazolam, flurazepam, quazepam, temazepam and triazolam; however, any agent of this class will likely have a similar pharmacologic effect. Nonbenzodiazepine benzodiazepine-receptor agonists (the term for a newer class of sleep aid medications) include zaleplon, eszopiclone and zolpidem. Adverse effects of benzodiazepine-like agents are similar to the benzodiazepines. These agents must only be used at bedtime for up to two weeks except for eszopiclone, which is approved for long-term use. Patients must not drink alcohol with these agents as this combination can lead to excessive sedation and, possibly, death in certain circumstances.

Antidepressants used as sleep aids include amitriptyline, doxepin, trimipramine, SSRIs, trazodone and mirtazapine. Trazodone and amitriptyline are the most commonly used antidepressants for sleep. When used for this indication, they are dosed much lower than when they are used to treat depression.

When antihistamines, such as doxylamine and diphenhydramine, are used to treat insomnia, they are dosed at the same levels used for allergies. Their side effects are also the same as those seen when these drugs are used to treat allergies. The most common side effects other than sedation (which is desirable in this case) are the anticholinergic side effects (e.g., dry eyes, dry mouth, dry skin, tachycardia, blurred vision, constipation and urinary retention).

Barbiturates, such as pentobarbital and butabarbital (not to be confused with butalbital), were often used for sleep in the past; however, they have been replaced by benzodiazepines and newer hypnotics due to the risk of death in overdose with barbiturates.

Hypersomnia and narcolepsy are problems associated with excessive or uncontrollable sleep. Therefore, stimulant drugs are used to treat these conditions. Dextroamphetamine, amphetamines, methylphenidate and modafinil are FDA-approved for narcolepsy. They can also be used for hypersomnia. Many of these agents have significant addiction liability and potential for dependence. For this reason, most of the agents mentioned in this section are classified as controlled substances, as detailed in Table 4.[39]

Table 4
Drugs Used to Treat Psychiatric Disorders

Drug Class(es)	Generic Name(s)**	Brand Name(s)**	Indication(s)	Available Dose Form(s)
Anti-Anxiety	Buspirone	BuSpar	Depression, Generalized Anxiety Disorder, Premenstrual Syndrome	Tablet
Anti-Anxiety	Meprobamate (Schedule 4)	Miltown	Anxiety, Muscle Spasms	Tablet
Anti-Anxiety: Anti-Nausea, Benzodiazepine	Diazepam (Schedule 4)	Diastat, Diastat Accudial, Valium	Ethanol Withdrawal, Generalized Anxiety Disorder, Muscle Relaxant, Nausea, Panic Disorder, Sedation, Seizures, Vomiting	Injectable, Rectal Gel, Solution (Concentrate), Tablet
Anti-Anxiety: Anti-Nausea, Benzodiazepine	Lorazepam (Schedule 4)	Ativan	Agitation, Ethanol Detoxification, Generalized Anxiety Disorder, Insomnia, Nausea, Seizures, Status Epilepticus, Vomiting	Drops, Injectable, Tablet
Anti-Anxiety: Benzodiazepine	Alprazolam (Schedule 4)	Niravam, Xanax, Xanax XR	Generalized Anxiety Disorder, Panic Disorder	Orally-Disintegrating Tablet, Tablet Solution (Concentrate)
Anti-Anxiety: Benzodiazepine	Chlordiazepoxide (Schedule 4)	Librium	Ethanol Withdrawal, Generalized Anxiety Disorder	Capsule, Gel Cap
Anti-Anxiety: Benzodiazepine	Clonazepam (Schedule 4)	Klonopin, Klonopin Wafers	Bipolar Disorder, Generalized Anxiety Disorder, Nerve Pain, Panic Disorder, Restless Leg Syndrome, Seizures	Orally-Disintegrating Tablet, Tablet
Anti-Anxiety: Benzodiazepine	Clorazepate (Schedule 4)	Tranxene SD Half-Strength, Tranxene T-Tab	Ethanol Withdrawal, Generalized Anxiety Disorder, Seizures	Tablet

Table 4 cont.
Drugs Used to Treat Psychiatric Disorders

Drug Class(es)	Generic Name(s)**	Brand Name(s)**	Indication(s)	Available Dose Form(s)
Anti-Anxiety: Benzodiazepine	Oxazepam (Schedule 4)	Serax	Generalized Anxiety Disorder, Seizures	Capsule
Anticonvulsant	Carbamazepine	Carbatrol, Epitol, Equetro, Tegretol, Tegretol XR	Alcohol Withdrawal, Bipolar Disorder, Post-Traumatic Stress Disorder, Restless Leg Syndrome, Schizophrenia, Seizures	Capsule, Chewable Tablet, Suspension, Tablet
Anticonvulsant	Divalproex Sodium or Valproic Acid or Valproate Sodium	Depacon, Depakene, Depakote, Depakote ER, Depakote Sprinkles, Stavzor	Behavior Disorders in Alzheimer's Disease, Bipolar Disorder Mania, Migraine Prophylaxis, Seizures, Status Epilepticus	Capsule (Sprinkles), Gel Cap, Injectable, Syrup, Tablet
Anticonvulsant	Gabapentin	Neurontin	Bipolar Disorder, Chronic Pain, Peripheral Neuropathy, Post-Herpetic Neuralgia, Seizures, Social Anxiety Disorder	Capsule, Solution, Tablet
Anticonvulsant	Lamotrigine	Lamictal, Lamictal ODT, Lamictal Starter Kit, Lamictal XR	Bipolar Disorders, Seizures	Orally-Disintegrating Tablet, Tablet
Anticonvulsant	Levetiracetam	Keppra, Keppra XR	Bipolar Disorder, Migraine Prevention, Seizures	Extended-Release Tablet, Injectable, Solution, Tablet
Anticonvulsant	Oxcarbazepine	Trileptal	Bipolar Disorder, Seizures	Suspension, Tablet
Anticonvulsant	Phenytoin	Dilantin, Dilantin Infatabs, Phenytek	Seizures	Capsule, Chewable Tablet, Injectable, Suspension
Anticonvulsant	Pregabalin (Schedule 5)	Lyrica	Fibromyalgia, Nerve Pain, Peripheral Neuropathy	Capsule

Drug Class(es)	Generic Name(s)**	Brand Name(s)**	Indication(s)	Available Dose Form(s)
Anticonvulsant	Topiramate	Topamax, Topamax Sprinkles	Bipolar Disorder, Cluster Headache, Migraine Prophylaxis, Neuropathic Pain, Seizures	Capsule (Sprinkles), Tablet
Antidepressant: Mono-Amine Oxidase Inhibitor	Phenelzine	Nardil	Depression, Panic Disorder	Tablet
Antidepressant: Mono-Amine Oxidase Inhibitor	Tranylcypromine	Parnate	Depression, Post-Traumatic Stress Disorder	Tablet
Antidepressant: Norepinephrine Antagonist	Mirtazapine	Remeron, Remeron SolTab	Depression	Tablet
Antidepressant: Norepinephrine / Dopamine Reuptake Inhibitor	Budeprion or Buproprion	Aplenzin, Wellbutrin, Wellbutrin SR, Wellbutrin XL, Zyban	Attention Deficit Hyperactivity Disorder, Depression, Smoking Cessation	Extended-Release Tablet, Tablet
Antidepressant: Selective Serotonin Reuptake Inhibitor	Citalopram	Celexa	Depression, Obsessive Compulsive Disorder	Solution, Tablet
Antidepressant: Selective Serotonin Reuptake Inhibitor	Escitalopram	Lexapro	Depression, Generalized Anxiety Disorder	Solution, Tablet
Antidepressant: Selective Serotonin Reuptake Inhibitor	Fluoxetine	Prozac, Prozac Weekly, Sarafem, Selfemra	Bulimia Nervosa, Depression, Fibryo-myalgia, Obsessive Compulsive Disorder, Panic Disorder, Pre-menstrual Dysphoric Disorder	Capsule, Gel Cap, Solution, Tablet
Antidepressant: Selective Serotonin Reuptake Inhibitor	Fluvoxamine	Luvox, Luvox CR	Depression, Generalized Anxiety Disorder, Obsessive Compulsive Disorder, Panic Disorder	Capsule, Tablet

Table 4 *cont.*
Drugs Used to Treat Psychiatric Disorders

Drug Class(es)	Generic Name(s)**	Brand Name(s)**	Indication(s)	Available Dose Form(s)
Antidepressant: Selective Serotonin Reuptake Inhibitor	Paroxetine	Paxil, Paxil CR, Pexeva	Depression, Eating Disorders, Impulse Control, Obsessive Compulsive Disorder, Panic Disorder, Post-Traumatic Stress Disorder, Pre-menstrual Dysphoric Disorder, Social Anxiety Disorder	Suspension, Tablet
Antidepressant: Selective Serotonin Reuptake Inhibitor	Sertraline	Zoloft	Depression, Eating Disorders, Generalized Anxiety Disorder, Impulse Control, Obsessive Compulsive Disorder, Panic Disorder, Post-Traumatic Stress Disorder, Premenstrual Dysphoric Disorder, Social Anxiety Disorder	Solution (Concentrate), Tablet
Antidepressant: Selective Serotonin Reuptake Inhibitor / Antipsychotic: Second Generation	Fluoxetine / Olanzapine	Symbyax	Depressive Episodes from Bipolar Disorder	Capsule
Antidepressant: Serotonin Agonist and Reuptake Inhibitor	Nefazodone	Serzone	Depression, Post-Traumatic Stress Disorder	Tablet
Antidepressant: Serotonin Agonist and Reuptake Inhibitor	Trazodone	Desyrel, Oleptro ER	Depression, Insomnia	Extended-Release Tablet, Tablet
Antidepressant: Serotonin / Norepinephrine Reuptake Inhibitor	Amoxapine	Ascendin	Depression	Tablet
Antidepressant: Serotonin / Norepinephrine Reuptake Inhibitor	Desvenlafaxine	Pristiq	Depression	Tablet

Drug Class(es)	Generic Name(s)**	Brand Name(s)**	Indication(s)	Available Dose Form(s)
Antidepressant: Serotonin / Norepinephrine Reuptake Inhbitor	Maprotiline	Ludiomil	Depression	Tablet
Antidepressant: Serotonin / Norepinephrine Reuptake Inhibitor	Milnacipran	Savella	Fibromyalgia	Tablet
Antidepressant: Serotonin / Norepinephrine Reuptake Inhibitor	Venlafaxine	Effexor, Effexor XR, Venlafaxine ER Tablets	Attention Deficit Hyperactivitiy Disorder, Autism, Chronic Fatigue Syndrome, Depression, General Anxiety Disorder, Hot Flashes, Obsessive Compulsive Disorder, Pain from Neuropathy, Social Anxiety Disorder	Extended-Release Capsule, Extended-Release Tablet, Tablet
Antidepressant: Tricyclic	Amitriptyline	Elavil	Depression, Fibromyalgia, Insomnia, Migraine, Pain, Prophylaxis	Tablet
Antidepressant: Tricyclic	Clomipramine	Anafranil	Chronic Pain, Depression, Obsessive Compulsive Disorder, Panic Disorder	Capsule
Antidepressant: Tricyclic	Desipramine	Norpramin	Attention Deficit Hyperactivity Disorder, Depression, Pain, Peripheral Neuropathy, Substance Abuse Disorders	Tablet
Antidepressant: Tricyclic	Doxepin	Prudoxin, Silenor, Sinequan, Zonalon	Anxiety, Depression, Pain	Capsule, Solution (Concentrate), Tablet, Topical Cream
Antidepressant: Tricyclic	Imipramine	Tofranil, Tofranil-PM	Attention Deficit Hyperactivity Disorder, Bed-Wetting, Depression, Pain, Panic Disorder	Capsule, Tablet

Table 4 *cont.*
Drugs Used to Treat Psychiatric Disorders

Drug Class(es)	Generic Name(s)**	Brand Name(s)**	Indication(s)	Available Dose Form(s)
Antidepressant: Tricyclic	Notriptyline	Pamelor	Anxiety Disorders, Attention Deficit Hyperactivity Disorder, Depression, Enuresis, Pain, Smoking Cessation	Capsule, Solution
Antidepressant: Tricyclic	Protriptyline	Vivactil	Depression	Tablet
Antidepressant: Tricyclic	Trimipramine	Surmontil	Depression	Capsule
Antihistamine	Cyproheptadine	Periactin	Allergies, Appetite Stimulation, Bed-Wetting, Migraine Prophylaxis, Nightmares, Post-Traumatic Stress Disorder	Syrup, Tablet
Antihistamine	Doxylamine	Aldex AN, Doxytex, Unisom	Allergies, Insomnia	Chewable Tablet, Solution, Tablet
Antihistamine	Hydroxyzine	Atarax, Vistaril	Allergies, Anxiety, Insomnia, Itching	Capsule, Injection, Suspension, Syrup, Tablet
Antihistamine: Anti-Nausea	Diphenhydramine	Benadryl, Unisom	Allergies, Insomnia, Motion Sickness (Nausea), Vomiting	Aerosol, Capsule, Cream, Dissolving Strip, Elixir, Gel, Gel Cap, Injectable, Solution, Syrup, Tablet
Antihypertensive: Alpha-2 Agonist (Centrally Acting)	Guanfacine	Intunix, Tenex	Attention Deficit Hyperactivity Disorder, High Blood Pressure	Extended-Release Capsule, Tablet
Antihypertensive: Alpha-2 Blocker	Clonidine	Catapres, Catapres-TTS, Duraclon	Attention Deficit Hyperactivity Disorder, Dysmenorrhea, Ethanol Dependence, High Blood Pressure, Impulse Control Problems, Severe Pain	Injectable, Patch, Tablet

Drug Class(es)	Generic Name(s)**	Brand Name(s)**	Indication(s)	Available Dose Form(s)
Antihypertensive: Beta Blocker, Antidysrhythmic	Propranolol	Inderal, Inderal LA, Innopran XL	Acute Coronary Syndrome, Aggressive Behavior, Angina, Anxiety, Dysrhythmias, Heart Attack Prevention, High Blood Pressure, Migraine Prophylaxis, Parkinson's Tremor	Injectable, Patch, Tablet
Anti-Migraine	Acetaminophen / Butalbital / Caffeine	Fioricet	Migraines	Capsule, Tablet
Anti-Migraine	Sumatriptan	Imitrex, Imitrex Stat-Dose	Migraines	Injectable, Nasal Spray, Tablet
Anti-Parkinson's Disease	Carbidopa / Levodopa	Sinemet, Sinemet CR	Parkinson's Disease	Extended-Release Tablet
Anti-Parkinson's Disease	Ropinirole HCl	Requip, Requip XL	Parkinson's Disease, Restless Leg Syndrome	Extended-Release Tablet, Tablet
Antipsychotic: Neuroleptic	Fluphenazine	Prolixin	Pervasive Development Disorder, Schizophrenia	Elixir, Injectable Solution (Concentrate), Tablet
Antipsychotic: Neuroleptic	Haloperidol	Haldol	Agitation, Behavior Problems in Children, Ethanol Dependence, Nausea, Schizophrenia, Tourette's Syndrome, Vomiting	Injectable, Solution (Concentrate), Tablet
Antipsychotic: Neuroleptic	Loxapine	Loxitane	Schizophrenia	Capsule
Antipsychotic: Neuroleptic	Thioridazine	Mellaril	Schizophrenia	Tablet
Antipsychotic: Neuroleptic	Thiothixene	Navane	Schizophrenia	Capsule
Antipsychotic: Neuroleptic	Trifluoperazine	Stelazine	Schizophrenia	Tablet

Table 4 *cont.*
Drugs Used to Treat Psychiatric Disorders

Drug Class(es)	Generic Name(s)**	Brand Name(s)**	Indication(s)	Available Dose Form(s)
Antipsychotic: Neuroleptic, Anti-Nausea	Chlorpromazine	Thorazine	Acute Intermittent Porphyria, Hiccups, Mania, Schizophrenia, Vomiting	Injectable, Tablet
Antipsychotic: Neuroleptic, Anti-Nausea	Perphenazine	Trilafon	Dementia, Ethanol Withdrawal, Huntington's Chorea, Nausea, Reye's Syndrome, Schizophrenia, Spasmodic Torticollis, Tourette's Syndrome, Vomiting	Tablet
Antipsychotic: Second-Generation	Aripiprazole	Abilify, Abilify Discmelt	Mania, Schizophrenia	Injectable, Orally-Disintegrating Tablet, Solution, Tablet
Antipsychotic: Second-Generation	Asenapine	Saphris	Bipolar Disorder, Schizophrenia	Sublingual Tablet
Antipsychotic: Second-Generation	Clozapine	Clorazil, Fazaclo	Bipolar Disorder, Obsessive Compulsive Disorder, Schizo-Affective Disorder, Schizophrenia	Orally-Disintegrating Tablet
Antipsychotic: Second-Generation	Iloperidone	Fanapt	Schizophrenia	Tablet
Antipsychotic: Second-Generation	Olanzapine	Zydis, Zyprexa, Zyprexa, Zyprexa Intramuscular, Zyprexa Relprevv	Acute Agitation (in Bipolar Disorder or Schizophrenia), Bipolar Disorder, Chronic Pain, Mania, Schizophrenia	Injectable, Orally-Disintegrating Tablet
Antipsychotic: Second-Generation	Paliperidone	Invega, Invega Sustenna	Schizophrenia	Injectable, Tablet
Antipsychotic: Second-Generation	Quetiapine	Seroquel, Seroquel XR	Autism, Mania, Schizophrenia	Tablet

Drug Class(es)	Generic Name(s)**	Brand Name(s)**	Indication(s)	Available Dose Form(s)
Antipsychotic: Second-Generation	Risperidone	Risperdal, Risperdal Consta, Risperdal M-Tab	Autism, Behavioral Problems from Dimenta, Mania, Mixed Bipolar Disorder, Schizophrenia, Tourette's Syndrome	Injectable, Orally-Disintegrating Tablet, Solution, Tablet
Antipsychotic: Second-Generation	Ziprasidone	Geodon	Acute Agitation in Schizophrenia, Mania, Schizophrenia, Tourette's Syndrome	Capsule, Injectable
Cholinesterase Inhibitor	Galantamine	Razadyne	Alzheimer's Disease	Extended-Release Capsule, Solution, Tablet
Dopamine Receptor Agonist (Long-Acting)	Cabergoline	Dostinex	Low Prolactin Levels	Tablet
Hormone	Desmopressin Acetate	DDAVP	Bed-Wetting	Injectable, Nasal Spray, Tablet
Hormone	Levothyroxine	Levothroid, Levoxyl, Synthroid, Tirosint, Unithroid	Hypothyroidism	Injectable, Tablet
Melatonin Receptor Agonist	Ramelteon	Rozerem	Insomnia	Tablet
Methylxanthines	Theophylline	Theo-24, Uniphyl	Asthma	Capsule, Liquid, Tablet
Norepinephrine Reuptake Inhibitor	Atomoxetine	Strattera	Attention Deficit Hyperactivity Disorder, Depression	Capsule
Pain Reliever	Methadone (Schedule 2)	Dolophine, Methadone Diskets	Drug Addiction, Pain	Injectable, Liquid, Orally-Disintegrating Tablets, Solution (Concentrate), Tablet
Peripherally-Acting Opioid Antagonist	Methylnaltrexone	Relistor	Constipation	Injectable

Table 4 *cont.*
Drugs Used to Treat Psychiatric Disorders

Drug Class(es)	Generic Name(s)**	Brand Name(s)**	Indication(s)	Available Dose Form(s)
Sedative-Hypnotic	Chloral Hydrate (Schedule 4)	Somnote	Insomnia	Capsule, Syrup
Sedative-Hypnotic	Eszopiclone (Schedule 4)	Lunesta	Insomnia	Tablet
Sedative-Hypnotic	Zaleplon (Schedule 4)	Sonata	Insomnia	Capsule
Sedative-Hypnotic	Zolpidem (Schedule 4)	Ambien, Ambien CR, Edluar	Insomnia	Tablet
Sedative-Hypnotic: Barbiturate	Butabarbital (Schedule 3)	Butisol	Insomnia	Elixir, Tablet
Sedative-Hypnotic: Barbiturate	Pentobarbital (Schedule 2)	Nembutal	Anesthesia	Injectable
Sedative-Hypnotic: Benzodiazepine	Estazolam (Schedule 4)	ProSom	Insomnia	Tablet
Sedative-Hypnotic: Benzodiazepine	Flurazepam (Schedule 4)	Dalmane	Insomnia	Capsule
Sedative-Hypnotic: Benzodiazepine	Quazepam (Schedule 4)	Doral	Insomnia	Tablet
Sedative-Hypnotic: Benzodiazepine	Temazepam (Schedule 4)	Restoril	Anxiety, Insomnia, Panic Disorder	Capsule
Sedative-Hypnotic: Benzodiazepine	Triazolam (Schedule 4)	Halcion	Insomnia	Tablet
Stimulant	Amphetamine Salt Combo (Schedule 2)	Adderall, Adderall XR	Attention Deficit Disorder, Narcolepsy	Extended-Release Capsule, Tablet
Stimulant	Armodafinil (Schedule 4)	Nuvigil	Narcolepsy, Shift-Work Sleep Disorder, Sleep Apnea	Tablet
Stimulant	Dexmethylpheni-date (Schedule 2)	Focalin, Focalin XR	Attention Deficit Hyperactivity Disorder	Capsule, Tablet
Stimulant	Dextroamphet-amine (Schedule 2)	Dexedrine, DextroStat, Procentra	Attention Deficit Hyperactivity Disorder, Narcolepsy, Obesity	Capsule, Solution, Tablet

Drug Class(es)	Generic Name(s)**	Brand Name(s)**	Indication(s)	Available Dose Form(s)
Stimulant	Methylphenidate (Schedule 2)	Dexedrine, DextroStat, Procentra	Attention Deficit Hyperactivity Disorder, Narcolepsy, Obesity	Capsule, Solution, Tablet
Stimulant	Modafinil (Schedule 4)	Provigil	Attention Deficit Hyperactivity Disorder, Depression, Narcolepsy	Capsule, Chewable Tablet, Patch, Solution, Tablet
Stimulant	Phentermine (Schedule 4)	Adipex-P, Ionamin, Pro-Fast HS	Attention Deficit Disorder, Obesity	Capsule, Tablet

**All rights to all brand names and trademarks are held by their respective owners. There may be additional brand names for some of the products listed.*

References

1. World Health Organization, www.who.int/about/definition/en/, Aug. 3, 2005.
2. National Institute of Health, Substance Abuse and Mental Health Services Administration, www.healthypeople.gov/document/pdf/Volume2/18Mental.pdf, Aug. 3, 2005.
3. American Psychiatric Association, Diagnostic and Statistical Manual of Mental Disorders, 4th edition, Washington, D.C., 2000.
4. Kando, J.C., Wells, B.G., Hayes, P.E., "Chapter 69, Depressive Disorders," Pharmacotherapy: A Pathophysiologic Approach, 5th edition, New York, NY, 2002, pp. 1243-1264.
5. Crismon, M., Dorson, P.G., "Chapter 68, Schizophrenia," Pharmacotherapy: A Pathophysiologic Approach, 5th edition, New York, NY, 2002, pp. 1219-1242.
6. Fankhauser, M.P., "Chapter 70, Bipolar Disorder," Pharmacotherapy: A Pathophysiologic Approach, 5th edition, New York, NY, 2002, pp. 1265-1287.
7. Kirkwood, C.K., Melton, S.T., "Chapter 71, Anxiety Disorders," Pharmacotherapy: A Pathophysiologic Approach, 5th edition, New York, NY, 2002, pp. 1289-1310.
8. Gibbons, R.D., Hur, K., Bhaumik, D.K., Mann, J.J., "The Relationship Between Antidepressant Medication Use and Rate of Suicide," Archives of General Psychiatry, Chicago, IL, Vol. 62, No. 2, pp. 165-172, 2005.
9. Olfson, M., Shaffer, D., Marcus, S.C., Greenberg, T., "Relationship Between Antidepressant Medication Treatment and Suicide in Adolescents," *Archives of General Psychiatry*, Chicago, IL, Vol. 60, No. 10, pp. 978-982, 2003.
10. Facts and Comparisons, www.efactsonline.com.libcat.ferris.edu/Fac/servlet/MainPage, July 11, 2005.
11. Grunebaum, M.F., Ellis, S.P., Li, S., Oquendo, M.A., Mann, J.J., "Antidepressants and Suicide Risk in the United States," *The Journal of Clinical Psychiatry*, Memphis, TN, Vol. 65, No. 11, pp. 1456-1462, 2004.
12. Stahl, S.M., Essential Psychopharmacology of Depression and Bipolar Disorder, New York, NY, 2000.
13. Stahl, S.M., "Basic Psychopharmacology of Antidepressants, Part 1: Antidepressants Have Seven Distinct Mechanisms of Action," *The Journal of Clinical Psychiatry*, Memphis, TN, Vol. 59, No. 4, pp. 5-14, 1998.
14. Blumenthal, M., "German Federal Institute for Drugs and Medical Devices. Commission E. The Complete German Commission E Monographs: Therapeutic Guide to Herbal Medicines, 1st edition," Austin, TX, 1998.
15. Mannel, M., "Drug Interactions with St. John's Wort: Mechanisms and Clinical Implications," *Drug Safety*, Vol. 27, No. 11, pp. 773-797, November 2004.
16. Merriam-Webster's Collegiate Dictionary, 10th edition, Springfield, MA, 1996, p. 408.
17. "Treatment of Bipolar Disorder, The Expert Consensus Panel for Bipolar Disorder," *The Journal of Clinical Psychiatry*, Memphis, TN, Vol. 57, No. 12A, pp. 3-88, 1996.
18. Wittchen, H.U., Hoyer, J., "Generalized Anxiety Disorder: Nature and Course," *The Journal of Clinical Psychiatry*, Memphis, TN, Vol. 62, No. 11, pp. 20-21, 2001.
19. Eaton, W.W., Kessler, R.C., Wittchen, H.U., Magee, W.J., "Panic and Panic Disorder in the United States," *American Journal of Psychiatry*, Vol. 151, No. 3, pp. 413-420, March 1994.
20. Sandford, J.J., Argyropoulos, S.V., Nutt, D.J., "The Psychobiology of Anxiolytic Drugs. Part I: Basic Neurobiology, " *Pharmacology & Therapeutics*, Orlando, FL, Vol. 88, No. 3, pp. 197-212, 2000.
21. Wells, B.G., Hayes, P.E., "Chapter 72, Obsessive-Compulsive Disorder," Pharmacotherapy: A Pathophysiologic Approach, 5th edition, New York, NY, 2002, pp. 1311-1322.
22. Ereshefsky, L., Lacombe, S., "Pharmacological Profile of Risperidone," *Canadian Journal of Psychiatry*, Ottawa, Ontario, Vol. 38, No. 3S, pp. 80-88, 1993.

23. Richelson, E., "Interactions of Antidepressants with Neurotransmitter Transporters and Receptors and Their Clinical Relevance," *Journal of Clinical Psychiatry*, Memphis, TN, Vol. 64, No. 12, pp. 5-12, 2003.

24. Sareen, J., Kirshner, A., Lander, M., Kjernisted, K.D., Eleff, M.K., Reiss, J.P., "Do Antipsychotics Ameliorate or Exacerbate Obsessive-Compulsive Disorder Symptoms? A Systematic Review," *Journal of Affective Disorders*, San Diego, CA, Vol. 82, No. 2, pp. 167-174, 2004.

25. Greist, J.H., Bandelow, B., Hollander, E., et. al., "WCA Recommendations for the Long-Term Treatment of Obsessive-Compulsive Disorder in Adults," *CNS Spectrums*, New York, NY, Vol. 8, No. 8, pp. 7-16, 2003.

26. Ackerman, D.L., Greenland, S., "Multivariate Meta-Analysis of Controlled Drug Studies for Obsessive-Compulsive Disorder," *The Journal of Clinical Psychopharmacology*, Vol. 22, No. 3, pp. 309-317, 2002.

27. Greist, J.H., Jefferson, J.W., Kobak, K.A., Katzelnick, D.J., Serlin, R.C., "Efficacy and Tolerability of Serotonin Transport Inhibitors in Obsessive-Compulsive Disorder. A Meta-Analysis," *Archives of General Psychiatry*, Chicago, IL, Vol. 52, No. 1, pp. 53-60, 1995.

28. Piccinelli, M., Pini, S., Bellantuono, C., Wilkinson, G., "Efficacy of Drug Treatment in Obsessive-Compulsive Disorder. A Meta-Analytic Review," *British Journal of Psychiatry*, London, England, Vol. 166, No. 4, pp. 424-423, April 1995.

29. Crismon, M., Buckley, P., "Chapter 63, Schizophrenia," Pharmacotherapy: A Pathophysiologic Approach, 6th edition, New York, NY, 2005, pp. 1209-1233.

30. Remington, G., "Understanding Antipsychotic 'Atypicality': A Clinical and Pharmacological Moving Target," *Journal of Psychiatry and Neuroscience*, New York, NY, Vol. 28, No. 4, pp. 275-284, 2003.

31. Jeste, D.V., Okamoto, A., Napolitano, J., Kane, J.M., Martinez, R.A., "Low Incidence of Persistent Tardive Dyskinesia in Elderly Patients with Dementia Treated with Risperidone," *American Journal of Psychiatry*, Arlington, VA, Vol. 157, No. 7, pp. 1150-1155, 2000.

32. Tollefson, G.D., Beasley, C.M., Jr., Tamura, R.N., Tran, P.V., Potvin, J.H., "Blind, Controlled, Long-Term Study of the Comparative Incidence of Treatment-Emergent Tardive Dyskinesia with Olanzapine or Haloperidol," *American Journal of Psychiatry*, Arlington, VA, Vol. 154, No. 9, pp. 1248-1250, 1997.

33. Tran, P.V., Dellva, M.A., Tollefson, G.D., Beasley, C.M., Jr., Potvin, J.H., Kiesler, G.M., "Extrapyramidal Symptoms and Tolerability of Olanzapine Versus Haloperidol in the Acute Treatment of Schizophrenia," *Journal of Clinical Psychiatry*, Memphis, TN, Vol. 58, No. 5, pp. 205-211, 1997.

34. "Consensus Development Conference on Antipsychotic Drugs and Obesity and Diabetes," *Diabetes Care*, Alexandria, VA, Vol. 27, No. 2, pp. 596-601, 2004.

35. Montgomery, J., Winterbottom, E., Jessani, M., et. al., "Prevalence of Hyperprolactinemia in Schizophrenia: Association with Typical and Atypical Antipsychotic Treatment," *Journal of Clinical Psychiatry*, Memphis, TN, Vol. 65, No. 11, pp. 1491-1498, 2004.

36. Brown, C.S., Markowitz, J.S., Moore, T.R., Parker, N.G., "Atypical Antipsychotics: Part II: Adverse Effects, Drug Interactions and Costs," *Annals of Pharmacotherapy*, Cincinnati, OH, Vol. 33, No. 2, pp. 210-217, 1999.

37. Dopheide, J.A., Theesen, K.A., "Childhood Disorders" Pharmacotherapy: A Pathophysiologic Approach, 5th edition, New York, NY, 2002, pp. 1145-1154.

38. Curtis, J.L., Jermain, D.M., "Chapter 73, Sleep Disorders," Pharmacotherapy: A Pathophysiologic Approach, 5th edition, New York, NY, 2002, pp. 1323-1333.

39. Lexi-Comp, Inc., Lexi-Drugs™, July 11, 2005.

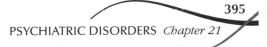

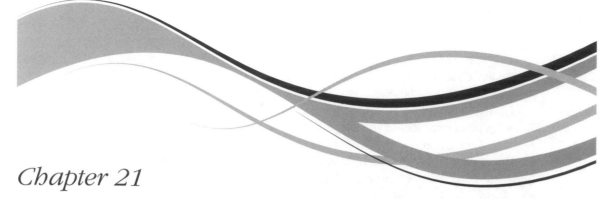

Chapter 21

REVIEW QUESTIONS

1. Which of the following neurotransmitters is not a target of the currently available antidepressants?
    a. Dopamine
    b. Norepinephrine
    c. Acetylcholine
    d. Serotonin

2. Schizophrenia is currently attributed to imbalances in which of these neurotransmitters?
    a. Norepinephrine
    b. Acetylcholine
    c. Epinephrine
    d. Dopamine

3. Which of the following is/are disadvantages of using the SSRIs?
    a. SSRIs are only effective in treating depression
    b. SSRIs are effective if used on a "prn" basis
    c. SSRIs are safer in overdose than TCAs
    d. None of the above

4. Which of the following is a first-choice agent in the treatment of bipolar disorder?
    a. Sertraline
    b. Fluoxetine
    c. Quetiapine
    d. Alprazolam
    e. None of these are agents of first choice

5. Which of the following is true about ADHD?
    a. When diagnosed in adults, it is referred to as attention deficit disorder (ADD)
    b. It is usually seen in childhood
    c. The three hallmark signs are hyperactivity, impulsivity and inattention
    d. Genetics play a significant role in the disorder
    e. All of the above

6. Which of the following medications requires routine lab draws that must be monitored and reported before dispensing to the patient?
    a. Quetiapine
    b. Valproic acid
    c. Clozapine
    d. Risperdal Consta

7. Which of the following medications are not used much anymore due to potentially dangerous food/drug interactions?
    a. TCAs
    b. SSRIs
    c. SNRIs
    d. MAOIs

8. Which of the following is an advantage of the benzodiazepines?
    a. They can help sleep problems associated with anxiety disorders
    b. They can be used on an as needed basis
    c. They are effective for a broad range of anxiety disorders
    d. All of the above are advantages

9. Which of the following statements is false?
    a. All of the antipsychotics are FDA-approved for the treatment of schizophrenia
    b. The term "dystonia" refers to a constant need to be in motion
    c. Clozapine is usually reserved for only the most severely ill schizophrenic patients
    d. Hallucinations and delusions are classified as "positive" symptoms

10. Which of the following combinations is correct?
    a. Clomipramine – SSRI
    b. Olanzapine – FGA
    c. Methylphenidate – stimulant
    d. Lorazepam – SNRI

Chapter 22

CENTRAL AND PERIPHERAL NERVOUS SYSTEM

By   Hannah M. Bursiek, Pharm.D.
    Victoria A. Gates, Pharm.D.
    Kari L. Vavra, Pharm.D.

Learning Objectives

This chapter seeks to prepare a pharmacy technician to:

■   describe the components and functions of the central and peripheral nervous systems.

■   differentiate between the actions of the sympathetic and parasympathetic systems.

■   identify commonly utilized medications affecting the peripheral nervous system.

■   discuss the differences between acute and chronic pain.

■   describe the mechanism of action of commonly-utilized nonsteroidal anti-inflammatory drugs (NSAIDs) and opioid analgesics for the treatment of pain disorders.

■   identify common side effects associated with all of the pharmacologic agents for treating pain.

■   differentiate between acute and preventative pharmacologic therapies for the management of migraine headaches.

■   discuss the disease-modifying therapies available for multiple sclerosis.

■   describe the signs and symptoms of Parkinson's disease.

■   list the different classes of medication used in the treatment of Parkinson's disease.

■   identify common adverse effects from anti-epileptic (anticonvulsant) medication use.

Introduction

Upon touching one's hand to a stove, the reality that the brain is communicating with the rest of the body (including through pain signals) becomes quite clear. Instinctively, the hand that is now burned pulls away from the heat before becoming even more damaged. Although this reaction seems instantaneous, and it nearly is, there are many processes that must occur to make this reaction happen. Any of these processes can fail or work improperly, leading to unfortunate consequences. This chapter seeks to briefly overview how the nervous system works normally, how it can fail or work improperly, and what treatment options are available for conditions resulting from the improper functioning of the nervous system.

Function of the Nervous System

The major functions of the **nervous system** include detecting information, analyzing information and transmitting information. This information is initially gathered by the sensory system through a person's five senses: sight, sound, taste, smell and touch. In the example of a hand touching a stove, nerves are activated in the skin, via the sense of touch, that indicate that a heat source is in close proximity to the hand. Then, a message is sent from the skin to the brain notifying the brain of the sensation of growing heat. The sensation grows as the hand approaches contact with the stove until the system reaches the threshold where the system has to take action; and, as a result of this stimulus, the brain sends a message back to the hand telling the muscles in the hand to pull away from the stove. This information sharing is done through the body's information superhighway – **neurons**. See Figure 1 below for more information on how the nervous system is organized.

Figure 1
Organization of the Nervous System

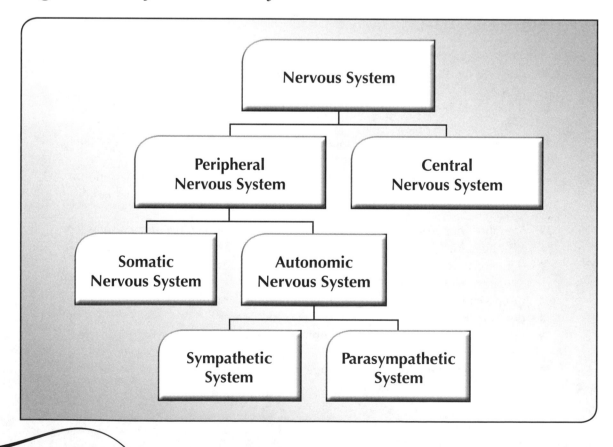

The **central nervous system** contains the brain and the spinal cord. The **brain** serves as the computer of the body; the brain is responsible for processing outside sensory information. The **spinal cord** acts as the conducting cables for the computer's input and output. The **peripheral nervous system** contains all of the neurons outside of the central nervous system. Neurons in the peripheral nervous system allow communication to occur between the central nervous system and outside stimuli. **Sensory (afferent or incoming) neurons** deliver stimuli from skin and other organs to the central nervous system. **Motor (efferent or outgoing) neurons** carry information from the central nervous system to terminals found in the muscles and glands via the peripheral nervous system. The peripheral nervous system is further broken down based on the functions that are being controlled. Voluntary movements associated with skeletal muscle and the sensory neurons of the skin are controlled by the **somatic nervous system**. Involuntary components of the nervous system, such as those innervated by smooth muscles, cardiac muscles and glands, are controlled by the **autonomic nervous system**. The autonomic nervous system is further broken down into the sympathetic and parasympathetic systems. The sympathetic and parasympathetic systems often run in opposition to each other in the body. In response to a stressful situation, the body is programmed to respond with either a fight response or a flight response; either way, the response is executed by the **sympathetic system**. During the activation of the sympathetic system, many systems are stimulated to prepare the individual to move: heart rate increases, senses become heightened, blood flow increases to most areas of the body and all unnecessary functions are shut down. Neurotransmitters involved in the sympathetic system include norepinephrine, epinephrine and dopamine. In contrast to the "fight or flight" response, the **parasympathetic system** prepares the body for rest. The neurotransmitter involved in communication between neurons in the parasympathetic system is acetylcholine. Acetylcholine exerts its effect in the parasympathetic system through its **agonist** (stimulatory) effects at both muscarinic and nicotinic receptors. Further effects of the autonomic system are included in Table 1; notice that the effects of the parasympathetic system can be arranged into the mnemonic code SLUDGE, which is appropriate for a system that is active during unexciting periods of rest. Notice that secretion of the various body fluids occurs during parasympathetic stimulation and that production of these secretions (which are nonessential for short-term survival) is stopped if the sympathetic system is activated; it would be quite a problem for someone running from a threat to life or limb to be crying or feeling the need to use a bathroom.

Table 1
Parasympathetic and Sympathetic Nervous System Effects: SLUDGE

Parasympathetic Effect	Sympathetic Effect	Organ Affected
Salivation (Production of Saliva)	Dry Mouth (Xerostomia)	Mouth
Lacrimation (Tear Production) / Pupil Constriction	Dry Eyes / Pupil Dilation	Eye
Urination	Urinary Retention	Urinary Tract
Defecation	Constipation	Bowels
Gastrointestinal Upset **E**mesis (Vomiting)	Decreased Peristalsis and Relaxed Intestines	Gastrointestinal Tract

Pain

Roughly 50 million people are disabled by pain in the United States. Although **pain** may be experienced differently by every patient, it is generally defined as a distressing and/or unpleasant sensation in a particular area of the body resulting from tissue damage. When an injury occurs, cellular damage leads to the release of substances, including bradykinins, prostaglandins, histamine, leukotrienes, serotonin and substance P. These substances stimulate **nociceptors** (pain/sensory receptors) in **somatic** (skin, bone, joint, muscle or connective tissue) and **visceral** (internal organ) structures. Upon nociceptor activation, pain signals are transmitted from the site of injury, along nerve fibers, to the spinal cord and brain, resulting in a painful sensation (known as **nociceptive pain**). Nociceptive pain may range from dull and aching (somatic) to deep and pressure-like (visceral). Other types of pain include neuropathic and functional pain. **Neuropathic pain** (e.g., diabetic neuropathy) results from damage to nerves, and **functional pain** (e.g., fibromyalgia) results from nervous system dysfunction. Neuropathic and functional pain disorders produce burning, tingling and/or stabbing sensations.

Pain can further be classified as acute or chronic. **Acute pain** has a sudden onset, is usually nociceptive in nature and generally has a clear cause (e.g., surgery, broken bones, dental/medical procedures, burns, cuts, childbirth and/or other trauma). This type of pain generally resolves quickly once the damage has healed or has been treated. If the acute pain continues beyond the healing phase, then it becomes chronic pain. **Chronic pain** may be nociceptive and/or neuropathic/functional in nature. Unlike acute pain, chronic pain doesn't always have a clear cause, and it is often accompanied by sleep disturbances, depression, impaired mobility and/or other problems. Examples of chronic pain include low back pain, osteoarthritis and some headache pain. Not all types of pain, however, are distinctly divided into acute or chronic; for instance, cancer pain often has components of both. Depending on the type of pain (nociceptive vs. neuropathic/functional), the classification (acute vs. chronic) and the severity, a variety of pharmacologic treatment options are currently available. One class of drugs commonly used for mild pain, fever reduction and inhibition of inflammation, is the NSAID. Acetaminophen, which does not have any anti-inflammatory action, is also commonly used for mild pain and to reduce a fever. All of these agents may be combined with opioid analgesics to increase pain relief and to reduce the amount of opioids needed to control pain. NSAIDs block cyclooxygenase-1 (COX-1) and/or cyclooxygenase-2 (COX-2) enzyme activity in the body which leads to inhibition of prostaglandin formation in response to injury, and subsequent activation of the nociceptors responsible for pain. Although NSAIDs provide similar pain relief regardless of the agent selected (at equipotent doses), patient response may vary greatly between agents. Further, there is a psychosomatic response with pain therapy, such that if the patient believes that an agent will work then it has a much better chance of providing pain relief than an agent that the patient feels less favorable about for whatever reason. Common NSAID side effects include nausea, abdominal pain, diarrhea, stomach/intestinal ulcers and bleeding. The gastrointestinal side effects result from inhibiting COX-1; COX-1 normally produces prostaglandins that protect the stomach from ulcers. Selective COX-2 inhibitors were developed in an effort to reduce gastrointestinal side effects. These agents have a far-greater affinity for COX-2 than COX-1 and thus allow COX-1 activity and stomach-protecting prostaglandins to remain intact. Although the full extent of the risk increase is not completely understood, all NSAIDs carry some increased risk of causing a heart attack or stroke. Anyone using NSAID therapy for more than a short course must discuss the potential increase in these risks with a physician or pharmacist. Unlike other salicylates (a type of NSAID), aspirin permanently inhibits COX activity in platelets, which prevents platelets from sticking together and forming a blood clot. Therefore, aspirin (but not other salicylates or NSAIDs) is commonly utilized for clot-based heart attack and clot-based stroke prevention.

The drug that most commonly leads to hospitalization for drug overdose (intentional or unintentional) is acetaminophen. Patients using acetaminophen must be made aware of the limits of acetaminophen use. Those patients without complicating factors may use up to 4,000 mg in a 24-hour period without being concerned about liver damage; however, those patients with a dysfunctional liver (or who are also consuming alcohol) must be restricted to 2,000 mg in a 24-hour period. Further, those taking some other medications, such as warfarin, must also limit their acetaminophen intake. Although patients must be aware of all of the acetaminophen that they are taking, pharmacy technicians can assist in preventing acetaminophen overdose. Many prescription pain relievers are combination products that contain acetaminophen, and many over-the-counter (OTC) products also contain acetaminophen. Asking patients who are getting a prescription product containing acetaminophen if they are also using an OTC product that contains acetaminophen can be very helpful. Further, adding daily limits to prescription labels, after the instructions provided by the physician, can be helpful (e.g., a prescription written for hydrocodone/acetaminophen 7.5 mg/750 mg with directions to take one tablet, by mouth, every four to six hours could reasonably have the statement "Maximum of five tablets in 24 hours" added to the end of the directions for a patient known to be able to take up to 4,000 mg/day of acetaminophen).

Opioid analgesics, also known as narcotic analgesics, are commonly utilized for the treatment of moderate to severe pain. These agents provide analgesia, or pain relief, through stimulation of opioid receptors in the brain, spinal cord and smooth muscle. Patients using opioids generally still have pain; however, opioids provide the patient with a greater tolerance to their pain and generally decrease their perception of being in pain. Morphine, and its derivates hydromorphone and oxymorphone, is considered the drug of choice for the treatment of severe pain; however, morphine must be used with caution in patients with renal (kidney) impairment, as the drug is eliminated from the body by the kidneys. Codeine is commonly combined with acetaminophen for the treatment of moderate pain but is also available as a stand-alone product for the treatment of more severe pain. Derivatives of codeine, including hydrocodone and oxycodone, are most effective for moderate to severe pain when combined with NSAIDs or acetaminophen. Meperidine is no longer widely used because its metabolite (normeperidine) may accumulate (especially in the elderly and in patients with renal impairment), causing seizures. Fentanyl is available as a transdermal (through the skin) patch, as well as in other forms, for the treatment of severe chronic (not acute) pain. When applied to the skin, the patch provides pain relief for 72 hours in most patients (some patients find that relief subsides sooner). A fentanyl patch begins working 12-24 hours after being first applied and must be accompanied by other pain therapies while it is being initiated. Finally, methadone has a very long duration of action, is useful for acute and/or chronic (including neuropathic) pain and requires careful dose initiation and titration.

For acute pain, opioids are usually initiated on a scheduled basis (e.g., every four hours) with irregular availability as needed for breakthrough pain (pain that occurs despite the use of pain-relieving medications). Once the pain decreases in severity, the patient may be switched to only an "as-needed" regimen and then may transition off of the pain medications, if appropriate, after the acute pain subsides. To manage chronic pain, patients must be given both a long-acting pain medication that is used to provide round-the-clock pain relief, and then the patient must also be provided with a short-acting medication for breakthrough pain episodes. From a therapeutic perspective, there are no maximum doses of opioids; doses are titrated up or down based on the patient's response to a given dose. If a patient is in pain, or is using their breakthrough therapy too often, then the long-acting medication dose will be increased to control the patient's pain. If the patient is experiencing side effects that are limiting their functionality, then doses are decreased until a balance is reached between pain control and side effect tolerance. Common side effects include nausea, vomiting, constipation and sedation. Respiratory depression may also occur with opioid use; however, it is extremely rare and is generally associated with rapidly escalating doses of opioids that go well beyond what the patient needs for pain control. Excluding constipation, tolerance to these side effects generally develops with repeated drug use. Constipation is nearly guaranteed with opioid use, especially chronic use, and therefore all patients using opioids must be counseled by a pharmacist on the use of combination stool-softener/stimulant laxative products. Multiple routes of administration are available for opioid products, including oral, rectal, intravenous, subcutaneous, intramuscular, transdermal and transmucosal (through the cavity between the cheek and gum). For patients with opioid-related allergies, switching to a different opioid may be possible. When switching from one opioid, or route of administration, to another, **equianalgesic** (providing the same pain relief) or **equipotent** (relative doses that produce an equivalent effect) dosing charts are available to help guide the conversion. A pharmacist or physician must always take into consideration patient-specific factors, as well as the incomplete cross-tolerance of opioids, when calculating the proper dose of a new opioid for someone who is on an opioid currently. See Table 2 below for an equianalgesic dosing chart.

Table 2
Equianalgesic Dosing Chart

Drug	Route of Administration	Equivalent Doses*
Codeine	IM / IV / SQ	120 mg
	PO	200 mg
Fentanyl	IM / IV	0.1-0.2 mg
Hydrocodone	PO	20-30 mg
Hydromorphone	IM / IV / SQ	1.3-1.5 mg
	PO	7.5 mg
Meperidine (Acute Dosing Only)	IM / IV / SQ	75 mg
	PO	300 mg
Methadone	IM / IV / SQ	Acute Use: 5-10 mg Chronic Use: 1-4 mg
	PO	Acute Use: 20 mg Chronic Use: 2-4 mg
Morphine	IM / IV / SQ	10 mg
	PO	Acute Dosing (Opioid-Naive): 60 mg Chronic Dosing: 30 mg
Oxycodone	PO	15-30 mg

Some correction may be necessary for incomplete opioid cross-tolerance; a pharmacist or physician will make patient-specific dosing determinations when converting between narcotics.

Similar to opioid analgesics, tramadol stimulates opioid receptors in the central nervous system; however, an additional mechanism of the inhibition of serotonin and norepinephrine reuptake is also seen with tramadol use. Tramadol is often used for moderate to severe acute and chronic (including neuropathic) pain. Seizures and other opioid side effects (constipation) may occur with tramadol. Dosage adjustments are necessary for those with renal impairment and elderly patients. Also, tramadol is not a controlled substance and is, therefore, often preferred by both patients and physicians due to it not having the restrictions present with controlled substances. Tapentadol, a new opioid analgesic, is similar to tramadol. In addition to being an opioid analgesic, tapentadol also inhibits norepinephrine reuptake. In clinical studies, it appears that tapentadol is associated with less gastrointestinal side effects (nausea, vomiting and constipation) than tramadol.

In addition to nonopioid and opioid analgesics, adjuvant analgesics may be essential for successful pain management. **Adjuvant analgesics** are medications that are typically used to treat diseases other than pain, but that also help relieve pain or work with true analgesics to provide greater relief from pain. Examples include the following:

- Antidepressants: tricyclic antidepressants (e.g., amitriptyline and nortriptyline), selective serotonin reuptake inhibitors (e.g., fluoxetine), serotonin-norepinephrine reuptake inhibitors (e.g., venlafaxine and duloxetine)
- Anticonvulsants (e.g., gabapentin, pregabalin)
- Corticosteroids (e.g., dexamethasone, prednisone)
- Muscle relaxants (e.g., baclofen, carisoprodol or cyclobenzaprine)

Although nonopioid and opioid analgesics are the mainstay of treatment for pain, nonpharmacologic therapies may play a role in relieving pain. A variety of strategies are available to help reduce pain, including acupuncture, chiropractic care, breathing exercises, yoga exercises, Tai-Chi exercises, distraction techniques, meditation and/or prayer, electrical nerve stimulation, heat/cold application, medical massage, music and physical therapy. These strategies may be utilized by themselves or with pharmacologic therapies for pain control. Patient attitude is also important; patients who feel confident that they will control their pain (rather than be controlled by it) generally have more success in achieving pain control. Further, those who remain as active as their body will allow (continuing to exercise) do better at maintaining pain control. Pain control is much more than responding to a stimulus with a drug of a reasonable dose; pain control truly involves the whole person, including body, mind and spirit.

Migraine Headache Disorder

Migraines, a very common and painful type of headache, affect 18.2 percent of women and 6.5 percent of men in the United States each year. Migraine headaches typically start during adolescence or early adulthood and greatly impair family, school, social and/or work activities. Head pain and other associated symptoms (e.g., nausea) result from activation of the **trigeminal nerve** (a major sensory facial nerve) that releases substances that stimulate dilation and inflammation of brain blood vessels. As the blood vessels swell, they squeeze neighboring nerves and cause pain. The migraine attack may have different phases, starting with **premonitory symptoms** (difficulty concentrating, food cravings, irritability) in the hours or days before the migraine. Following premonitory symptoms, one-third of patients experience an **aura** (temporary visual, sensory or speech symptoms, such as flickering lights, flickering spots, vision loss, feeling of pins and needles or numbness) immediately prior to the migraine. Next, the **headache phase** involves unilateral (one-sided), throbbing, moderate-to-severe pain. This phase generally lasts for four to 72 hours and may be accompanied by nausea, vomiting or sensitivity to light, sound and/or movement. Finally, the **resolution phase** (feelings of tiredness, exhaustion and/or irritability) occurs after the headache. The phases and the symptoms experienced may differ from patient to patient and from attack to attack.

Two different medication strategies exist for the management of migraine headaches: acute and preventative therapy. Acute therapy is administered at the onset of the migraine attack to help relieve pain, whereas preventative therapy is taken every day to help prevent or decrease the number and/or the severity of attacks. Much like in pain control, patients using preventative therapies will still need access to acute therapies for breakthrough episodes. Acute therapy agents are taken immediately at the onset of migraine pain to increase their effectiveness and to reduce disruption of daily activities. Often, nausea and vomiting occur during a migraine attack (or may be a side effect of drug treatment). This may limit the use of oral drugs and may delay pain relief. **Antiemetics** (agents used to relieve nausea and vomiting) are often given prior to ingestion of acute therapy when appropriate. Another option is to use an acute therapy that is not given by the oral route of administration. Products are available as inejctables, nasal sprays and rectal suppositories.

Medications for the treatment of migraine pain include acetaminophen, NSAIDs, opioids, combination analgesics, ergot alkaloids, local anesthetics and serotonin receptor agonists (the triptans). Some of these therapies are used to treat the pain associated with going through a migraine; some of these therapies, specifically the triptans, are designed to actually stop a migraine from progressing (and thereby preventing the pain from initiating). There are seven commercially-available triptans that each have slightly different properties and available dose forms. Sumatriptan has a short onset of action and is available as a tablet, a nasal spray and as an injectable product. Frovatriptan has a longer onset of action (than sumatriptan) but lasts for up to 72 hours, whereas sumatriptan is relatively short-lived in terms of its effects on the body. It is important that a pharmacist or physician take these specific considerations into account when recommending or prescribing a triptan. The triptans constrict blood vessels in the brain, block the release of inflammatory substances, inhibit pain transmission and, therefore, relieve pain associated with migraines. Common side effects include fatigue, dizziness, flushing, abnormal skin sensations (burning or tingling), drowsiness and taste disturbances (generally only seen when an intranasal formulation is used). Due to the varying properties of the seven available agents, patients may need to try all seven before settling on a regimen that works to control their migraines. One limitation for the triptans is that patients who overuse them may experience rebound headaches. Rebound headaches occur when the blood vessels in the brain cannot sustain the constriction caused by the triptans and relax in exhaustion, leading to severe headaches that may not respond to repeated triptan doses (however, patients often continue to take more and more of the triptan in order to attempt to find relief). Thus, each product has a maximum dose that may be used in a single day or in a single month without causing rebound headaches (exceptions exist, however, and a pharmacist or physician must be consulted before a prescription is determined to be inappropriate). These limits are included in Table 3.

Migraine prevention may be appropriate in the following situations: persistent, severe migraines despite acute therapy; the presence of side effects, contraindications and/or unresponsiveness to acute therapy; and/or the use of acute therapy three or more times per week (when there is a risk of rebound headaches). A variety of medications, which are typically used to treat other disorders, are utilized for migraine prevention. Examples include the following:

- Antihypertensives: beta-adrenergic blockers (e.g., atenolol, metoprolol, nadolol, propranolol and timolol), calcium channel blockers (e.g., verapamil)
- Antidepressants: tricyclic antidepressants (e.g., amitriptyline and nortriptyline), selective serotonin reuptake inhibitors (e.g., fluoxetine) or mono-amine oxidase inhibitors (e.g., phenelzine)
- Anticonvulsants (e.g., gabapentin, topiramate, valproic acid/divalproex sodium)

Nonpharmacologic interventions for the prevention of migraine involve lifestyle changes and the identification and avoidance of migraine triggers. Examples of lifestyle changes include adhering to a regular sleep, exercise and meal schedule and staying away from excess caffeine and/or tobacco consumption. Migraine sufferers may also be able to identify **migraine triggers** (factors that promote, or worsen, a migraine attack). Common triggers are certain foods (e.g., alcohol, aspartame, caffeine, chocolate, monosodium glutamate, nitrates and tyramine), certain environmental irritants (e.g., perfume, tobacco smoke, weather changes), lifestyle changes (e.g., skipping meals, increasing stress, irregular sleep pattern) and hormonal changes (e.g., a point in the menstrual cycle of women, menopause, decreased testosterone in men). Other nonpharmacologic interventions for the management of migraines include applying ice packs to the painful area and/or seeking a dark, quiet, room to relax/sleep during the headache phase.

Table 3
Migraine Medications and Dosing Limitations

Generic Name	Dose / Unit	Route of Administration	Max Dose in 24 Hours	Max Dose in 30 Days
Almotriptan	6.25 mg	Oral	4 Tablets	16 Tablets
	12.5 mg	Oral	2 Tablets	8 Tablets
Eletriptan	20 mg	Oral	4 Tablets	12 Tablets
	40 mg	Oral	2 Tablets	6 Tablets
Frovatriptan	2.5 mg	Oral	3 Tablets	12 Tablets
Naratriptan	1 mg	Oral	5 Tablets	20 Tablets
	2.5 mg	Oral	2 Tablets	8 Tablets
Rizatriptan	5 mg	Oral	6 Tablets	24 Tablets
	10 mg	Oral	3 Tablets	12 Tablets
Sumatriptan	25 mg	Oral	8 Tablets	32 Tablets
	50 mg	Oral	4 Tablets	16 Tablets
	100 mg	Oral	2 Tablets	8 Tablets
	4 mg	SQ	3 Injections	12 Injections
	6 mg	SQ	2 Injections	8 Injections
	5 mg	Nasal	8 Sprays	32 Sprays
	20 mg	Nasal	2 Sprays	8 Sprays
Sumatriptan / Naproxen	85 mg / 500 mg	Oral	2 Tablets	10 Tablets
Zolmitriptan	2.5 mg	Oral	4 Tablets	12 Tablets
	5 mg	Oral	2 Tablets	6 Tablets
	5 mg	Nasal	2 Sprays	6 Sprays

Multiple Sclerosis

Multiple sclerosis (MS) is an inflammatory disease that affects between 250,000 and 350,000 people in the United States. MS is usually diagnosed in patients between the ages of 15 and 45 years of age, with women more commonly affected than men. The exact cause of MS is unknown, but it is believed to be caused by an autoimmune process that results in the stripping of the myelin sheath surrounding CNS axons. Patients with MS present with a wide variety of symptoms that are categorized based on how directly they are related to the nerve damage experienced by the patient. Primary symptoms are a direct consequence of conduction disturbances produced by demyelination and axonal damage. These symptoms include visual problems, parasthesias, cognitive changes, muscle spasticity, tremor, weakness and fatigue. Secondary symptoms are complications resulting from primary symptoms (e.g., recurrent urinary tract infections caused by a lack of nerve control on the muscles surrounding the bladder leading to urinary retention and bacterial growth in the urinary tract). Tertiary symptoms relate to the effect the disease has on a patient's everyday life and can include personal, social and emotional disturbances. There are four distinct types of MS that have been described. Many patients have attacks (new symptoms lasting at least 24 hours and separated from other symptoms by at least 30 days), followed by remissions. This course is called **relapsing-remitting multiple sclerosis (RRMS)**. Most RRMS patients will eventually worsen and enter a progressive phase in which it is difficult to differentiate between attacks and remissions because the attacks seem to be nearly constant. This is referred to as **secondary-progressive multiple sclerosis (SPMS)**. It is referred to as secondary because this phase is always secondary to some period of RRMS during the patient's life. Some patients never cycle between attacks and remissions; these patients have symptoms that are constant and progressively worsen over time. This is called **primary-progressive multiple sclerosis (PPMS)** and referred to as primary because it does not come after another phase but is the only phase that the patient experiences. A few patients experience attacks that last so long that they present as being progressive but are part of a prolonged relapsing-remitting cycle; this very rare form of MS is called **progressive-relapsing multiple sclerosis (PRMS)**. Regardless of the type of MS, treatment includes: treatment of acute exacerbations, disease-modifying therapies that seek to prevent progression of the attacks and symptomatic support. Acute attacks of MS, which affect a person's functional ability, are treated with high-dose IV corticosteroids. Unless another agent must be used, 500-1,000 mg of Methylprednisolone are generally given daily for three to five days to control acute attacks. This therapy can not only reduce the duration of the attack, but also quickly improve the patient's symptoms. Disease-modifying therapies alter the course of MS and slow the patient's progression toward disability. As soon as a diagnosis of MS is made, an interferon product, or glatiramer, is recommended. Mitoxantrone and natalizumab are reserved for patients who have not had an adequate response to previous therapies or who continue to rapidly progress despite the use of interferon. All these medications have been shown to reduce the attack rate in patients with MS and slow disease progression; however, these therapies are not curative and individual patients may experience the entire range from successful suppression of attacks for long periods of time to complete failure of the therapy. The annual cost for these medications is between $10,000 and $30,000. This is just one of the many economic costs associated with MS. The most common adverse events with these products are injection-site reactions. Many symptoms of MS do not require or respond to pharmacologic treatment; but for those that do, appropriate treatment is of the utmost importance to maintain a patient's quality of life. **Spasticity**, or involuntary muscle contractions, which can cause problems walking and result in falls, can be successfully managed with pharmacologic treatments. Baclofen is the preferred agent for spasticity, with tizanidine being an effective alternative. Patients with MS frequently complain of bowel and bladder symptoms (e.g., incontinence, urgency, frequency and nocturia). Anticholinergic agents are the most commonly used agents to treat mild bladder symptoms. Tricyclic antidepressants and newer antimuscarinic medications have also been used to treat mild bladder symptoms. Numbness and paresthesia are frequent sensory complaints that do not usually require treatment, but some patients may develop acute or chronic pain syndromes for which treatment is necessary. One of the most common complaints in patients is fatigue. Amantadine, methylphenidate, dextroamphetamine and modafinil have all been used successfully to offer relief.

See Table 4 on the next page for a list of treatment options for common symptoms of MS.

Table 4
Treatment of Multiple Sclerosis Symptoms

Spasticity	Bladder Symptoms	Sensory Symptoms	Fatigue
Baclofen, Botulinum Toxin Type A, Dantrolene, Diazepam, Gabapentin, Pregabalin, Tiagabine, Tizanidine	Amitriptyline, Botulinum Toxin Type A, Darifenacin, Desmopressin, Dicyclomine, Hyoscyamine, Imipramine, Oxybutynin, Prazosin, Propantheline, Self-Catheterization, Solifenacin, Trospium	Carbamazepine, Gabapentin, Lamotrigine, Phenytoin, Pregabalin, Tricyclic Antidepressants	Amantadine, Antidepressants, Dextroamphetamine, Methylphenidate, Modafinil

Many patients with MS use **complementary and alternative medicine (CAM)**. Common CAM therapies include high doses of antioxidants (including vitamin A and E), high doses of water-soluble vitamins, high doses of vitamin D supplementation (as prevention and as treatment), magnesium supplementation and marijuana use (smoked or ingested orally). There is a growing body of evidence that having adequate vitamin D levels can be preventative for MS; however, the studies seem to show that the effect may be genetically influenced, with Caucasians seeing a greater prevention effect from vitamin D supplementation. Further, cannabinoids, found in marijuana, seem to be effective at reducing the spasticity effects and tremors that are associated with MS. The other therapies mentioned either have little or no evidence to support their use. Pharmacy technicians can assist their pharmacists by asking patients with MS if they are using, or have used, any of these CAM therapies as significant drug interactions need to be screened. Further, changes in counseling requirements when pharmacists discuss traditional medications may be warranted for patients using these other therapies.

Parkinson's Disease

Up to one million Americans have been diagnosed with Parkinson's disease, with the highest incidence occurring in persons over the age of 85 years. **Parkinson's disease** is characterized by a slow and progressive loss of dopamine-producing neurons in the brain. This decrease in dopamine is responsible for the hallmark signs of Parkinson's disease: resting tremor, rigidity, **bradykinesia** (muscles that are slow to respond) and postural instability. Resting tremor is often the only complaint when patients are diagnosed. It is seen most commonly in the hands with a characteristic "pill-rolling" motion. Rigidity most often affects the extremities, but it can also affect facial muscles causing reduced facial expressions. Bradykinesia refers to slowed movement throughout an action, including freezing at the initiation of a movement. Postural instability is seen in the advanced stages of Parkinson's disease. It is one of the most disabling symptoms because it increases a patient's risk for falls and does not usually respond to pharmacologic therapy. Other symptoms of Parkinson's disease can include **dysarthria** (slurred speech), **dysphagia** (difficulty swallowing) and **micrographia** (reduction of handwritten letter size). There are no proven neuroprotective agents available for Parkinson's disease, so the current therapies are referred to as symptomatic treatment. Generally, initial pharmacologic therapy begins with a mono-amine oxidase type B (MAO-B or MAOI) inhibitor or, if a patient is physiologically young, a dopamine agonist. MAO-B inhibitors interfere with the degradation of dopamine in the brain, resulting in prolonged dopaminergic activity, while dopamine agonists enhance the activity of dopamine. When more symptomatic control is needed, levodopa, the immediate precursor to dopamine, is usually supplemented. All patients will require treatment with levodopa at some point, as it is the most effective drug for Parkinson's disease. Catechol-o-methyltransferase (COMT) inhibitors can be added to levodopa to extend its effects and manage symptoms that occur as tolerance develops to levodopa supplementation (referred to as "wearing off" symptoms). Anticholinergics can be effective against the tremor that is usually seen with Parkinson's disease. These drugs may be used alone or in combination with other classes to provide symptomatic relief. Patients taking dompaminergic agents may complain of side effects, including nausea, hypotension, hallucinations and motor complications (dyskinesias).

Nonpharmacologic therapy is encouraged for all patients with Parkinson's disease. Physical therapy, support groups, occupational therapy, speech therapy and exercise are all viable treatment options for patients with Parkinson's disease that may help to improve their overall quality of life. Some patients may also consider the following CAM therapies:

- Caffeine (usually from tea or coffee) ingested daily has been shown to reduce a patient's risk of developing Parkinson's disease.
- Co-enzyme Q10 may be effective during the early stages of the disease at delaying progression to more advanced stages of the disease.
- Creatine may aid patients in the early stages of the disease to delay progression to more advanced disease. It may also help those in more advanced stages of the disease lower their dosage of levodopa to experience symptom control.

Epilepsy

Epilepsy is a chronic disorder characterized by recurrent and unprovoked seizures that are a result of abnormal or excessive excitation of cortical neurons. There are many different types of seizures that may present with a wide spectrum of severity, appearance, cause and management requirements. The International League Against Epilepsy classifies seizures into two main groups: partial seizures and generalized seizures. **Partial seizures** begin locally in one hemisphere of the brain and can cause somatosensory (i.e., sense of pain and sense of touch) or motor symptoms. Partial seizures with no loss of consciousness are classified as simple, whereas partial seizures with an alteration of consciousness are described as complex. **Generalized seizures** have involvement of both hemispheres of the brain and therefore manifest with bilateral symptoms and loss of consciousness. Generalized seizures can be further classified into absence, myoclonic, atonic and tonic-clonic seizures. Generalized tonic-clonic seizures are what many people think of as epilepsy. They are characterized by a sharp tonic contraction of muscles, followed by a period of rigidity and clonic movements.

The goal of treatment for epilepsy is to decrease the number of seizures while minimizing drug side effects. Antiepileptic pharmacotherapy is highly individualized and depends on the type of seizure diagnosed. Approximately 50-70 percent of patients can be maintained on one medication; however, if the therapeutic goal is not achieved with monotherapy, a second medication can be added. The mechanism of action for most antiepileptic drugs (AEDs) can be categorized as either effecting sodium channels, effecting calcium channels, increasing concentrations of inhibitory neurotransmitters (e.g., GABA), or decreasing concentrations of inhibitory neurotransmitters (e.g., glutamate and aspartate). Some of the most widely-used medications are older, first generation, AEDs, including carbamazepine, phenobarbital, phenytoin and valproic acid. There are also many newer, second generation AEDs used for the treatment of epilepsy. All AEDs are likely to cause central nervous system side effects, such as sedation, dizziness, blurred vision, difficulty with concentration and **ataxia** (a loss of coordination causing significant impairment).

Nonpharmacologic therapy for epilepsy includes: vagus nerve stimulation (VNS), modifications to a patient's diet, and identification and avoidance of seizure triggers (if any exist). Some centers have found a ketogenic diet, high in fat and low in carbohydrates and protein, to be beneficial in epileptic patients; however, it is poorly tolerated by many patients and can cause long-term adverse effects not related to epilepsy. A vagal nerve stimulator is an implanted medical device that can be used along with medications to help reduce the frequency of seizures. Avoiding seizure triggers, such as sleep deprivation and alcohol, may also be beneficial for patients. Some triggers are very specific and can be hard to identify. There have been reports of patients with triggers, such as summer sunlight reflecting off from a large body of water, sunlight reflecting off from snow in winter, watching movies or TV in 3-D, observing flashing lights (such as strobe lights) and smelling certain scents.

Table 5
Drugs Associated with the Central and Peripheral Nervous System and Related Disorders

Drug Class(es)	Generic Name(s)**	Brand Name(s)**	Indication(s)	Available Dose Form(s)
Anti-Cancer: Enyzme Inhibitor	Mitoxantrone	Novantrone	Leukemia, Multiple Sclerosis, Prostate Cancer	Injectable
Anticholinergic	Atropine	Isopto Atropine, Sal-Tropine	Intestinal Spasms, Mydriasis, Over-Production of Saliva, Parkinson's Disease	Injectable, Ophthalmic, Tablet, Topical
Anticholinergic	Benztropine	Cogentin	Parkinson's Disease	Injectable, Tablet
Anticholinergic	Trihexyphenidyl	Artane	Parkinson's Disease	Liquid, Tablet
Anticholinergic, Anti-Nausea	Scopolamine	Isopto Hyoscine, Scopace, Transderm Scop	Motion Sickness, Nausea, Vomiting	Injectable, Ophthalmic, Patch, Tablet
Anticonvulsant	Carbamazepine	Carbatrol, Epitol, Equetro, Tegretol, Tegretol XR	Alcohol Withdrawal, Bipolar Disorder, Post-Traumatic Stress Disorder, Restless Leg Syndrome, Schizophrenia, Seizures	Capsule, Chewable Tablet, Suspension, Tablet
Anticonvulsant	Divalproex Sodium or Valproic Acid or Valproate Sodium	Depacon, Depakene, Depakote, Depakote ER, Depakote Sprinkles, Stavzor	Behavior Disorders in Alzheimer's Disease, Bipolar Disorder Mania, Migraine Prophylaxis, Seizures, Status Epilepticus	Capsule (Sprinkles), Gel Cap, Injectable, Syrup, Tablet
Anticonvulsant	Ethosuximide	Zarontin	Seizures	Capsule, Liquid

Table 5 *cont.*
Drugs Associated with the Central and Peripheral Nervous System and Related Disorders

Drug Class(es)	Generic Name(s)**	Brand Name(s)**	Indication(s)	Available Dose Form(s)
Anticonvulsant	Felbamate	Felbatol	Seizures	Suspension, Tablet
Anticonvulsant	Gabapentin	Neurontin	Bipolar Disorder, Chronic Pain, Peripheral Neuropathy, Post-Herpetic Neuralgia, Seizures, Social Anxiety Disorder	Capsule, Solution, Tablet
Anticonvulsant	Lamotrigine	Lamictal, Lamictal ODT, Lamictal Starter Kit, Lamictal XR	Bipolar Disorder, Seizures	Extended-Release Tablet, Orally-Disintegrating Tablet, Tablet
Anticonvulsant	Levetiracetam	Keppra, Keppra XR	Bipolar Disorder, Migraine Prevention, Seizures	Injectable, Solution, Tablet
Anticonvulsant	Oxcarbazepine	Trileptal	Bipolar Disorder, Seizures	Suspension, Tablet
Anticonvulsant	Phenytoin	Dilantin, Dilantin Infatabs, Phenytek	Seizures	Capsule, Chewable Tablet, Injection, Suspension
Anticonvulsant	Pregabalin (Schedule 5)	Lyrica	Fibromyalgia, Nerve Pain, Peripheral Neuropathy	Capsule
Anticonvulsant	Primidone	Mysoline	Seizures	Tablet
Anticonvulsant	Tiagabine	Gabitril	Seizures	Tablet
Anticonvulsant	Topiramate	Topamax, Topamax Sprinkles	Bipolar Disorder, Cluster Headache, Migraine Prophylaxis, Neuropathic Pain, Seizures	Capsule (Sprinkles), Tablet
Anticonvulsant	Zonisamide	Zonegran	Migraine Prophylaxis, Seizures	Capsule
Anticonvulsant: Barbiturate	Phenobarbital (Schedule 4)	Not Available	Seizures	Injectable, Liquid, Tablet

Drug Class(es)	Generic Name(s)**	Brand Name(s)**	Indication(s)	Available Dose Form(s)
Antihypertensive: Beta Blocker	Timolol	Betimol, Blocadren, Istalol, Timoptic, Timoptic Ocudose, Timoptic-XE	Acute Coronary Syndrome, Heart Failure, High Blood Pressure, Migraine Prophylaxis	Ophthalmic, Tablet
Antihypertensive: Beta Blocker, Antidysrhythmic	Propanolol	Inderal, Inderal LA, Innopran XL	Acute Coronary Syndrome, Aggressive Behavior, Angina, Anxiety, Dysrhythmias, Heart Attack Prevention, High Blood Pressure, Migraine Prophylaxis, Parkinson's Tremor, Portal Hypertension	Extended-Release Capsule, Injectable, Solution, Tablet
Anti-Migraine	Almotriptan	Axert	Migraines	Tablet
Anti-Migraine	Butalbital / Acetaminophen / Caffeine with or wtihout Codeine (some are Schedule 3)	Esgic-Plus, Fioricet, Fiorinal	Migraines	Capsule, Liquid, Tablet
Anti-Migraine	Dihydoergotamine	DHE-45, Migranal	Migraines	Injectable, Nasal Spray
Anti-Migraine	Eletriptan	Relpax	Migraines	Tablet
Anti-Migraine	Ergotamine	Ergomar	Migraines	Sublingual Tablet
Anti-Migraine	Ergotamine / Caffeine	Cafergot, Migergot	Migraines	Suppository, Tablet
Anti-Migraine	Frovatriptan	Frova	Migraines	Tablet
Anti-Migraine	Isometheptene / Acetaminophen / Caffeine	Prodrin	Migraines	Tablet
Anti-Migraine	Isometheptene / Acetaminophen / Dichloralphenazone	Epidrin, Midrin, Migrazone	Migraines	Capsule
Anti-Migraine	Naratriptan	Amerge	Migraines	Tablet

Table 5 *cont.*
Drugs Associated with the Central and Peripheral Nervous System and Related Disorders

Drug Class(es)	Generic Name(s)**	Brand Name(s)**	Indication(s)	Available Dose Form(s)
Anti-Migraine	Rizatriptan	Maxalt, Maxalt-MLT	Migraines	Orally-Disintegrating Tablet, Tablet
Anti-Migraine	Sumatriptan	Alsuma, Imitrex, Imitrex Stat-Dose, Sumavel Dosepro	Migraines	Injectable, Nasal Spray, Tablet
Anti-Migraine	Zolmitriptan	ZOMIG, ZOMIG-ZMT	Migraines	Orally-Disintegrating Tablet, Nasal Spray, Tablet
Anti-Migraine / Nonsteroidal Anti-Inflammatory Drug	Sumatriptan / Naproxen	Treximet	Migraines	Tablet
Anti-Parkinson's Disease	Carbidopa / Levodopa	Parcopa, Sinemet, Sinemet CR	Parkinson's Disease	Extended-Release Tablet, Orally-Disintegrating Tablet, Tablet
Anti-Parkinson's Disease	Entacapone / Levodopa / Carbidopa	Stalevo	Parksinson's Disease	Tablet
Anti-Parkinson's Disease	Ropinirole	Requip, Requip XL	Parkinson's Disease, Restless Leg Syndrome	Extended-Release Tablet, Tablet
Cholinergic	Bethanechol	Urecholine	Urinary Retention	Tablet
Cholinergic	Pilocarpine	Isopto Carpine, Pilopine HS, Salagen	Dry Mouth, Glaucoma	Ophthalmic, Tablet
COMT Inhibitor	Entacapone	Comtan	Parkinson's Disease	Tablet
COMT Inhibitor	Tolcapone	Tasmar	Parkinson's Disease	Tablet
Dopamine Agonist	Amantadine	Symmetrel	Parkinson's Disease	Capsule, Liquid, Tablet
Dopamine Agonist	Apomorphine	Apokyn	Parkinson's Disease	Injectable
Dopamine Agonist	Pramipexole	Mirapex, Mirapex ER	Parkinson's Disease, Restless Leg Syndrome	Extended-Release Tablet, Tablet
Dopamine Receptor Agonist	Bromocriptine	Cycloset, Parlodel	Acromegaly, Diabetes (Type 2), Parkinson's Disease	Capsule, Tablet

Drug Class(es)	Generic Name(s)**	Brand Name(s)**	Indication(s)	Available Dose Form(s)
Immunomodulator	Glatiramer	Copaxone	Multiple Sclerosis	Injectable
Immunomodulator	Interferon Beta-1a with or without Albumin	Avonex, Rebif	Mutliple Sclerosis	Injectable
Immunomodulator	Interferon Beta-1b	Betaseron, Extavia	Multiple Sclerosis	Injectable
Immunomodulator	Natalizumab	Tysabri	Multiple Sclerosis	Injectable
Mono-Amine Oxidase Inhibitor	Rasagiline	Azilect	Parkinson's Disease	Tablet
Mono-Amine Oxidase Inhibitor	Selegiline	Eldepryl, Emsam, Zelapar	Parkinson's Disease	Capsule, Orally-Disintegrating Tablet, Patch, Tablet
Nonsteroidal Anti-Inflammatory Drug	Mefenamic Acid	Ponstel	Inflammation, Pain	Capsule
Nonsteroidal Anti-Inflammatory Drug	Oxaprozin	Daypro	Inflammation, Pain	Tablet
Nonsteroidal Anti-Inflammatory Drug: COX-2 Selective	Celecoxib	Celebrex	Osteoarthritis, Rheumatoid Arthritis	Capsule
Nonsteroidal Anti-Inflammatory Drug: COX-2 Selective	Etodolac	Lodine, Lodine XL	Inflammation	Extended-Release Tablet, Tablet
Nonsteroidal Anti-Inflammatory Drug: COX-2 Selective	Herpagophytum Procumbens	Devil's Claw (Herbal)	Inflammation, Pain	Capsule, Liquid, Tablet
Nonsteroidal Anti-Inflammatory Drug: COX-2 Selective	Meloxicam	Mobic	Osteoarthritis, Rheumatoid Arthritis	Suspension, Tablet
Nonsteroidal Anti-Inflammatory Drug: Nonselective	Diclofenac	Cambia, Cataflam, Flector, Pennsaid, Voltaren, Zipsor	Osteoarthritis, Rheumatoid Arthritis	Capsule, Patch, Tablet, Topical Gel, Topical Solution
Nonsteroidal Anti-Inflammatory Drug: Nonselective	Fenoprofen	Nalfon	Inflammation, Pain	Capsule, Tablet

Table 5 *cont.*
Drugs Associated with the Central and Peripheral Nervous System and Related Disorders

Drug Class(es)	Generic Name(s)**	Brand Name(s)**	Indication(s)	Available Dose Form(s)
Nonsteroidal Anti-Inflammatory Drug: Nonselective	Flurbiprofen	Ansaid, Ocufen	Inflammation, Pain	Ophthalmic, Tablet
Nonsteroidal Anti-Inflammatory Drug: Nonselective	Ibuprofen	Advil, Motrin	Gout, Osteoarthritis, Rheumatoid Arthritis	Capsule, Chewable Tablet, Liquid, Tablet
Nonsteroidal Anti-Inflammatory Drug: Nonselective	Ketoprofen	Orudis, Orudis KT	Inflammation, Pain	Capsule, Extended-Release Capsule
Nonsteroidal Anti-Inflammatory Drug: Nonselective	Ketorolac	Acular, Acular LS, Aculvail, Toradol	Inflammation, Pain	Extended-Release Tablet, Injectable, Nasal Spray, Ophthalmic, Tablet
Nonsteroidal Anti-Inflammatory Drug: Nonselective	Meclofenamate	Meclomen	Inflammation, Pain	Capsule
Nonsteroidal Anti-Inflammatory Drug: Nonselective	Nabumetone	Relafen	Inflammation	Tablet
Nonsteroidal Anti-Inflammatory Drug: Nonselective	Naproxen	Aleve, Anaprox, Mediproxen, Naprelan, Naprosyn, Pamprin	Gout, Osteoarthritis, Rheumatoid Arthritis	Capsule, Extended-Release Tablet, Suspension, Tablet
Nonsteroidal Anti-Inflammatory Drug: Nonselective	Piroxicam	Feldene	Gout, Osteoarthritis, Rheumatoid Arthritis	Capsule
Nonsteroidal Anti-Inflammatory Drug: Nonselective	Sulindac	Clinoril	Gout, Osteoarthritis, Rheumatoid Arthritis	Tablet
Nonsteroidal Anti-Inflammatory Drug: Nonselective	Tolmetin	Tolectin	Inflammation, Pain	Capsule, Tablet

Drug Class(es)	Generic Name(s)**	Brand Name(s)**	Indication(s)	Available Dose Form(s)
Nonsteroidal Anti-Inflammatory Drug: Nonselective, Anti-Gout	Indomethacin	Indocin, Indocin SR	Gout, Osteoarthritis, Rheumatoid Arthritis	Capsule, Extended-Release Capsule, Suppository, Suspension
Nonsteroidal Anti-Inflammatory Drug: Salicylate	Choline Magnesium Trisalicylate	Trisilate	Inflammation, Pain	Liquid, Tablet
Nonsteroidal Anti-Inflammatory Drug: Salicylate	Diflunisal	Dolobid	Inflammation, Pain	Tablet
Nonsteroidal Anti-Inflammatory Drug: Salicylate	Magnesium Salicylate	DeWitt's Pain Reliever, Doan's Extra-Strength, Momentum Muscular Backache, MST 600, Percogesic	Inflammation, Pain	Tablet
Nonsteroidal Anti-Inflammatory Drug: Salicylate	Salsalate	Salflex	Inflammation, Pain	Tablet
Nonsteroidal Anti-Inflammatory Drug: Salicylate, Antiplatelet	Apsirin	Bayer, Ecotrin, St. Joseph's	Acute Coronary Syndrome, Coronary Artery Disease, Fever, Heart Attack Prevention, Osteoarthritis, Pain, Rheumatoid Arthritis, Stroke	Capsule, Chewable Tablet, Delayed-Release Tablet, Effervescent Tablet, Gum, Suppository, Tablet
Pain Reliever	Acetaminophen / Codeine (Schedule 3 or 5)	Tylenol with Codeine	Pain	Liquid, Tablet
Pain Reliever	Acetaminophen / Oxycodone (Schedule 2)	Endocet, Magnacet, Percocet, Primlev, Roxicet, Tylox, Xolox	Pain	Capsule, Liquid, Tablet
Pain Reliever	Codeine (Schedule 2)	Codeine	Pain	Injectable, Tablet

Table 5 *cont.*
Drugs Associated with the Central and Peripheral Nervous System and Related Disorders

Drug Class(es)	Generic Name(s)**	Brand Name(s)**	Indication(s)	Available Dose Form(s)
Pain Reliever	Fentanyl (Schedule 2)	Actiq, Duragesic, Fentora, Onsolis, Sublimaze	Pain	Buccal Film, Buccal Tablet, Injectable, Lollipop, Patch
Pain Reliever	Hydrocodone / Acetaminophen (Schedule 3)	Hycet, Lortab, Norco, Vicodin	Pain	Elixir, Tablet
Pain Reliever	Hydromorphone (Schedule 2)	Dilaudid, Dilaudid-HP, Exalgo	Pain	Extended-Release Tablet, Injectable, Suppository Liquid, Tablet
Pain Reliever	Meperidine (Schedule 2)	Demerol, Meperitab	Pain	Injectable, Liquid, Tablet
Pain Reliever	Methadone (Schedule 2)	Dolophine, Methadone Diskets	Drug Addiction, Pain	Injectable, Liquid, Orally-Disentigrating Tablets, Solution (Concentrate), Tablet
Pain Reliever	Morphine (Schedule 2)	Astramorph, Avinza, DepoDur, Infumorph, Kadian, MSContin, MSIR, Oramorph, Roxanol	Pain	Extended-Release Capsule, Extended-Release Tablet, Injectable, Solution (Concentrate), Suppository, Tablet
Pain Reliever	Oxycodone (Schedule 2)	OxyContin, OxyIR, Roxicodone	Pain	Capsule, Extended-Release Tablet, Liquid, Solution (Concentrate), Tablet
Pain Reliever	Oxymorphone	Opana, Opana ER	Pain	Extended-Release Tablet, Injectable, Tablet
Pain Reliever	Tapentadol	Nucynta	Pain	Tablet
Pain Reliever	Tramadol	Rybix ODT, Ryzolt, Ultram, Ultram ER	Pain	Extended-Release Tablet, Orally-Disintegrating Tablet, Tablet

Drug Class(es)	Generic Name(s)**	Brand Name(s)**	Indication(s)	Available Dose Form(s)
Pain Reliever	Tramadol / Acetaminophen	Ultracet	Pain	Tablet
Pain Reliever, Fever Reducer	Acetaminophen	Tylenol	Fever, Osteoarthritis, Pain	Capsule, Chewable Tablet, Drops, Gel Cap, Gel Tab, Suppository, Tablet
Pain Reliever / Nonsteroidal Anti-Inflammatory Drug	Hydrocodone / Ibuprofen (Schedule 3)	Ibudone, Reprexain, Vicoprofen	Inflammation, Pain	Tablet
Pain Reliever / Nonsteroidal Anti-Inflammatory Drug	Oxycodone / Aspirin (Schedule 2)	Endodan, Percodan	Inflammation, Pain	Tablet
Pain Reliever / Nonsteroidal Anti-Inflammatory Drug	Oxycodone / Ibuprofen (Schedule 2)	Combunox	Inflammation, Pain	Tablet

**All rights to all brand names and trademarks are held by their respective owners. There may be additional brand names for some of the products listed.*

Conclusion

The nervous system interprets everyday stimuli through the brain and transduces this information to the body's organs for action. Neurons communicate with each other at synapses through chemicals known as neurotransmitters. Neurons in the central nervous system are found in the brain and spinal cord. All of the other neurons are located in the peripheral nervous system. The peripheral nervous system is broken down into the voluntary control of the somatic nervous system and the involuntary control of the autonomic nervous system. The autonomic nervous system is further broken down into the parasympathetic and sympathetic nervous systems. Medications targeted at the autonomic nervous system allow us to mitigate an abhorrent problem, such as emesis, by augmenting or decreasing the effect of the autonomic nervous system in the body. Common central nervous system disorders include pain, migraine headache disorder, multiple sclerosis, Parkinson's disease and epilepsy. These diseases affect many Americans and, while they are not generally curable, there are many pharmacologic and nonpharmacologic therapies to treat symptoms and slow the progression of these diseases.

Bibliography

- Bainbridge, J.L., Corboy, J.R., "Chapter 57, Multiple Sclerosis," Pharmacotherapy: A Pathophysiologic Approach, 7th edition, New York, NY, 2008.
- Barrett, K.E., Barman, S.M., Boitano, S., Brooks, H., "Chapter 17, The Autonomic Nervous System," Ganong's Review of Medical Physiology, 23rd edition, New York, NY, 2009.
- Baumann, T.J., "Chapter 62, Pain Management," Pharmacotherapy: A Pathophysiologic Approach, 7th edition, New York, NY, 2008.
- Chen, J.J., Nelson, M.V., Swope, D.M., "Chapter 61, Parkinson's Disease," Pharmacotherapy: A Pathophysiologic Approach, 7th edition, New York, NY, 2008.
- Elmhurst College, http://elmhurst.edu/~chm/vchembook/661nervoussys.html, Aug. 30, 2010.
- Lomen-Hoerth, C., Messing, R.O., "Chapter 7, Nervous System Disorders," Pathophysiology of Disease: An Introduction to Clinical Medicine, 6th edition, New York, NY, 2010.
- Minor, D.S., Wofford, M.R., "Chapter 63, Headache Disorders," Pharmacotherapy: A Pathophysiologic Approach, 7th edition, New York, NY, 2008.
- Rogers, S.J., Cavazos, J.E., "Chapter 58, Epilepsy," Pharmacotherapy: A Pathophysiologic Approach, 7th edition, New York, NY, 2008.
- Opioid Analgesic Converter, www.globalrph.com/narcoticonv.htm, Feb. 5, 2011.
- Natural Medicine's Comprehensive Database, http://naturaldatabase.therapeuticresearch.com, Feb. 5, 2011.

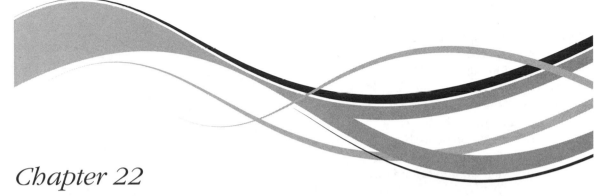

Chapter 22
REVIEW QUESTIONS

1. Sensory neurons are responsible for:
   a. outgoing transmissions from the central nervous system.
   b. incoming transmissions to the central nervous system.
   c. controlling motor neurons.
   d. None of the above

2. Which of the following does not comprise the autonomic nervous system?
   a. Somatic nervous system
   b. Parasympathetic nervous system
   c. Sympathetic nervous system
   d. None of the above

3. Atropine can be utilized in ophthalmic exams to dilate the pupils. Atropine works on muscarinic receptors to cause pupil dilation. Based upon its mechanism of action, atropine would best be classified as which of the following?
   a. Muscarinic agonist
   b. Antimuscarinic agent
   c. A beta blocker
   d. None of the above

4. Which of the following statements is false regarding chronic pain?
   a. Chronic pain has an obvious cause
   b. Chronic pain is nociceptive and/or neuropathic/functional in nature
   c. Chronic pain may be accompanied by other disorders (e.g., depression)
   d. Chronic pain continues even after the injury has healed

5. CJ is a 68-year-old man with chronic back pain. His doctor has prescribed oxycodone to help relieve his pain. Which of the following is true regarding oxycodone?
   a. This agent relieves pain through cyclooxygenase inhibition
   b. This agent may cause nausea, vomiting and/or constipation
   c. This agent is available as an oral tablet and as a transdermal patch
   d. This agent is not to be administered with an "as-needed" regimen

6. Which of the following would not be an appropriate agent for migraine preventative therapy?
   a. Propranolol
   b. Amitriptyline
   c. Almotriptan
   d. Topiramate

7. Which of the following is not a disease-modifying therapy for multiple sclerosis?
   a. Interferon beta-1a
   b. Interferon beta-1b
   c. Glatiramer
   d. Methylprednisolone

8. Which of the following is not a symptom of Parkinson's disease?
   a. "Freezing" at initiation of movements
   b. Generalized convulsions
   c. Microphagia
   d. "Pill-rolling" motion of the hands

9. Which of the following is not a class of medication used for the treatment of Parkinson's disease?
   a. Anticonvulsant
   b. COMT inhibitor
   c. Dopamine agonist
   d. MAO-B inhibitor

10. Which of the following is a common adverse effect of AEDs?
    a. Dry eyes
    b. Muscle rigidity
    c. Nausea/vomiting
    d. Sedation

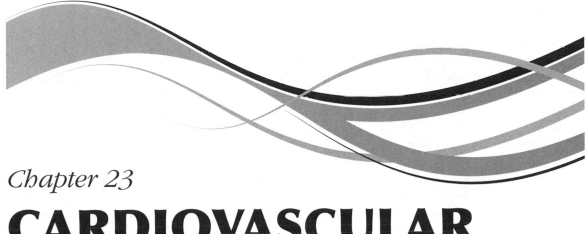

Chapter 23

CARDIOVASCULAR SYSTEM

By Douglas L. Jennings, Pharm.D., BCPS (AQ Cardiology)

Learning Objectives

This chapter seeks to prepare a pharmacy technician to:

- explain the basic purpose of the cardiac system.
- describe the structure of the heart and great vessels.
- discuss the normal function of the cardiovascular system.
- describe the electrophysiology of the heart.
- describe the significance of common diseases of the heart.
- list the brand/generic equivalents, indications, mechanism of action, adverse drug reactions and important drug interactions for the medications used to treat disorders of the cardiovascular system.

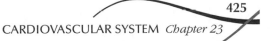

Introduction[1]

The **cardiovascular system** is comprised of the heart and the blood vessels. The **heart** is basically a pump that moves blood throughout the blood vessels of the body. By doing so, the cardiovascular system is able to provide all of the other systems of the body with fresh, oxygen-rich blood. Just as we are dependent on a highway system to move vital goods around the country, every organ and tissue in the body is dependent on the cardiovascular system for supply of nutrients and removal of waste products. For this reason, diseases of the cardiovascular system are particularly devastating, since every other organ is dependent upon the heart.

Cardiovascular disease (CVD) remains the No. 1 killer of Americans, accounting for more than one in three deaths in this country. In fact, since 1900, CVD has been the leading cause of death in America every year except 1918. With obesity rates on the rise annually, it is unlikely that deaths from CVD will significantly decrease in the near future. This is distressing given that obesity and other risk factors for CVD like high cholesterol are preventable and treatable conditions.

The focus of this chapter will be on the cardiovascular system. First, it will describe the basic function of the heart and blood vessels, and then it will explore each of the risk factors and treatments for common cardiovascular disorders in detail.

Anatomy and Physiology

The human heart has four chambers: two **atria** and two **ventricles**. The atria are the top chambers of the heart, and they receive blood from other parts of the body. The ventricles, which are much bigger and thicker than the atria, are the bottom chambers of the heart. The main role of the ventricles is to squeeze blood back out to the body through the great blood vessels (see Figure 1). In addition to the four chambers and all of the blood vessels, the heart also has four main valves. These valves open to allow blood to move between the chambers of the heart, and close to prevent the blood from flowing backward where it doesn't belong. The movement of blood through these chambers, valves and vessels occurs in a cyclic or repetitious fashion, and it is, therefore, called the **cardiac cycle**.

Figure 1
Anatomy of the Heart

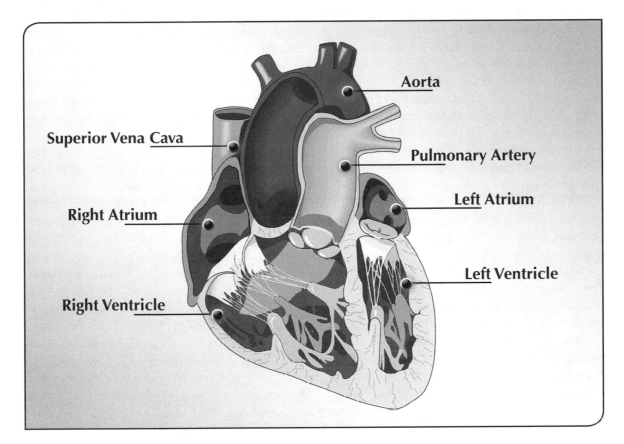

The cardiac cycle occurs through the stages of the heartbeat, which are called **diastole** and **systole**. Diastole is when the heart is relaxed, and the flow of blood is passive and due only to the force of gravity. Systole is when the heart muscle contracts (squeezes) and blood is being moved by the force of this contraction.

Before discussing the heart further, the **vasculature**, the blood vessels of the body, must briefly be discussed. The blood vessels that carry blood to the heart are called **veins**, while the blood vessels that carry blood away from the heart are called **arteries**. Generally, the pressure inside of arteries is much higher than it is in veins.

Back to the cardiac cycle, blood first enters the heart in the right atrium, arriving from two big veins called the **superior vena cava** and the **inferior vena cava**. The blood collects in the right atrium during diastole, and then travels down through the **tricuspid valve** into the right ventricle. From the right ventricle, the next move occurs during systole when this blood is pumped through the **pulmonary valve** and into the pulmonary artery and off to the lungs. In the lungs, the blood obtains fresh oxygen and expels waste products, like carbon dioxide, out into the atmosphere. After the lungs, the blood travels back to the heart through the pulmonary veins and arrives in the left atrium. The blood collects in the left atrium during diastole, and then moves into the left ventricle by passing through the **bicuspid valve**. In the left ventricle (which is the biggest and strongest chamber of the heart), the blood is pumped out of the heart through the **aortic valve** during systole. From the **aorta**, which is the body's largest artery, the blood flows out to every tissue in the body, eventually returning to the heart from either vena cava, ready to repeat the whole process again.

The cardiac cycle is a very complex process and requires a great deal of coordination. This coordination is achieved by the electrical system of the heart. The cardiac cycle begins when an electrical signal is released from the heart's pacemaker, which is called the **sinoatrial (SA) node**. The signal released by the SA node propagates throughout the heart like a wave, and this wave is what causes all of the muscles of the heart to contract in an organized and efficient manner. There are many other electrically active areas that help transmit the signal throughout the heart, such as the **atrioventricular (AV) node**. The electrical activity of the heart can be measured and visualized with a test called an **electrocardiogram (ECG)**, also still sometimes referred to as EKG from the German word elektrokardiogramm. The ECG can confirm that the heart is beating normally, or it can reveal abnormal heartbeats, which are called **dysrhythmias**. Dysrhythmias can be deadly; because, if the heartbeat isn't coordinated, then the flow of blood throughout the body is effectively halted.

The heart rate is the number of full cardiac cycles (systole and diastole) that occurs each minute. A normal heart rate is between 60 and 100 beats per minute (bpm). A heart rate of less than 60 bpm is called **bradycardia**, while a heart rate higher than 100 bpm is called **tachycardia**. It's important to point out that having a low or high heart rate doesn't necessarily indicate that a disease is present. For example, anyone who is performing intense exercise will be tachycardic. Abnormal heart rates are only bad if they are causing symptoms (e.g., a tachycardia that results in a patient feeling palpitations or lightheadedness).

The amount of blood that the heart pumps out with each heartbeat is called the **stroke volume**. The usual stroke volume is roughly half of the blood contained in the heart, or about 70 milliliters (just over two ounces). The **cardiac output**, which is a measure of the volume of blood that the heart delivers to the body in one minute, can be calculated by multiplying the stroke volume and the heart rate. The normal cardiac output is around four liters per minute, although it does vary somewhat depending on the size of the person. Cardiac output is a very good way to measure how effectively the heart is pumping blood to the rest of the tissues in the body (e.g., if the heart is failing and the cardiac output drops too low, then the body's energy needs will not be met and the patient will feel sick). One way in which cardiac output is described is with the **ejection fraction (EF)**. A normal EF is around 55 percent, while someone with a failing heart will have an EF of less than 40 percent.

While cardiac output is an accurate method for describing how well the heart is pumping, it is difficult to measure without advanced techniques. One easy way to get a sense of how the heart is working is **blood pressure (BP)**, which is a measure of the pressure that exists within the arteries. This pressure is actually composed of two separate forces: the force of the heartbeat against the blood vessels when the heart contracts **(systolic)**, and the force in the vessels during rest **(diastolic)**. These two forces together denote the blood pressure, with the systolic being represented over the diastolic (e.g., systolic/diastolic or 120/80 mmHg). The units of "mmHg" seen on a blood pressure reading refer to the millimeters of mercury (atomic symbol Hg) that can be measured on older BP monitors that use mercury in a glass tube to measure BP. If the BP is too low, like when the heart is failing or when someone is dehydrated, the organs of the body will not get enough blood and the person will feel sick. High BP, on the other hand, can be very dangerous, especially for a long period of time. Elevated BP can damage many organs and tissues, resulting in a wide array of different diseases like heart attack (i.e., myocardial infarction or M.I.) and stroke.

The **autonomic nervous system (ANS)**, consisting of the sympathetic and parasympathetic nervous systems, exerts a very strong effect on the cardiac system. The **sympathetic nervous system** raises blood pressure and heart rate in times of stress, while the **parasympathetic nervous system** lowers heart rate during periods of rest. For more information on the nervous system, see Chapter 22.

Hypertension[1-4]

Hypertension, or BP higher than 140/90 mmHg, is a very prevalent condition, affecting about 50 million Americans and approximately one billion people worldwide. The risk of developing hypertension increases with age, and data suggest that individuals who have normal blood pressure at age 55 have a 90 percent lifetime risk of developing high blood pressure. While getting older obviously cannot be avoided, there are many other risk factors for hypertension that people can modify. These include obesity, high salt intake, poor diet and lack of exercise. Patients with one or more of these risk factors may eventually develop hypertension; however, a small percentage of patients without any of these risk factors may develop high blood pressure. These patients may have an identifiable cause of their hypertension (e.g., sleep apnea, thyroid disease or endocrine problems). Certain medications, including some over-the-counter cold products, can also cause elevated blood pressure.

Over time, hypertension is an extremely dangerous disease because it can damage many different organs and tissues. Hypertension can damage the arteries around the heart and in the brain, which can lead to heart attacks and strokes. When the heart has to work against the elevated pressures in the blood vessels over a period of years, it can eventually weaken and begin to fail. Finally, hypertension can damage the eyes and the kidneys, leading to blindness and kidney failure. The one reason that hypertension is so dangerous is that most people will not have any symptoms until organ damage has already occurred. Because hypertension can do so much harm, and, is virtually without symptoms, it is often referred to as the "silent killer."

Patients can have various stages of hypertension, ranging from pre-hypertension to stage 2 hypertension. Generally, the higher the BP, the greater the risk of organ damage over time. The Seventh Report of the Joint National Committee on Prevention, Detection, Evaluation and Treatment of High Blood Pressure (JNC-7) provides a detailed classification of the various stages of hypertension (see Table 1). Extremely elevated BP (>180/110 mmHg) can be a life-threatening emergency and can lead to imminent heart attack, stroke, heart failure or kidney failure. This condition is called **hypertensive emergency** and requires hospitalization for acute control of BP.

Table 1
JNC-7 Classifications

Classification	Systolic BP (mmHg)	Diastolic BP (mmHg)
Normal	< 120	< 80
Prehypertension	120-139	80-89
Stage 1 Hypertension	140-159	90-99
Stage 2 Hypertension	> 160	> 100

Treatment of Hypertension[2-4]

Thankfully, most of the risk factors for hypertension are modifiable; so, patients are able to lower their BP by making healthy lifestyle decisions. Patients with hypertension should be instructed to attain and then maintain a healthy body weight, eat a diet rich in fruits and vegetables, restrict their salt intake, increase their physical activity and moderate their alcohol consumption. Smoking cessation is also important if the patient is a smoker. These changes to a patient's way of life can have a dramatic influence on his or her hypertension. For instance, a 10 kg (22 lb) weight loss can produce a 5 mmHg to 20 mmHg drop in BP. Restricting one's salt to a maximum of 1,600 mg per day, combined with a diet rich in fruits and vegetables, can be as effective as taking medication for lowering BP.

Unfortunately, most patients are unwilling or unable to make sufficient lifestyle modifications to reduce their BP to a safe range. When lifestyle modifications are insufficient to maintain a blood pressure less than 140/90 mmHg, drug therapy is recommended. There are many different classes of medications used to treat hypertension. **Diuretics**, or "water pills," work in the kidneys to alter reabsorption of water and electrolytes, which ultimately reduces blood volume and lowers blood pressure. There are actually three different sub-classes of diuretics, which are called the loop, thiazide and potassium-sparing diuretics (see Table 2). The thiazide diuretics are the preferred agents for treating hypertension, while the loop diuretics are used primarily to treat heart failure. The potassium-sparing diuretics are not usually used to treat the hypertension itself, rather they are used to reduce the likelihood of dangerously low serum potassium from loop or thiazide diuretics. Since diuretics work to lower BP, the main adverse drug reaction experienced by patients is low BP (**hypotension**). Some patients don't have any symptoms of low BP; others may report mild symptoms like dizziness or lightheadedness, or more severe symptoms like fainting. The other main side effect of diuretics is electrolyte deficiencies, such as low magnesium and low potassium (though usually not with the potassium-sparing diuretics). Patients may increase their dietary intake of these electrolytes to avoid deficiencies (bananas are a common source of potassium for patients taking a thiazide diuretic). Other, less common side effects of diuretics include increases in blood sugar, increases in uric acid (associated with gout) and kidney injury.

Two other closely related classes of medications used to treat hypertension are the **angiotensin converting enzyme (ACE) inhibitors** and the **angiotensin receptor blockers (ARB)**. Both of these classes of agents work to reduce the effects of a powerful **vasoconstrictor** called angiotensin II. By antagonizing angiotensin II, these agents can relax the blood vessels and reduce blood pressure. These medications are good choices for patients who have heart disease or heart failure. As with all BP medications, the main adverse drug reaction from these agents is hypotension. Other potential side effects for both agents include reduced kidney function; **hyperkalemia** (increased blood potassium); and swelling of the lips, mouth and tongue. In addition, ACE inhibitors can also produce a bothersome cough. Patients will often describe this cough as dry and persistent. Switching to an ARB will generally relieve the cough. It is very important to mention that neither ACE inhibitors nor ARB should be used in women who are pregnant or who could become pregnant, as they have the potential to cause serious birth defects. The available ACE inhibitors and ARB are listed in Table 2; note that the ACE inhibitors all end in "pril" and the ARB all end in "sartan."

There is a new class of BP medications, called the direct renin inhibitors, which works similarly to ACE inhibitors and ARB. Currently, only one direct renin inhibitor (aliskiren) is available on the market. As this medication is fairly new, it is not yet prescribed very often to treat hypertension.

Another class of medications used in the treatment of hypertension is the **calcium channel blocker (CCB)**. The muscles in the heart and around the blood vessels need calcium ions in order to contract; by blocking the influx of calcium ions, CCB can cause a relaxation of the heart muscles and the blood vessels. This results in a slower heart rate and a reduction in BP. There are actually two different sub-classes of CCB, the dihydropyridines and the nondihydropyridines. The dihydropyridines work mostly to lower BP, while the nondihydropyridines not only lower BP but also decrease the heart rate. As with the other antihypertensives, the main side effect of these medications is hypotension. Additional adverse drug reactions can include flushing, headache and swelling of the feet and ankles. The nondihydropyridines can also cause bradycardia and are generally not recommended for patients with heart failure. The CCB are listed in Table 2; notice that most of these medications end with "ipine."

Yet, another class of medications used to treat hypertension is the **beta receptor antagonists**, otherwise referred to as **beta blockers**. Beta receptors are part of the sympathetic nervous system, and the beta-receptors on the heart are responsible for making the heart beat faster and stronger. Although it is still not clear exactly how beta blockers lower BP, it is believed that they **antagonize** (interfere with) beta receptors on the heart, which leads to a reduction in heart rate and cardiac output. Since the beta blockers can lower BP, the main side effects are dizziness, lightheadedness and hypotension.

In addition, beta blockers can cause bradycardia, fatigue and a reduced ability to exercise. Because the sympathetic nervous system is involved in many body tissues, there are many other side effects that beta blockers can cause. Therefore, patients who have lung conditions (like asthma or emphysema), severe diabetes, peripheral vascular disease or depression should use beta blockers with caution. There can also be serious drug-interactions with beta blockers as a result of their ability to block beta-receptors anywhere in the body. An important drug interaction exists between the beta blockers and many medications used to treat asthma; since these medicines work to stimulate beta receptors in the lungs, administering a drug that blocks beta receptors can work to cancel out the effects of both drugs. It is important to note that some beta blockers are more likely to interfere with asthma medications (e.g., propranolol interferes more than metoprolol). There are many different beta blockers on the market; some important differences between these drugs include the frequency of administration, the affinity for different beta receptors and the route of elimination from the body (see Table 2). Notice that all of the beta blockers end in "lol."

Some drugs work to lower blood pressure by directly dilating (widening) the blood vessels (see Table 2). These medications are capable of producing rapid and significant reductions in blood pressure. To visualize how these drugs work, think of water passing through a narrow garden hose vs. a wide hose. The pressure in the narrow hose is much greater than that of the wide hose, and the same is true for constricted versus dilated blood vessels. Since these **vasodilators** are so powerful, they are usually used on an emergency basis for treating dangerously high blood pressure or on a long-term basis for patients who have failed to respond to other therapies. Vasodilators can produce tachycardia and swelling, which can be counteracted with beta blockers and diuretics. Special toxicities for these medications include cyanide poisoning for nitroprusside, drug-induced lupus for hydralazine and excessive hair growth for minoxidil.

All of the drugs discussed thus far for treating hypertension have worked on the heart or blood vessels. The site of action for the final class of antihypertensives is in the central nervous system (see Table 2). These centrally-acting agents decrease the activity of the sympathetic nervous system, which lowers blood pressure by producing vasodilation and bradycardia. These medications have many side effects, so they are generally reserved for patients who fail to adequately respond to other therapies. Drugs in this class can cause dizziness, drowsiness, dry mouth, fatigue and lack of concentration. In addition, patients who stop clonidine abruptly can have an acute spike in BP. This "rebound" effect can be so severe that patients have to be admitted to the hospital for intensive monitoring of BP. Patients should therefore always taper off clonidine slowly to avoid this dangerous effect.

The choice of which blood pressure medication to use for any given patient is complex. The side effects of each medication are unique, and the patient's wishes should be incorporated into the decision making process. The old recommendations were to start a diuretic or a beta blocker in most patients who didn't have other medical problems; however, newer recommendations advocate that most patients should receive an ACE inhibitor, a calcium channel blocker or a diuretic. For patients with stage 2 hypertension, two of these medications should be started at nearly the same time (leaving only a few days in between to ensure that an allergic reaction to one of the medications is not going to happen). As we will discuss in greater detail in the following sections, patients with heart failure or coronary artery disease require specific BP medications.

Table 2
Drugs Used to Treat Cardiac System Disorders

Drug Class(es)	Generic Name(s)**	Brand Name(s)**	Indication(s)	Available Dose Form(s)
ACE Inhibitors	Benazepril	Lotensin	ACS, Heart Failure, Hypertension	Tablet
ACE Inhibitors	Captopril	Capoten	ACS, Heart Failure, Hypertension	Tablet
ACE Inhibitors	Enalapril	Vasotec	ACS, Heart Failure, Hypertension	Tablet
ACE Inhibitors	Fosinopril	Monopril	ACS, Heart Failure, Hypertension	Tablet
ACE Inhibitors	Lisinopril	Prinivil, Zestril	ACS, Heart Failure, Hypertension	Tablet
ACE Inhibitors	Moexipril	Univasc	ACS, Heart Failure, Hypertension	Tablet
ACE Inhibitors	Perindopril	Aceon	ACS, Heart Failure, Hypertension	Tablet
ACE Inhibitors	Quinapril	Accupril	ACS, Heart Failure, Hypertension	Tablet
ACE Inhibitors	Ramipril	Altace	ACS, Heart Failure, Hypertension	Capsule
ACE Inhibitors	Trandolapril	Mavik	ACS, Heart Failure, Hypertension	Tablet
ADP Receptor Antagonist	Clopidogrel	Plavix	ACS	Tablet
ADP Receptor Antagonist	Prasugrel	Effient	ACS	Tablet
Anticoagulants	Bivalirudin	Angiomax	ACS	Injection
Anticoagulants	Dalteparin	Fragmin	ACS	Injection
Anticoagulants	Enoxaparin	Lovenox	ACS	Injection
Antidysrhythmic Drugs	Amiodarone	Cordarone, Pacerone	Dysrhythmias	Injection, Tablet
Antidysrhythmic Drugs	Disopyramide	Norpace	Dysrhythmias	Capsule, Extended-Release Capsule, Extended-Release Tablet
Antidysrhythmic Drugs	Dofetilide	Tikosyn	Dysrhythmias	Capsule
Antidysrhythmic Drugs	Dronedarone	Multaq	Dysrhythmias	Tablet

Drug Class(es)	Generic Name(s)**	Brand Name(s)**	Indication(s)	Available Dose Form(s)
Antidysrhythmic Drugs	Flecainide	Tambocor	Dysrhythmias	Tablet
Antidysrhythmic Drugs	Ibutilide	Corvert	Dysrhythmias	Injection
Antidysrhythmic Drugs	Lidocaine	Xylocaine	Dysrhythmias	Film-Forming Gel, Ointment, Other Noncardiac Formulations
Antidysrhythmic Drugs	Mexiletine	Mexitil	Dysrhythmias	Capsule
Antidysrhythmic Drugs	Procainamide	Procabid, Pronestyl	Dysrhythmias	Capsule, Extended-Release Tablet, Injection, Tablet
Antidysrhythmic Drugs	Propafenone	Rythmol, Rythmol SR	Dysrhythmias	Extended-Release Tablet, Tablet
Antidysrhythmic Drugs	Quinidine	Cardioquin, Quinaglute, Quinidex	Dysrhythmias	Extended-Release Tablet, Injection, Tablet
Antidysrhythmic Drugs	Sotalol	Betapace	Dysrhythmias	Tablet
ARB	Candesartan	Atacand	Heart Failure, Hypertension	Tablet
ARB	Eprosartan	Tevetan	Heart Failure, Hypertension	Tablet
ARB	Irbesartan	Avapro	Heart Failure, Hypertension	Tablet
ARB	Losartan	Cozaar	Heart Failure, Hypertension	Tablet
ARB	Olmesartan	Benicar	Heart Failure, Hypertension	Tablet
ARB	Telmisartan	Micardis	Heart Failure, Hypertension	Tablet
ARB	Valsartan	Diovan	Heart Failure, Hypertension	Tablet
Beta Blockers	Acebutolol	Sectral	ACS, Heart Failure, Hypertension	Capsule
Beta Blockers	Atenolol	Tenormin	ACS, Heart Failure, Hypertension	Tablet

Table 2 *cont.*
Drugs Used to Treat Cardiac System Disorders

Drug Class(es)	Generic Name(s)**	Brand Name(s)**	Indication(s)	Available Dose Form(s)
Beta Blockers	Betaxolol	Kerlone	ACS, Heart Failure, Hypertension	Tablet
Beta Blockers	Bisoprolol	Zebeta	ACS, Heart Failure, Hypertension	Tablet
Beta Blockers	Carteolol	Cartrol	ACS, Heart Failure, Hypertension	Tablet
Beta Blockers	Esmolol	Brevibloc	ACS, Heart Failure, Hypertension	Injection
Beta Blockers	Metoprolol	Lopressor, Toprol XL	ACS, Heart Failure, Hypertension	Extended-Release Tablet, Tablet
Beta Blockers	Nadolol	Corgard	ACS, Heart Failure, Hypertension	Tablet
Beta Blockers	Penbutolol	Levatol	ACS, Heart Failure, Hypertension	Tablet
Beta Blockers	Pindolol	Visken	ACS, Heart Failure, Hypertension	Tablet
Beta Blockers	Propranolol	Inderal	ACS, Heart Failure, Hypertension	Extended-Release Capsules, Oral Solution, Tablets
Beta Blockers	Timolol	Blocadren	ACS, Heart Failure, Hypertension	Tablet
Bile Acid Sequestrants	Cholestyramine	Questran	Hyperlipidemia	Oral Powder
Bile Acid Sequestrants	Colesevelam	WelChol	Hyperlipidemia	Tablet
Bile Acid Sequestrants	Colestipol	Colestid	Hyperlipidemia	Granules
Combined Alpha / Beta Blockers	Carvedilol	Coreg, Coreg CR	Hypertension	Extended-Release Capsule, Tablet
Combined Alpha / Beta Blockers	Labetalol	Normodyne, Trandate	Hypertension	Tablet
Dihyrdropyridine CCB	Amlodipine	Norvasc	Hypertension	Tablet
Dihyrdropyridine CCB	Felodipine	Plendil	Hypertension	Tablet
Dihyrdropyridine CCB	Isradipine	Dynacirc, Dynacirc CR	Hypertension	Capsule, Extended-Release Tablet
Dihyrdropyridine CCB	Nicardipine	Cardene	Hypertension	Capsule, Extended-Release Tablet

Drug Class(es)	Generic Name(s)**	Brand Name(s)**	Indication(s)	Available Dose Form(s)
Dihyrdropyridine CCB	Nifedipine	Adalat, Procardia	Hypertension	Capsule, Extended-Release Tablet
Dihyrdropyridine CCB	Nimodipine	Nimotop	Hypertension	Capsule
Dihyrdropyridine CCB	Nisoldipine	Sular	Hypertension	Extended-Release Tablet
Fibrates	Fenofibrate	Antara, Lofibra, Tricor	Hyperlipidemia	Capsule, Tablet
Fibrates	Gemfibrozil	Lopid	Hyperlipidemia	Tablet
Glycoprotein IIb/IIIa Receptor Antagonists	Abciximab	Reopro	ACS	Injection
Glycoprotein IIb/IIIa Receptor Antagonists	Eptifibatide	Integrilin	ACS	Injection
Glycoprotein IIb/IIIa Receptor Antagonists	Tirofiban	Aggrastat	ACS	Injection
Heparin	Heparin	Not Available	ACS	Injection
HMG-CoA Reductase Inhibitors (Statins)	Atorvastatin	Lipitor	ACS, Hyperlipidemia	Tablet
HMG-CoA Reductase Inhibitors (Statins)	Fluvastatin	Lescol, Lescol XL	ACS, Hyperlipidemia	Capsule, Extended-Release Tablet
HMG-CoA Reductase Inhibitors (Statins)	Lovastatin	Altoprev, Mevacor	ACS, Hyperlipidemia	Extended-Release Tablet, Tablet
HMG-CoA Reductase Inhibitors (Statins)	Pravastatin	Pravachol	ACS, Hyperlipidemia	Tablet
HMG-CoA Reductase Inhibitors (Statins)	Rosuvastatin	Crestor	ACS, Hyperlipidemia	Tablet
HMG-CoA Reductase Inhibitors (Statins)	Simvastatin	Zocor	ACS, Hyperlipidemia	Tablet
Loop Diuretics	Bumetanide	Bumex	Heart Failure, Hypertension	Injection, Tablet
Loop Diuretics	Ethacrynic Acid	Edecrin	Heart Failure, Hypertension	Injection, Oral Solution, Tablet

Table 2 *cont.*
Drugs Used to Treat Cardiac System Disorders

Drug Class(es)	Generic Name(s)**	Brand Name(s)**	Indication(s)	Available Dose Form(s)
Dihyrdropyridine CCB	Nifedipine	Adalat, Procardia	Hypertension	Capsule, Extended-Release Tablet
Dihyrdropyridine CCB	Nimodipine	Nimotop	Hypertension	Capsule
Dihyrdropyridine CCB	Nisoldipine	Sular	Hypertension	Extended-Release Tablet
Fibrates	Fenofibrate	Antara, Lofibra, Tricor	Hyperlipidemia	Capsule, Tablet
Fibrates	Gemfibrozil	Lopid	Hyperlipidemia	Tablet
Glycoprotein IIb/IIIa Receptor Antagonists	Abciximab	Reopro	ACS	Injection
Glycoprotein IIb/IIIa Receptor Antagonists	Eptifibatide	Integrilin	ACS	Injection
Glycoprotein IIb/IIIa Receptor Antagonists	Tirofiban	Aggrastat	ACS	Injection
Heparin	Heparin	Not Available	ACS	Injection
HMG-CoA Reductase Inhibitors (Statins)	Atorvastatin	Lipitor	ACS, Hyperlipidemia	Tablet
HMG-CoA Reductase Inhibitors (Statins)	Fluvastatin	Lescol, Lescol XL	ACS, Hyperlipidemia	Capsule, Extended-Release Tablet
HMG-CoA Reductase Inhibitors (Statins)	Lovastatin	Altoprev, Mevacor	ACS, Hyperlipidemia	Extended-Release Tablet, Tablet
HMG-CoA Reductase Inhibitors (Statins)	Pravastatin	Pravachol	ACS, Hyperlipidemia	Tablet
HMG-CoA Reductase Inhibitors (Statins)	Rosuvastatin	Crestor	ACS, Hyperlipidemia	Tablet
HMG-CoA Reductase Inhibitors (Statins)	Simvastatin	Zocor	ACS, Hyperlipidemia	Tablet
Loop Diuretics	Bumetanide	Bumex	Heart Failure, Hypertension	Injection, Tablet
Loop Diuretics	Ethacrynic Acid	Edecrin	Heart Failure, Hypertension	Injection, Oral Solution, Tablet

Drug Class(es)	Generic Name(s)**	Brand Name(s)**	Indication(s)	Available Dose Form(s)
Potassium-Sparing Diuretics	Amiloride	Midamor	Hypertension	Tablet
Potassium-Sparing Diuretics	Eplerenone	Inspra	Hypertension	Tablet
Potassium-Sparing Diuretics	Spironolactone	Aldactone	Hypertension	Tablet
Potassium-Sparing Diuretics	Triamterene	Dyrenium	Hypertension	Capsule, Tablet
Salicylate (NSAID)	Aspirin	Bayer, Ecotrin, St. Joseph's	ACS, CAD	Capsule, Chewable Tablet, Coated Tablet, Effervescent Tablet, Extended-Release Tablet, Gum, Suppository, Tablet
Thiazide and Thiazide-like Diuretics	Chlorothiazide	Diuril	Hypertension	Liquid, Tablet
Thiazide and Thiazide-like Diuretics	Chlorthalidone	Hygroton, Thalitone	Hypertension	Tablet
Thiazide and Thiazide-like Diuretics	Hydrochloro-thiazide	Esidrix, HydroDIURIL, Microzide, Oretic	Hypertension	Liquid, Tablet
Thiazide and Thiazide-like Diuretics	Indapamide	Lozol	Hypertension	Tablet
Thiazide and Thiazide-like Diuretics	Methyclothiazide	Enduron	Hypertension	Tablet
Thiazide and Thiazide-like Diuretics	Metolazone	Mykrox, Zaroxolyn	Hypertension	Tablet
Thrombolytics	Alteplase	Activase	ACS	Injection
Thrombolytics	Reteplase	Retavase	ACS	Injection
Thrombolytics	Streptokinase	Kabikinase	ACS	Injection
Thrombolytics	Tenecteplase	TNKase	ACS	Injection
Vasodilators	Hydralazine	Apresoline	Heart Failure, Hypertension	Injection, Oral Solution, Tablet

Table 2 *cont.*
Drugs Used to Treat Cardiac System Disorders

Drug Class(es)	Generic Name(s)**	Brand Name(s)**	Indication(s)	Available Dose Form(s)
Vasodilators	Minoxidil	Loniten	Heart Failure, Hypertension	Tablet
Vasodilators	Sodium Nitroprusside	Nitropress	Heart Failure, Hypertension	Injection

ACS=acute coronary syndrome, ADP=adenosine diphosphate, CAD=coronary artery disease, CCB=calcium channel blocker

**All rights to all brand names and trademarks are held by their respective owners. There may be additional brand names for some of the products listed.

Heart Failure[1,5]

Heart failure is an extremely expensive and devastating disease. Overall costs for the treatment of heart failure rose to almost $39 billion in the United States in 2010. More than 1.1 million people were hospitalized for heart failure in 2006, and nearly one in five people diagnosed with heart failure will die within one year. **Heart failure** is a condition in which the heart muscle is unable to pump effectively enough to meet the body's energy demands. This usually occurs as a result of damage to the muscle. Unfortunately, the most common causes of heart failure (i.e., heart attack and hypertension) are preventable. Other causes, like infections, pregnancy and valve disease, are largely unpreventable. Medications, like certain chemotherapy and illicit substances (i.e., heroin), can also damage the heart muscle and cause heart failure. Many times, the exact cause for a patient's heart failure is never determined.

Patients with heart failure will feel very fatigued as a result of the inability of their heart to adequately deliver blood to the rest of the body. Patients may also experience shortness of breath and swelling of the hands, feet, ankles and abdomen. This swelling, which is also called **edema**, is the result of fluid backing up into the body's tissue due to the failure of the heart to move it forward. The symptoms of heart failure can completely incapacitate a patient, leading to an inability to work or care for oneself, a reduced quality of life and repeated hospitalizations. Eventually, other organs (e.g., the kidneys) will start to fail as a result of the heart's inability to supply them with enough nutrients and oxygen.

Patients with heart failure either die slowly from progression of their disease or suddenly from a lethal dysrhythmia. In fact, heart failure patients are at a six to nine times higher risk of dying from sudden dysrhythmia than patients without heart failure. This high risk of death, combined with the debilitating symptoms, make heart failure a truly terrible disease.

Treatment of Heart Failure[5]

Once the heart muscle is damaged, it cannot be repaired with drug therapy. Cardiac transplant is the only way to cure a patient from heart failure; however, medications can be used to help relieve the symptoms of heart failure and prolong survival. Since patients with heart failure often accumulate fluid and develop edema, loop diuretics are often necessary to remove the excess fluid (see Table 2). These medications are essential for relieving the symptoms of shortness of breath and edema in patients with heart failure. Unfortunately, loop diuretics can injure the kidneys and, over time, patients may stop responding to these medications and re-accumulate fluid.

Beta blockers are very important medications for patients with heart failure. Beta blockers have been shown to reduce the risk of dying and alleviate some symptoms of the disease. This benefit is due to the ability of beta blockers to slow the heart rate and decrease the risk of life-threatening dysrhythmias. Unfortunately, beta blockers can make a patient's heart failure worse when the medication is first started, so patients must be watched closely when initiating or titrating these medications. All patients with heart failure should be on a beta blocker unless a contraindication is present.

Since the fundamental problem in patients with heart failure is a weak heart muscle, one of the main treatment goals for this disease is to reduce how hard the heart has to work. This can be accomplished by lowering BP with an ACE inhibitor, an ARB or a direct-acting vasodilator (see Table 2). Like the beta blockers, ACE inhibitors have been shown to improve survival and relieve symptoms in patients with heart failure. All patients with heart failure are recommended to be taking an ACE inhibitor unless a contraindication is present. Patients who experience a cough with an ACE inhibitor are recommended to be treated with an ARB. Patients who cannot tolerate either an ACE inhibitor or an ARB are recommended to be treated with the direct-acting vasodilator hydralazine (usually in combination with a nitrate-like isosorbide dinitrate).

In addition to diuretics, beta blockers and ACE inhibitors, patients with heart failure may be treated with digoxin (Lanoxin®), spironolactone or eplerenone. Digoxin is a very old medication that has been shown to improve symptoms and reduce hospitalizations in patients with heart failure. Digoxin, however, should be avoided in elderly patients or those with renal disease, as it can accumulate in these patients and cause potentially life-threatening toxicity. Also, unlike ACE inhibitors and beta blockers, digoxin does not reduce mortality in patients with heart failure. The potassium-sparing diuretics spironolactone and eplerenone have been shown to improve survival and relieve the symptoms of heart failure. These medications, like ACE inhibitors, can increase potassium levels in the blood and therefore must be used cautiously when combined with an ACE inhibitor.

Despite the use of drug therapy, heart failure is a progressive disease. Many patients experience flare ups or exacerbations of their disease; and, those near the end of their lives usually require the use of powerful intravenous medications to help sustain their heart function. Examples of these drugs include dobutamine (Dobutrex®), milrinone (Primacor®) and nesiritide (Natrecor®). It is important to note that these medications actually increase mortality, so they must only be used when no other options exist.

Because the number of donor hearts for transplantation is very small compared to the number of patients with heart failure, many people die each year waiting on the transplant list. One solution for these patients is a mechanical heart, otherwise known as a left-ventricular assist device. These devices are implanted inside of the patient's chest, and they can help bridge patients to a heart transplant. Because these devices are so new, very little is known about how to optimally manage the drug therapy of patients who receive them.

Hyperlipidemia[1,6]

Hyperlipidemia, or high cholesterol, affects approximately 37 million Americans. Like hypertension, hyperlipidemia is asymptomatic (without symptoms) and dangerous. There are several types of cholesterol in the blood. **Low density lipoprotein (LDL)** is often referred to as "bad" cholesterol, since high levels of LDL are associated with an increased risk of heart disease and stroke. **High density lipoprotein (HDL)**, on the other hand, is "good" cholesterol, as high HDL levels have been shown to be protective against heart disease. Triglycerides are also considered bad, since, like LDL, they raise the risk of heart disease when they are elevated. The blood test for cholesterol is called the **lipid panel**; it includes measuring at least the LDL, HDL and triglyceride levels in the blood. Patients have **dyslipidemia** when they have more than one type of cholesterol outside the normal ranges (e.g., if the patient's LDL is high and the patient's HDL is low). There are many factors that contribute to hyperlipidemia and dyslipidemia (e.g., poor diet, lack of exercise and genetic factors).

Treatment of Hyperlipidemia[5,6]

Lifestyle modification is the first step in the treatment of hyperlipidemia. Patients should be instructed to reduce their dietary intake of saturated fats and cholesterol, increase dietary intake of fiber, attain and maintain a healthy body weight, exercise and moderate alcohol intake (generally two drinks per day or less). Some patients are able to stick to these strict recommendations. Most patients, however, cannot adhere to such a strict regimen. Other patients may have a genetic or inherited cause for their hyperlipidemia, in which case, diet and exercise modifications will not be effective. In these cases, drug therapy is required.

The National Cholesterol Education Program Adult Treatment Panel III (ATP III) guidelines provide health care providers with recommendations for initiating drug therapy in patients with high cholesterol. Ultimately, how high a person's LDL has to be before drug therapy is determined by the patient's risk for cardiac disease. Patients are considered to be high risk if they have had a previous heart attack or stroke, if they have diabetes or if they have disease in the blood vessels in their legs or abdomen. Moderately high, moderate and low risk categories are determined by the patient's number of risk factors, which is used to calculate their 10-year risk of developing cardiac disease. Cardiac risk factors include smoking, having hypertension, having a family history of premature heart disease, increased age and having low HDL. Generally, a 10-year risk of greater than 20 percent is considered high risk, while a risk greater than 10 percent is considered moderate risk. The ATP III recommendations are summarized in Table 3.

Table 3
ATP III Guidelines[7]

Risk Category	LDL Goal (mg/dL)	Initiate TLC* (mg/dL)	Consider Drug Therapy (mg/dL)
High	< 100 (< 70 optional)	> 100	> 100
Moderately High	< 130	> 130	> 130
Moderate	< 130	> 130	> 160
Low	< 160	> 160	> 190

*TLC=therapeutic lifestyle changes

There are four main classes of medications used in the therapy of hyperlipidemia. The first, and most widely utilized, group of drugs is the **HMG-CoA reductase inhibitors**. These medications, otherwise referred to as **statins**, are the first line agents for treating most patients with hyperlipidemia. Statins work by blocking an essential step in the formation of cholesterol by the liver. While statins primarily reduce LDL, some patients may see some reduction in their triglycerides and a small increase in their HDL. In addition to their effect on cholesterol, statins have been shown to improve outcomes in a wide array of patients, and they are routinely used in patients with high cholesterol to prevent a first heart attack and, in patients with a previous heart attack, to prevent a second one. The reason statins are so beneficial is that they may also decrease the amount of inflammation in the arteries, which is believed to ultimately reduce the risk of heart disease.

Statins are very well-tolerated; the most frequent side effects of statin use include: mild nausea, headaches and abdominal pain. Some patients may complain of muscle pains after starting a statin. These pains are related to the dose of the medication, so decreasing the dose may help to relieve the symptoms. Some statins, like pravastatin, are less likely to cause muscle pains and can be used in patients who have failed to tolerate other statins. Most of the time, this muscle pain is harmless; however, in extremely rare cases, it could be a symptom of a potentially dangerous toxicity called rhabdomyolysis. **Rhabdomyolysis**, or breakdown of skeletal muscle, can cause death or significant kidney damage if not caught early. Patients taking statins should therefore be counseled to report any muscle pains or weakness to their physician or pharmacist. It is also very important for patients to tell their physician or pharmacist about all other medications that they are taking, including over-the-counter and herbal therapies, as drug interactions with statins are usually to blame for the development of rhabdomyolysis. Finally, statins can also cause liver irritation, so patients taking these medications should have their liver function monitored regularly with a simple blood test. The statins are listed in Table 2.

Another group of medications used to treat hyperlipidemia is the **fibrates**. The exact mechanism of how fibrates lower cholesterol is not fully known; it is thought that they alter the body's production, and elimination, of triglyceride-rich lipoproteins. Fibrates are very effective at lowering triglycerides and may produce a moderate increase in HDL; however, fibrates can increase LDL and therefore should not be used in patients whose primary problem is elevated LDL. Unlike the statins, fibrate agents have not been shown to reduce mortality in any studies, so they are generally considered to be second-line drugs. The main side effects of fibrates include headache, nausea, vomiting, diarrhea, abdominal pain and rash. Furthermore, the fibrates can also cause liver irritation and rhabdomyolysis; so, patients taking these drugs, especially with statins, should be closely monitored. The fibrates are also listed in Table 2.

In addition to the statins and fibrates, another class of medications used to treat hyperlipidemia is the **bile acid sequestrants** (see Table 2). These drugs take advantage of the body's requirement for bile to be present in order to manufacture cholesterol. By binding to bile in the intestines, and preventing its reabsorption, these medications force the body to use its cholesterol to replace its depleted bile stores, which ultimately lowers LDL. There are several drawbacks to bile acid sequestrants. They can cause significant nausea, bloating, constipation and flatulence (which many patients will not tolerate). Furthermore, they can raise triglycerides, which is undesirable for most patients. Finally, bile acid sequestrants interfere with the absorption of many other drugs; therefore, they must be dosed away from the patient's other medications. Newer bile acid sequestrants, like colesevelam, seem to have fewer side effects and drug interactions than other drugs in this class. Nevertheless, because of the side effects and potential drug interactions, these medications are not commonly used to treat hyperlipidemia.

Niacin, which is vitamin B_3, is very effective for treating hyperlipidemia. Niacin lowers LDL and triglycerides and raises HDL, which means that niacin is a very good choice for patients with dyslipidemia; however, adverse drug reactions from niacin often limit its use. Niacin produces intense flushing, and often itching, shortly after it is administered, which is very uncomfortable and can be embarrassing for the patient. Administration of aspirin, or another nonsteroidal anti-inflammatory drug (NSAID), such as ibuprofen, 30 minutes before the dose of niacin, or utilizing an extended-release dosage form, may reduce these unpleasant side effects. Other side effects of niacin include headache, stomach upset, liver irritation, elevated blood sugar and exacerbation of gout. Often, the occurrence of these side effects is related to the type of niacin being administered. Many different preparations are available and they all differ based on how fast they are absorbed. The immediate-release preparations cause more flushing, while the slow-release preparations cause more liver irritation. A newer prescription form of niacin named Niaspan® seems to be fairly well tolerated when compared to earlier preparations. While there seems to be a renewed interest in niacin lately, as evidenced by several new clinical trials, this agent will likely remain a second-line choice for managing hyperlipidemia due to its side effect profile.

One final medication used to treat hyperlipidemia is ezetimibe (Zetia®). Ezetimibe blocks the absorption of cholesterol from the intestines and it has been shown to be effective at lowering LDL when combined with statins. Ezetimibe is available in a combination product with simvastatin, which is called Vytorin®. Ezetimibe has a good safety profile, with many patients reporting only minimal adverse drug reactions; however, recent studies suggest that while ezetimibe is able to lower cholesterol, patients who take this drug do not have lower rates of heart attack or stroke. This evidence has called into question the value of ezetimibe, and many physicians are now reluctant to prescribe it to patients with hyperlipidemia unless other therapies are contraindicated.

Most of the new drug development with dyslipidemia has focused on therapies that will raise the HDL. One of these medications, torcetrapib, seemed promising based on early clinical trial data; however, eventually it was discovered that patients who received this medication had higher death rates than those who received placebo (sugar tablet). Development of this drug was subsequently terminated. Clinical trials of other drugs in this class are ongoing.

Coronary Artery Disease[1,8]

The heart, like any tissue in the body, requires a constant supply of oxygen-rich blood in order to stay alive. This blood supply comes from an intricate system of arteries called the **coronary arteries**. Disease of these arteries is called **coronary artery disease (CAD)**. CAD is very common in the United States, affecting more than 18 million people in 2006. CAD occurs as a result of the slow buildup of a plaque in the coronary arteries, which is called **atherosclerosis**. A **plaque** is made up of cholesterol and other blood components, and, as it grows, it has the potential to block the delivery of oxygen rich blood to the heart muscle. The process of atherosclerosis is very complex, and involves many factors like dyslipidemia and vascular inflammation. There are actually many different risk factors for developing CAD. Some of these risk factors are not modifiable, like age and a family history of cardiac disease. Others are modifiable, like smoking, dyslipidemia, hypertension, obesity and diabetes.

Ischemia occurs if this obstruction becomes significant enough to deprive the heart muscle of oxygen. When heart muscle is ischemic, the patient will usually develop symptoms, like chest pain, shortness of breath or dizziness. If heart muscle is deprived of oxygen for a long enough period of time, it will actually start to die. This death of heart muscle tissue is called **infarction**. Dead heart muscle will not grow back.

Stable angina (chest pain) occurs when a plaque in the coronary artery grows large enough to produce ischemia. This ischemia manifests as chest pain and discomfort during periods of exercise or exertion, and it usually requires a plaque big enough to obstruct more than 70 percent of the artery. The chest pain that occurs during stable angina is predictable and fairly consistent in nature. An acute change in the frequency or intensity of the chest pain that a patient experiences is called **unstable angina**. Unstable angina is often very hard to distinguish from a heart attack without blood tests or an ECG; so, patients who have a significant change in their chest pain must go to the hospital.

Heart attack, or **acute coronary syndrome (ACS)**, occurs when a plaque ruptures and causes a blood clot (thrombus) to form in the coronary artery. During an ACS, patients can experience chest pain, shortness of breath, dizziness, nausea, profuse sweating or palpitations. This blood clot can grow and further block the flow of blood, and it may even obstruct the entire artery. A complete obstruction of the coronary artery will result in death of heart muscle. When this happens, a patient will have an **acute myocardial infarction (AMI)**. Signs and symptoms of an AMI are usually more severe than ACS, and include severe, crushing chest pain; nausea and vomiting; sweating; dizziness; fainting; and a feeling of impending doom. An AMI is usually diagnosed with specific ECG findings and positive blood tests for certain enzymes. AMI is an acute, life-threatening condition, and patients who do not receive prompt treatment can die or become permanently disabled.

Treatment of Coronary Artery Disease[8]

CAD is a preventable condition, in most cases, by modifying risk factors that lead to the development of CAD and subsequent ACS. Examples of risk factor modification include: smoking cessation, weight loss and aggressive treatment of hypertension, high cholesterol and diabetes.

Regardless of the stage of the disease, all patients with CAD are recommended to receive several key medications. For instance, all patients with CAD are recommended to take 75-325 mg of aspirin every day. Aspirin has been shown to reduce the risk of having another AMI.

All patients with CAD should also carry sublingual nitroglycerin with them at all times (either as tablets or as a spray). Nitroglycerin works to dilate the coronary arteries, which improves the supply of blood to the heart muscles. This medication is used to relieve chest pain in patients with stable angina, as well as in patients experiencing an ACS. Patients are instructed to place one tablet or one spray under the tongue every five minutes for a total of three doses or until their chest pain resolves. If the pain fails to resolve within five minutes after the first dose, patients should seek emergency attention and continue to take the second and third doses with five minutes in between each dose. Intravenous nitroglycerin is also used to relieve chest pain in patients experiencing ACS. Oral and transdermal forms of nitroglycerin are used to prevent chest pain in patients with CAD. The various forms of nitroglycerin are listed in Table 2.

Patients experiencing an ACS are at a much greater risk of dying or developing a lethal dysrhythmia, or heart failure, than those patients with stable CAD. Because of this increased risk, ACS patients are treated aggressively with powerful intravenous medications and invasive procedures. These patients should receive nitroglycerin and morphine (if necessary) to relieve their chest pain. In addition, multiple blood thinners are often given to reduce the formation of blood clots since blood clots are the main underlying problem in ACS. Examples of these medications include aspirin, clopidogrel, heparin, low-molecular weight heparins and glycoprotein IIb/IIIa receptor antagonists. In AMI, these medications will not be strong enough to open a completely blocked artery. Most patients experiencing an AMI will go for cardiac catheterization where the blocked artery will be manually opened up by a small balloon that is floated into the coronary artery (usually by going through a blood vessel in the arm or leg). Patients may also receive a "clot buster" medication to open the blocked artery. These drugs, called **thrombolytics**, are specially designed to dissolve the clot and reopen the artery. These medications are not used in most major U.S. hospitals due to a high risk of bleeding and the proven superiority of invasive procedures. The blood thinners and thrombolytics that are used for ACS and AMI are listed in Table 2.

After an ACS or AMI, patients are at an increased risk of dying or experiencing a subsequent heart attack. Aspirin, beta blockers, ACE inhibitors and statins have all been shown to improve survival and reduce the risk of a second ACS in these patients.

Dysrhythmias

Dysrhythmias are disorganized or abnormal heart rhythms. Common causes of dysrhythmias include hypertension, ACS and heart failure. Dysrhythmias are diagnosed by electrocardiography. There are many different kinds of dysrhythmias, and any of the chambers of the heart can be affected. Some dysrhythmias only reduce the ability of the heart to pump blood to the body (e.g., atrial fibrillation and supraventricular tachycardia). These dysrhythmias are not acutely life threatening, but they can make patients feel dizziness or palpitations. Atrial fibrillation also greatly increases a patient's risk of stroke. Other abnormal rhythms, like ventricular tachycardia or ventricular fibrillation, can completely stop the pumping of the heart. These dysrhythmias are medical emergencies that are often fatal without immediate medical attention.

Treatment of Dysrhythmias

Antidysrhythmic medications can be used to bring a patient out of an abnormal heart rhythm (cardioversion) or they can be used to maintain a patient in a normal rhythm who is at risk of reverting back into an abnormal rhythm. These medications can produce many adverse drug reactions, the most threatening being the development of new or more serious dysrhythmias. Because of these dangerous side effects, antidysrhythmic medications should only be used when the benefit outweighs the risk of treatment. Antidysrhythmic medications are classified according to how they affect the electrical activity of the heart. These drugs are listed in Table 2.

Conclusion

With the projected increase in incidence of cardiovascular disease in the United States, the pharmacy technician will encounter many patients with heart disease and other cardiovascular system disorders. Its important for technicians to familiarize themselves with the cardiovascular system, the diseases and disorders affecting the system, and the medications used for treatment that are being dispensed from the pharmacy to comprehend how medications will affect functions of the heart.

References

1. American Heart Association, www.americanheart.org, July 13, 2010.
2. Chobanian, A.V., Bakris, G.L., Black, H.R. et. al., "The Seventh Report of the Joint National Committee on Prevention, Detection, Evaluation, and Treatment of High Blood Pressure," *Journal of the American Medical Association*, Vol. 289, No. 19, pp. 2560-2572, 2003.
3. The National Institute for Clinical Excellence, "Hypertension: Management in adults in primary care: pharmacological update," www.nice.org.uk, July 13, 2010.
4. Straka, R.J., Burkhardt, R.T., Parra, D. "Hypertension," *Pharmacotherapy: A Pathophysiologic Approach*, 6th edition, New York, NY, 2008, pp. 9-31.
5. Hunt, S.A., Baker, D.W., Chin, M.H. et al., "ACC/AHA Guidelines for the Evaluation and Management of Chronic Heart Failure in the Adult," www.acc.org.
6. Ito, M.K. "Hyperlipidemia," *Pharmacotherapy: A Pathophysiologic Approach*, 6th edition, New York, NY, 2008, pp. 175-193.
7. Grundy, S.M., Cleeman, J.I., Bairey Merz, C.N. et. al., "Implications of Recent Clinical Trials for the National Cholesterol Education Program Adult Treatment Panel III Guidelines," *Circulation*, Vol. 110, pp. 227-239, 2004.
8. Spinler, S.A., de Denus, S., "Acute Coronary Syndromes," *Pharmacotherapy: A Pathophysiologic Approach*, 6th edition, New York, NY, 2008, pp. 83-105.

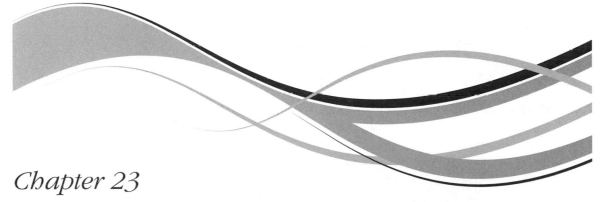

Chapter 23

REVIEW QUESTIONS

1. What is the strongest chamber of the heart that is responsible for pushing the blood out to the body?
    a. Right atrium
    b. Left atrium
    c. Left ventricle
    d. Right ventricle

2. What is the main purpose of the heart valves?
    a. Push blood forward
    b. Prevent blood from flowing backward in the heart
    c. Trigger the heartbeats
    d. Slow the heart rate

3. Tachycardia is defined as:
    a. a heart rate greater than 100 beats per minute.
    b. a heart rate less than 60 beats per minute.
    c. a cardiac output less than four liters per minute.
    d. a blood pressure less than 120/80 mmHg.

4. ACE inhibitors usually end in:
    a. "lol."
    b. "pril."
    c. "pine."
    d. "sartan."

5. The main, often limiting, side effect of niacin is:
    a. muscle pain.
    b. flushing.
    c. cough.
    d. depression.

6. Which of the following is a calcium channel blocker?
   a. Zestril®
   b. Lopressor®
   c. Norvasc®
   d. Zocor®

7. Which of the following drugs would be a good first choice for treating hypertension?
   a. Enalapril
   b. Clonidine
   c. Hydralazine
   d. Terazosin

8. Which of the following drugs should be used in a patient with ACS?
   a. Heparin
   b. Aspirin
   c. Clopidogrel®
   d. All of the above

9. What is the generic name of Lopressor®?
   a. Lisinopril
   b. Metoprolol
   c. Carvedilol
   d. Hydrochlorothiazide

10. Which of the following is a drug used to treat irregular heart rhythms?
    a. Dofetilide
    b. Clopidogrel
    c. Simvastatin
    d. Isosorbide dinitrate

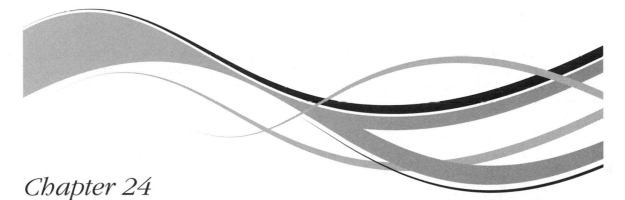

Chapter 24

UPPER RESPIRATORY SYSTEM

By Stephanie L. Freed, Pharm.D.
Jennifer K. Hagerman, Pharm.D., AE-C

Learning Objectives

This chapter seeks to prepare a pharmacy technician to:

- explain the anatomy and function of the upper respiratory tract.
- discuss the symptoms, common causes and appropriate treatment of the common cold, rhinitis, pharyngitis and sinusitis.
- describe the mechanism of action, uses and adverse effects of the following medication classes: antihistamines, antitussives, decongestants, expectorants, leukotriene receptor blockers, mast cell stabilizers and nasal corticosteroids.

Introduction

The upper respiratory tract is comprised of structures that work together to filter, warm and humidify air during inhalation (see Figure 1).[1] When air is inhaled through the nostrils, it travels to the nasal cavity, where it collides with the **turbinates**.[2] The turbinates create a turbulent air flow within the nasal cavity allowing particles (i.e., dust, pollen, bacteria or viruses) to stick to mucus within the sinuses.[2,3] **Sinuses** are air-filled spaces located throughout the skull that work together to perform three main functions: insulate the skull, decrease the weight of the skull and resonate the sound of a person's voice.[4] There are four main sinus systems: frontal, maxillary, ethmoid and sphenoid; infection or inflammation of these is known as **sinusitis**.[4] After colliding with the tubinates, air travels to the pharynx (throat). The **pharynx** is a tube-like structure that connects the upper respiratory cavities to the larynx (voicebox).[1] Located within the pharynx, adenoids and tonsils help protect against respiratory infections by releasing immune cells.[1] Lastly, before reaching the lower respiratory tract, air travels through the **larynx,** a tube-like structure that connects to the lungs. The upper respiratory tract also contains tiny hair-like structures called **cilia** that are constantly moving mucus down the tract for eventual removal by the gastrointestinal system.[2,5]

[handwritten: Untreated Cold]

[handwritten: An inflammation of mucous membranes of the sinuses and nose]

Figure 1
Upper Respiratory Tract

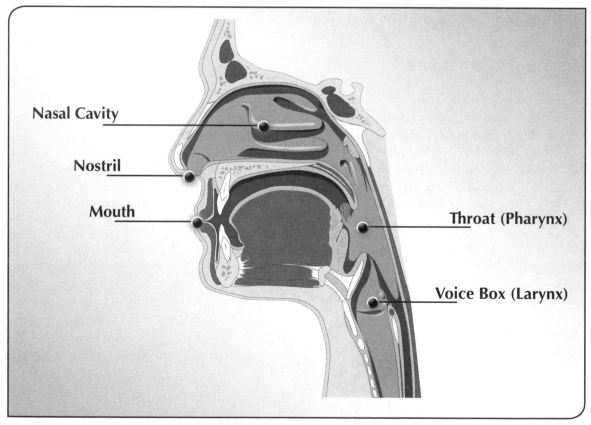

Disorders of the Upper Respiratory Tract

Infections of the upper respiratory tract are extremely common and a leading cause of missed days of school and work. These disorders are also one of the most frequent reasons why patients visit their primary care provider or seek over-the-counter products (OTC) for relief of related symptoms.[6] In a 2007 survey, almost a third of responding pharmacists said that they counseled 16-22 patients per week on various cough and cold products.[6] This chapter will cover the presentation of and therapy used for the management of the common cold, rhinitis, pharyngitis and sinusitis.

Common Cold

The "common cold" is a viral illness. More than 200 viruses can cause cold symptoms, but the most common cause (implicated in up to half of all cases) is the rhinovirus.[7] Although the common cold can affect persons of all ages, infants and young children are disproportionately affected. On average, young children are affected with six to eight colds per year compared to two to four per year in adults.[7,8] The common cold can occur throughout the year, with peak incidence in the fall and winter months. Initial symptoms of a cold commonly include sore throat (**pharyngitis**), **malaise** (a feeling of tiredness, weakness or fatigue) and a low-grade fever. These symptoms are often followed by **rhinorrhea** (runny nose), congestion of the nose and cough.[8] Peak symptoms usually occur three to four days after the onset of symptoms, and symptoms typically subside around day seven.[8] The virus causing the common cold can be spread via direct contact with infected secretions or via inhalation of infected particles. Infected patients are strongly encouraged to cover coughs and sneezes, and to wash their hands or use hand sanitizers frequently to decrease transmission of the offending virus.

There are no available medications to cure the common cold. As a result, when treatment is utilized, it is aimed at symptomatic relief. Numerous OTC products, including decongestants, antihistamines, cough suppressants and expectorants, have been utilized for management of cold symptoms. In infants and children under two years of age, the Food and Drug Administration (FDA) recommends against the use of OTC cough and cold products, citing a lack of benefit and the risk of potentially dangerous adverse effects.[9] The FDA is currently reviewing the data for use of these products in children two to 11 years of age. In infants and young children, nonpharmacological methods, such as intake of adequate fluids, saline nasal drops, gentle suction of mucus from the nose with a bulb syringe and use of humidified air, can be utilized in an effort to decrease symptoms.[8,10] **Antipyretics**, such as acetaminophen and ibuprofen, can be utilized by those older than six months if a fever is present.[10] Aspirin may not be given to children due to the risk of a rare, but serious, disease called Reye's syndrome. Parents must follow the instructions that accompany medications and not exceed the maximum recommended dose.

Oral or nasal-administered decongestants, either alone or in combination with an antihistamine, may provide some relief of nasal obstruction.[8] First-generation antihistamines, such as diphenhydramine, may decrease rhinorrhea. Second-generation antihistamines, however, have not been shown in clinical studies to effectively treat common cold symptoms. Due to the cold being a viral illness, antibiotics have no effect on decreasing cold symptom severity or duration and must not be used for this indication when bacterial complications are absent. When used inappropriately, antibiotics can cause adverse effects and increase the risk of bacterial resistance. Numerous complementary therapies, such as echinacea, vitamin C and zinc, have been marketed to alleviate symptoms related to the common cold; however, scientific evidence that these therapies provide significant benefit is lacking.[8]

Rhinitis

Rhinitis is defined as inflammation of the mucous membranes of the nose. Rhinitis can be characterized as allergic or nonallergic.[11] It is estimated that nearly 40 million Americans are afflicted with allergic rhinitis.[3] In comparison, approximately 17 million Americans are afflicted with nonallergic rhinitis.[3] Many types of non-allergic rhinitis exist, including infectious, drug-induced or vasomotor rhinitis.[11] Rhinitis encompasses a constellation of symptoms including: runny or itchy nose, sneezing, nasal congestion, and itchy or watery eyes. In **allergic rhinitis**, symptoms are triggered by a host's

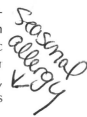

exposure to airborne allergens, such as dust, pollen or mold.[2] The body responds to the allergen-releasing chemicals, such as histamine, that leads to inflammation and mucus production. Patients with allergic rhinitis may suffer from seasonal or **perennial** symptoms. Seasonal allergic rhinitis may also be referred to as hay fever. A complete patient history can help differentiate between the types of rhinitis.[11] A proper history focuses on symptom type, timing and duration, triggers, medical history and family history.

Patients suffering from allergic rhinitis must limit allergen exposure. This can be done through avoidance and environmental control measures. Several classes of medications are utilized for management of the symptoms of allergic rhinitis. Patient factors, such as age, cause of rhinitis and description of symptoms, must be taken into consideration when a therapy is selected. Antihistamines are often utilized first in the management of allergic rhinitis and can relieve nasal symptoms such as runny or itchy nose and sneezing; however, they are ineffective for relieving nasal congestion. Second-generation antihistamines are preferred over first-generation antihistamines due to a lower risk of sedation. Oral or topical decongestants can be utilized in combination with an antihistamine, if needed, to reduce nasal congestion (alone they are ineffective for treatment of other symptoms related to allergic rhinitis). It is important to note that the use of topical decongestants must be limited to a maximum of three consecutive days to prevent **rebound congestion** from occurring. Intra-nasal corticosteroids, available only with a prescription, are the most effective therapy for allergic and nonallergic rhinitis.[3,12] Corticosteroids are effective at suppressing key symptoms of allergic rhinitis, including runny or itchy nose, sneezing and nasal congestion. Intra-nasal cromolyn, oral montelukast or inhaled ipratropium can also work on facets of allergic rhinitis symptoms, but these options are less effective then intra-nasal corticosteroids.[3,12] In select cases of allergic rhinitis, immunotherapy may also be utilized.[2]

Pharyngitis

A sore throat can occur secondary to inflammation of the pharynx (pharyngitis). Common causes for pharyngitis include infection by a virus (such as the viruses that causes the common cold, influenza or infectious mononucleosis) or infection by a bacteria.[13] Other noninfectious conditions, such as allergies or irritants, may also cause a sore throat. A patient's history, a physical exam and a rapid diagnostic test or throat culture may help differentiate between the types of pharyngitis. A frequent cause of bacterial pharyngitis is group A streptococci; this type of pharyngitis is commonly referred to as strep throat.[14] A typical presentation of strep throat includes a sudden onset of sore throat and pain upon swallowing. Additional symptoms may include fever, redness and swelling of the throat, swollen lymph nodes (small glands of the lymphatic system that help fight infection) in the neck and fluid from the tonsils.[14] Cough is generally absent with pharyngitis not accompanied by a secondary infection (such as a cold or influenza). Antibiotics can be utilized to shorten the time that a patient is contagious, decrease the presence of symptoms by approximately one day and reduce the likelihood that complications from the infection will occur.[13] When treating strep throat, penicillin is the antibiotic of choice (e.g., oral penicillin or a one-time intramuscular injection). Alternative antibiotics may include other penicillins, such as amoxicillin, a cephalosporin or erythromycin.[14] Factors such as medication allergies, patient age, regimen convenience and tolerability must be taken into consideration when a medication is selected. Patients must be instructed to complete the full course of the prescribed antibiotic, even if symptoms improve, to prevent a relapse and bacterial resistance.

If the etiology of the sore throat is viral, patients may also complain of **conjunctivitis**, fatigue or a low-grade fever.[13] Viral pharyngitis is typically self-limiting. Antibiotics are not effective for a sore throat caused by a virus and must not be prescribed in this case. OTC medications, such as acetaminophen and ibuprofen, may be utilized to decrease pain associated with pharyngitis.[15] Various topical analgesics (e.g., throat spray and lozenges) are also marketed to help alleviate sore throat pain. It must be noted, however, that throat lozenges must not be utilized in young children due to the risk of choking. Non-pharmacological measures such as rest, adequate fluid intake or gargling with warm salt water may help ease symptoms.[15]

Sinusitis

Sinusitis is described as inflammation of the mucous membranes of the sinuses surrounding the nasal cavity.[5,15] It may also be referred to as **rhinosinusitis** due to the frequency of coexisting rhinitis. Rhinosinusitus is classified as acute when symptoms last for less than four weeks.[5] Symptoms commonly include nasal congestion, post-nasal drip and facial pain or pressure (the location of the pain may vary depending on which sinus is involved). Additional symptoms may include a sore throat, cough, a headache or fatigue. Causes of sinus inflammation may include infection (viral or bacterial), allergies or other irritants. It is common for sinusitis to occur following a cold or other viral upper respiratory tract infection. It is important for a physician to attempt to differentiate between the kinds of sinusitis to prevent unnecessary utilization of antibiotics; approximately 65 percent of patients with acute sinusitis will get better without therapy.[15] If symptoms are severe or persist for longer than seven days, bacteria may be the cause of the sinusitis, and antibiotics may be prescribed.[5,15] A number of antibiotics may be utilized to treat bacterial sinusitis. Amoxicillin is commonly utilized first for uncomplicated cases of bacterial sinusitis. Other antimicrobial options include trimethoprim-sulfamethoxazole, doxycycline, azithromycin, clarithromycin and an oral cephalosporin. Supportive therapy can also be utilized to reduce the severity of symptoms. Oral or nasal decongestants, or a nasal saline wash, can lessen nasal congestion. In patients with a history of allergies, nasal corticosteroids may also be utilized.[5,15] Chronic sinusitis is defined as symptoms lasting for more than 12 weeks and can be difficult to treat.[5] Patients with chronic bacterial sinusitis may need three to four weeks of treatment with antibiotics. Administration of intranasal corticosteroids, or saline nasal wash, may also be utilized to reduce symptoms. In select cases, sinus surgery may be required.

Cough and Cold Preparation Use in Children

From 2004-2005, it was reported that more than 1,500 emergency room visits resulted from adverse effects (including overdoses) of cough and cold products in children less than two years of age.[16] Adverse effects from overdose include mental status changes, increases in blood pressure, changes in heart rate, changes in respiratory rate, lethargy and death.[17] As a result of growing safety concerns, and lack of data supporting efficacy in this patient population, the FDA, through a 2007 public advisory committee, recommended against the use of OTC cough and cold preparations for children under two years of age.[9] Subsequently, drug manufacturers voluntarily withdrew more than 20 cough and cold products that were labeled with directions specifically for this young population.[10] The FDA is investigating the use of cough and cold medications in children ages two to 11 years of age. For symptomatic relief of cough and cold symptoms in children less than two years of age, the FDA advises that health care professionals may recommend nonpharmacological interventions, such as using a humidifier or vaporizer, instilling saline nasal drops, the removal of nasal mucus with a bulb syringe and fluid hydration.[10,18]

Local and Systemic Antihistamines

Histamine is a compound that is widely distributed throughout the human body; it is stored inside immune cells known as basophils and mast cells.[19] When an **allergen** is introduced into a body, these immune cells release histamine that leads to an allergic response. There are four types of receptors that histamine binds to; however, histamine type-1 receptors (H_1) are most commonly involved with allergic reactions.[19] Within two minutes after histamine's release, capillary permeability, contraction of bronchial and vascular smooth muscle and hypersecretion of mucous can occur.[2] To prevent or lessen existing symptoms, antihistamines can be used to block histamine from binding to the body's H_1 receptors.[19] For the prevention of allergies, patients may administer antihistamines one to two hours before being exposed to a known allergen.[2] Local (intranasal sprays) and systemic (oral) antihistamine formulations are currently available (see Tables 1 and 2). Antihistamines are further classified into two categories: first generation (nonselective) and second-generation (selective). First-generation antihistamines (e.g., diphenhydramine) act on both central and peripheral H_1-receptors; second-generation antihistamines (e.g., loratidine) only exert their effects on peripheral H_1-receptors. Thus, the second-generation antihistamines cause less sedation and anticholinergic effects as these effects are mediated by the central nervous system. Other than sedation, antihistamines tend to be well-tolerated. Additional side effects include nausea, vomiting and weight loss. If tolerance occurs with one antihistamine, it is appropriate to recommend the use of another.[2]

Leukotriene Receptor Blockers

Leukotrienes are stored and released from basophils and eosinophils. In contrast to histamine, leukotrienes have a longer duration of action and a slower onset of action.[2] Leukotrienes play a major role in allergic rhinitis because they increase inflammation and bronchoconstriction within the respiratory tract.[2] Of the available leukotriene receptor blockers, also called leukotriene modifiers, only montelukast is approved for allergic rhinitis. Montelukast helps relieve sneezing, congestion and a runny nose by binding to leukotriene receptors and inhibiting the effects of leukotrienes.[20] Montelukast is available in three different formulations: tablets, chewable tablets and granules. The granules are approved for use in children as young as six months of age and can be placed directly into the mouth, dissolved in a teaspoon of baby formula or breast milk, or mixed into a selected number of food items. When used for allergic rhinitis, patients must be instructed to take montelukast on a daily basis, even on asymptomatic days. Montelukast is generally well-tolerated; side effects include gastrointestinal upset, cough, headache and tiredness.[20]

Systemic and Local Decongestants

Nasal congestion occurs when the nasal mucosa becomes swollen and the local vasculature becomes dilated. Decongestants, such as pseudoephedrine, are **sympathomimetics** that act on receptors to cause constriction within blood vessels. Due to the vasoconstrictor effect of the decongestants, it is advised to use these medications with caution in patients with cardiovascular problems, such as coronary artery disease, peripheral vascular disease or hypertension.[20] Decongestants are currently available for oral and intranasal administration. Orally-administered decongestants tend to last longer and cause less irritation to the nasal mucosa. In contrast to oral decongestants, topical formulations work more quickly to relieve nasal congestion; however, if nasal decongestants are utilized for more than three consecutive days, patients may develop rebound congestion. Options to treat rebound congestion include slow withdrawal of the topical decongestant or use of an oral decongestant until the nasal mucosa is relieved. Adverse effects of decongestants may include increased heart rate, insomnia, nervousness and dizziness. Topical decongestants may also cause stinging in the nose and sneezing.[20]

Pseudoephedrine Laws

Recently, an increase in the number of home laboratories used to make methamphetamine (an addicting stimulant drug) have been found and seized. In a 2009 survey, the number of new users greater than or equal to 12 years of age rose by 62 percent.[21] One major ingredient used to prepare methamphetamine illegally is pseudoephedrine, or its close relative ephedrine. In an attempt to reduce the illegal manufacturing of methamphetamine, most states, as well as the federal government, have restricted sales of OTC pseudoephedrine and ephedrine.[22] Any products containing either of these two chemicals must now be kept either behind a counter or in a locked case. Although state laws may be more strict, the federal law states that no more than 3.6 g may be sold in a single purchase, and no more than 9 g may be sold within a 30-day period to any one person. In addition, the person making the purchase must be at least 18 years of age, have appropriate government-issued identification and sign a logbook.[21,22] This signature logbook must be available for law enforcement to review upon request.[21] In April 2011, the federal Combat Methamphetamine Enhancement Act of 2010 went into effect.[21] This new act mandates all retailers to use the National Association of Drug Diversion Investigator's (NADDI) electronic database . The National Precursor Log Exchange (NPLEx) database will allow the federal government to meticulously monitor pseudoephedrine sales beginning Jan. 1, 2012.[23] If a purchaser attempts to obtain an additional amount of pseudoephedrine than allowed by law, a stop alert will appear; this alert will allow the retailer to immediately terminate the sale.[23] There are many more requirements in the federal statute; and with each state having additional pseudoephedrine laws, a pharmacy technician would do well to investigate the rules in his or her state and read the federal law on pseudoephedrine before entering a pharmacy for the first time.

Mast Cell Stabilizers

Mast cell stabilizers prevent histamine from being released into the body by stabilizing mast cell membranes. Current mast cell stabilizers available for allergic rhinitis include cromolyn nasal spray and nedocromil eye drops.[20] The inhaled mast cell stabilizer works by relieving the symptoms of allergic rhinitis. When using cromolyn nasal spray, patients begin therapy one week prior to allergen exposure. Before each use, patients blow their nose to ensure proper application. It is notable that it may take up to two weeks to see an effect from cromolyn nasal spray. Similar to topical decongestants, topical mast cell stabilizers may cause stinging and sneezing.[20] Nedocromil eye drops, if used properly, may prevent allergic conjunctivitis. It is recommended to use one or two drops in each eye twice daily throughout the patient's allergy season.[20] Forty percent of patients using the ophthalmic drops reported a headache with other side effects, including ocular burning, eye redness, local irritation and unpleasant taste.

Antitussives over The counter

Cough is a complex mechanism used by the body to expel foreign material located within the respiratory tract.[19] Cough can be considered **productive** or nonproductive. Codeine and dextromethorphan are opioid-derived compounds that may be used to suppress cough in adults.[19] In children, data demonstrating opioid-like antitussive (anti-cough) effectiveness in cough suppression is lacking.[8] Codeine and dextromethorphan work centrally and peripherally to increase the cough threshold in an unknown way.[19] Dextromethorphan is available in a variety of OTC products. Dextromethorphan tends to be the drug of choice because it lacks analgesic and addictive properties when used at recommended dosages. When ingested in large amounts, dextromethorphan may cause central nervous system (CNS) depression; however, in the 10-30 mg needed for cough suppression, these effects are unlikely.[19] Commonly associated side effects of dextromethorphan and codeine include stomach upset, dizziness and drowsiness.[20] In overdose, codeine can also cause CNS and respiratory depression. Codeine generally requires a prescription from a physician; however, most states still allow a pharmacist to dispense up to 120 mL of a codeine-based cough syrup, if it is listed as a Schedule 5 controlled substance and is combined with other ingredients that do not require a prescription (e.g., guaifenesin), to a patient with a legitimate medical need without a physician's authorization. Patients with a chronic cough associated with smoking or asthma must not use either of these drugs due to the increased risk of infection from uncleared mucus.[20]

Expectorants

The most commonly recommended cough expectorant drug in the pharmacy is guaifenesin. Guaifenesin is available in a wide variety of OTC products in many dosage formulations, including tablets, granules, syrup and liquid.[20] Guaifenesin is believed to produce its effect by increasing respiratory secretions, loosening phlegm and thinning mucus, leading to an increase in ciliary action and a more effective, productive cough. Guaifenesin is taken with 240 mL of water; these together help thin the mucus within the respiratory tract. This medication is usually well-tolerated. Side effects may include gastrointestinal effects, dizziness, headache and rash. When given in high doses, guaifenesin may increase the risk for kidney stones.[20]

Intranasal Corticosteroids

Intranasal corticosteroids work locally in the nasal mucosa by decreasing inflammation and increasing vascular constriction.[2] In addition, there are other underlying mechanisms that are involved, making intranasal corticosteroids superior to topical decongestants for the management of allergic rhinitis.[2,20] When intranasal corticosteroids are used for prophylaxis, administration begins two to three weeks prior to any anticipated symptom onset. If congestion is already present, a patient may use a decongestant or saline irrigation five to 10 minutes prior to administering the corticosteroid to open nasal passageways and allow for greater tissue penetration of the corticosteroid.[2] Prior to administration, patients must gently shake the intranasal corticosteroid device, with a rocking side-to-side motion, to avoid the formation of air bubbles in the solution.[20] After administering the dose, patients must avoid blowing their nose for 10-15 minutes.[2] The intranasal corticosteroids differ in their approved age ranges. Triamcinolone and mometasone are approved for patients as young as two years of age.[20] Unlike systemic corticosteroids, the effects of intranasal corticosteroids on growth suppression in children are unclear.[2,20] Growth during therapy must be monitored in children by the health care team.[20] Additional side effects include increased chance for a local fungal infection, sneezing, stinging inside the nose and a bloody nose (**epistaxis**).[2] With the use of intranasal flunisolide, permanent and temporary loss of smell and taste has also been reported.[20] If a patient does not experience any improvement of symptoms within three weeks after starting an intranasal corticosteroid, he/she must be referred back to the prescribing physician.[20]

Table 1
Drugs Associated with the Upper Respiratory System and Related Disorders

Drug Class(es)	Generic Name(s)**	Brand Name(s)**	Indication(s)	Available Dose Form(s)
Anti-Cough	Codeine / Guaifenesin (Schedule 5)	Robitussin AC	Cough	Liquid
Anti-Cough	Dextro-methorphan	Delsym	Cough	Capsule, Elixir, Extended-Release Suspension, Liquid, Lozenge, Solution, Suspension, Syrup, Tablet

Drug Class(es)	Generic Name(s)**	Brand Name(s)**	Indication(s)	Available Dose Form(s)
Antihistamine	Azelastine	Astelin, Astepro	Allergies	Nasal Spray
Antihistamine	Brompheniramine	Bromax, Lohist-12	Allergies	Chewable Tablet, Extended-Release Capsule, Extended-Release Tablet, Liquid, Tablet
Antihistamine	Cetirizine	Zyrtec	Allergies	Chewable Tablet, Liquid, Orally-Disintegrating Tablet, Tablet
Antihistamine	Chlorpheniramine	Chlortrimeton	Allergies	Capsule, Liquid, Tablet
Antihistamine	Clemastine	Tavist Allergy, Tavist-1	Allergies	Tablet
Antihistamine	Cyproheptadine	Periactin	Allergies, Appetite Simulation, Bed-Wetting, Migraine, Nightmares, Post-Traumatic Stress Disorder, Prophylaxis	Syrup, Tablet
Antihistamine	Desloratadine	Clarinex	Allergies	Orally-Disintegrating Tablet, Tablet
Antihistamine	Doxylamine	Aldex AN, Doxytex, Unisom	Allergies, Insomnia	Chewable Tablet, Solution, Tablet
Antihistamine	Fexofenadine	Allegra	Allergies	Liquid, Tablet
Antihistamine	Hydroxyzine	Atarax, Vistaril	Allergies, Anxiety, Insomnia, Itching	Capsule, Injectable, Suspension, Syrup, Tablet
Antihistamine	Levocetirizine	Xyzal	Allergies	Liquid, Tablet
Antihistamine	Loratadine	Alavert, Claritin	Allergies	Injectable, Orally-Disintegrating Tablet, Solution, Tablet

Table 1 cont.
Drugs Associated with the Upper Respiratory System and Related Disorders

Drug Class(es)	Generic Name(s)**	Brand Name(s)**	Indication(s)	Available Dose Form(s)
Antihistamine	Olopatadine	Pataday, Patanase, Patanol	Allergies	Nasal Spray, Ophthalmic
Antihistamine	Dimenhydrinate	Dramamine	Allergies, Nausea, Vomiting	Chewable Tablet, Injectable, Tablet
Antihistamine, Anti-Nausea	Diphenhydramine	Benadryl	Allergies, Insomnia, Motion Sickness (Nausea), Vomiting	Aerosol, Capsule, Cream, Dissolving Strip, Elixir, Gel, Gel Cap, Injectable, Solution, Syrup, Tablet
Antihistamine, Anti-Nausea	Meclizine	Antivert, Dramamine	Nausea, Vertigo, Vomiting	Chewable Tablet, Tablet
Antihistamine, Anti-Nausea: Phenothiazine	Promethazine	Phenergan	Allergies, Nausea, Vomiting	Injectable, Suppository, Tablet
Corticosteroid	Beclomethasone	Beconase AQ, Qvar	Allergies, Asthma	Aerosol, Nasal Spray
Corticosteroid	Budesonide	Entocort, Pulmicort, Rhinocort Aqua	Allergies, Asthma, Bowel Inflammation	Extended-Release Capsule, Nasal Spray, Powder for Inhalation, Suspension for Inhalation
Corticosteroid	Flunisolide	Nasarel	Allergies, Asthma	Aerosol, Nasal Spray
Corticosteroid	Fluticasone	Cutivate, Flonase, Flovent Diskus, Flovent HFA, Veramyst	Allergies, Asthma	Aerosol, Cream, Lotion, Nasal Spray, Ointment, Powder for Inhalation
Corticosteroid	Mometasone	Asmanex Twisthaler, Elocon, Nasonex	Allergies, Asthma, Skin Inflammation	Cream, Lotion, Nasal Spray, Ointment, Powder for Inhalation, Solution

Drug Class(es)	Generic Name(s)**	Brand Name(s)**	Indication(s)	Available Dose Form(s)
Corticosteroid	Triamcinolone	Aristopan, Kenalog, Nasacort AQ	Allergies, Inflammation, Osteoarthritis	Cream, Dental Paste, Injectable, Nasal Spray, Ointment
Expectorant	Guaifenesin	Mucinex, Robitussin	Cough	Capsule, Elixir, Extended-Release Capsule, Extended-Release Tablet, Liquid, Packet, Solution, Syrup, Tablet
Leukotriene Modifier	Montelukast	Singulair	Allergic Rhinitis, Asthma	Chewable Tablet, Granules, Tablet
Leukotriene Modifier	Zafirlukast	Accolate	Asthma	Tablet
Mast Cell Stabilizer	Cromolyn	Intal, NasalCrom	Allergies, Asthma	Aerosol, Nasal Spray
Mast Cell Stabilizer	Nedocromil	Alocril	Allergic Conjunctivitis	Ophthalmic
Nasal Decongestant	Naphazoline	Naphcon, Privine	Nasal Congestion	Nasal Spray, Ophthalmic
Nasal Decongestant	Oxymetazoline	Afrin	Nasal Congestion	Nasal Spray
Nasal Decongestant	Phenylephrine	Sudafed PE	Nasal Congestion	Liquid, Tablet
Nasal Decongestant	Propylhexedrine	Vicks Vapor Inhaler	Nasal Congestion	Nasal Spray
Nasal Decongestant	Pseudophedrine	Sudafed	Nasal Congestion	Capsule, Chewable Tablet, Extended-Release Capsule, Extended-Release Tablet, Liquid, Solution, Suspension, Syrup
Nasal Decongestant	Tetrahydrozoline	Tyzine	Nasal Congestion	Nasal Spray
Nasal Decongestant	Xylometazoline	Triaminic Nasal and Sinus Congestion	Nasal Congestion	Liquid, Nasal Spray

*All rights to all brand names and trademarks are held by their respective owners. There may be additional brand names for some of the products listed.

Conclusion

Upper respiratory tract disorders are extremely prevalent, and numerous prescription and OTC medications are available for symptomatic management. To effectively treat signs and symptoms, it is important to understand the basic pathophysiology of upper respiratory tract disorders and be familiar with available medications. Before recommending any OTC cough and cold medication, a detailed patient history, including the age of the patient, a description of the patient's symptoms and any concurrent medical problems, must be obtained. Lastly, it is important to note that many OTC products contain more than one active ingredient. Labels must be carefully reviewed to determine the appropriate product for each patient.

References

1. Zieve, D., Anatomy and function of the respiratory system, A.D.A.M. 2008, http://adam.about.com/care/asthma/asthma_respsyst.html, Aug. 26, 2010.

2. May, R., Smith, P.H., "Chapter 98, Allergic rhinitis," in Pharmacotherapy: A Pathophysiologic Approach, 7th edition, www.accesspharmacy.com/content.aspx?aID=3214703, Aug. 21, 2010.

3. Inamdar, S.R., "Chapter 37, Allergic and nonallergic rhinitis," in Pharmacotherapy in Primary Care, www.accesspharmacy.com/content.aspx?aID=3604241, Aug. 21, 2010.

4. Kantz, B., Sinus infection, www.webmd.com/allergies/sinus-infection, Sept. 3, 2010.

5. Inamdar, S.R., Best, B.M., "Chapter 38, Otitis media and sinusitis," in Pharmacotherapy in Primary Care, www.accesspharmacy.com/content.aspx?aID=3604318, Aug. 21, 2010.

6. Levy, S., "Pharmacist knows best: OTC recommendation survey 2007," Drug Topics, http://drugtopics.modernmedicine.com/drugtopics/article/articleDetail.jsp?id=423918, Aug. 21, 2010.

7. Pratter, M.R., "Cough and the common cold: ACCP evidence-based clinical practice guidelines," CHEST, 2006, Vol. 129, pp. 72S-74S.

8. Simasek, M., Blandino, D.A., "Treatment of the common cold," American Family Physician, 2007, Vol. 75, pp. 515-20, 522.

9. FDA, Public Health Advisory: Nonprescription cough and cold medicine use in children, www.fda.gov/Drugs/DrugSafety/PostmarketDrugSafetyInformationforPatientsandProviders/DrugSafetyInformationforHeathcareProfessionals/PublicHealthAdvisories/UCM051282, Sept. 6, 2010.

10. FDA, OTC cough and cold products: Not for infants and children under 2 years of age, www.fda.gov/ForConsumers/ConsumerUpdates/ucm048682.htm, Sept. 6, 2010.

11. Quillen, D.M., Feller, D.B., "Diagnosing rhinitis: Allergic vs. nonallergic," American Family Physician, 2006, Vol. 73(9), pp. 1583-1590.

12. Management of allergic and nonallergic rhinitis, Summary, Evidence Report/Technology Assessment: No. 54, May 2002, Agency for Healthcare Research and Quality, Rockville, MD, www.ahrq.gov/clinic/epcsums/rhinsum.htm.

13. Vincent, M.T., Celestin, N., Hussain, A.N., "Pharyngitis," American Family Physician, 2004, Vol. 69, pp. 1465-1470.

14. Choby, B.A., "Diagnosis and treatment of Streptococcal pharyngitis," American Family Physician, 2009, Vol. 79(5), pp. 383-390.

15. Yasmin, K., Forgie, S., Zhanel, G., "Chapter 112, Upper respiratory tract infections," in Pharmacotherapy: A Pathophysiologic Approach, 7th edition, www.accesspharmacy.com/content.aspx?aID=3184661, Aug. 21, 2010.

16. CDC, "Infant deaths associated with cough and cold medications — two states, 2005," Morbidity and Mortality Weekly Report, 2007, Vol. 56, pp. 1-4.

17. Gunn, V.L., Taha, S.H., Liebelt, E.L., Serwint, J.R., "Toxicity of over-the-counter cough and cold medications," *Pediatrics*, 2001, Vol. 108(3), p. e52.

18. Aguilera, L., "Pediatric OTC cough and cold product safety," U.S. Pharmacist, July 20, 2009, Vol. 34(7), pp. 39-41, www.uspharmacist.com/content/d/feature/i/765/c/14137.

19. Skidgel, R.A., Erdös, E.G., "Histamine, bradykinin, and their antagonists," Brunton, L.L., Lazo, J.S., Parker, K.L., Goodman & Gilman's The Pharmacological Basis of Therapeutics, 11th edition, www.accesspharmacy.com/content.aspx?aID=941777, Aug. 21, 2010.

20. Drug Facts and Comparisons, Indianapolis, IN, Wolters Kluwer Health Inc, 2009, Various monographs, http://online.factsandcomparisons.com, July 25, 2010.

21. Michigan Department of Community Health, "Ephedrine sales restricted beginning Dec. 15, 2005," www.michigan.gov/mdch/0,1607,7-132-2941_4871-129470--,00.html, Aug. 21, 2010.

22. Carpenter, L., "Pseudoephedrine sales and reporting laws," Drug Store News, www.ce-drugstorenews.com/userapp//lessons/page_view_ui.cfm?lessonuid=&pageid=4F62201816 22094C1508312801292F81, Aug. 21, 2010.

23. Michigan Pharmacists Association, "Gov. Snyder Signs New Pseudoephedrine Bills into Law," www.michiganpharmacists.org/news/articles.php?x=2237, Aug. 21, 2011.

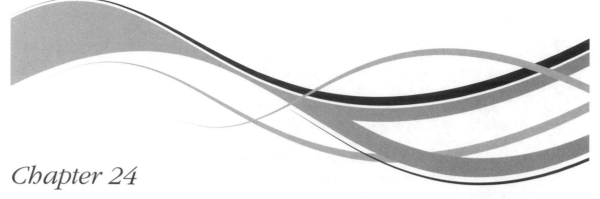

Chapter 24

REVIEW QUESTIONS

1. Which of the following structures can be described as air-filled spaces within the skull?
   a. Turbinates
   b. Larynx
   c. Sinuses
   d. Cilia

2. A mother comes into the pharmacy with her one-year-old daughter who is experiencing nasal congestion due to the common cold. Which of the following is an appropriate, FDA-supported recommendation for this child?
   a. Loratadine
   b. Naphazoline
   c. Pseudoephedrine
   d. Saline nasal drops

3. Which of the following medications is classified as a sedating antihistamine?
   a. Cetirizine
   b. Montelukast
   c. Diphenhydramine
   d. Mometasone

4. How much pseudoephedrine can be sold in a single purchase under federal law?
   a. 2 grams
   b. 3.6 grams
   c. 9 grams
   d. 48 grams

5. Which of the following medications is available OTC and would be appropriate to recommended for an adult with a dry, nonproductive cough?
   a. Guaifenesin
   b. Codeine
   c. Dextromethorphan
   d. Ciclesonide

6. In which of the following instances would an antibiotic, such as amoxicillin, be an appropriate therapy?
   a. Allergic rhinitis
   b. Bacterial sinusitis
   c. Common cold
   d. Viral sinusitis

7. Which of the following antibiotics is commonly utilized first for the management of strep throat?
   a. Penicillin
   b. Moxifloxacin
   c. Erythromycin
   d. Trimethoprim-sulfamethoxazole

8. Which of the following medications is approved for the management of perennial allergic rhinitis in children as young as six months of age?
   a. Montelukast
   b. Pseudoephedrine
   c. Oxymetazoline
   d. Triamcinolone nasal

9. To which of the following drug classes does guaifenesin belong?
   a. Antihistamine
   b. Corticosteroid
   c. Decongestant
   d. Expectorant

10. Which of the following medications may cause rebound nasal congestion if used intranasally for greater than three days?
    a. Oxymetazoline nasal
    b. Azelastine nasal
    c. Fluticasone nasal
    d. Cromolyn nasal

Chapter 25

LOWER RESPIRATORY SYSTEM

By Tracey L. Mersfelder, Pharm.D., BCPS
Kali M. VanLangen, Pharm.D., BCPS

Learning Objectives

This chapter seeks to prepare a pharmacy technician to:

- describe the anatomy and function of the lower respiratory system.
- describe common causes and symptoms of asthma, chronic obstructive lung disease, pneumonia and influenza.
- identify the indications and common adverse effects associated with each of the following medication classes: bronchodilators, anti-inflammatory drugs, antileu kotrienes, mast cell stabilizers, antibiotics and antivirals.
- describe how to properly use a metered-dose inhaler.

Introduction

The lower respiratory system consists primarily of the lungs, airways and air sacs, along with many blood vessels. These structures allow oxygen (O_2) to be taken into the body, and they facilitate breathing. Direct contact with the environment allows the lungs to be damaged by substances, such as smoke, air pollution, allergens and humidity, which prevent them from working properly. Asthma, chronic obstructive lung disease, pneumonia and influenza are a few diseases that affect the lungs and will be discussed in further detail throughout this chapter. A variety of medications are used to treat these disease states; many of the medications used to treat these diseases are used by patients for more than one breathing disorder. A pharmacy technician is expected to understand the basic function of these body tissues, the use of the drugs associated with the lower respiratory system and how to use some of the devices that patients will employ to get drugs into the lungs.

Anatomy and Physiology

The lower respiratory system is a series of airways that begins with the **trachea** and ends with the smallest **alveoli** in the lungs (see Figure 1). Once air carrying oxygen passes through the upper respiratory system, it enters the **trachea**, which then divides into two main **bronchi** (one for each lung). Each bronchus divides further into many smaller airways called **bronchioles** and delivers the oxygen-rich air to millions of air sacs, referred to as alveoli. The wall thickness of these structures gets progressively thinner as air moves through the lower respiratory tract so that once it reaches the alveoli; there is only a thin layer of cells surrounded by capillaries. This allows for the exchange of gases to occur. Oxygen from the air enters the blood through the capillaries in exchange for carbon dioxide (CO_2). The oxygen-carrying blood then travels to the heart to be delivered to other organs in the body. In addition to the structures mentioned above, other features of the lower respiratory system that are important include **smooth muscle**, **mucus** and **cilia**. The airway structures have layers of smooth muscle that surround them. The muscles gradually get thinner as they progress toward the alveoli and help control the diameter of the airways. When the muscles constrict, the diameter becomes smaller and less air can pass through. When they relax, air is able to pass through more easily due to the larger diameter. Mucus-producing glands are also found in the airway. Mucus in the airway is responsible for humidifying incoming air as well as trapping pollutants, dust and other unwanted substances. The airways are also lined with hair-like structures called cilia. The cilia aid in the removal of foreign substances from the lungs by moving mucus up from the lower respiratory system in a waving motion.

Figure 1
Lower Respiratory System

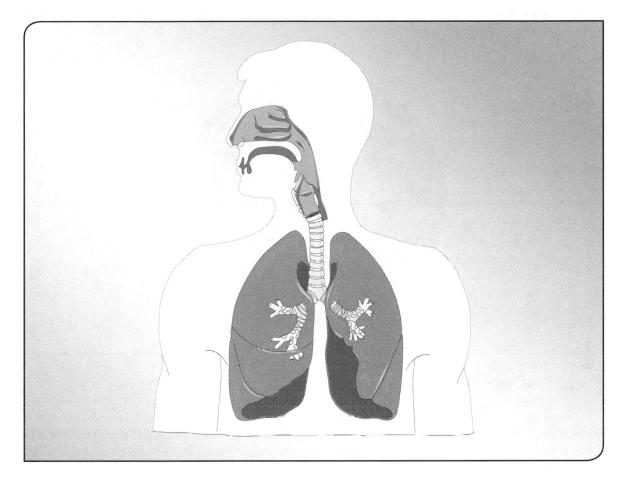

The primary function of the lower respiratory system is to deliver O_2 to the blood and remove CO_2. During inhalation, oxygen in the air is delivered to the alveoli and transported to the capillaries, where the oxygen then enters the blood. Carbon dioxide is transported from capillaries to the alveoli and then removed from the body during exhalation (see Figure 2). Breathing is automatically controlled by the "respiratory center" located in the brain. When increased amounts of carbon dioxide are present, the brain sends a message to the **diaphragm** and other respiratory muscles. When the diaphragm goes down, air can more freely move into the lungs and air is inhaled. During exhalation, the diaphragm goes back up and air is forced out of the lungs. The average adult at rest moves about 500 mL of air in and out of the body with each breath. Respiratory stimulants, including low oxygen and emotions, such as fear or increased oxygen demand from exercise, can cause the respiration rate to vary.

Figure 2
Gas Exchange in the Lungs

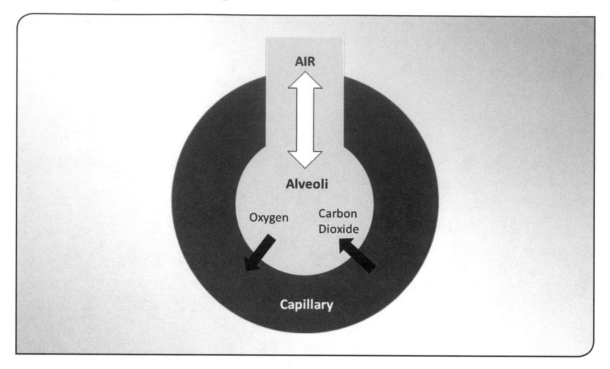

Drug Delivery Devices

A variety of medications are used in the treatment of lower respiratory diseases. Many of the medications discussed below are administered using medical devices designed to deliver a drug directly to the lungs; understanding how these devices work is important for every pharmacy technician. Patients must be extensively counseled by a pharmacist when receiving the first prescription for any of these devices; but, that does not mean that important information cannot be shared by a pharmacist when a patient is picking up a refill of these medications. It is important to remind patients of the proper technique for using their device to ensure that the treatment is most effective. Failure to use good technique may result in a poor response to the therapy. The most commonly used devices to aid in delivering drugs to the lungs include the following:

- **Metered-dose inhaler (MDI)**
- **Dry powder inhaler (DPI)**
- **Nebulizer**
- **Spacer**

The MDI is the most commonly used device to deliver medications to the lungs. A recent ban on the use of chlorofluorocarbons (CFCs) in the production of MDIs is resulting in the development of new devices. Figure 3 illustrates three ways an MDI can be used. With the first method, the mouthpiece is placed into the patient's mouth. The patient must not put their tongue over the mouthpiece while it is in their mouth as this will block the medication from reaching the lungs. The second method allows the patient to keep the mouthpiece two finger widths in front of their mouth. This requires the patient to have good coordination and cannot be done by many patients, especially young children or the elderly. The third and most preferred technique uses a spacer device that is designed to attach to the MDI. Spacers are helpful for patients with poor coordination and can help improve efficacy significantly; unfortunately, spacers can be costly for the patient.

Figure 3
Metered-Dose Inhaler Use

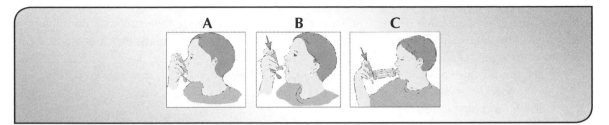

Regardless of the method used, these steps must always be followed with each use of an MDI:
1. Remove the cap and hold the inhaler upright
2. Shake the inhaler for five seconds
3. Tilt the head back slightly and breathe out as completely as possible
4. Position the inhaler inside the mouth, two finger widths outside of mouth (with the mouth open), or with a spacer
5. Press down on the inhaler to release medication while breathing in deeply over three to five seconds
6. Hold one's breath for 10 seconds to allow the medication to settle into the lungs
7. Breathe out very slowly to avoid expelling the medication
8. If a second dose is needed, wait one to two minutes before repeating steps 1-6
9. Replace the cap on the mouthpiece and store the inhaler upright
10. Rinse one's mouth with water (especially if using an inhaled corticosteroid) and do not swallow the water

DPIs require a slightly different technique than the technique used for MDIs. To use a DPI, the patient is to place his/her mouth tightly around the mouthpiece and rapidly inhale. Many DPIs, and now some MDIs, include a dose counter so patients are aware of the number of doses remaining and when a refill is needed. Rinsing the mouth after each use is recommended for both MDIs and DPIs.

Asthma

Asthma is a chronic, long-term disease that affects the lungs. More than 22 million people in the United States, including an estimated six million children, are affected by asthma, and these numbers continue to rise. The National Asthma Education and Prevention Program (NAEPP) and Global Initiative For Asthma (GINA) define asthma as a lung disease characterized by:
- variable airflow obstruction that is often reversible either spontaneously or with treatment.
- increased airway responsiveness to various stimuli, including allergens or irritants.
- chronic airway inflammation.

A patient with asthma may experience wheezing, breathlessness (trouble breathing), chest tightness and coughing. These symptoms typically occur at night or in the early morning. Patients with well-controlled asthma can avoid these troublesome symptoms and lead active and productive lives. When asthma is well controlled, air can move more freely through the airways; however, when asthma is not controlled, the airways are thick and swollen and more responsive to specific triggers that allow an asthma attack to happen easily.

During an acute asthma attack, the airways become narrowed due to constriction of the surrounding smooth muscle, and less air is able to travel in and out of the lungs. Increased inflammation also contributes to further narrowing of the airways and mucus production. During severe asthma episodes, the airways can become extremely narrow; this severe constriction can prevent airflow and lead to death if not treated by emergency medical professionals . One way to prevent an acute asthma attack is to be aware of one's asthma triggers. Since not all patients experience the same asthma triggers, it is important that each patient is aware of his or her triggers. Some common asthma triggers that can precipitate an attack include the following:

- Smoke from any source (tobacco smoke, including secondhand, smoke from burning wood or grass, etc.)
- House dust mites
- Mold
- Plant pollen
- Strong odors from cleaners or perfumes
- Animals with fur (dogs, cats, etc.)
- Changes in the weather (thunderstorms or high humidity)
- Air pollution
- Exercise
- Strong emotions

Although there is no cure for asthma, it can be controlled. The goal of current asthma therapy is to eliminate acute attacks and allow patients to live normal lives without restrictions. Although complete elimination of acute attacks and symptoms is the goal, it is not always achievable; current therapies can, if used correctly, significantly reduce symptoms and attacks even when such effects from the disease cannot be eliminated. Drug treatment for asthma involves two types of medications: drugs providing quick-relief during symptoms or an attack and drugs for long-term control that are used even when symptoms are not present. Quick-relief (also called rescue) medications are primarily used during an acute asthma attack to reverse airway constriction. Bronchodilators, such as short-acting beta agonists, are essential in the treatment of an acute attack and may be used in combination with anticholinergic agents and systemic (oral or intravenous) corticosteroids. In the event of a mild episode, the patient may be treated at home with a short-acting beta agonist. More severe attacks may require a visit to the emergency department or even hospitalization. Depending on the severity of the acute attack, treatment with rescue medications may vary from a single dose of a short-acting beta agonist to more aggressive treatment with three to 10 or more days of systemic corticosteroids.

Long-term control medications are used on a daily basis to prevent acute asthma attacks. It is important that patients with asthma are counseled to take these medications even in the absence of symptoms. Medications that are commonly used for long-term control include anti-inflammatory agents, long-acting beta-2 agonists, leukotriene modifiers and mast cell stabilizers. In some cases of persistent asthma, theophylline or omalizumab, an immunomodulating agent, may also be used.

Based on the severity of the patient's asthma, there are established guidelines that help physicians and pharmacists determine the most appropriate therapy for both short-term symptoms and long-term control. To determine the severity of a patient's asthma, a clinician will look at the frequency of symptoms and acute attacks, the frequency of rescue medication use, the dose of rescue medication used to control sudden symptoms, the level of interference that symptoms have on normal activity and measurements of respiratory function (pulmonary function tests). Upon assessing these factors for a patient, a clinician must place the patient into one of the following categories of asthma severity: mild intermittent asthma, mild persistent asthma, moderate persistent asthma or severe persistent asthma. The severity of a patient's asthma may change over time. When a patient's symptom severity changes, so, generally, must the patient's drug therapy. The aggressiveness of drug therapy may need to increase if symptoms become more frequent, and severe or the aggressiveness of drug therapy may need to decrease if symptoms become less bothersome or milder. Tables 1 and 2 illustrate this stepwise approach to the treatment of asthma, based on the NAEPP Expert Panel Report 3.

Table 1

Classification of Asthma Severity and Initiating Treatment in Youths ≥12 Years of Age and Adults

	Intermittent	Mild Persistent	Moderate Persistent	Severe Persistent
Recommended Step for Initiating Treatment	Step 1	Step 2	Step 3	Step 4
	In 2-6 weeks, evaluate level of asthma that is achieved and adjust therapy accordingly			
			Consider Adding Short Course of Oral Systemic Corticosteroids	

Table 2

Stepwise Approach for Managing Asthma in Youths ≥12 Years of Age and Adults

	Long-Term Control (Daily Treatment)	Rescue Medication
Step 1	No daily treatment needed	Short-Acting Bronchodilator as Needed for Symptoms
Step 2	*Preferred:* Low-Dose Inhaled Corticosteroids *Alternative:* Cromolyn / Nedocromil, Leukotriene Modifiers or Sustained-Release Theophylline	
Step 3	*Preferred:* Low-Dose Inhaled Corticosteroids plus Long-Acting Beta Agonist OR Medium-Dose Inhaled Corticosteroid (Alone) *Alternative:* Low-Dose Inhaled Corticosteroids plus either Leukotriene Modifier, Sustained-Release Theophylline or Zileuton	
Step 4	*Preferred:* Medium-Dose Inhaled Corticosteroids plus Long-Acting Beta Agonist *Alternative:* Medium-Dose Inhaled Corticosteroids plus either Leukotriene Modifier, Sustained-Release Theophylline or Zileuton	
Step 5	*Preferred:* High-Dose Inhaled Corticosteroids plus Long-Acting Beta Agonist AND Consider Omalizumab for patients who have allergies	
Step 6	*Preferred:* High-Dose Inhaled Corticosteroids plus Long-Acting Beta Agonist AND Consider Omalizumab for patients who have allergies	

Assessing the control of asthma symptoms and the response to therapy is important to patient care. Components that should be used to assess asthma control include the following:

- Frequency of symptoms
- Frequency of nighttime symptoms awakening the patient from sleep
- Frequency of short acting bronchodilator use for symptom relief (using more than two times per week suggests lack of control)
- Limitations of physical activity due to problems breathing
- Pulmonary function test results
- Medication adherence and tolerability

Discussing these components with patients during regular visits to the pharmacy helps stress the importance of symptom control and medication adherence. Pulmonary function tests are used in addition to symptom assessment to monitor lung function. The most common tests performed are **spirometry** and **peak flow monitoring**; pulmonary function tests are generally conducted in a physician's office. Some patients, typically those with more severe asthma or those who have difficulty detecting poor airflow, may use a peak flow meter on a daily basis at home to monitor their peak expiratory flow (PEF). Peak flow meters are dispensed by community pharmacies; pharmacists, sometimes with the aid of a pharmacy technician, must train patients on the use of a peak flow meter before dispensing one to a patient. The basic operation of a peak flow meter requires a patient to:

- take a deep breath and exhale forcefully into the device in a single breath.
- record the output value from the meter.
- repeat the process twice more.
- take the highest of the three readings; this is the patient's PEF.

The highest of the three readings, the patient's PEF, is then divided into three zones, with each zone being assigned a color from a traffic light (green, yellow and red) to tell the patient what action should be taken (see Table 3).

Table 3
Three-Zone Peak Expiratory Flow (PEF) System of Asthma Management

Zone	Personal Best Level	Action
Green	Greater than 80 percent of personal best	Go! Continue present activity and controller medication. No need for quick-relief medication.
Yellow	50-80 percent of personal best	Caution! Give quick-relief medication. Recheck PEF 15 minutes after medication use. PEF should return to green zone. If not, contact physician.
Red	Less than 50 percent of personal best	Stop! Get help! Give quick-relief medication. Contact physician or go to emergency department immediately.

Chronic Obstructive Pulmonary Disease

Chronic obstructive pulmonary disease (COPD) is the fourth leading cause of death in the United States; the only diseases accounting for more deaths are cancer, heart disease and cardiovascular accidents. It is the only cause of death that has increased over the past 30 years and is anticipated to be the third leading cause of death by 2020. Living with COPD can significantly impact a patient's daily activities and is currently the second leading cause of disability in the United States. A number of risk factors have been identified as contributing to the development of COPD, although tobacco smoke is believed to be the primary modifiable risk factor.

The Global Initiative for Chronic Obstructive Lung Disease (GOLD), as well as the American Thoracic Society, define COPD as a group of chronic lung diseases resulting in progressive airflow limitation, which is not reversible, associated with an abnormal inflammatory response to noxious particles or gases (tobacco smoke/air pollution). **Chronic bronchitis** (inflammation of the bronchi) and **emphysema** (enlarged and damaged alveoli, making gas exchange difficult) or a mixture of these diseases make up COPD. The first symptom a patient with COPD will experience is a cough that leads to increased sputum (saliva mixed with mucus) production. This cough is due to the increased amount of mucus needing to be cleared from the lungs. The increased presence of mucus in the lungs can also lead to an increased risk of infection. Over time, patients will develop shortness of breath (**dyspnea**) which causes them to seek medical attention. Other symptoms that patients may experience include chest tightness, fatigue and wheezing. Since COPD is a progressive disease, treatments are focused on slowing the progression and providing symptomatic relief.

Medications used to treat COPD are similar to those used in asthma. Most commonly, therapy for COPD includes bronchodilators (beta agonist, anticholinergics and theophylline) and anti-inflammatory agents (inhaled and oral corticosteroids). The main purpose of these medications is to relieve symptoms and improve airflow. More medications are needed to control symptoms as the disease progresses to more severe stages. The stages and severity of COPD are determined by pulmonary function tests, severity and frequency of symptoms, physical activity limitations and frequency of exacerbations that require hospitalization. These parameters are also used to monitor disease progression. Table 4 describes the recommended treatment at each stage of COPD according to the GOLD Guidelines.

Table 4

GOLD Guidelines for the Treatment of
Chronic Obstructive Pulmonary Disease

Stage	Recommended Treatment
All Stages	• Avoidance of risk factors • Influenza vaccination • Short-acting bronchodilator as needed
1: Mild COPD	• Short-acting bronchodilator as needed
2: Moderate COPD	• Regular treatment with one or more long-acting bronchodilators • Rehabilitation
3: Severe COPD	• Regular treatment with one or more long-acting bronchodilators • Inhaled corticosteroids if repeated exacerbations • Rehabilitation
4: Very Severe COPD	• Regular treatment with one or more long-acting bronchodilators • Inhaled corticosteroids if repeated exacerbations • Long-term oxygen if chronic respiratory failure • Rehabilitation • Consider surgical treatments

Medications Used in the Treatment of Asthma and COPD

■ Beta Agonists

Medications that are classified as beta agonists work primarily by stimulating the beta$_2$ (B$_2$) receptor. Stimulation of the B$_2$ receptor causes the smooth muscle surrounding the airways to relax. This allows the airways to dilate. Having dilated airways makes it easier for air to move in and out of the lungs. These agents also increase ciliary activity in the respiratory system. Increased ciliary activity helps clear mucus. The primary side effects seen with these agents are tachycardia (increased heart rate), nervousness and tremors. Beta agonists are available in a variety of dosage forms (e.g., MDI, solutions for nebulization, tablets and oral solutions). More side effects may be experienced when patients use tablets or liquids because the drugs must be absorbed and distributed throughout the body to have their effect on the lungs; although some portion of inhaled medications make it to the bloodstream, and therefore to the entire body, the chance for side effects that affect areas other than the lungs is smaller than for drugs absorbed through the gastrointestinal system.

Beta agonists can be broken down into two categories: short-acting and long-acting. Short-acting beta agonists (SABAs) are often used as rescue medications in asthma and COPD (when patients experience symptoms of wheezing, shortness of breath or chest tightness). Albuterol (Proventil®, Ventolin®, et al.), levalbuterol (Xoponex®), and pirbuterol (Maxair®) are all examples of short-acting beta agonists (see Table 5). These agents may also be used prior to strenuous physical activity in patients with exercise-induced bronchospasm. Given the quick onset of effectiveness (about 10 minutes), these agents are effective for controlling symptoms of wheezing and shortness of breath during an acute episode. These medications should primarily be used on an "as needed" basis, as frequent use indicates uncontrolled disease. In some patients with COPD, these agents may be used on a regular schedule to control symptoms and prevent progression of the disease.

Long-acting beta agonists (LABAs), such as salmeterol (Serevent®) and formoterol (Foradil®), are to be used on a regular basis in patients with COPD. Patients with asthma also benefit from the use of a LABA; however, combination therapy with an inhaled corticosteroid must be used because LABA alone in patients with asthma have been shown to increase the chance of death from asthma-related symptoms. Symbicort® and Advair® are both examples of combination products that include a long-acting beta agonist and an inhaled corticosteroid. These agents typically last 12 hours and are therefore given as two doses, 12 hours apart, each day. Some physicians have supported the use of such agents once daily in patients with mild and infrequent symptoms; although this may be appropriate for a patient, it is not a standard regimen and it should be brought to the attention of a pharmacist when seen by a pharmacy technician. The longer duration of action for LABA allows for better control of nighttime symptoms; however, these agents are not effective for managing acute episodes of wheezing and shortness of breath. In the event of an acute episode, additional doses of long-acting beta agonists should not be used; only short-acting agents are appropriate for controlling acute symptoms.

■ **Anticholinergic Medications**

The two anticholinergic medications currently available are ipratropium bromide (Atrovent®) and tiotropium (Spiriva®). These agents work by preventing the constriction of the smooth muscle surrounding the airway. By preventing this constriction, the airways are allowed to dilate. This dilation leads to air flowing more freely in and out of the lungs. These drugs are primarily used in the treatment of COPD, although ipratropium may be used to treat an acute asthma exacerbation. Due to the limited absorption into the blood, there is a low risk of systemic side effects with these medications. Side effects that may occur include dry mouth, nausea and a metallic taste experienced when eating or drinking. Tiotropium is administered as a dry powder for inhalation and may cause **pharyngitis** (sore throat). Ipratropium is normally dosed every four to six hours and reaches its maximum effect approximately 90 minutes after administration. The effects of tiotropium generally last for 24 hours; once daily dosing is recommended for tiotropium.

■ **Anti-inflammatory Agents**

Corticosteroids (anti-inflammatory agents) have multiple roles in lower respiratory diseases. In patients with asthma and COPD, inhaled corticosteroids are most commonly used as maintenance therapy to help reduce airway obstruction (by decreasing inflammation and airway hyperreactivity). When used in this way, the corticosteroids are delivered directly to the airways and little systemic absorption occurs (which helps to limit side effects). Inhaled corticosteroids do not work immediately; it takes approximately one to two weeks before any noticeable effect occurs from inhaled corticosteroids, and it may take up to eight weeks to see maximum improvement. It is important to recognize that, due to their slow onset of action, inhaled corticosteroids are not effective in the acute treatment of wheezing and shortness of breath. The side effects that are most common with low-to-moderate doses of inhaled corticosteroids include sore throat and a bad taste in the mouth. Another side effect from using inhaled corticosteroids is thrush; **thrush** is a fungal infection of the mouth and/or throat that can happen when the build up of corticosteroids in the mouth cause fungi and bacteria to grow much more rapidly than they could without the steroid. Patients should be advised to rinse their mouth out with water after each use of an inhaled corticosteroid to prevent the development of thrush. After rinsing, the water, which contains some level of the corticosteroid, should not be swallowed as swallowing the mixture could lead to systemic side effects. Patients who require higher doses of inhaled corticosteroids, or oral corticosteroids on a regular basis, may have more severe systemic side effects than those using lower doses of corticosteroids or those using only inhaled corticosteroids. Some systemic effects that patients may notice include weight gain, poor blood sugar control and glaucoma. Another possible systemic side effect of corticosteroid use that patients may not notice is an increased risk for osteoporosis (a weakening of the bones). Some patients may also start to look round or puffy in the face or start to experience excess growth of body hair. Since using corticosteroids orally is associated with more severe side effects, this route of administration is often reserved for patients with severe asthma or COPD, and the lowest effective dose is used for the shortest period of time possible.

Intravenous (IV) and oral corticosteroids are also used during an acute exacerbation of asthma or COPD. When used for this purpose, they are given for a short period of time (usually five to seven days). Short-term use of corticosteroids helps to limit the side effects; however, patients may still experience some weight gain from water retention, poor blood sugar control and stomach upset with short-term use of corticosteroids. These side effects will go away once the corticosteroids have been discontinued.

■ **Leukotriene Modifiers**
Leukotrienes are chemicals released from multiple inflammatory cells in the airways (including mast cells). They are known to be involved in bronchoconstriction, increased bronchial reactivity and mucus hypersecretion. The leukotriene modifiers montelukast (Singulair®) and zafirlukast (Accolate®) work by preventing leukotrienes from binding to specific receptors, while zileuton (Zyflo®) inhibits the production of leukotrienes. These agents are only available as oral therapy and must be taken on a scheduled basis to be effective. Montelukast is available as a tablet meant to be swallowed, a tablet meant to be chewed and as a packet of granules meant to be sprinkled over soft, cold or room-temperature food and swallowed; children who cannot yet swallow tablets may benefit from the chewable tablets or the granules. Zafirlukast and zileuton are only available as tablets meant to be swallowed. Even when used regularly, these agents are considered to be less effective than either systemic or inhaled corticosteroids. These agents are primarily used in patients with asthma.

■ **Mast Cell Stabilizers**
Cromolyn (Intal®) and nedocromil (Tilade®) are the only mast cell stabilizers currently available. These agents work by preventing mast cells from releasing histamine and other inflammatory substances. Due to this action, mast cell stabilizers are effective when used prior to exposure to an asthma trigger (e.g., exercise, cold air, environmental allergens). Similar to inhaled corticosteroids and LABAs, these agents should be used on a regularly scheduled basis. Patients receiving cromolyn or nedocromil should see improvement in their symptoms one to two weeks after the initiation of therapy; however, it may take much longer for patients to experience the maximum benefit from these drugs. Side effects of these two agents are minimal but include sore throat, cough and wheezing. Nedocromil has also been associated with a bad taste (causing some patients to not take it).

■ **Theophylline**
Theophylline has been used for many years in the treatment of asthma; but, its use is decreasing due to several factors, such as an increased risk of toxicity and drug interactions. Further, theophylline may not work as effectively as newer agents to control the frequency of acute asthma symptoms. Theophylline works in patients with asthma by relaxing the smooth muscle around the airways, similar to how beta agonists work. Theophylline is chemically related to caffeine; the side effects of taking theophylline are similar to taking caffeine, including nausea, vomiting, nervousness, tremors, insomnia, headache and increased heart rate. More

severe toxicities or side effects, such as heart arrhythmias, seizures and possibly death, can occur if a patient's blood level of theophylline goes, and stays, above the normal limit. It is therefore important that theophylline be monitored with periodic blood tests, leading to potential dose adjustments, to keep a patient's blood level in the acceptable range of 5 mcg/mL to 15 mcg/mL. Also complicating theophylline therapy, the drug has many interactions with other chemicals/drugs that can cause the levels in the body to fluctuate. Some example interactions with commonly-used medications include ciprofloxacin, cimetidine and clarithromycin. Further, patients experiencing disease states like liver failure and pneumonia or who are current smokers will all need more frequent monitoring to ensure that their theophylline blood levels remain in the normal range. All of these interactions require the dose of theophylline to be adjusted. Theophylline is typically administered as a sustained-release tablet for asthma maintenance therapy (although other preparations are available).

■ Immunomodulator

Omalizumab (Xolair®) is an immunomodulating agent currently approved for use in patients with allergic asthma that is poorly controlled by oral or inhaled corticosteroids. Omalizumab works by binding to receptors on mast cells and protecting those receptors from the immune system. This action prevents mast cells from releasing their contents in response to allergens. The content of mast cells is complex; however, many of the chemicals contained in a mast cell, including histamine, will exacerbate asthma. This agent is administered as a subcutaneous (just under the skin) injection every two or four weeks under medical supervision (in case anaphylaxis, an extremely rare event, occurs). Signs of anaphylaxis include wheezing, shortness of breath, tightness in the chest or throat, dizziness and tachycardia. Additional, more common, side effects include injection site reactions, upper respiratory infections and joint pain. Omalizumab is not to be used for the treatment of an acute asthma exacerbation.

Bacterial Pneumonia

Pneumonia is one of the most common infections of the lung and is currently the most common infectious cause of death in the United States. Pneumonia is typically either bacterial or viral; however, fungi or other lung irritants can also cause it. Although it can affect people of all ages, it is most severe in children less than five years of age, adults greater than 65 years of age and patients who are chronically ill. Pneumonia cases are classified based on the type of infection and the setting where the infection was acquired. The common classifications include the following:

- Community-acquired pneumonia (CAP)
- Hospital-acquired pneumonia
- Aspiration pneumonia
- Opportunistic pneumonia (affects people with a weakened immune system)

CAP is the most common type of pneumonia. The signs and symptoms associated with pneumonia depend on the organism causing the infection. Symptoms that are commonly seen with bacterial pneumonia are sudden onset of shortness of breath, productive cough, fever, chills and chest pain or chest tightness. Patients may also report fatigue, excessive sweating and confusion (especially in the elderly population). Treatment for pneumonia will depend on the type of pneumonia. Most patients with CAP can be treated at home. Patients who may require hospitalization for the treatment of pneumonia are those at risk for more severe symptoms, including the elderly, children and chronically ill patients.

Medications for Bacterial Pneumonia

Antibiotics are the mainstay of treatment for bacterial CAP. The duration of treatment varies; however, current guidelines recommend five to seven days of treatment (assuming symptoms improve over those five to seven days). The types of antibiotics typically used for bacterial CAP include the following:

- Beta-lactams: Penicillins (e.g., amoxicillin with or without clavulanate) and cephalosporins (e.g., cephalexin). Beta-lactams inhibit bacterial growth by disrupting cell wall synthesis.
- Macrolides: azithromycin, clarithromycin, etc. Macrolides inhibit the synthesis of bacterial proteins.
- Tetracycline D inhibits the synthesis of bacterial proteins.
- Fluoroquinolones (also known as respiratory fluoroquinolones): gatifloxacin, levofloxacin and moxifloxacin. Fluoroquinolones interfere with bacterial DNA replication.

The specific antibiotic used depends on many factors, including patient age, patient allergies, patient symptoms, the severity of the illness, health conditions and, ultimately, the organism causing the infection. If the exact organism is not known, a clinician will determine the antibiotic to use based on the most likely bacteria causing the infection. When possible and reasonable, a sample is obtained from the patient to culture the present bacteria to ensure that the chosen antibiotic is appropriate for the infection actually present.

Uncomplicated pneumonia (i.e., pneumonia without any other acute or chronic medical problems occurring in a patient who has not used antibiotics in the previous three months and does not need to be hospitalized) can be treated in the outpatient setting with doxycycline, azithromycin or clarithromycin. A respiratory fluoroquinolone (or combination therapy with a beta-lactam or cephalosporin plus a macrolide or doxycycline) can be used if patients have comorbid conditions (e.g., liver disease, kidney disease, diabetes mellitus, cancer, chronic obstructive pulmonary disease) or have recently used antibiotics.

Patients hospitalized for CAP in a non-ICU (intensive care unit) setting are recommended to have therapy initiated with either combination therapy (an intravenous cephalosporin plus a macrolide) or a respiratory fluoroquinolone. ICU patients are recommended to be started on both an intravenous cephalosporin and either azithromycin or a respiratory fluoroquinolone. Regardless of treatment setting, a broad-spectrum antibiotic is initiated and then, once a positive identification of the infecting bacteria is made, the antibiotic is changed to a more narrow-spectrum agent.

Viral Pneumonia

Bacterial pneumonia is commonly thought of when the generic term "pneumonia" is used; however, viral pneumonia needs to be considered as well. Viral pneumonia represents two to 35 percent of all pneumonia cases. Typically, viral pneumonia is caused by influenza A or respiratory syncytial virus (RSV); however, there are many other viruses that can cause viral pneumonia. During the 2009-2010 influenza season, H1N1 (also known as swine flu) had become a major concern due to its likelihood of causing pneumonia. There are two general types of influenza virus, A and B; within those types, there are subtypes; H1N1 is one of those subtypes. Approximately two to seven percent of patients who are infected with the influenza virus also have influenza pneumonia. For humans, influenza is generally spread from person to person; however, there are cases of the virus being spread between different species.

A few steps are recommended for the prevention of influenza. First, guidelines have been established to determine who should obtain an influenza vaccination. Vaccinations for seasonal influenza are recommended first for children, persons aged greater than 50 years, health care workers, those with close contact with immunocompromised persons, pregnant women, breastfeeding mothers, travelers and then anyone in the general population who would like to have one. The exact guidelines for who is recommended to receive an influenza vaccination are published each year by the Centers for Disease Control and Prevention (CDC). Patients who are 19 to 49 years of age have been recommended to obtain the H1N1 vaccination, in addition to the seasonal influenza vaccine, in past years. These two vaccines were available as a single injection during the 2010-11 flu season. Unfortunately, the influenza virus is one of the only viruses that currently can be vaccinated against, and it's not an easy process. The influenza vaccine has to be completely rebuilt each year to cover the strains of influenza expected for the upcoming flu season. Second, containment of the virus, is important to preventing influenza infection. Good hand-washing techniques are important to avoid the spread of the disease. Some patients will need to be placed in temporary isolation if infected. Other recommendations are available from the CDC at www.cdc.gov for specific situations. Lastly, if there is an isolated outbreak of influenza, antiviral medications can be utilized to minimize infection from the virus.

Typical symptoms of influenza include cough, shortness of breath and chest pain. One way to determine if a patient has influenza is by performing a rapid flu test. Results are available in less than 15 minutes and are very accurate at predicting a positive flu result; a negative result requires further tests that take longer. There are other tests that can confirm the rapid test that take two hours to two weeks for the results but are better at confirming a negative result on a rapid test.

A few medications exist that can lessen the severity and duration of an influenza virus infection. Neuraminidase inhibitors have been shown to be effective against both influenza A and B. For these medications to be effective, they need to be started within 48 hours from the first onset of symptoms the patient experiences. These medications shorten the duration of illness by an average of one to two days (compared to experiencing the infection without the drug) and may also help reduce the severity of the symptoms experienced from the influenza infection. Adamantanes (amantadine and rimantadine) were used for influenza in the past but are not as effective for influenza B and therefore are rarely used.

Medications Used for Influenza Pneumonia

■ **Neuraminidase Inhibitors**
Zanamivir and oseltamivir are neuraminidase inhibitors approved for the prevention and treatment of influenza A and B. Zanamivir is available as a powder that is inhaled. It is not to be used in patients with asthma or other breathing problems or heart disease. It can be used in adults and children seven years old and older. Side effects of zanamivir include dizziness, headache, nausea, diarrhea, runny nose and cough. Oseltamivir is available as a capsule and liquid. It can be used in adults and children one year old and older. If a child is less than one year old, they can receive oseltamivir for the H1N1 infection. Oseltamivir may cause nausea or vomiting but can be taken with food to lessen these side effects. Typically these medications are given for five days.

Table 5
Drugs Used With the Lower Respiratory System

Drug Class(es)	Generic Name(s)**	Brand Name(s)**	Indication(s)	Available Dose Form(s)
Anticholinergic	Ipratropium	Atrovent, Atrovent HFA	Allergies, Bronchospasm from Chronic Obstructive Pulmonary Disorder	Aerosol, Nasal Spray, Solution for Inhalation
Anticholinergic	Tiotropium	Spiriva Handihaler	Chronic Obstructive Pulmonary Disorder	Capsule for Inhalation
Anti-Cough	Benzonatate	Tessalon Perles	Cough	Capsule
Anti-Cough	Codeine / Guaifenesin (Schedule 5)	Robitussin AC	Cough	Liquid
Anti-Cough	Dextromethorphan	Delsym	Cough	Capsule, Elixir, Liquid, Lozenge, Solution, Suspension, Tablet
Anti-Cough Anti-Nausea: Phenothiazine / Pain Reliever	Promethazine / Codeine (Schedule 5)	Phenergan with Codeine	Cough	Syrup
Bronchodilator: Beta Agonist (Long-Acting)	Arformoterol	Brovana	Chronic Obstructive Pulmonary Disorder	Solution for Inhalation
Bronchodilator: Beta Agonist (Long-Acting)	Formoterol	Foradil Aerolizer	Asthma, Chronic Obstructive Pulmonary Disorder in Combination with Inhaled Corticosteroids, Exercise-Induced Bronchospasm	Capsule for Inhalation, Solution for Inhalation
Bronchodilator: Beta Agonist (Long-Acting)	Salmeterol	Serevent Diskus	Asthma, Chronic Obstructive Pulmonary Disorder, Exercise-Induced Bronchospasm in Combination with Inhaled Corticosteroids	Powder for Inhalation

Drug Class(es)	Generic Name(s)**	Brand Name(s)**	Indication(s)	Available Dose Form(s)
Bronchodilator: Beta Agonist (Short-Acting)	Albuterol	Accuneb, ProAir HFA, Proventil HFA, Ventolin HFA, Vospire	Exercise-Induced Bronchospasm, Shortness of Breath, Wheezing	Aerosol, Solution for Inhalation, Syrup, Tablet
Bronchodilator: Beta Agonist (Short-Acting)	Levalbuterol	Xopenex, Xopenex HFA	Shortness of Breath, Wheezing	Aerosol, Solution for Inhalation
Bronchodilator: Beta Agonist (Short-Acting)	Pirbuterol	Maxair Autohaler	Shortness of Breath, Wheezing	Aerosol
Bronchodilator: Beta Agonist (Short-Acting) / Anti-Anaphylaxis	Epinephrine	Adrenaclick, Adrenaline, Epi-Pen, Primatene Mist, TwinJect	Anaphylactic Reaction, Shortness of Breath, Wheezing	Aerosol, Injectable, Nasal Spray, Solution for Inhalation
Bronchodilator: Beta Agonist / Anticholinergic (Short-Acting)	Albuterol / Ipratropium	Combivent, DuoNeb	Chronic Obstructive Pulmonary Disorder	Aerosol, Solution for Inhalation
Bronchodilator: Beta Blocker (Long-Acting)	Budesonide / Formoterol	Symbicort	Asthma, Chronic Obstructive Pulmonary Disorder	Powder for Inhalation
Bronchodilator: Beta Blocker (Long-Acting)	Fluticasone / Salmeterol	Advair Diskus, Advair HFA	Asthma, Chronic Obstructive Pulmonary Disorder	Aerosol, Powder for Inhalation
Corticosteroid	Budesonide	Entocort, Pulmicort, Pulmicort Flexhaler, Pulmicort Respules, Rhinocort Aqua	Allergies, Asthma, Bowel Inflammation	Extended-Release Capsule, Nasal Spray, Powder for Inhalation, Suspension for Inhalation
Corticosteroid	Fluticasone	Cutivate, Flonase, Flovent Diskus, Flovent HFA, Veramyst	Allergies, Asthma	Aerosol, Cream, Lotion, Nasal Spray, Ointment, Powder for Inhalation

Table 5 *cont.*
Drugs Used With the Lower Respiratory System

Drug Class(es)	Generic Name(s)**	Brand Name(s)**	Indication(s)	Available Dose Form(s)
Corticosteroid	Methylpredniso-lone	Depo-Medrol, Medrol, Medrol Dosepak, Solu-Medrol	Acute Asthma Exacerbation, Gout, Osteoarthritis, Severe Asthma, Skin Inflammation	Injectable, Tablet
Corticosteroid	Mometasone	Asmanex Twisthaler, Elocon, Nasonex	Allergies, Asthma, Skin Inflammation	Cream, Lotion, Nasal Spray, Ointment, Powder for Inhalation, Solution
Corticosteroid	Prednisolone	Prelone	Acute Asthma Exacerbation, Severe Allergic Reaction, Severe Asthma	Liquid, Syrup, Tablet
Corticosteroid	Prednisone	Deltasone, Sterapred	Acute Asthma Exacerbation, Gout, Rheumatoid Arthritis, Severe Allergic Reaction, Severe Asthma	Liquid, Tablet
Corticosteroid, Anti-Nausea	Dexamethasone	Decadron	Edema, Nausea, Vomiting	Injectable, Liquid, Tablet
Expectorant	Guaifenesin	Mucinex, Robitussin	Cough	Granules, Liquid, Tablet
Immuno-modulator	Omalizumab	Xolair	Moderate-Severe Persistent Asthma	Injectable
Leukotriene Modifier	Montelukast	Singulair	Allergic Rhinitis, Asthma	Chewable Tablet, Granules, Tablet
Leukotriene Modifier	Zafirlukast	Accolate	Asthma	Tablet
Leukotriene Modifier	Zileuton	Zyflo, Zyflo CR	Asthma	Extended-Release Tablet, Tablet

All rights to all brand names and trademarks are held by their respective owners. There may be additional brand names for some of the products listed.

Conclusion

Diseases of the lower respiratory system can have a significant impact on a patient's life if not treated appropriately. A variety of medications can be used to help control these disease states and are delivered using a variety of methods. Patients with asthma lead relatively normal lives if they take their long-acting medications, as prescribed, to control the frequency of acute asthma attacks and use their rescue medications only for sudden symptoms. For those patients with COPD, treatment focuses more on symptomatic relief and delaying progression of the disease; however, the progression of the disease cannot yet be stopped entirely. Although patients with asthma or COPD are more likely to have respiratory-tract infections, anyone can catch a respiratory infection. Bacterial and viral pneumonia is common but can often be treated with antibiotics at home; more serious infections require hospitalization and may involve intravenous antibiotics. Clearly, there are many drugs involved with diseases of the lower respiratory system where pharmacists, and therefore pharmacy technicians, can greatly impact the quality of their patient's lives.

Bibliography

- Prendergast, T.J., Seeley, E.J., Ruoss, S.J., "Chapter 9, Pulmonary Disease," in McPhee, S.J., in Pathophysiology of Disease: An Introduction to Clinical Medicine, 6th edition, www.accesspharmacy.com/content.aspx?aID=5369033, Aug. 10, 2010.
- National Asthma Education and Prevention Program, Expert Panel Report 3: Summary Report 2007, Guidelines for the diagnosis and management of asthma, National Heart Lung and Blood Institute, National Institutes of Health, NIH Publication No. 08, p. 5846, October 2007.
- Global Initiative For Asthma: Global Strategy for Asthma Management and Prevention 2009 (Update), www.ginasthma.org, Aug. 14, 2010.
- Williams, D.M, Bourdet, S.V., "Chapter 29, Chronic Obstructive Pulmonary Disease," in Pharmacotherapy: A Pathophysiologic Approach, 7th edition, www.accesspharmacy.com./content.aspx?aID=3192403, Aug. 14, 2010.
- Global Initiative for Chronic Obstructive Lung Disease: Global Strategy for the Diagnosis, Management, and Prevention of Chronic Obstructive Pulmonary Disease Guidelines, updated 2009, www.goldcopd.com/Guidelineitem.asp?l1=2&l2=1&intId=2002, Aug. 14, 2010.
- Glover, M.L., Reed, M.D., "Chapter 111, Lower Respiratory Tract Infections," in DiPiro, J.T., Talbert, R.L., Yee, G.C., Matzke, G.R., Wells, B.G., Posey, L.M., Pharmacotherapy: A Pathophysiologic Approach, 7th edition, www.accesspharmacy.com/content.aspx?aID=3184352, Aug. 15, 2010.
- Community Acquired Pneumonia in Adults: Guidelines for Management, Clinical Infectious Diseases, 2007, Vol. 44, pp. S27–S72.
- CDC Seasonal Information for Health Professionals, www.CDC.gov/flu/professionals, Aug. 12, 2010.
- Marcos, A.M., Esperatti, M., Torres, A., "Viral Pneumonia," Current Opinion in Infectious Diseases, 2009, Vol. 22, pp. 143-147.

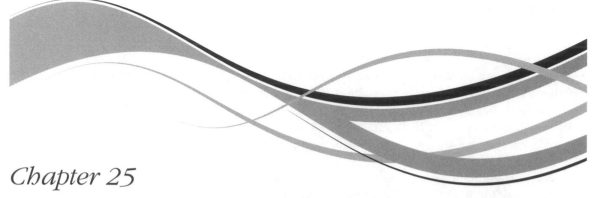

1. What is the main role of the lower respiratory system?
   a. Deliver CO_2 to the blood
   b. Deliver O_2 to the blood
   c. Remove O_2 from the blood
   d. A and C

2. In the event of an acute asthma attack, which of the following medications should be used?
   a. Albuterol
   b. Omalizumab
   c. Budesonide
   d. Theophylline

3. What is the goal of therapy in COPD?
   a. Prevent progression of the disease
   b. Reverse progression of the disease
   c. Manage symptoms of the disease
   d. Cure the disease

4. What is the most common risk factor for developing COPD?
   a. Tobacco smoke
   b. Air pollution
   c. Mold
   d. Exercise

5. Which of the following is the most common device used to administer medications in lower respiratory diseases?
   a. Intravenous infusion
   b. Metered-dose inhaler (MDI)
   c. Nebulizer
   d. Dry powder inhaler (DPI)

6. Which of the following agents is an inhaled corticosteroid?
    a. Albuterol
    b. Montelukast
    c. Tiotropium
    d. Fluticasone

7. When using a MDI, how long should a patient wait before the second dose of medication is administered?
    a. Do not wait, take the second dose immediately
    b. Wait 10-15 seconds
    c. Wait 30-45 seconds
    d. Wait 60-120 seconds

8. Which of the following statements regarding CAP is false?
    a. CAP is most common in the elderly population
    b. CAP must always be treated in the hospital
    c. Treatment for CAP lasts about five to seven days
    d. Treatment for CAP usually includes antibiotics

9. It is important to avoid giving zanamivir to anyone who:
    a. has influenza B.
    b. has asthma.
    c. is older than seven years of age.
    d. has had symptoms for 24 hours.

10. Which of the following can be used to prevent influenza pneumonia?
    a. Yearly vaccination
    b. Good hand-washing
    c. Prophylaxis with antiviral medications
    d. All of the above can be used to prevent influenza pneumonia

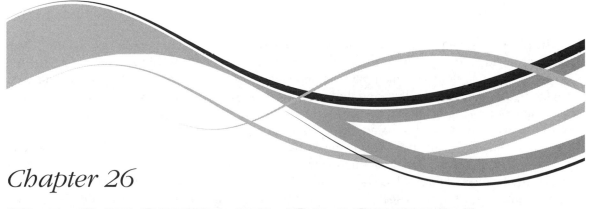

Chapter 26

DIGESTIVE SYSTEM

By Pramodini B. Kale-Pradhan, Pharm.D.
Kristin M. Verfaillie, Pharm.D.

Learning Objectives

This chapter seeks to prepare a pharmacy technician to:

- ■ understand which organs make up the digestive system and how they normally function to process food.
- ■ describe the actions of anti-flatulence and anti-diarrheal drugs.
- ■ explain the difference between laxatives and stool softeners.
- ■ describe the action of drugs used to treat irritable bowel syndrome.
- ■ list which antiemetic drugs are available over-the-counter (OTC) and which antiemetic drugs are available by prescription.
- ■ explain peptic ulcer formation and drug treatments for peptic ulcers.
- ■ describe the role of antibiotics in ulcer treatment.

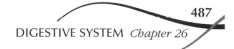

Introduction[1]

The digestive system is comprised of the gastrointestinal (GI) tract and accessory organs that secrete fluids to aid in digestion (see Figure 1). The organs that make up the GI tract include the mouth, pharynx, esophagus, stomach, small intestine and large intestine. The accessory organs include salivary glands, the pancreas, the liver and the gall bladder. All of these organs work together to process food using four basic principles: digestion, secretion, absorption and motility. When food is eaten, it is broken down into its smallest components. Food is broken down enough to be absorbed through the intestine and used by the body for energy. Also present in the GI tract are bacteria. These bacteria aid in the digestion of food and do not normally cause illness.

Disorders of the GI tract, which range from minor discomforts to serious ailments, are extremely common. Since they are often seen in the pharmacy, and treated with both OTC and prescription medications, it is important to be familiar with these disorders and the drugs that are used to treat them. In addition to normal GI tract function, this chapter will examine the most common disorders of the GI tract and the medications used for their treatment.

Figure 1
Digestive System

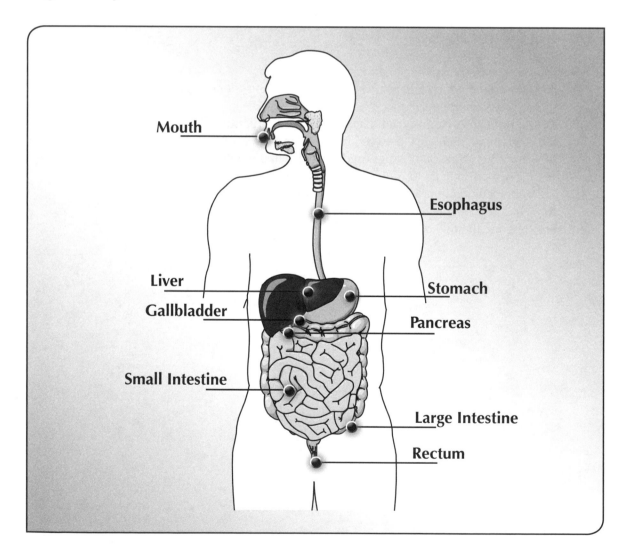

Anatomy of the GI Tract[1,2,3]

The process of the digestion of food begins in the mouth. Food is broken down into smaller pieces by chewing. **Salivary glands** located in the mouth secrete **saliva** that contain an enzyme called **amylase**. This enzyme helps to break down carbohydrates in food. Saliva also lubricates food, which makes it easier to swallow. The **pharynx** and **esophagus** provide a connection from the mouth to the stomach. The esophagus also secretes mucus to help lubricate food as it passes to the stomach.

The **stomach** is the next organ in the digestive system, which serves to store, break down and delay absorption of food that is eaten during a meal. The stomach is a sac-like organ located in the upper left portion of the abdomen. When food is introduced into the stomach, acid is secreted from the wall of the stomach, which helps to further break down the food. The stomach also moves the food around in a churning motion to help it mix with the acid. The food's progress is delayed in the stomach to allow it to be broken into smaller pieces and to be slowly released into the next section of the GI tract: the duodenum.

The **duodenum** is the first part of the **small intestine**. It breaks food down even more by using fluids secreted from the pancreas and liver. The **pancreas** is a long, glandular organ located near the stomach that secretes bicarbonate, insulin and enzymes to aid in the digestive process. The **liver** is a large organ located in the upper right portion of the abdomen that secretes substances called **bile salts** that also aid in the break down of foods (particularly fats). The liver works with another organ called the **gallbladder**, a small pouch-like organ located under the liver. The liver makes the bile salts and stores them in the gallbladder. The bile salts are kept there until food is consumed, and they are released into the duodenum.

Food leaves the duodenum and travels through the small intestine. The whole process is moved along by the **motility** of the GI tract. The contraction of the smooth muscles in the intestines pushes the food particles through the GI tract. The entire GI tract is approximately 24 feet long, and the small intestine is about 19 of those feet.[4,5] Once food particles are small enough, they are absorbed through the small intestine and then enter the bloodstream to be used for energy in the body.

The last section of the GI tract is the **large intestine**. All food particles that were not absorbed through the small intestine end up here as waste. Another large component of the waste in the large intestine is bacteria. Most of the bacteria located in the GI tract end up in the large intestine to be excreted as waste. The human GI tract processes about 9 L of fluids and food particles per day, and 99 percent of that is absorbed. Only around 100 mL of the 9 L is excreted as waste. That shows the great ability of the GI tract to absorb water and nutrients to assist with the body's functions. When the system is working properly, almost everything that is consumed is absorbed and only a small portion is excreted as waste. See Table 1 for a list of drugs commonly used to treat GI tract disorders.

Flatulence[1]

Flatulence is gas in the GI tract that can cause discomfort and pain. To treat flatulence, the OTC drugs alpha-galactosidase (Beano®) and simethicone (e.g., Mylicon®, Gas-X®, Phazyme®) are used.[6] Alpha-galactosidase is a natural enzyme that breaks down oligosaccharides, the sugars found in high-fiber foods, to make them more digestible. It must be taken before meals to be effective. Simethicone provides defoaming action by producing a film on the intestines that collapses the gas bubbles and prevents the trapping of these bubbles in the GI tract. It is available alone or in combination with antacid preparations. Simethicone may be used to treat conditions of excess gas, bloating and infant colic.

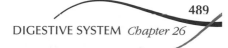

Diarrhea[1]

Diarrhea refers to the increased frequency and liquid nature of stools produced by rapid movement of fecal matter through the large intestine. Drugs to treat diarrhea are categorized as antimotility, adsorbent, antisecretory and other agents.

Antimotility agents include diphenoxylate with atropine (Lomotil®), loperamide (Imodium® A-D), paregoric and opium tincture. These are absorbed into the bloodstream and act systemically to depress **peristalsis** (contractions of the intestinal muscle). Diphenoxylate is related to meperidine (Demerol®) and is classified as a Schedule 5 controlled substance due to its potential for dependence and abuse. Atropine is combined with diphenoxylate to discourage abuse of the narcotic component. Some of its adverse effects include blurred vision, dry mouth and urinary hesitancy.

Adsorbents, such as polycarbophil (FiberCon®), act locally on the intestinal mucosa to bind with bacteria, toxins and other irritants that cause diarrhea. These products are given following a loose stool for symptomatic relief.

Antisecretory agents, such as bismuth subsalicylate (Pepto-Bismol®) and octreotide (Sandostatin®), work by inhibiting intestinal secretion (intestinal discharge which causes diarrhea) and by stimulating intestinal absorption. Bismuth subsalicylate is mainly used for travelers's diarrhea, which is caused by consuming food or water contaminated with bacteria, which generally occurs when visiting a foreign country. Bismuth subsalicylate may interfere with warfarin and some antibiotics (such as tetracyclines). Kaopectate® formerly contained an adsorbing agent called attapulgite; it has been reformulated and now contains bismuth subsalicylate. This is important to note because it was often used for treating diarrhea in children. With the new formulation containing salicylate, it should NOT be given to children because of the risk of developing a fatal brain condition called Reye's Syndrome. Octreotide is used to treat severe diarrhea and other symptoms caused by certain intestinal tumors.

Other agents used to treat diarrhea include lactase (Lactaid®) and bacterial replacement lactobacillus (Lactinex®). Lactase is an enzyme that digests carbohydrates. Individuals who are lactose intolerant are deficient in this enzyme, which leads to osmotic diarrhea when dairy products are consumed. Osmotic diarrhea occurs when too much water is drawn into the bowels, which results in diarrhea. Replacement of lactase prevents this type of diarrhea. Lactobacillus preparations replace normal colonic bacteria; therefore, supplementing lactobacillus aids in suppressing bacteria that cause disease. Lactobacillus may be replaced by eating yogurt containing live cultures of lactobacillus.

Constipation[1]

Constipation is the difficulty or infrequent passing of stool. Constipation may be treated with bulk-forming laxatives, emollients, stimulant laxatives and other agents. Taking bulk-forming laxatives, eating a high-fiber diet and drinking plenty of fluids are the most natural ways of preventing and treating constipation. In place of natural fiber, bulk-forming laxatives are available as OTC products. These may take up to three days for the desired effects to be seen. Bulk-forming laxatives include methylcellulose (Citrucel®), polycarbophil (FiberCon®) and psyllium (Metamucil®) and are used to treat simple constipation, to manage irritable bowel syndrome and to control diverticulitis (inflammation of a sac or pouch that has formed in the colon).

Stool softeners are emollients that work slowly over several days allowing for the absorption of water into the stool and making the formed stool soft and easier to pass. This helps to avoid straining during defecation. Stool softeners include mineral oil, glycerin suppositories and the different salts of docusate (Colace®).

Stimulant laxatives increase bowel movements by stimulating peristalsis; they include bisacodyl (Dulcolax®) and senna/sennosides (Senokot®). Senna also comes formulated as a combination product with docusate (Senokot-S®, Peri-Colace®). Peristalsis is stimulated within six to eight hours after oral administration. Stimulant laxatives are preferred for emptying the bowel in preparation for gastrointestinal surgery or tests. Habitual use may lead to dependence on laxatives. These laxatives are slightly absorbed and distributed to body tissues, including breast milk, and should be avoided when nursing.

Other laxatives include lactulose, magnesium salts (Milk of Magnesia®) and sodium phosphates (Fleet® Enema). These drugs draw water into the intestine causing the bowel to distend from fluid accumulation, which promotes peristalsis. This takes effect in one hour (or less) for sodium phosphates or in one day for lactulose.[7] Finally, other drugs that are involved with treating constipation include the following (see Table 1 for further examples):

- The 5-HT$_4$ (serotonin-4) partial receptor agonist tegaserod (Zelnorm®) was the first agent of this class of medications approved for the short-term treatment of constipation-predominant irritable bowel syndrome (IBS) in women. Tegaserod normalizes impaired GI motility, stimulates intestinal secretion and inhibits visceral sensitivity. It provides overall multisymptom relief of abdominal pain or discomfort, bloating and constipation for IBS sufferers. Tegaserod was withdrawn from the general market in 2007 due to reports of increased heart attacks and strokes in patients with pre-existing cardiovascular disease or cardiovascular risk factors.[8] It is now available for emergency use only.

- Lubiprostone (Amitiza®) is another agent used to treat IBS.[9] It acts as a chloride-channel activator in the GI tract. Activation of the chloride channel leads to an increase in intestinal fluid secretion and, thereby, the passage of stool and alleviation symptoms associated with constipation. Like tegaserod, it is approved for the treatment of IBS in women and for chronic constipation in adults. A pregnancy test and the use of contraceptives are recommended before starting lubiprostone due to the potential for early termination of a pregnancy, which was noted in animal studies.

- Methylnaltrexone (Relistor®) is a peripherally-acting opioid antagonist used for the treatment of opioid-induced constipation in patients with advanced disease receiving palliative care.[10] It acts in the GI tract to block the effects of opioids (including decreased GI motility and a delay in GI transit time) without affecting the central analgesic effects.

- Methscopolamine (Pamine®), hyoscyamine (Levbid®, Levsin®, et al.) and dicyclomine (Bentyl®) are anticholinergic agents that decrease gastrointestinal motility in IBS patients where abdominal pain or spasms are the primary complaints.

Nausea and Vomiting[1]

Nausea and vomiting (also called **emesis**) may occur for a variety of reasons including pregnancy onset, motion sickness, GI obstruction, ulcer development, drug toxicity, heart attack, kidney failure or chemotherapy initiation. Overall, the vomiting center in the brain integrates the nausea response and coordinates the resulting vomiting reflex. Antiemetics are used to control nausea and vomiting by acting on either the GI tract or the brain. Currently, nausea and vomiting can be treated with a multitude of drug classes, including antihistamines, phenothiazines, butyrophenones, cannabinoids, corticosteroids, benzodiazepines, selective serotonin receptor antagonists and other medications.

Antihistamines/anticholinergics are effective in decreasing nausea, vomiting, vertigo (dizziness) and motion sickness through effects on the nervous system. To prevent nausea from motion sickness, the patient takes the first dose 30 minutes before exposure to motion. These agents can cause sedation and include OTC products such as dimenhydrinate (Dramamine®), diphenhydramine (Benadryl®) and meclizine (Antivert®, Non-Drowsy Dramamine®). Others, including trimethobenzamide (Tigan®) and scopolamine (Transderm Scop®), require a prescription. Scopolamine is the most effective drug for

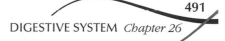

motion sickness; it is worn as a small patch behind the ear and is changed every 72 hours.

Phenothiazines are another class of antiemetics. This class works by blocking dopamine receptors. Prochlorperazine (Compazine®) and promethazine (Phenergan®) are the most commonly prescribed antiemetics in this class. Their use is limited due to the sedation they cause and the possible side effect of involuntary muscle jerking (dystonia).

Butyrophenones work by blocking the action of dopamine in the brain. Some examples of drugs in this class include droperidol (Inapsine®) and haloperidol (Haldol®). These agents may cause sedation and dystonic reactions. In addition, droperidol has a black box warning due to the potential for producing heart rhythm disturbances.

Cannabinoids such as dronabinol (Marinol®) and nabilone (Cesamet®) are derivatives of marijuana.[11] They are used to treat vomiting associated with chemotherapy. Adverse effects associated with this class include dizziness, memory loss, loss of motor coordination, hallucinations, euphoria, inappropriate fear, dry mouth, blurred vision, low blood pressure, palpitations and tachycardia (rapid heart rate). Caution should be taken in the elderly and patients with mental illness, liver disease or cardiovascular disease.

The corticosteroids, like dexamethasone (Decadron®), are used to treat chemotherapy-induced nausea and vomiting. Steroids are often used in combination with a selective serotonin receptor antagonist (5-HT$_3$ antagonist), such as ondansetron (Zofran®), granisetron (Kytril®, Sancuso®), dolasetron (Anzemet®) or palonosetron (Aloxi®), when patients receive chemotherapeutic agents with a high potential for inducing nausea/vomiting. The most common adverse effects include mood changes, metallic taste and mild drowsiness.

Benzodiazepines, such as lorazepam (Ativan®) or diazepam (Valium®), are used to treat anticipatory nausea and vomiting due to chemotherapy agents. They are given one to two hours before the course of treatment. The most common adverse effects of these agents include drowsiness, hypotension, urinary retention and hallucinations.

Miscellaneous antiemetics include metoclopramide (Reglan®) and phosphorylated carbohydrate solution (Emetrol®). Emetrol® is used for symptomatic relief of vomiting due to travel sickness, early pregnancy, gastric upset, nervous stomach and food poisoning. Another miscellaneous drug used to treat chemotherapy-induced nausea and vomiting is called aprepitant (Emend®).[12] Aprepitant and its injection form, fosaprepitant (Emend® for Injection), can be used in combination with other anti-nausea drugs to help prevent nausea both right after chemotherapy and nausea and vomiting delayed from chemotherapy. Aprepitant works differently than the other anti-nausea medications and is added to chemotherapy regimens that are highly emetogenic (producing severe nausea and vomiting). Common adverse effects include hiccups, constipation, diarrhea, loss of appetite, dizziness and headaches.

Gastroesophageal Reflux Disease[3]

Gastroesophageal reflux disease (GERD) is a chronic, but treatable condition that occurs as a result of stomach acid backing up into the esophagus and mouth. If left untreated, GERD may lead to esophageal erosion. Patients experiencing GERD will typically present with some, or all, of the following symptoms: heartburn, regurgitation, difficulty swallowing, asthma, noncardiac related chest pain, and water brash. Symptoms may worsen by bending over or laying flat. Patients may see relief of symptoms by lifestyle modifications including: weight loss, smoking cessation, eating smaller meals, refraining from lying down for three hours after eating, and avoiding certain foods (chocolate, alcohol, caffeinated beverages, and highly acidic beverages).

Patients that do not see a resolution of symptoms from dietary modification might have either an endoscopy, barium esophagram, or esophageal pH monitoring test to confirm or refute the diagnosis of GERD. If a patient is unresponsive to dietary and lifestyle modifications, there are a variety of medication treatment options. Antacids are valuable in treating patients with mild symptoms and are available without a prescription. Mucosal protective agents, like sucralfate, are available by prescription and are used for moderate to severe GERD. Promotility agents, like metoclopromide are available by prescription and can be helpful in reducing stomach acid and subsequent reflux as a result of decreased stomach emptying time. Perhaps the most advertised and successful treatment option for GERD are the acid suppressing agents in the H_2 receptor antagonists and proton pump inhibitor class that are available OTC and by prescription.

Acid-Peptic Disease[1]

An open lesion, or ulcer, in the lining of the lower esophagus, stomach or intestines is called a **peptic ulcer**. The GI tract has mechanisms in place to prevent the acid and digestive enzymes from damaging its lining. When the protective mechanisms fail, or are overcome, peptic ulcers can form. Factors that encourage ulcer formation include an excess of acid, the presence of the bacteria *Helicobacter pylori*, and the use of aspirin, nonsteroidal anti-inflammatory drugs (NSAIDs) and corticosteroids. Neutralizing the acidic nature of the stomach, and treating *Helicobacter pylori*, have been shown in studies to lead to the healing of ulcers and preventing ulcer recurrence.

Acid-Peptic Disease Treatments

■ **Antacids[1]**
Eating a meal will stimulate an outpouring of gastric acid. A dose of an antacid, given an hour after a meal, will neutralize the already-produced acid for about two hours. Antacids are effective in healing ulcers when the dose is sufficient and when they are given one to three hours after each meal and at bedtime. Most antacids contain magnesium or aluminum. Magnesium may cause diarrhea, and aluminum may cause constipation. A combination of these two drugs (Maalox®) helps offset the side effects. Calcium carbonate (Tums®) is another antacid that may cause constipation. Magnesium-containing and calcium-containing products must be used cautiously in patients with kidney failure, as they may cause toxicities.

Antacids are available as oral suspensions, swallowable tablets, chewable tablets and soft chews that resemble gum. These drugs are also used to relieve symptoms of refluxing acid into the esophagus, acid indigestion, heartburn and upset stomach. Antacids mostly stay in the GI tract and are eliminated in the stool. They often absorb other drugs, reducing their effect, therefore, spacing the doses of other drugs far apart from antacids is important. Patients may be reluctant to use antacids due to frequent dosing, their chalky taste and their consistency.

■ **Histamine-2 Receptor Antagonists[1]**
Cimetidine (Tagamet®), famotidine (Pepcid®, Pepcid® AC), ranitidine (Zantac®) and nizatidine (Axid®, Axid® AR) are included in the group of histamine-2 (H_2) receptor antagonists. These drugs promote the healing of ulcers by blocking the H_2 receptors in the GI tract and, in turn, reducing the production of acid from other cells. Many studies have proven the effectiveness of H_2 receptor antagonists in the healing of stomach and duodenal ulcers; with continued use, H_2 receptor antagonists have been shown to prevent recurrence of ulcers. All are equally effective and capable of more than a 90 percent reduction in food-stimulated, resting and nocturnal acid production. These drugs may also be prescribed to treat conditions of acid hypersecretion (Zollinger-Ellison Syndrome), to prevent stress-related ulcers in severely ill patients, to prevent upper GI bleeding and to prevent acid reflux into the esophagus.

The H$_2$ receptor antagonists are well-tolerated with few side effects. This tolerability profile has led to H$_2$ antagonists being available as OTC products, as well as by prescription; in some cases, the OTC version is of a lower strength than the prescription version. Recently, however, the Food and Drug Administration (FDA) has approved OTC H$_2$ antagonists with the same strength as the lowest prescription-requiring dose of these drugs. Original dosing recommendations for this class of medications were to take one dose at least twice per day but studies show that a single bedtime dose may be effective for ulcer healing and may result in better compliance. This class of drugs interacts with many drugs. Cimetidine is known to interact and cause increased blood levels of the target drug, such as with warfarin, theophylline, diazepam, and phenytoin, to name a few.

■ **Proton Pump Inhibitors**[1]
By inhibiting the hydrogen-ion pump (the last step in the production of gastric acid), omeprazole (Prilosec®, Prilosec OTC®), esomeprazole (Nexium®), lansoprazole (Prevacid®, Prevacid® 24 HR), rabeprazole (Aciphex®) and pantoprazole (Protonix®) can block almost 100 percent of gastric acid secretion. Dexlansoprazole (Dexilant®), the newest addition to this class, has a unique dual, delayed-release formulation that releases drug at two points in time, allowing it to stay in the body for longer periods.[13] Proton pump inhibitors (PPIs) are better than the H$_2$ receptor antagonists at reducing acid production. These drugs are given once or twice daily for the treatment of an ulcer and are effective for patients with acid reflux into the esophagus. They also are used in combination with antibiotics to treat the ulcer-producing bacteria, *Helicobacter pylori*. In addition, an injectable formulation of pantoprazole is available for short-term treatment of GERD/Zollinger-Ellison syndrome in patients who are unable to tolerate oral medications. FDA released new safety information in May 2010 regarding a possible increased risk of fractures of the hip, wrist and spine with the use of PPIs.[14] It is recommended that patients receiving this class of drug and who are at risk for osteoporosis must also receive Vitamin D supplementation, calcium supplementation and bone-density scans. In addition, health care providers should consider a lower dose or shorter duration of therapy to lessen the impact from decreased vitamin and mineral absorption.

■ **Miscellaneous Drugs**[1]
Misoprostol (Cytotec®) protects the lining of the GI tract and is used to prevent ulcers caused by NSAIDs. The most frequent side effect is diarrhea, especially in higher doses. It can also cause menstrual disorders and miscarriage of pregnancy. A pregnancy test must be conducted, and contraceptives begun, before starting misoprostol in a woman of child-bearing age.

Sucralfate (Carafate®) works by binding to the ulcer forming a protective barrier and it is minimally absorbed. It requires an acid media to form a paste-like substance to be effective. Therefore, sucralfate should not be given with antacids, H$_2$ receptor antagonists or PPIs.

Helicobacter pylori has been implicated as the cause of gastric ulcers in some patients. Eradication of this bacteria may be the focus of ulcer treatment. The most current recommendations for the treatment of this infection include a combination of antibiotics and a PPI. Antibiotics shown to be effective include amoxicillin, metronidazole and clarithromycin.

Bismuth, like sucralfate, also binds to an ulcer, which coats it and protects it from further acid damage. Bismuth subsalicylate has been successful, in combination with other drugs, in the treatment of *Helicobacter pylori* bacterial infections. See Table 1 below for more examples of drugs used to treat acid-peptic disease.

Table 1

Drugs Used to Treat Common GI Tract Disorders[1,15]

Drug Class(es)	Generic Name(s)**	Brand Name(s)**	Indication(s)	Available Dose Form(s)
Adsorbant, Bulk-Forming Laxative	Polycarbophil	FiberCon	Constipation, Diarrhea	Powder, Tablet
Antacid	Aluminum Hydroxide	Alternagel	Heartburn	Suspension
Antacid	Aluminum / Magnesium	Maalox, Mylanta	Heartburn	Chewable Tablet, Liquid
Antacid, Mineral	Calcium Carbonate	Maalox, Oyst-Cal 500, Rolaids, Tums	Heartburn, Osteomalacia, Osteoporosis	Chewable Tablet, Powder, Tablet
Anti-Anxiety: Anti-Nausea, Benzodiazepine	Diazepam (Schedule 4)	Diastat, Diastat Accudial, Valium	Ethanol Withdrawal, Generalized Anxiety Disorder, Muscle Relaxant, Nausea, Panic Disorder, Sedation, Seizures, Vomiting	Injectable, Rectal Gel, Solution, Tablet
Anti-Anxiety: Anti-Nausea, Benzodiazepine	Lorazepam (Schedule 4)	Ativan	Agitation, Ethanol Detoxification, Generalized Anxiety Disorder, Insomnia, Nausea, Seizures, Status Epilepticus, Vomiting	Injectable, Solution, Tablet
Anticholinergic, Anti-Nausea	Scopolamine	Isopto Hyoscine, Scopace, Transderm Scop	Motion Sickness, Nausea, Vomiting	Injectable, Ophthalmic, Patch, Tablet
Anticholinergic, Anti-Nausea	Trimethobenza-mide	Tigan	Nausea, Vomiting	Capsule, Injectable
Anti-Diarrhea: Anti-Motility	Atropine / Diphenoxylate	Logen, Lomonate, Lomotil, Lonox	Diarrhea	Tablet
Anti-Diarrhea: Anti-Motility	Loperamide	Imodium	Diarrhea	Capsule, Liquid, Tablet
Anti-Diarrhea: Anti-Secretory	Bismuth Subsalicylate	Kaopectate, Pepto-Bismol	Diarrhea	Chewable Tablet, Liquid
Anti-Diarrhea: Anti-Secretory	Octreotide	Sandostatin	Diarrhea	Injectable

Table 1 *cont.*
Drugs Used to Treat Common GI Tract Disorders[1,15]

Drug Class(es)	Generic Name(s)**	Brand Name(s)**	Indication(s)	Available Dose Form(s)
Anti-Gas	Simethicone	Gas-X, Mylicon, Phazyme	Flatulence	Capsule, Chewable Tablet, Liquid, Orally-Disintegrating Strips
Antihistamine, Anti-Nausea	Dimenhydrinate	Dramamine	Allergies, Nausea, Vomiting	Chewable Tablet, Injectable, Tablet
Antihistamine, Anti-Nausea	Meclizine	Antivert	Nausea, Vertigo, Vomiting	Chewable Tablet, Tablet
Antihistamine, Anti-Nausea	Diphenhydramine	Benadryl, Unisom	Allergies, Insomnia, Motion Sickness (Nausea), Vomiting	Aerosol, Capsule, Cream, Dissolving Strip, Elixir, Gel, Gel Cap, Injectable, Solution, Syrup, Tablet
Anti-Nausea	Droperidol	Inapsine	Nausea, Vomiting	Injectable
Anti-Nausea: Cannabinoid	Dronabinol	Marinol	Loss of Appetite, Nausea, Vomiting	Capsule
Anti-Nausea: Cannabinoid	Nabilone	Cesamet	Nausea, Vomiting	Capsule
Anti-Nausea, Corticosteroid	Dexamethasone	Decadron	Edema, Nausea, Vomiting	Injectable, Liquid, Tablet
Anti-Nausea: Phenothiazine	Prochlorperazine	Compazine	Nausea, Vomiting	Injectable, Suppository, Tablet
Anti-Nausea: Phenothiazine	Promethazine	Phenergan	Nausea, Vomiting	Injectable, Suppository, Tablet
Anti-Nausea: Phenothiazine / Pain Reliever, Anti-Cough	Promethazine / Codeine (Schedule 5)	Phenergan with Codeine	Cough	Syrup
Anti-Nausea: Prokinetic	Metoclopramide	Reglan	Nausea, Various Bowel Disorders, Vomiting	Injectable, Liquid, Tablet
Anti-Nausea: Serotonin Antagonist	Dolasetron	Anzemet	Nausea, Vomiting	Injectable, Tablet
Anti-Nausea: Serotonin Antagonist	Granisetron	Kytril, Sancuso	Nausea, Vomiting	Injectable, Liquid, Patch, Tablet

Drug Class(es)	Generic Name(s)**	Brand Name(s)**	Indication(s)	Available Dose Form(s)
Anti-Nausea: Serotonin Antagonist	Ondansetron	Zofran	Nausea, Vomiting	Injectable, Liquid, Orally-Disintegrating Tablet, Tablet
Anti-Nausea: Serotonin Antagonist	Palonosetron	Aloxi	Nausea, Vomiting	Injectable
Anti-Nausea: Substance P / Neurokinin-1 Receptor Antagonist	Aprepitant	Emend	Nausea, Vomiting	Capsule
Anti-Nausea: Substance P / Neurokinin-1 Receptor Antagonist	Fosaprepitant	Emend	Nausea, Vomiting	Injectable
Antipsychotic: Anti-Nausea, Neuroleptic	Chlorpromazine	Thorazine	Acute Intermittent Porphyria, Hiccups, Mania, Schizophrenia, Vomiting	Injectable, Tablet
Antipsychotic: Anti-Nausea, Neuroleptic	Perphenazine	Trilafon	Dementia, Ethanol Withdrawal, Huntington's Chorea, Nausea, Reye's Syndrome, Schizophrenia, Spasmodic Torticollis, Tourette's Syndrome, Vomiting	Tablet
Biguanide	Metformin	Glucophage, Glucophage XR	Diabetes	Extended-Release Tablet, Tablet
Biguanide / Sulfonylurea	Glyburide / Metformin	Glucovance	Diabetes	Tablet
Bulk-Forming Laxative	Methylcellulose	Citrucel	Constipation	Powder, Wafer
Bulk-Forming Laxative	Polyethylene Glycol	Miralax	Constipation	Powder

Table 1 *cont.*

Drugs Used to Treat Common GI Tract Disorders[1,15]

Drug Class(es)	Generic Name(s)**	Brand Name(s)**	Indication(s)	Available Dose Form(s)
Bulk-Forming Laxative	Psyllium	Metamucil	Constipation	Capsule, Powder, Wafer
Chloride Channel Activator	Lubiprostone	Amitiza	Constipation	Capsule
Corticosteroid	Budesonide	Entocort, Pulmicort Flexhaler, Pulmicort Respules, Rhinocort Aqua	Allergies, Asthma, Bowel Inflammation	Extended-Release Capsule, Nasal Spray, Powder for Inhalation, Suspension for Inhalation
Corticosteroid	Methylprednis-olone	Depo-Medrol, Medrol, Medrol Dosepak, Solu-Medrol	Acute Asthma Exacerbation, Gout, Osteoarthritis, Rheumatoid Arthritis, Severe Asthma, Skin Inflammation	Injectable, Tablet
Corticosteroid	Prednisolone	Prelone	Acute Asthma Exacerbation, Severe Allergic Reaction, Severe Asthma	Liquid, Syrup, Tablet
Corticosteroid	Prednisone	Deltasone, Sterapred	Acute Asthma Exacerbation, Gout, Rheumatoid Arthritis, Severe Allergic Reaction, Severe Asthma	Liquid, Tablet
Digestive Enzyme	Lactase	Lactaid	Lactose Intolerance (Diarrhea, Gas)	Chewable Tablet, Granules, Milk-Like Products, Tablet
Gastrointestinal Protectant	Sucralfate	Carafate	Gastroesophageal Reflux Disease, Heartburn	Liquid, Tablet
Gastrointestinal Protectant, Uterine Contractant	Misoprostol	Cytotec	Gastroesophageal Reflux Disease, Ulcer Prevention	Tablet
H$_2$ Blocker	Cimetidine	Tagamet	Heartburn	Liquid, Tablet

Drug Class(es)	Generic Name(s)**	Brand Name(s)**	Indication(s)	Available Dose Form(s)
H₂ Blocker	Famotidine	Pepcid	Heartburn	Chewable Tablet, Injectable, Powder Tablet
H₂ Blocker	Nizatidine	Axid, Axid AR	Heartburn	Capsule, Liquid, Tablet
H₂ Blocker	Ranitidine	Zantac	Gastroesophageal Reflux Disease, Heartburn	Capsule, Effervescent Tablet, Injectable, Liquid, Tablet
Hormone	Megestrol	Megace, Megace ES	Loss of Appetite	Liquid, Tablet
Laxative: Hyperosmotic	Lactulose	Kristalose	Constipation, Hepatic Encephalopathy	Powder, Solution
Osmotic	Magnesium Salts	Milk of Magnesia	Constipation	Liquid
Osmotic	Sodium Phosphates	Fleet Enema	Constipation	Enema
Proton Pump Inhibitor	Dexlansoprazole	Dexilant	Gastroesophageal Reflux Disease, Heartburn	Capsule
Proton Pump Inhibitor	Esomeprazole	Nexium	Gastroesophageal Reflux Disease, Heartburn	Capsule, Granules, Injectable
Proton Pump Inhibitor	Lansoprazole	Prevacid, Prevacid 24 HR	Gastroesophageal Reflux Disease, Heartburn	Capsule, Orally-Disintegrating Tablet
Proton Pump Inhibitor	Omeprazole	Prilosec, Prilosec OTC	Gastroesophageal Reflux Disease, Heartburn	Capsule, Granules, Tablet
Proton Pump Inhibitor	Pantoprazole	Protonix	Gastroesophageal Reflux Disease, Heartburn	Granules, Injectable, Tablet
Proton Pump Inhibitor	Rabeprazole	Aciphex	Acid-Peptic Disease	Tablet
Serotonin Agonist	Tegaserod	Zelnorm	Constipation	Tablet
Stimulant Laxative	Bisacodyl	Dulcolax	Constipation	Suppository, Tablet
Stimulant / Laxative Stool Softener	Docusate / Senna	Peri-Colace, Senokot-S	Constipation	Capsule, Tablet
Stool Softener	Docusate	Colace	Constipation	Capsule, Liquid

Table 1 *cont.*

Drugs Used to Treat Common GI Tract Disorders[1,15]

Drug Class(es)	Generic Name(s)**	Brand Name(s)**	Indication(s)	Available Dose Form(s)
Systemic Alkalizer	Sodium Bicarbonate	Neut	Antacid, Systemic or Urinary Inappropriate Acidity	Tablet
Vitamin: Water-Soluble	Cyanocobalamin (Vitamin B_{12})	Nascobal	Vitamin B_{12} Deficiency	Extended-Release Tablet, Injectable, Lozenge, Nasal Spray, Solution, Sublingual Tablet, Tablet

**All rights to all brand names and trademarks are held by their respective owners. There may be additional brand names for some of the products listed.*

Conclusion

The GI tract is affected not only by what the body consumes, but also by disease states in the body and the treatment of those diseases. Pharmacy technicians in all practice settings need to be knowledgeable about how the normal GI tract functions and the types of medications used to treat the disorders affecting the digestive system.

References

1. Michigan Pharmacists Association, Pharmacy Certified Technician Training Manual, 9th edition, Lansing, MI, 2004.

2. Vander, A., Sherman, J., Luciano, D., "The Digestion and Absorption of Food," Human Physiology, The Mechanisms of Body Function, New York, NY, 2001, pp. 553-591.

3. Chisholm, M., Jackson, M., "Chapter 31, Evaluation of the Gastrointestinal Tract," Pharmacotherapy: A Pathophysiologic Approach, 5th edition, New York, NY, 2002, pp. 575-584.

4. Intestine, World Book Encyclopedia Millennium 2000, Chicago, IL, 2000, p. 353.

5. Avraham, R., "The Digestive System," Chelsea House, 2000, p. 52.

6. Ganiats, T.G., Norcross, W.A., Halverson, A.L. et al, "Does Beano prevent gas?: a double-blind crossover study of oral alpha-galactosidase to treat dietary oligosaccharide intolerance," *Journal of Family Practice*, San Diego, Vol. 39, N5, pp. 441-445, November 1994.

7. Spruill, W.J., Wade, W.E., "Chapter 38, Diarrhea, Constipation, and Irritable Bowel Syndrome," Pharmacotherapy: A Pathophysiologic Approach, 7th edition, New York, NY, 2008, p. 627.

8. U.S. Food and Drug Administration, "Zelnorm (tegaserod maleate) Information," www.fda.gov, Aug. 2, 2010.

9. Amitiza prescribing information, Bethesda, MD, Sucampo Pharmaceuticals, Inc., May 2009.

10. Relistor prescribing information, Philadelphia, PA, Wyeth Pharmaceuticals, Inc., May 2010.

11. Ashton, C.H., "Adverse effects of cannabis and cannabinoids," *British Journal of Anaesthesia*, Newcastle upon Tyne, United Kingdom, Vol. 83, N4, pp. 637-649, 1999.

12. Aprepitant prescribing information, Whitehouse Station, NJ, Merck and Company, Inc., March 2010.

13. Abel, C., Desilets, A.R., Willett, K., "Dexlansoprazole in the treatment of esophagitis and gastroesophageal reflux disease," *The Annals of Pharmacotherapy*, Vol. 44, pp. 871-877, May 2010.

14. U.S. Food and Drug Administration, "FDA Drug Safety Communication: Possible increased risk of fractures of the hip, wrist, and spine with the use of proton pump inhibitors," www.fda.gov, Aug. 2, 2010.

15. Lexi-Comp, Inc. (Lexi-Drugs™), July 26, 2010.

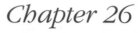

Chapter 26
REVIEW QUESTIONS

1. What is the purpose of the digestive system?
   a. To break down food and store nutrients in the liver
   b. To break down food and absorb nutrients
   c. To break down food and excrete nutrients
   d. To break down food and stimulate growth

2. What is the action of the anti-flatulent simethicone?
   a. It acts by some unknown means
   b. It produces a film that collapses gas bubbles and prevents the bubbles from being trapped in the GI tract
   c. It stimulates intestinal absorption
   d. It binds with bacteria on the intestinal mucosa

3. Which of the following drugs used to treat diarrhea should not be given to children?
   a. Any drug containing bismuth subsalicylate
   b. Pepto-Bismol®
   c. Kaopectate®
   d. All of the above

4. Which of the following is a drug that acts systematically to treat diarrhea by suppressing peristalsis?
   a. Diphenoxylate
   b. Methylnaltrexone
   c. Tegaserod
   d. Octreotide

5. Which is true regarding stimulant laxatives?
   a. They take several days to work
   b. They work by drawing water into the intestine
   c. They can be used frequently over a long period of time
   d. They cause a rapid evacuation of the bowel

6. Which of the following is an emollient laxative (stool softener)?
   a. Senna
   b. Bisacodyl
   c. Docusate sodium
   d. Lubiprostone

7. Which of the following drugs used as an antiemetic requires a prescription?
   a. Dimenhydrinate
   b. Diphenhydramine
   c. Emetrol
   d. Scopolamine

8. Which of the following drugs is not used to treat chemotherapy-induced nausea and vomiting?
   a. Metoclopramide
   b. Methylnaltrexone
   c. Aprepitant
   d. Dexamethasone

9. Which of the following has not been shown to encourage peptic ulcer formation?
   a. Excess of gastric acid
   b. Aspirin
   c. Spicy foods
   d. *Helicobacter pylori*

10. Which of the following drugs does not decrease gastric acid?
    a. Sucralfate
    b. Ranitidine
    c. Calcium carbonate
    d. Omeprazole

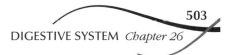

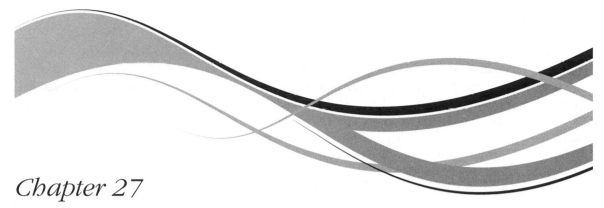

Chapter 27

HEPATIC SYSTEM

By Linda J. Stuckey, Pharm.D., BCPS

Learning Objectives

This chapter seeks to prepare a pharmacy technician to:

- describe the structure of the liver.
- understand the role of the different cells that comprise the liver.
- identify the functions of the liver.
- define cirrhosis and understand the complications from cirrhosis.
- list the drugs that are commonly used to treat the complications of cirrhosis.
- explain the differences between the forms of viral hepatitis.

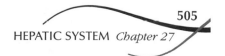

Introduction

The **liver** is the largest visceral organ in the body, weighing about three pounds, with its size and shape depending on body shape (see Figure 1). The liver is located on the right side of the abdomen, just under the lower rib cage and the diaphragm. It is partially protected by the rib cage and it partially covers the stomach. The liver is anchored in the abdomen by the falciform ligament, which attaches to both the diaphragm and the abdominal wall. The liver consists of two lobes: a large right lobe and smaller left lobe. Each lobe contains hundreds of cells, a network of blood vessels and channels. These components, which will be further discussed in the next section, intertwine with each other to provide the functions of the liver.[1]

Figure 1
Liver Anatomy

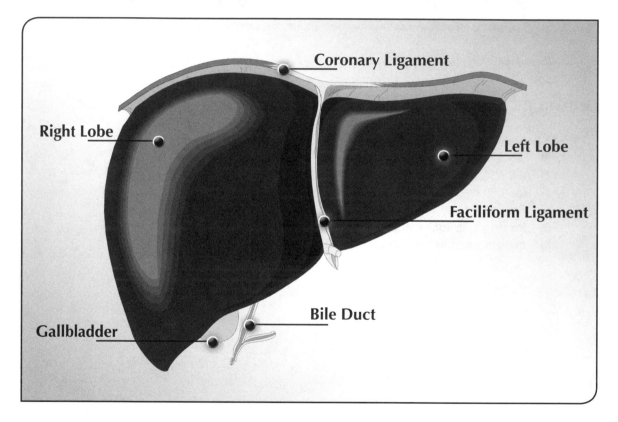

Microscopic Level

Hepatocytes are the main worker cells of the liver, and there are about 100 billion hepatocytes in an adult liver (accounting for about 66 percent of the total weight of the organ). Since they are the worker cells, they control many of the functions of the liver, such as synthesizing essential proteins, producing bile, regulating nutrients and breaking down chemicals. Hepatocytes have the ability to regenerate if a portion of the liver is lost, or surgically removed, as in those undergoing living-donor liver transplantation.

Hepatic sinusoids are channels between the hepatocytes that receive oxygenated blood from the hepatic artery and nutrient-rich blood, which does not contain oxygen, from the portal vein. Sinusoids connect and bring the blood to the central vein, which then flows into hepatic veins leading to the inferior vena cava.

Kupffer cells are responsible for defense; they are killer cells that destroy worn-out red and white blood cells, bacteria and other foreign matter that present to the liver from the blood flow draining from the upper gastrointestinal tract. Kupffer cells are present in the sinusoids.

Endothelial cells line the hepatic sinusoids. These cells are different from other endothelial cells that are located in other areas of the body since they are perforated by larger pores that allow passage of molecules out of the blood into the liver. Albumin and lipoproteins are the main molecules that pass through these pores, while formed elements such as white blood cells, red blood cells and platelets are denied passage.

Bile is a yellow-green product that is produced in the hepatocytes. It is a mixture of bile salts, bile pigments known as bilirubin, cholesterol, phospholipids and electrolytes. Bile salts and cholesterol mechanically break up and emulsify fats. **Bile canaliculi** are small ducts between hepatocytes that collect bile. The bile then travels through the bile ducts that carry it away from the hepatocytes to the small intestine. Bile drains from the right and left hepatic ducts that form the **common bile duct**.

The portal vein, hepatic artery and the common bile duct form the **portal triad**.[2]

Blood Supply

The liver receives blood from the hepatic artery and the portal vein. The hepatic artery supplies approximately 20 percent of the liver's blood supply, while the portal vein supplies approximately 80 percent. The hepatic portal vein receives blood from the capillaries of the digestive organs and delivers blood to the sinusoids. The venous blood from the capillaries contains nutrients from the gastrointestinal tract. The hepatic artery delivers oxygen-rich blood to the sinusoids. The sinusoids allow for a place for the nonoxygen-rich and the oxygen-rich blood to mix, which allows certain chemical reactions to occur that are necessary for nutrient processing, and then the mixed blood, which is now deoxygenated, exits the liver through the **hepatic veins**. Hepatic veins connect into the inferior vena cava; the inferior vena cava connects directly into the heart.

Physiology

The liver provides many functions that support life. One of the main functions is its ability to metabolize, or break down, nutrients and substances that are ingested. Three nutrients in particular that are metabolized by the liver are carbohydrates, lipids and proteins. The liver performs **carbohydrate metabolism** with the goal of maintaining normal blood glucose levels (especially after a meal has been ingested). This occurs, in part, by breaking down stored glucose (stored as **glycogen** in the liver) to **glucose** and then releasing that glucose into the bloodstream. The liver also converts glucose found in the blood, above what is needed by the body, into glycogen stores for when they are needed. Further, the liver uses many other substances found in food to make many other chemicals that the body uses (e.g., triglycerides).

The goal of **lipid metabolism** is generating energy and storing fats. The liver breaks down fatty acids to generate **adenosine triphosphate (ATP)**; ATP is the base energy molecule used by most cells in the body. The liver also synthesizes cholesterol, bile salts and lipoproteins.

Protein metabolism provides energy and stores nutrients that may be used later. The liver removes amino acid from the blood that can be utilized for ATP production (or be converted into carbohydrates or fats). The liver's protein metabolism also converts toxic ammonia into urea, which is less toxic, for excretion in the urine. In addition, the liver synthesizes blood proteins (such as albumin, prothrombin and fibrinogen). **Albumin** maintains blood volume, while **prothrombin** and **fibrinogen** are essential clotting proteins.

Along with the metabolism of the above nutrients, the liver breaks down drugs and other substances, such as alcohol, in order to protect the body from toxic injury. The body also regularly cycles the circulating hormones, such as estrogen, thyroid hormones and aldosterone, and the liver functions to remove hormones that are no longer needed from the system. The liver also secretes drugs, such as penicillin and erythromycin, into bile to be eliminated from the system.

The liver is responsible for the excretion of bilirubin. **Bilirubin** is a waste product from red blood cells and is absorbed by the liver from the blood and secreted into bile. Bilirubin is eventually metabolized by bacteria in the small intestine and eliminated in feces.[3]

The liver is also a storage place for chemicals other than glucose (e.g., vitamins and minerals). In particular, the fat-soluble vitamins (vitamins A, D, E and K), vitamin B_{12}, iron and copper are all stored there and released from the liver when needed. The liver is one place where vitamin D is activated from vitamin D precursors stored in the body.

Liver Disorders

Because the liver has many important functions for life, and because many complex processes occur there, any failure of the liver to perform can be devastating. Liver failure is the 12th leading cause of death in the United States.[4] Liver disorders can be divided according to the type of injury that has led to the dysfunction of the liver. Diseases of the cells of the liver, such as viral hepatitis and alcoholic liver disease, cause injury by inappropriate, persistent inflammation leading to cells no longer functioning normally and therefore dying off (called **necrosis**). Disease of the processes surrounding bile (formation, storage, flow, etc.) cause injury by building up chemicals that are meant to be excreted from the body through the bile-intestinal elimination process. Drug-induced liver disease often shows signs of both cellular damage and a breakdown in the bile process. Initial symptoms of liver disease can present as **jaundice** (yellowing of the skin and/or whites of the eyes), fatigue, itching, right upper quadrant pain, abdominal distention and intestinal bleeding. Many times, patients may have no symptoms of liver disease; a diagnosis of liver disease is often made based on repeated abnormal laboratory values from routine blood draws.

Chronic liver disease, or chronic exposure to liver toxins (including alcohol), can cause cirrhosis. **Cirrhosis** occurs when tough, nonfunctional, fibrous tissue replaces liver cells that have died from being exposed to toxic substances. Even though liver cells can regenerate, it takes a long time, and many repeated cell deaths in an area, for a section of the liver to become cirrhotic. With fewer functioning liver cells available to do the liver's work, complications develop because the liver fails to process all of the chemicals that it needs to; this can ultimately lead to death if the buildup of toxins in the body overwhelm the system. Complications from cirrhosis, and from other chronic liver diseases, will be the focus of the rest of this section.

■ **Portal Hypertension**
Portal hypertension is increased resistance (pressure) to blood flowing from the intestines through the liver and into the inferior vena cava. The resistance may be caused by a blockage in the liver, by a decrease in liver function or by an unmanageable increase in blood coming from the intestines. When the blood traveling through the portal vein reaches the peak capacity of sinusoids available to process that blood, the excess blood pools until it finds alternate routes back to the systemic circulation. Portal hypertension, by itself, is a concern, but it is not directly life-threatening; how the body deals with portal hypertension can be far worse, and that is why it is important to treat portal hypertension. The treatment goal is to prevent the formation of **varices** (covered below). Nonselective beta blockers are the first line in preventing variceal bleeding in patients with small varices.[5,6] Beta blockers will reduce the portal pressure and may delay variceal growth. The most common beta blockers (see Table 1) used for portal hypertension are nadolol and propranolol; however, carvedilol has been recently studied for this use.[6] Beta blockers must be titrated up according to heart rate, with the goal rate of 55-60 beats/minute. Other side effects from beta blockers include fatigue and shortness of breath. Nitrates are no longer recommended for primary prevention of varices due to

insufficient evidence of effectiveness compared to beta blockers, which have significant evidence of effectiveness.[7] Patients who have larger varices may need surgery in addition to drug therapy.

Table 1
Portal Hypertension Medications

Drug Class(es)	Generic Name(s)**	Brand Name(s)**	Indication(s)	Available Dose Form(s)
Antidysrhythmic, Antihypertensive: Beta Blocker	Propranolol	Inderal, Inderal LA, Innopran XL	Acute Coronary Syndrome, Aggressive Behavior, Angina, Anxiety, Dysrhythmias, Heart Attack Prevention, High Blood Pressure, Migraine Prophylaxis, Parkinson's Tremor, Portal Hypertension	Extended-Release Capsule, Injectable, Solution, Tablet
Antihypertensive: Alpha / Beta Blocker	Carvedilol	Coreg, Coreg CR	High Blood Pressure, Portal Hypertension	Extended-Release Capsule, Tablet
Antihypertensive: Beta Blocker	Nadolol	Corgard	Acute Coronary Syndrome, Heart Failure, High Blood Pressure, Portal Hypertension	Tablet

**All rights to all brand names and trademarks are held by their respective owners.

■ Gastroesophageal Varices

When portal hypertension becomes too great or goes untreated for too long, the body will actually grow new blood vessels to relieve the pressure. Often, these vessels grow in such a way as to avoid the liver so that the blood can flow back into systemic circulation. These "bypass" vessels are known as varices. Varices can form between any points along the gastro-intestinal tract; however, a common place for varices to form is to and from the esophagus. As portal hypertension increases and persists, the demand on these varices grows; the body, in response, grows the varices to accommodate its blood flow needs. A measure that can be used to predict when varices will grow is the comparison of the portal venous pressure to the vena cava pressure. Portal pressure is normally 9 mmHg, and pressure in the inferior vena cava is normally between 2 and 6 mmHg. Normally, therefore, the difference is 3 mmHg to 7 mmHg; if the difference exceeds 7 mmHg, or the portal pressure exceeds 12 mmHg, then it is expected that any varices are growing in response to the body's blood flow demands. Growing varices increase the risk of bleeding internally into places, such as the stomach or intestines, where blood is not usually found; bleeding occurs in about 25-40 percent of patients with cirrhosis. A bleeding episode in a patient with cirrhosis has a 25-30 percent chance of being fatal.[4] Patients who experience one episode of variceal bleeding have a 60

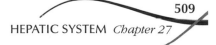

percent chance of having a second episode.[6] Considering the fatality rate and the seriousness of such a bleed, acute variceal hemorrhage is considered a medical emergency. The first major sign of a bleeding episode is often vomiting blood or finding blood in the stool. Management of an acute bleed is generally done in an intensive care setting and includes IV fluids to maintain systemic blood flow, blood products to promote clotting and replace blood lost from the systemic circulation, vasoconstrictor agents to minimize blood loss and antibiotics to prevent infections from entering the systemic circulation through the bleeding location.[7] Vasoconstrictor agents available in the U.S. include octreotide and vasopressin. Both agents can decrease portal blood flow and pressure; however, octreotide does not cause systemic vasoconstriction or elevation in systemic blood pressure, due to its selectivity for the portal system. Vasopressin is less selective and, therefore, leads to an increase in systemic blood pressure. Octreotide may be given as either an intravenous infusion or as a subcutaneous injection (see Table 2). Once the patient is stabilized, then endoscopic intervention, such as sclerotherapy or band ligation, is often recommended. Patients who present with a bleeding episode have a high risk of infection (especially sepsis). Broad-spectrum antibiotics must be used to prevent such infections. After the bleeding episode is under control, therapies must be initiated to prevent a second bleed from occurring. Isosorbide mononitrate is currently being studied, in combination with beta blockers, for prevention of a second variceal bleed.[6]

Table 2
Gastroesophageal Varices Medications

Drug Class(es)	Generic Name(s)**	Brand Name(s)**	Indication(s)	Available Dose Form(s)
Anti-Anginal: Nitrate	Isosorbide Mononitrate	ImDur, ISMO, Monoket	Acute Coronary Syndrome, Chest Pain, Coronary Artery Disease, Variceal Bleeding	Extended-Release Capsule, Injectable, Solution, Tablet
Anti-Diarrhea: Anti-Secretory	Octreotide	Sandostatin	Diarrhea, Variceal Bleeding	Injectable
Hormone	Vasopressin	Pitressin	Cardiac Arrest, Shock, Traumatic Brain Injury, Variceal Bleeding	Tablet

**All rights to all brand names and trademarks are held by their respective owners.

■ Ascites

The term **ascites** comes from the Greek word askos, meaning wineskin (or water bag).[8] It is the accumulation of serous fluid within the abdominal cavity, resulting from portal hypertension. Portal hypertension can cause increased systemic blood pressure; the body's natural response to try and lower that pressure is to dilate the arteries. However, since the increase in pressure is accompanied by a decrease in circulating blood (the opposite of what the body is geared for), this causes a significant decrease in blood pressure in the body's arteries. This is a more serious threat to the body, and so the body reacts to correct this problem. The body seeks to keep the arteries dilated, but it calls for more fluid to enter the blood stream. This is done by activating the systems in the kidneys that hold back both sodium and water, and that leads to more fluid being left in the blood and less going to the urine. Further, to try to restore an overall balance, the body, after realizing that all of these actions were probably overreactions, will spill excess hepatic lymph fluid into the abdominal cavity to reduce the overall fluid excess created by the previous actions.[8] Development of ascites can be an early sign of cirrhosis and has led to a poor prognosis. Symptoms of ascites include abdominal pain, shortness of breath, loss of appetite and leg swelling. Ascites can be classified according to severity: grade 1 (mild), grade 2 (moderate) and grade 3 (severe).[8]

Treatment of ascites is usually a combination of lifestyle modification and pharmacological therapy. Abstinence from alcohol and sodium restriction are important lifestyle modifications that can improve ascites. Sodium must be limited to less than 2,000 mg/day.[6] If lifestyle modifications are failing, then the addition of diuretic therapy can be utilized to reduce the swelling and ascites. Aldosterone receptor antagonists, specifically spironolactone, are the first-line therapy (see Table 3).[9] These agents work at the kidneys to increase sodium excretion, leading to decreased edema (swelling). Spironolactone, however, has several potential side effects that can complicate therapy: high blood potassium, **gynecomastia** (growth of male mammary glands) and headaches. Eplerenone is another aldosterone receptor antagonist that could be used; it has a lower incidence of gynecomastia than seen with aldosterone. Eplerenone, though, has not been studied in liver failure, so it is not routinely recommended. If spironolactone cannot be tolerated, amiloride is the second-line option.[8] It is less effective than spironolactone, but it does not cause gynecomastia.[6]

Loop diuretics, such as furosemide or bumetanide, are other agents used for ascites management in combination with spironolactone. Together, they provide greater fluid removal than furosemide alone;[6] however, the combination places the patient at higher risk of developing kidney failure. Furosemide and bumetanide can cause low potassium, low sodium and kidney failure.

When ascites becomes classified as grade 3, the abdominal distention and discomfort can interfere with activities of daily living. Patients not only require high-dose diuretic therapy (up to spironolactone 400 mg daily and furosemide 100 mg daily) but also large-dose paracentesis. **Paracentesis** is an invasive procedure that drains fluid from the abdomen. This procedure, to alleviate symptoms, does not address the underlying cause, but it can allow a short-term improvement of a patient's condition. During a large volume paracentesis (removing greater than 5 L), intravenous albumin is infused while the fluid is removed. Since albumin helps maintain blood volume, the patient will have a lower risk of developing circulatory dysfunction due to the lack of fluid now present after the procedure.[6] Albumin is derived from large pools of human albumin, and it is classified as a biological agent and available in concentrations of either 5 or 25 percent.[10] Since it is from human sources, albumin can cause allergic reactions, including severe (anaphylactic) reactions, during the infusion. Albumin must be inspected visually for turbidity (cloudiness) and discoloration prior to administration.[10]

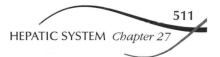

Table 3
Ascites Medications

Drug Class(es)	Generic Name(s)**	Brand Name(s)**	Indication(s)	Available Dose Form(s)
Diuretic: Aldosterone Antagonist, Potassium-Sparing	Eplerenone	Inspra	High Blood Pressure	Tablet
Diuretic: Aldosterone Antagonist, Potassium-Sparing	Spironolactone	Aldactone	Edema, Heart Failure, High Blood Pressure	Tablet
Diuretic: Loop Diuretic	Bumetanide	Bumex	Edema, Heart Failure, High Blood Pressure	Injectable, Solution, Tablet
Diuretic: Loop Diuretic	Furosemide	Lasix	Edema, High Blood Pressure	Injectable, Solution, Tablet
Diuretic: Potassium-Sparing	Amiloride	Midamor	High Blood Pressure	Tablet
Plasma Volume Expander	Albumin	Albumar-5, Albumar-25, Buminate, Flexbumin 25%	Low Plasma Volume	Injectable

**All rights to all brand names and trademarks are held by their respective owners.*

■ **Spontaneous Bacterial Peritonitis**

A complication from ascites is an infection in pre-existing ascitic fluid with no other source of infection. This is called **spontaneous bacterial peritonitis (SBP)**. It can occur in 10-30 percent of patients who have cirrhosis and can have a mortality rate as high as 30-50 percent.[11] SBP is thought to be caused by a combination of processes: altered gut permeability, bacterial overgrowth and suppression of the defense cells. Bacteria present in the intestine migrate across the intestinal walls into the abdominal cavity, leading to the infection. These bacteria are primarily gram-negative organisms, specifically *Escherichia coli* and *Klebsellia pneumonia*. Signs and symptoms of SBP include fever, increased white blood cell count, abdominal pain, altered mental status and rebound tenderness. If SBP is not treated promptly, it can cause sepsis, leading to death. Antibiotic choices (see Table 4) will initially be empiric (i.e., based on the expectation that the bacteria causing the problem is a typical bacteria that is susceptible to the typical antibiotics usually used for that organism). Third-generation cephalosporins, such as ceftriaxone and cefotaxime, are the first-line antibiotics for SBP since they are highly potent against *Escherichia coli* and *Klebsellia pneumonia*.[9] Then, after a culture is grown from fluid collected from the patient's abdomen, a more selective antibiotic is usually chosen to complete the total therapy of five to 10 days that is usually required to clear this type of infection.[9] Since ceftriaxone and cefotaxime are both intravenous therapies, patients may not be able to be at home during this phase of the treatment; either someone able to establish an IV must come to the patient's home or the patient must stay in a facility with skilled nurses to receive these drugs. An oral fluoroquinolone, such as ciprofloxacin, is an alternative treatment for SBP. SBP treatment can be switched to ciprofloxacin after three to five days of intravenous antibiotics to finish the course.[8] Ciprofloxacin is well tolerated by patients; renal function must be closely monitored, in addition to monitoring for tendon rupture, in all patients receiving ciprofloxacin.

Within one year of a first instance of SBP, patients are at a 70 percent risk of having a second episode; it is generally recommended to use prophylactic antibiotics for any patient who has experienced a single episode of SBP.[10] Patients who are at a high risk for recurrence have the following risk factors: prior SBP episode, variceal hemorrhage and low-protein ascites.[9] Oral antibiotic therapy includes norfloxacin 400 mg daily or sulfamethoxazole/trimethoprim daily.[10] Both of these therapies are successful in preventing against SBP.[9] Alternative therapies include ciprofloxacin 750 mg weekly and sulfamethoxazole/trimethoprim (double strength) daily for five of seven days each week.[10] Administering intermittent antibiotic regimens may be successful in preventing SBP, but these courses could also increase the risk of bacterial resistance.[9]

Table 4
Spontaneous Bacterial Peritonitis Medications

Drug Class(es)	Generic Name(s)**	Brand Name(s)**	Indication(s)	Available Dose Form(s)
Antibiotic: Antiprozal, Sulfonamide	Sulfamethoxazole, Trimethoprim	Bactrim, Septra	Bacterial Infection, Pneumocystis, Pneumonia Prophylaxis	Injectable, Suspension, Tablet
Antibiotic: Cephalosporin	Cefotaxime	Claforan	Bacterial Infection	Injectable
Antibiotic: Cephalosporin	Ceftriaxone	Rocephin	Bacterial Infection	Injectable
Antibiotic: Fluoroquinolone	Ciprofloxacin	Cetraxal, Ciloxan, Cipro, Cipro XR, Proquin XR	Bacterial Infection	Injectable, Ophthalmic, Otic, Suspension, Tablet
Antibiotic: Fluoroquinolone	Norfloxacin	Noroxin	Bacterial Infection	Tablet

**All rights to all brand names and trademarks are held by their respective owners.

■ **Hepatic Encephalopathy**
Hepatic encephalopathy (HE) is a central nervous system disturbance resulting in many neuropsychiatric symptoms associated with liver disease or failure. It occurs in 20-60 percent of patients with liver disease.[12] Symptoms may range from forgetfulness and mild confusion to disorientation, amnesia and coma.[13] The proposed mechanism of hepatic encephalopathy is the accumulation of gut-derived nitrogenous substances in the systemic circulation.[13] The most common substance is ammonia; however, other substances, such as manganese and gamma-aminobutyric acid (GABA), can also accumulate.[4] Zinc deficiency has also been linked to the development of HE.[13] Ammonia is released from the kidney and muscles, and is

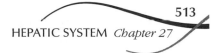

usually metabolized in the liver to a nontoxic substance. Ammonia accumulation can lead to swelling of **astrocytes**, which are the primary cells that metabolize ammonia in the brain.[13] Acute HE is defined as symptoms occurring for less than four weeks and can occur because of short-term stressors. Stressors that commonly lead a patient with liver disease to experience HE include gastrointestinal bleeding, infection, electrolyte abnormalities, sedative ingestion, dietary excesses, constipation and renal insufficiency.[4]

Treatment of HE includes avoidance of stressors, modification of lifestyle and management with medications. Since animal proteins are converted to ammonia at a greater rate than vegetable proteins, patients are encouraged to reduce their overall dietary protein intake if they are at risk for HE, and to make plant proteins their main source of dietary protein.[14] The mainstays of treatment are nonabsorbable disaccharides and nonabsorbable antibiotics (see Table 5). What is meant by "nonabsorbable" is that these drugs do not pass from the intestines into the body; rather, these agents simply pass through the intestinal tract and take unwanted chemicals with them. The most common disaccharide is lactulose. **Lactulose** inhibits ammonia production and traps available ammonia for excretion.[15] Lactulose can be dosed orally or rectally as a solution. Lactulose rectal enemas are made by mixing 300 mL (200 g) of lactulose into 700 mL of saline. Lactulose enemas are given every four hours as needed. Lactulose is given orally at a starting dose of 30-60 mL every one to two hours, and then the dose is adjusted to achieve two to four regular (semi-soft) stools every 24 hours. Lactulose has demonstrated efficacy for HE, and it is the first-line therapy for HE.[15] Some patients find the abdominal bloating, cramping, diarrhea and flatulence that may accompany the use of lactulose to be intolerable.

Nonabsorbable antibiotics are utilized when patients are intolerant or are not responding to lactulose. These antibiotics can reduce the population of enteric bacteria that produce ammonia.[12] Neomycin is the most common antibiotic used for this treatment since it has good gram-negative coverage. Neomycin is administered orally by giving 1 g every six hours. Side effects of neomycin can be severe (such as renal failure and hearing loss); however, these effects are less likely to occur when neomycin is given orally (rather than parenterally) due to the limited absorption of the drug into the systemic circulation.[15] Other antibiotics that have been studied include metronidazole and vancomycin. Metronidazole was found to have similar efficacy when compared to neomycin in small studies; however, toxicities of metronidazole include gastrointestinal side effects and neurotoxicity.[15] Using oral vancomycin for HE is more likely to lead to bacterial resistance to vancomycin than using intravenous vancomycin, therefore, it is not recommended for use in HE unless all other therapy options have failed or are inappropriate.[15] Another antibiotic that has been used more frequently for HE is rifaximin. Rifaximin is an oral antibiotic that has minimal systemic absorption, resulting in minimal side effects (such as headache, flatulence, abdominal pain, constipation, nausea and rash). It has been studied in comparison to lactulose and neomycin, and has similar efficacy in HE.[16] Other alternative therapies for HE include branched-chain amino acids (BCAA), zinc supplementation, acarbose and probiotics.[15]

Table 5
Hepatic Encephalopathy Medications

Drug Class(es)	Generic Name(s)**	Brand Name(s)**	Indication(s)	Available Dose Form(s)
Antibiotic	Rifaximin	Xifaxan	Hepatic Encephalopathy, Traveler's Diarrhea	Tablet
Antibiotic	Vancomycin	Vancocin	Bacterial Infection	Capsule, Injectable
Antibiotic: Aminoglycoside	Neomycin	Neo-Fradin	Bacterial Infection	Solution, Tablet
Antibiotic: Anti-Anaerobe	Metronidazole	Flagyl, Flagyl ER	Bacterial Infection	Capsule, Extended-Release Tablet, Injectable, Tablet
Laxative: Hyperosmotic	Lactulose	Kristalose	Constipation, Hepatic Encephalopathy	Powder, Solution

**All rights to all brand names and trademarks are held by their respective owners.*

■ **Coagulation**

One of the functions of the liver is to synthesize clotting factors. Liver failure can cause a reduction in the synthesis of **coagulation** factors, increased consumption of factors and Vitamin K deficiency.[17] These factors result in an increased prothrombin and, thus, an increased risk of bleeding. Prothrombin time prolongation is related to the severity of the liver disease and decreased synthetic activity in the liver. Management of coagulopathy must be considered if bleeding is present or if an invasive procedure or surgery is in the immediate future.[18] Treatments include fresh frozen plasma, cryoprecipitate, recombinant activated factor VII and plasmapheresis.[17]

■ **Viral Hepatitis**

Hepatitis is an inflammation in the liver. It can cause hepatocellular injury, leading to liver injury, inflammation and necrosis. Viral hepatitis is the leading cause of liver failure and liver cancer, and is one of the most common causes of acute liver disease.[19] Roughly 4.4 million Americans are living with chronic hepatitis; most of them are unaware that they have it.[19] The most common viruses in the U.S. that cause liver disease are hepatitis A, hepatitis B and hepatitis C. Hepatitis A is the only virus that does not lead to chronic infection, while hepatitis C is the leading indication for liver transplantation. Table 6 compares hepatitis A, B and C, while Table 7 lists medications utilized to treat hepatitis.[20-25]

Table 6

Comparison of Hepatitis A, B and C

	Hepatitis A Virus (HAV)	Hepatitis B Virus (HBV)	Hepatitis C Virus (HCV)
U.S. Statistics	~25,000 new infections in 2007 -HAV rates decreased by 92 percent with vaccine	~43,000 new infections in 2007 ~1.2 million with chronic HBV infections	~17,000 new infections in 2007 ~3.2 million with chronic HCV infections
Routes of Transmission	Oral-fecal route: -Person-to-person contact -Sexual contact -Ingestion of contaminated food / drinks	Infected blood and bodily fluids: -Birth to an infected mother -Sexual contact -Sharing needles, syringes -Needle sticks	Infected blood: -Sharing needles, syringes -Sexual contact -Birth to an infected mother -Needle sticks
Persons at Risk	-Travelers to regions with high rates of HAV -Men who have sex with men -Illegal drug users (injection and non-injection)	-Infants born to infected mothers -Sex partners of infected partners -Persons with multiple sex partners -Men who have sex with men -Injection drug users -Household contacts of persons with chronic HBV -Health care and public safety workers -Hemodialysis patients -Residents and staff of facilities for developmentally disabled persons -Travelers to regions with high HBV	-Current or former drug users -Recipients of clotting factor concentrates before 1987 -Recipients of blood transfusions or transplants before 1992 -Chronic hemodialysis patients -Health care workers after needle sticks -HIV-infected persons -Children born to HCV infected mothers

	Hepatitis A Virus (HAV)	Hepatitis B Virus (HBV)	Hepatitis C Virus (HCV)
Signs and Symptoms of Acute Infection	-Asymptomatic in young children (< 6 yrs) -Fever -Fatigue -Loss of appetite -Nausea/vomiting -Abdominal pain -Dark urine -Clay-colored bowel movements -Joint pain -Jaundice	-Fever -Fatigue -Loss of appetite -Nausea/vomiting -Abdominal pain -Dark urine -Clay-colored bowel movements -Joint pain -Jaundice	-Fever -Fatigue -Loss of appetite -Nausea/vomiting -Abdominal pain -Dark urine -Clay-colored bowel movements -Joint pain -Jaundice
Treatment	-No medication available -Supportive care	-Acute: supportive care -Chronic: regular monitoring of antivirals (see Table 7)	-Acute: supportive care -Chronic: regular monitoring of antivirals (see Table 7)
Vaccine is Recommended for:	-All children at 1 year -Travelers going to regions with high rates of HAV -Men who have sex with men -Illegal drug users -Persons with occupational risk -Persons with chronic liver disease -Persons with clotting-factor disorders	-All infants at birth -Older children who were not vaccinated -Susceptible sex partners -Persons with multiple sex partners -Men who have sex with men -Injection drug users -Susceptible household contacts of infected persons -Health care and public safety workers -Persons with end-stage renal disease -Residents and staff of facilities for developmentally disabled -Travelers going to regions with high rates of HBV -Persons with chronic liver disease	-No HCV vaccine available

Table 6 *cont.*

Comparison of Hepatitis A, B and C

	Hepatitis A Virus (HAV)	Hepatitis B Virus (HBV)	Hepatitis C Virus (HCV)

Vaccine	-2 doses given 6 months apart
	-HAV vaccines in U.S.
	  -Single:
	  HAVRIX®
	  VAQTA®
	  -Combination:
	  TWINRIX® contains HBV vaccine
		-Infants and children: 3-4 doses over 6 to 18-month period
		-Adults: 3 doses given over 6-month period
		-HBV vaccines in U.S.
		  -Single:
		  ENGERIX-B®
		  RECOMBIVAX HB®
		  -Combination:
		  COMVAX® contains haemophilus influenza type b (Hib)
		  PEDIARIX® contains diphtheria, tetanus, pertussis (DTAP)
		  TWINRIX® contains HAV vaccine
			-No vaccine available

Table 7

Hepatitis Medications

Drug Class(es)	Generic Name(s)**	Brand Name(s)**	Indication(s)	Available Dose Form(s)
Antiviral	Adefovir	Hepsera	Hepatitis B Infection	Tablet
Antiviral	Entecavir	Baraclude	Hepatitis B Infection	Solution, Tablet
Antiviral	Ribavirin	Copegus, Rebetol, Virazole	Hepatitis C Infection	Capsule, Solution, Solution for Inhalation, Tablet
Antiviral: Nucleoside Reverse Transcriptase Inhibitor	Lamivudine	Epivir	Hepatitis B Infection, Human Immuno-deficiency Virus / Acquired Immune Deficiency Syndrome	Tablet

Drug Class(es)	Generic Name(s)**	Brand Name(s)**	Indication(s)	Available Dose Form(s)
Antiviral: Nucleoside Reverse Transcriptase Inhibitor	Telbivudine	Tyzeka	Hepatitis B Infection	Solution, Tablet
Antiviral: Nucleoside Reverse Transcriptase Inhibitor	Tenofovir	Viread	Hepatitis B Infection, Human Immunodeficiency Virus / Aquired Immune Deficiency Syndrome	Tablet
Antiviral: Protease Inhibitor	Boceprevir	Victrelis	Hepatitis C Infection	Capsule
Antiviral: Protease Inhibitor	Telaprevir	Incivek	Hepatitis C Infection	Tablet
Immunomodulator	Interferon Alfa-2b	Intron-A	Chronic Hepatitis B, Chronic Hepatitis C, Human Immunodeficiency Virus-Associated Kaposi's Sarcoma	Injectable
Immunomodulator	Peginterferon Alfa-2a	Pegasys	Hepatitis B Infection, Hepatitis C Infection	Injectable

**All rights to all brand names and trademarks are held by their respective owners. There may be additional brand names for some of the products listed.

■ Liver Transplantation

End-stage liver disease can only be treated by liver transplantation. Liver transplantation has increased patient survival to 85 percent at one year and 70 percent at five years post-transplant.[26] Evaluation for transplantation is an extensive process that requires a multidisciplinary team. Candidates for listing are evaluated for etiology of liver disease, complications of cirrhosis, exclusion criteria and psychosocial assessment.[26] Deceased and living donor transplants are preformed in the U.S. After transplant, patients are at risk for rejection, infection, malignancy and recurrence of native disease. Post-transplant patients require lifetime immunosuppression. Currently, approximately 16,000 people await liver transplantation in the U.S.[27]

Conclusion

The liver is a complex organ that performs many vital functions to maintain life. A complex network of blood vessels connects the liver to the rest of the systemic circulation. Since the liver is the main center for metabolism, it may receive repeated exposure to substances and viruses that can cause damage. The damage eventually becomes irreversible, and cirrhosis can develop. Cirrhosis has many unavoidable complications that can lead to significant illness and death. The only true cure for cirrhosis is liver transplantation; however, the need for transplants is greater than the available organs. It's important for pharmacy technicians to be well-versed in knowledge of the hepatic system, including liver functions, to assist pharmacists in specialized monitoring of disease states, such as dosing drugs in hepatic failure.

References

1. Tortora, G.J., Derrickson, B., Introduction to the Human Body, 8th edition, John Wiley & Sons, New York, NY, 2010, pp. 499-501.

2. Thibodeau, G.A., Pattan, K.T., Structure & Function of the Body, 13th edition, Mosby Elsevier, St. Louis, MO, 2008, pp. 424-428.

3. Marieb, E.N., Essentials of Human Anatomy & Physiology, 7th edition, Benjamin Cummings, San Francisco, CA, 2003, pp. 462-464.

4. Sease, J.M., Timm, E.G., Stragand, J.J. "Chapter 39, Portal Hypertension and Cirrhosis," Pharmacotherapy: A Pathophysiologic Approach, 7th edition, www.accesspharmacy.com/content.aspx?aID=3193101, July 29, 2010.

5. Franchis, R., "Evolving consensus in portal hypertension report of the Baveno IV consensus workshop on methodology of diagnosis and therapy in portal hypertension," *Journal of Hepatology*, 2005, Vol. 44, pp. 167-176.

6. Garcia-Tsao, G., Bosch, J., "Management of varices and variceal hemorrhage in cirrhosis," *New England Journal of Medicine*, 2010, Vol. 362, pp. 823-832.

7. Garcia-Tsao, G., Sanyal, A.J., Grace, N.D., Carey, W., Practice Guidelines Committee of the American Association for the Study of Liver Diseases, Practice Parameters Committee of the American College of Gastroenterology, "Prevention and management of gastroesophageal varices and variceal hemorrhage in cirrhosis," *Hepatology*, 2007, Vol. 46(3), pp. 922-938.

8. Hou, W., Sanyal, A.J., "Ascites: diagnosis and management," *Medicine Clinics of North America*, 2009, Vol. 93, pp. 801-817.

9. Runyon, B.A., "Management of adult patients with ascites due to cirrhosis: an update," *Hepatology*, 2009; Vol. 49, pp. 2087-2107.

10. Saab, S., Hernandez, J.C., Chi, A.C., Tong, M.J., "Oral antibiotic prophylaxis reduces spontaneous bacterial peritonitis occurrence and improves short-term survival in cirrhosis: a meta-analysis," *American Journal of Gastroenterology*, 2009, Vol. 104, pp. 993-1049.

11. Food and Drug Administration, www.fda.gov/downloads/BiologicsBloodVaccines/BloodBloodProducts/ApprovedProducts/LicensedProductsBLAs/FractionatedPlasmaProducts/UCM056844.pdf, Nov. 13, 2010.

12. Eroglu, Y., Byrne, W.J., "Hepatic Encephalopathy," *Emergency Medicine Clinics of North America*, 2009, Vol. 27, pp. 401-414.

13. Cash, W.J., McConville, P., McDermott, E., McCormick, P.A., Callender, M.E., McDougall, N.I., "Current Concepts in the Assessment and Treatment of Hepatic Encephalopathy," *The Quarterly Journal of Medicine*, 2010, Vol. 103, pp. 9-16.

14. Merli, M., Riggio, O., "Dietary and Nutritional Indications in Hepatic Encephalopathy," *Metabolic Brain Disease*, 2009, Vol. 24, pp. 211-221.

15. Phongsamran, P.V., Kim, J.W., Abbott, J.C., Rosenblatt, A., "Pharmacotherapy for Hepatic Encephalopathy," *Drugs*, 2010, Vol. 70, pp. 1131-1148.

16. Maclayton, D.O., Eaton-Maxwell, A., "Rifaximin for Treatment of Hepatic Encephalopathy," *The Annals of Pharmacotherapy*, 2009, Vol. 43, pp. 77-84.

17. Munoz, S.J., Stravitz, R.T., Gabriel, D.A., "Coagulopathy of Acute Liver Failure," *Clinics in Liver Disease*, 2009, Vol. 13, pp. 95-107.

18. Trotter, J.F., "Coagulation Abnormalities in Patients who have Liver Disease," *Clinics in Liver Disease*, 2006, Vol. 10, pp. 665-678.

19. Centers for Disease Control and Prevention, www.cdc.gov/hepatitis, Nov. 2, 2010.

20. Centers for Disease Control and Prevention, www.cdc.gov/hepatitis/Resources/Professionals/PDFs/ABCTable.pdf, Nov. 2, 2010.

21. Centers for Disease Control and Prevention, www.cdc.gov/hepatitis/HAV/HAVfaq.htm, Nov. 2, 2010.

22. Centers for Disease Control and Prevention, www.cdc.gov/hepatitis/HBV/HBVfaq.htm, Nov. 2, 2010.

23. Lok, A.S., McMahon, B.J. "Chronic hepatitis B: update 2009," *Hepatology*, 2009, Vol. 50, pp. 661-662.

24. Centers for Disease Control and Prevention, www.cdc.gov/hepatitis/HCV/HCVfaq.htm, Nov. 2, 2010.

25. Ghany, M.G., Strader, D.B., Thomas, D.L., Seeff, L.B., American Association for the Study of Liver Diseases, "Diagnosis, management, and treatment of hepatitis C: an update," *Hepatology*, 2009, Vol. 49, pp. 1335-1374.

26. Poordad, F., McCone, J., Bacon, B.R., et al., "Boceprevir for untreated chronic HCV genotype 1 infection," *New England Journal of Medicine*, 2011, Vol. 364, pp. 1195-1206.

27. Jacobson, I.M., McHutchison, J.G., Dusheiko, G. et al., "Telaprevir for previously untreated chronic hepatitis C virus infection," *New England Journal of Medicine*, 2011, Vol. 364, pp. 2405-2416.

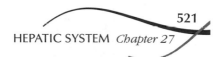

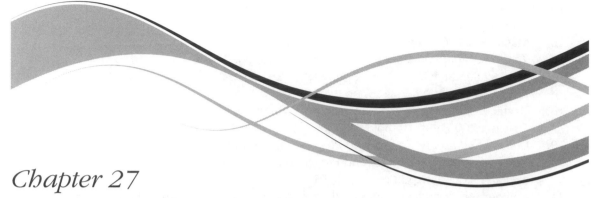

Chapter 27

REVIEW QUESTIONS

1. Which of the following accurately describes the liver?
    a. It contains two lobes of equal size.
    b. It contains a smaller right lobe and larger left lobe.
    c. It contains three lobes of varying sizes.
    d. It contains a larger right lobe and a smaller left lobe.

2. Which cells are responsible for the production of bile?
    a. Kupffer cells
    b. Endothelial cells
    c. Hepatocytes
    d. Bile canaliculi

3. Which function of the liver helps maintain normal blood glucose in the body?
    a. Protein metabolism
    b. Lipid metabolism
    c. Carbohydrate metabolism
    d. Excretion of bilirubin

4. What therapy is first-line in preventing variceal bleeding in patients with small varices?
    a. Propanolol
    b. Furosemide
    c. Spironolactone
    d. Isosorbide mononitrate

5. What is accumulation of fluid in the abdominal cavity called?
    a. Portal hypertension
    b. Spontaneous bacterial peritonitis
    c. Cirrhosis
    d. Ascites

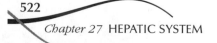

6. What antibiotic is used as secondary prophylaxis for spontaneous bacterial peritonitis?
    a. Ceftriaxone
    b. Norfloxacin
    c. Neomycin
    d. Cefotaxime

7. Which substance is the most common cause of hepatic encephalopathy?
    a. Ammonia
    b. Zinc
    c. Manganese
    d. Protein

8. Which viral hepatitis does not lead to chronic infection?
    a. Hepatitis B
    b. Hepatitis C
    c. Hepatitis E
    d. Hepatitis A

9. Which disease listed below does not have a vaccine available?
    a. Hepatitis A
    b. Pertussis
    c. Hepatitis C
    d. Hepatitis B

10. After liver transplant, what is the recipient at risk of developing that he or she was not at risk of developing before the transplant?
    a. Hepatic encephalopathy
    b. Portal hypertension
    c. Rejection
    d. Cirrhosis

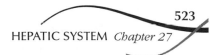

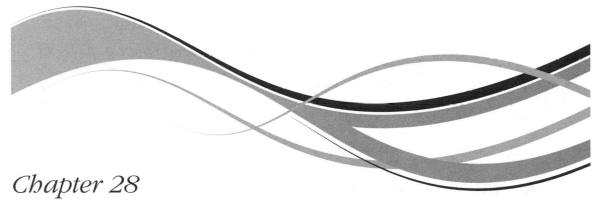

Chapter 28

REPRODUCTIVE SYSTEM

By   Dianne E. Miller, R.Ph.
Reta E. Naoum, Pharm.D.
Gregg S. Potter, Ph.D., R.Ph.

Learning Objectives

This chapter seeks to prepare a pharmacy technician to:

- ■ describe the components of the male and female reproductive systems and understand the function of the components.
- ■ understand how erectile dysfunction is different from normal function and how it is treated.
- ■ describe the causes of primary and secondary male hypogonadism (testosterone deficiency) and explain the various pharmacological treatments.
- ■ identify the phases and hormones involved in the normal menstrual cycle.
- ■ list examples of different types of contraceptive methods and understand how they work, including the mechanisms of action of estrogen and progesterone in contraception.
- ■ define menopause and list signs and symptoms commonly observed.
- ■ explain the advantages and disadvantages of drugs used in hormone replacement therapy.
- ■ describe endometriosis and the different medications used to treat it.
- ■ define infertility and describe how medications are used in the treatment of infertility.
- ■ list the causative agent for each of the sexually transmitted infections and identify the type of infectious agent involved.

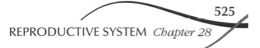

Introduction

There are two primary functions of the reproductive systems: to facilitate the production of off-spring and to facilitate sexual activities. The same structures responsible for these functions may also operate in the urinary system, which is discussed in Chapter 29. There are four main categories of diseases or disorders that are related to this system: those affecting reproduction, those affecting hormone expression, those affecting sexual function and infectious diseases. Beyond the obvious structures involved in this system, there is also a neurological component and a connection to numerous chemicals (e.g., hormones) related to the proper and improper functioning of this system.

Male Reproductive System

There are two distinct, but connected, parts to the male reproductive anatomy: the external and internal components (see Figure 1). The external components are the **penis**, **scrotum** and **testes** (inside the scrotum); the internal components are more complex and include many ducts and glands. The scrotum is a sack of loose skin that expands and contracts based on temperature to allow the testes to move closer or further from the torso to achieve the optimal temperature for sperm production. **Sperm**, the male sex cell, are produced in the testes and are produced most efficiently between 95-97 degrees Fahrenheit (with the average internal body temperature being around 98.6 degrees). Unlike all other cells of the body that contain 46 chromosomes (23 pairs), a sex cell contains 23 unpaired chromosomes. When a male sex cell (sperm) and female sex cell (ovum) merge, the 23 chromosomes provided by each will pair to create a nonsex cell. The penis consists of the **glans penis**, a region of densely-packed nerves near the tip, foreskin (unless removed by circumcision) and a shaft housing special blood vessels (called the **corpus cavernosum**) that fill and retain blood to sustain an erection. The internal structures include the **epididymis**, **vas deferens**, ejaculatory duct, **urethra**, **seminal vesicle** and **prostate**. Although each of these structures has a specific function, the main function is to produce the nonsperm components of semen and then store them, as well as sperm that are still maturing. **Semen** is a fluid that contains sperm, proteins, sugars and many other chemicals that allow sperm to more efficiently and effectively reach their target. Having a liquid vehicle for the delivery of sperm allows the same structures that are used for urination (namely the penis and the urethra that runs through the penis) to be used for the delivery of this other liquid vehicle. It must be noted, however, that the urethra cannot carry both urine and semen at the same time; a muscle closes off the junction of the urethra with the bladder during ejaculation and then opens again after ejaculation is complete.

Figure 1
Male Reproductive System

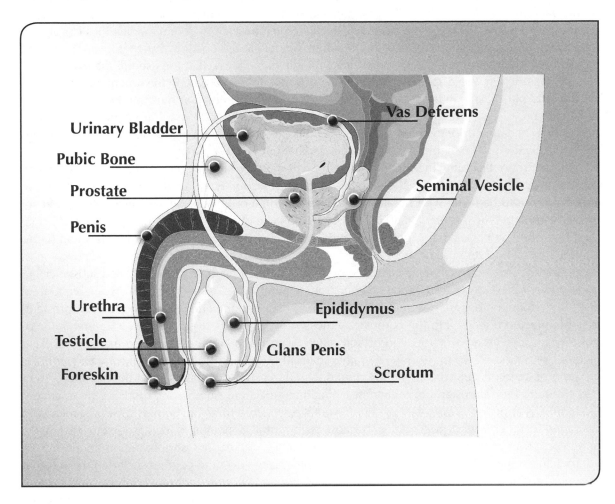

Erectile Dysfunction

To understand erectile dysfunction, one must first understand what physiologic actions are involved in producing and sustaining an erection. When an erection is achieved and maintained normally, penile blood flow increases, the penis engorges with blood and this causes swelling and elongation. This increased blood flow is due to the release of neurotransmitters, such as acetylcholine and nitric oxide, in the penis. An enzyme in the penis decreases the effects of acetylcholine and nitric oxide over time, and the penis then becomes **flaccid**. In males, testosterone is responsible for normal sexual characteristic development and sexual desire. During aging, many males experience decreased **testosterone** production, referred to as **hypogonadism**. This decreased testosterone production can lead to a loss of sexual desire and erectile dysfunction. **Erectile dysfunction** (previously known as impotence) is the failure to achieve a penile erection suitable for sexual activity. The causes of erectile dysfunction may exist without any other disorder; however, erectile dysfunction is often a result of another condition or the presence of a drug. Conditions such as decreased blood flow (often due to cardiovascular disease or diabetes), abnormal nerve function, hormone imbalances or deficiencies and psychological conditions can all lead to erectile dysfunction. Drugs, such as beta blockers and antidepressants, as well as smoking and excessive alcohol consumption, can also lead to erectile dysfunction.

Due to the multitude of causes for erectile dysfunction, the treatments are equally as diverse. In general, patients are encouraged to initiate and maintain a heart-healthy lifestyle (including physical fitness, a low-cholesterol diet and not smoking). Many nondrug therapies, such as psychosexual counseling, vacuum erection medical devices, penile prostheses and penile pump implants are available, but these are utilized far less often than drug therapy. The introduction of oral medications has greatly increased the recognition and successful treatment of erectile dysfunction. Sildenafil, vardenafil and tadalafil are orally available phosphodiesterase-5 inhibitors (PDE-5) that are used in the treatment of erectile dysfunction; these agents increase blood flow due to an increase in the functioning of acetylcholine and nitric oxide in the penis. Some amount of sexual stimulation must be present to achieve and maintain an erection when taking these drugs. Sildenafil and vardenafil are typically taken one half-hour to one hour prior to sexual activity, and their effects can last up to four hours. These two drugs are not to be used more than once in 24 hours. Tadalafil has a duration of action averaging 36 hours, allowing for more flexibility in initiating sexual activity. Further, tadalafil may be taken once each day to provide continuous coverage, allowing for the greatest flexibility in initiating sexual activity. These agents are not to be taken with nitrates (e.g., nitroglycerine) or alpha-blockers because a significant drop in blood pressure can result and lead to fainting or a heart attack. Due to the significant potential for abuse, the Food and Drug Administration (FDA) and the Drug Enforcement Administration (DEA) continue to monitor the use of these drugs; however, they are not scheduled controlled substances. Some pharmacies, however, have taken the precaution of treating them like controlled substances to try to prevent these drugs from being diverted from legitimate use. Other agents are available to treat erectile dysfunction but are not routinely used due to their nonoral administration routes. Alprostadil may be injected directly into the corpus cavernosum or may be delivered via an intra-urethral suppository to achieve an erection. Alprostadil differs from the oral agents in three main ways. First, its onset of action is five to 10 minutes rather than 30-60 minutes for the oral agents. Secondly, its duration of action is approximately 60 minutes. Thirdly, sexual stimulation from the nervous system is not required for alprostadil to initiate or maintain an erection. Another approach to the treatment of erectile dysfunction is testosterone supplementation. Testosterone can be prescribed for men who are found to suffer from hypogonadism because testosterone is thought to increase sex drive. Finally, nonprescription products claiming to improve the quality of erections are commonly found on the Internet and sometimes in the herbal sections of a pharmacy's over-the-counter shelves. Products that contain L-arginine have been suggested for erectile dysfunction; however, more clinical studies need to be done before L-arginine is recommended on a routine basis. Patients using 5 g of L-arginine per day subjectively believed that the quality of their sexual function was better than a placebo group.

Male Hypogonadism

The inability of the testes to produce testosterone, sperm or both, is hypogonadism in males. Testosterone is a hormone important in the development and maintenance of male physical characteristics and genitals. **Primary hypogonadism** results from an abnormality in the testes; **secondary hypogonadism** results from a defect in the brain, usually at the pituitary gland, that leads to a decrease in testosterone production. Common causes of primary hypogonadism include undescended testicles (in children), injury to one or both testes, cancer treatments and normal aging. Secondary hypogonadism can be caused by disorders of the pituitary gland, inflammatory diseases, HIV/AIDS and some medications (e.g., certain pain medications and hormone therapies).

Symptoms of testosterone deficiency during puberty include decreased development of muscle mass, impaired growth of the penis and testicles, development of breast tissue and a lack of voice deepening. Testosterone deficiency in adult males can be apparent by erectile dysfunction, infertility, increased body fat, decreased testicles size, decreased testicle firmness and decreased muscle mass. Mental and emotional changes can also accompany the physical symptoms of testosterone deficiency.

Treatment of testosterone deficiency involves hormone replacement therapy. Testosterone is available as a patch, an injection or a gel. Common side effects of testosterone therapy include **edema** (swelling), **hirsutism** (inappropriate hair growth) and aggressive behavior. It must also be noted that men have, and need, estrogen as well as testosterone; however, testosterone is the predominant sex hormone in men.

Female Reproductive System

There are three distinct parts of the female reproductive system: the **mammary glands** and surrounding tissues, the external genitalia and the internal structures (see Figure 2). The mammary glands are located in the breasts and produce milk to feed a newborn. The external genitalia in a female are referred to as the **vulva**, which includes the **mons pubis**, the **labia majora**, the **labia minora** and the **clitoris**. The mons pubis refers to the tissue present at the junction of the thighs and torso. The labia (majora and minora) refer to the folds of skin surrounding the vagina that function to protect the more internal structures (such as the vagina). The clitoris is a bundle of nerves that are positioned and designed to be stimulated during sexual activity. The internal structures include the **ovaries**, the **Fallopian tubes**, the **uterus**, the **vagina** and the **cervix**. The ovaries produce **ovum** (egg cells), and unlike all other cells of the body that contain 46 chromosomes (23 pairs), a sex cell contains 23 unpaired chromosomes. As previously stated in the chapter, when a male sex cell (sperm) and female sex cell (ovum) merge, the 23 chromosomes provided by each will pair to create a nonsex cell. The ovaries also produce hormones (such as estrogen and progesterone). The Fallopian tubes connect the ovaries to the uterus. In the Fallopian tubes, fertilization occurs if a sperm is able to merge with the egg. An unfertilized ovum will degenerate in the Fallopian tubes and never make it to the uterus. The uterus is the structure that nourishes and houses a growing fetus during development. The cervix is the connective tissue between the uterus and the vagina. The vagina connects the uterus (with the cervix in-between) to the outside of the body. The vagina serves both sexual and reproductive functions, including providing a structure for semen to be deposited during heterosexual intercourse, providing a means for menstrual tissue to exit the body, contracting and secreting fluids during sexual activity and facilitating a fetus to go from the uterus to outside the mother's body during birth. The vagina and the uterus can both expand considerably from their normally constricted states; this allows for a growing child to have an expanding space in which to grow and for a child to have an expanding canal from which to be birthed.

Figure 2
Female Reproductive System

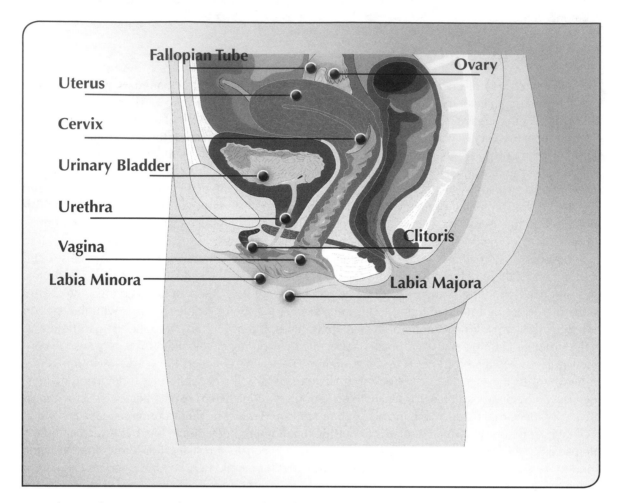

The predominant sex hormones produced in the female body are **estrogen** and **progesterone**. The body actually produces a variety of estrogens, such as estradiol, estrone and estriol. They are most commonly and collectively referred to as estrogen. Most of this production occurs in the ovaries, yet the stimulus for secretion is in the hypothalamus (in the brain). The network of organs involved in hormone production is referred to as the **hypothalamic-pituitary-ovarian (HPO) axis**. The hypothalamus secretes **gonadotropin-releasing hormone (GnRH)**, which acts on receptors in the pituitary gland. In response to GnRH, the pituitary gland secretes **luteinizing hormone (LH)** and **follicular stimulating hormone (FSH)** into the blood. LH and FSH travel to the ovaries and then stimulate the production and release of estrogen and progesterone. These hormones are responsible for development of the female reproductive organs and secondary sexual characteristics (e.g., hair growth and breast development). Estrogen and progesterone play a crucial role, beginning at puberty, in maintaining the menstrual cycle. They have additional effects in many tissues all over the body and are involved in normal female physiology throughout life. For example, estrogen aids in the maintenance of healthy skin, heart and bones. Likewise, progesterone influences insulin levels and promotes mammary gland development. It must also be noted that women have and need testosterone; however, estrogen is the primary sex hormone found in women.

Menstrual Cycle

The average menstrual cycle lasts 28 days, though some women find that this is truly an average and does not describe every cycle throughout their lives (and sometimes none of the cycles during their lives). When counting the days of a cycle, always begin with the first day of menstrual flow and count until the last day before menstrual flow begins again. Egg release from the ovaries is called **ovulation**. Ovulation usually occurs on day 13-14 of a menstrual cycle but may occur at any time during the cycle; further, the day of ovulation varies from one woman to another and may vary from one cycle to the next. Ovulation separates the cycle into two phases that also correspond to significant differences in the levels of hormones secreted by the ovaries. The **follicular phase** lasts from the beginning of the cycle until ovulation and is dominated by the production of estrogen from the ovum preparing to be released from the ovary. This special ovum is called the **dominant follicle**. The amount of estrogen being produced increases throughout the phase and peaks just before ovulation. This spike in plasma estrogen concentration just prior to ovulation initiates the secretion of GnRH from the hypothalamus. This stimulates the HPO axis, which eventually signals the ovaries to release an ovum into the Fallopian tubes. If a sperm is able to come into contact with this ovum released into the Fallopian tubes and gain entry into the ovum, the ovum is referred to as fertilized. A fertilized ovum is able to implant itself in the endometrial lining of the uterus to grow and continue development. Fertilized ovum that implant somewhere other than in the uterus (such as in the Fallopian tubes) may develop but will be a danger to both mother and fetus; this type of pregnancy is known as an **ectopic pregnancy**. During the luteal phase, which follows ovulation, progesterone secretion dramatically increases. Progesterone prepares the uterus for implantation and the 40 weeks of gestation that it takes for a human child to fully develop. If fertilization does not occur, the egg regresses and the lining of the uterus sheds. This process is known as **menses**, or menstrual bleeding, and begins the next menstrual cycle.

Pregnancy

When trying to have a baby, many prospective parents will visit the pharmacy in search of a pregnancy test. Many different types of pregnancy tests are available (e.g., Clearblue Easy®, E.P.T.®, First Response®), and all measure **human chorionic gonadotropin (hCG)** in the urine. Approximately one week after fertilization, hCG is produced in sufficient amounts to be detectable by pregnancy tests. Typically, females are expected to sample from the first morning urine and test immediately after collection. Most tests have a high degree of accuracy (greater than 95 percent), but positive results must be followed by a physician visit. When advising patients on the selection and use of these products, some degree of professionalism and discretion for the patient's privacy is warranted. Pregnant mothers experience a wide variety of issues related to the growth of the fetus that may require visits to the pharmacy. Alterations in normal gastrointestinal function can lead to complaints of nausea and vomiting, constipation, gastroesophageal reflux and hemorrhoids. Pharmacists can aid in reducing these pregnancy-induced issues through recommending changes in lifestyle or through the use of over-the-counter products. Pregnancy-induced diseases, such as gestational diabetes mellitus, preeclampsia and urinary tract infections, cause the future mother to initiate lifestyle changes and often require drug therapy. In general, however, it is recommended that pregnant mothers avoid taking medications, both prescription and nonprescription, during pregnancy, unless a health care provider has been consulted. Many drugs have a long history of being used safely during pregnancy; however, most drugs do not have adequate safety data to evaluate the relative risks to the developing fetus. In situations where prescriptions are written during pregnancy, the physician may deem the benefit of drug therapy to outweigh the potential risks to the mother and fetus. On the other hand, some drugs have a well-established history of causing problems during pregnancy and must always be avoided. It is absolutely essential that a physician, a pharmacist and the patient all collaborate on discussing the benefits and risks of using any medication during pregnancy. Table 1 gives a partial list of drugs known to cause developmental abnormalities in a fetus during pregnancy.

Table 1
Drugs to Avoid During Pregnancy

Drug Class(es)	Generic Name(s)**	Brand Name(s)**	Indication(s)	Available Dose Form(s)
Anti-Acne: Retinoid	Isoretinoin	Accutane, Amnesteem, Claravis, Sotret	Severe Acne	Capsule
Antibiotic: Tetracycline	Doxycycline	Adoxa, Periostat, Vibramycin, Vibra-Tabs	Bacterial Infection	Capsule, Extended-Release Capsule, Extended-Release Tablet, Injectable, Suspension, Tablet
Antibiotic: Tetracycline	Tetracycline	Achromycin V, Sumycin	Acne, Bacterial Infection	Capsule
Anti-Cancer: Alkylating Agent, Anti-Rheumatic: Disease-Modifying Anti-Rheumatic Drug	Cyclophosphamide	Cytoxan	Multiple Cancers, Rheumatoid Arthritis	Injectable, Tablet
Anti-Cancer: Antimetabolite, Anti-Rheumatic: Disease-Modifying Anti-Rheumatic Drug	Methotrexate	Folex, Rheumatrex, Trexall	Multiple Cancers, Rheumatoid Arthritis, Psoriasis	Injectable, Tablet
Anticoagulant: Vitamin K Epoxide Reductase Inhibitor	Warfarin	Coumadin, Jantoven	Deep Vein Thrombosis, Pulmonary Embolism	Solution, Tablet
Anticonvulsant	Carbamazepine	Carbatrol, Epitol, Equetro, Tegretol, Tegretol XR	Alcohol Withdrawal, Bipolar Disorder, Post-Traumatic Stress Disorder, Restless Leg Syndrome, Schizophrenia, Seizures	Capsule, Chewable Tablet, Suspension, Tablet
Anticonvulsant	Phenytoin	Dilantin, Dilantin Infatabs, Phenytek	Seizures	Capsule, Chewable Tablet, Injectable, Suspension

Drug Class(es)	Generic Name(s)**	Brand Name(s)**	Indication(s)	Available Dose Form(s)
Antidepressant: Selective Serotonin Reuptake Inhibitor	Paroxetine	Paxil, Paxil CR, Pexeva	Depression, Eating Disorders, Impulse Control, Obsessive Compulsive Disorder Panic Disorder, Post-Traumatic Stress Disorder, Premenstrual Dysphoric Disorder, Social Anxiety Disorder	Suspension, Tablet
Antihypertensive: Angiotensin-Converting Enzyme Inhibitor	Enalapril	Vasotec	Acute Coronary Syndrome, Heart Failure, High Blood Pressure	Tablet
Antihypertensive: Angiotensin-Converting Enzyme Inhibitor	Lisinopril	Zestril, Prinivil	Acute Coronary Syndrome, Heart Failure, High Blood Pressure	Tablet
Antihypertensive: Angiotensin Receptor Blocker	Losartan	Cozaar	Heart Failure, High Blood Pressure	Tablet
Antihypertensive: Angiotensin Receptor Blocker	Valsartan	Diovan	Heart Failure, High Blood Pressure	Tablet
Anti-Rheumatic: Disease-Modifying Anti-Rheumatic Drug	Leflunomide	Arava	Rheumatoid Arthritis	Tablet
Hormone	Conjugated Estrogens, Estradiol, Estrogen	Alora, Climara, Delestrogen, Depo-Estradiol, Divigel, Elestrin, Esclim, Estrace, Estraderm, Estrasorb, Estratab, Estring, Evamist, Femring, Femtrace, Menostar, Ogen, Ortho-Est, Premarin, Vagifem, Vivelle-Dot	Osteoporosis, Perimenopausal Symptoms, Post-Menopausal Symptoms	Gel, Injectable, Intravaginal Ring, Patch, Tablet, Vaginal Cream, Vaginal Tablet

Table 1 *cont.*
Drugs to Avoid During Pregnancy

Drug Class(es)	Generic Name(s)**	Brand Name(s)**	Indication(s)	Available Dose Form(s)
Hormone	Testosterone or Methyltestosterone	Androderm, Androgel, Android, Delatestryl, Depo-Testosterone, Methitest, Striant, Testopel, Testrid	Erectile Dysfunction, Low Testosterone	Cream, Gel, Injectable, Lozenge, Patch
Immunomodulator	Thalidomide	Thalomid	GI Bleeding, Multiple Myeloma, Nausea, Vomiting	Capsule
Nonsteroidal Anti-Inflammatory Drug: Nonselective	Ibuprofen	Advil, Motrin	Gout, Osteoarthritis, Rheumatoid Arthritis	Capsule, Chewable Tablet, Liquid Gel, Suspension
Nonsteroidal Anti-Inflammatory Drug: Nonselective	Naproxen	Aleve, Anaprox, Mediproxen, Naprelan, Naprosyn, Pamprin	Gout, Osteoarthritis, Rheumatoid Arthritis	Capsule, Extended-Release Tablet, Suspension, Tablet

**All rights to all brand names are held by their respective owners. There may be additional brand names for some of the products listed.

Contraception

There are many forms of **contraception** available to females who wish to avoid pregnancy. Barrier methods, such as condoms, diaphragms and vaginal sponges, are available in the pharmacy; but, these are associated with a higher rate of pregnancy than hormonal contraceptives. Hormonal contraceptives are available in oral and nonoral forms and contain synthetic derivatives of estrogen and/or progesterone. The most common estrogen derivative used in hormonal contraceptives is ethinyl estradiol. Progestins are the class of drugs that mimic progesterone that is normally produced by the ovaries. Common progestins include norgestrel, levonorgestrel and norethindrone. When taken daily, ethinyl estradiol and/or the progestins exert a contraceptive effect. The constant blood level of these agents inhibits the release of the pituitary gonadotropins and prevents the surge of LH and FSH that normally comes right before ovulation. Without the gonadotropin surge, the dominant follicle does not develop and the egg is not released. Since there is no dominant follicle, ovulation does not occur and there is little chance for pregnancy. Progestins also exert contraceptive actions by increasing vaginal mucous secretions, leading to a decrease in sperm movement and to an inhibition of egg implantation into the endometrial lining of the uterus. Hormonal contraceptives are also used for indications other than contraception, such as regulating monthly menstrual cycles, decreasing symptoms of endometriosis and in the treatment of acne.

Contraceptive Products

Side effects associated with estrogen excess include nausea, bloating, migraine headaches and weight gain. Progestin excess can result in hair loss, fatigue and acne. Depending on the individual needs of the patient and the occurrence of side effects, differing estrogen and progestin products and their concentrations can be selected to achieve the proper hormonal balance and desired effects. Most oral contraceptives include some length of either placebo or iron-containing tablets that are taken during some part of the menstrual cycle to allow for menstrual bleeding (maintaining high hormone levels prevents menstrual bleeding). Some women find that monophasic products work best for them; a monophasic contraceptive delivers the same amount of hormones throughout the cycle. There are also biphasic and triphasic options. Each product will use a different estrogen and progesterone combination and at a different strength, so some effort may go into finding exactly the right combination for a particular patient. Further, options other than tablets exist; a plastic ring that is inserted vaginally for 21 days and releases hormones, injectable hormones, patches and intrauterine devices are all options to chemically achieve contraception.

Table 2
Relative Activity of Selected Hormonal Contraceptives

Brand Name**	Ethinyl Estradiol Content	Estrogen Activity	Progestin Content	Progestin Activity
Monophasic Combination				
Alesse	20 mcg	Very Low	Levonogestrel 0.1 mg	Low
Levlen	30 mcg	Low	Levonogestrel 0.1 mg	Intermediate
Ortho Cyclen	35 mcg	Intermediate	Norgestimate 0.25 mg	Low
Ovcon	50 mcg	High	Norethindrone 1.0 mg	Intermediate
Biphasic Combination				
Mircette Days 1-21 Days 22-28	20 mcg 10 mcg	Very Low	Desogestrel 0.15 mg None	High
Triphasic Combination				
Ortho-Novum 7/7/7 Days 1-7 Days 8-14 Days 15-21 Days 22-28	35 mcg 35 mcg 35 mcg None	Intermediate	Norethindrone 0.5 mg Norethindrone 0.75 mg Norethindrone 1.0 mg None	Low Low Intermediate
Seasonale Days 1-84	30 mcg	Low	Levonorgestrel 0.15 mg	Intermediate
TriPhasil Days 1-7 Days 8-14 Days 15-21 Days 22-28	30 mcg 40 mcg 30 mcg None	Low Intermediate Low	Levonorgestrel 0.05mg Levonorgestrel 0.075 mg Levonorgestrel 0.125 mg None	Low Low Intermediate

Table 2 *cont.*

Relative Activity of Selected Hormonal Contraceptives

Brand Name**	Ethinyl Estradiol Content	Estrogen Activity	Progestin Content	Progestin Activity
Progestin-Only				
Micronor	None	Not Available	Norethindrone 0.35 mg	Very Low
Ovrette	None	Not Available	Norgestrel 0.075 mg	Very Low
Emergency Contraception				
Plan B	None	Not Available	Levonorgestrel 0.75 mg	Very High
Preven	50 mcg	High	Levonorgestrel 0.25 mg	High

**All rights to all brand names and trademarks are held by their respective owners.

Progestin-only oral contraceptives (e.g., minipills) are available for women who cannot take estrogen. These products have the disadvantage of having an increased rate of pregnancy compared to the combination products (3 vs. 1 percent). Nonoral products are designed to minimize adverse effects and/or increase compliance rates. Ortho-Evra® (norelgestromin) patches are changed weekly for three weeks and then a patch is left off for one week to allow for menses. This option is good for patients who struggle to remember to take a daily tablet; especially since the oral tablets must be taken at exactly the same time each and every day to be fully effective. Depo-Provera® (medroxyprogesterone) injection exerts a contraceptive action for up to three months and is generally injected in a physician's office. This allows for even less need for the patient to remember to take the product. Taking hormonal contraceptives as prescribed is very important in preventing pregnancy. Missing even one active tablet can increase the chances of getting pregnant. If an active tablet is missed, the tablet needs to be taken when the missed tablet is discovered or two tablets may be taken at the regular dosing time the next day. If two active tablets are missed consecutively, the patient needs to take two tablets when remembered or take two tablets daily for the next two days. Additionally, if two consecutive days of a contraceptive tablet are missed, the patient must add an alternate form of contraception for the remainder of the cycle (such as a barrier method, like using a condom with each occurrence of sexual activity where pregnancy could result). Besides preventing pregnancy, hormonal contraceptives have been shown to decrease the risk of pelvic inflammatory disease, ovarian cancer, endometrial cancer and ovarian cysts. Hormonal contraceptives increase the risk of blood clots and elevate blood pressure. Therefore, they must be used cautiously in patients who currently are experiencing, recently experienced or are at an increased risk for stroke or coronary artery disease. Cigarette smoking must be avoided in patients who take hormonal contraceptives that contain estrogen because both smoking and estrogen increase the risk of developing a blood clot; the combination makes it more likely that a dangerous blood clot will develop. Many drugs interact with hormonal contraceptives and can cause a decreased contraceptive effect. There are also other drugs that interact with hormones to prevent their contraceptive effects. Since hormones are recycled in the body through a system that involves the natural bacteria found in the intestines, any drug that kills or disrupts these bacteria could have an effect on the blood level of hormones. For this reason, many antibiotics have a warning that they might interrupt the contraceptive effects of hormone-containing products. Although the chance of this occurring is slim, patients must be made aware of the potential for these effects when taking antibiotics so that sexual activity is avoided or another contraceptive method is used if this is a concern for the patient. Other drugs simply inhibit the natural activities of these hormones. A selection of the commonly-encountered drugs that may counteract the contraceptive effect of hormones include ampicillin/penicillin antibiotics, griseofulvin, phenytoin, sulfonamides/sulfa antibiotics, tetracycline antibiotics, theophylline and topiramate.

Emergency Contraception

Pregnancy can also be prevented after intercourse by administering estrogens and/or progestins in high doses around the time of ovulation. The effectiveness of such emergency options greatly diminishes 72 hours after intercourse. In some states, pharmacists have the authority to dispense emergency contraceptive tablets without a prescription written by a physician. Further, in some states, a pharmacy may refuse to carry emergency contraception or may be compelled by law to carry it. Pharmacy technicians are strongly encouraged to review their state's laws on emergency contraception. Emergency contraceptive tablets are intended to be used following unprotected intercourse or after a suspected contraceptive failure (e.g., condom rupture) and are not to be used as a woman's routine form of contraception. This method of contraception will not terminate a pregnancy (where a fertilized ovum is implanted in the endometrial lining) but may prevent a pregnancy from occurring altogether. Nausea and vomiting are more common with emergency contraception than with lower doses of these hormones used in daily oral contraceptives. A progesterone antagonist is available for the medical termination of a pregnancy within the first 49 days after conception. Mifepristone (Mifeprex®) blocks the effects of progesterone and causes the endometrial lining of the uterus to shed; along with the endometrial lining, the developing fetus is also expelled from the uterus. Nausea, vomiting and vaginal pain occur in more than 50 percent of patients taking mifepristone. Due to the potential for conflicts between individual beliefs and pharmacy policies, all pharmacy personnel are encouraged to discuss the pharmacy's policies on emergency contraception before beginning employment to ensure that any conflict between the pharmacy's policies and the individual's beliefs are handled professionally.

Menopause

Estrogen and progesterone production from the ovaries plays a significant role in the normal functioning of females throughout life. As women age, a loss of ovarian function occurs that usually starts in the fifth decade of life and can last for many years. **Menopause** is the term for this loss of ovarian function that results in the loss of the monthly menstrual cycle along with the loss of estrogen and progesterone production by the ovaries. The decrease in female hormone production during and after menopause produces a wide variety of symptoms and potentially increases the risk of developing certain diseases. Middle-aged women undergoing menopause often complain of **vasomotor symptoms** (e.g., hot flashes, night sweats), psychological symptoms (e.g., mood swings, insomnia, anxiety) and disturbances in sexual behavior (e.g., vaginal dryness, loss of libido). Loss of ovarian function has been associated with an increased occurrence of various diseases, including osteoporosis, colorectal cancer and heart disease.

Historically, health care providers have recommended the use of estrogenic substances and progestins to replenish the diminished concentrations of endogenous hormones in the body. These therapies, which have included both herbal and synthetic compounds, have been used for decades and have provided good relief of symptoms with the presumption of a disease benefit to the patient. Recent clinical evidence has cast doubt on the proposed benefit of many of these previously accepted therapies and has actually demonstrated increased risk of developing some diseases. The issue of initiating hormonal therapy for the symptoms of menopause and preventing disease is currently quite controversial and, at a minimum, must be assessed on an individual basis to identify therapeutic benefits vs. risks in each patient. The reasons for replacing hormones in women who are undergoing menopause are to decrease the occurrence of symptoms and to slow down or eliminate diseases that may depend on hormonal loss. Similarly to oral contraceptives, there is a wide variety of estrogen-only and progestin-only products, along with hormonal combinations. Adding to the complexity of determining appropriate therapy are the variations in routes of drug administration. Products used for hormonal replacement therapy are available orally, transdermally (e.g., patches, creams, gels), intravaginally (e.g., creams, rings), intramuscularly and in implanted pellets. The choices of hormone therapy, along with the routes of administration, provide many options for the patient to ensure acceptability and enhance compliance. Conjugated estrogens are the most commonly used source of estrogens for replacement therapy. These are derived from the purified urine of pregnant horses (Premarin®) or plant sources (Cenestin®). Synthetic estrogens, such as ethinyl estradiol, are available orally and in transdermal patches. Premarin® and Estrace® are available in vaginal cream preparations for the relief of vaginal dryness associated with menopause.

Hormone replacement in postmenopausal women has advantages and disadvantages. For the reduction of symptoms of menopause, estrogen therapy is the most effective with no evidence that one estrogenic compound is more effective than another. Also, estrogens have been shown to increase bone mineral density and decrease the risk of osteoporosis-related fractures. Progestin-only products are available for hormone replacement therapy in those patients where estrogen use is contraindicated. More commonly, progestins are prescribed as a complementary therapy to estrogens, either as individual (e.g., medroxyprogesterone—Provera®) or combination products (e.g., conjugated estrogens/medroxyprogesterone—Prempro®). The combination products are also available in transdermal patches (e.g., estradiol/norethindrone—Combipatch®). Progestins are added to estrogen therapy to decrease the risk of endometrial cancer that occurs with unopposed estrogen replacement therapy. Women who have undergone a **hysterectomy** (removal of the uterus) typically do not require progestin therapy. Continuous combined estrogen and progestin treatment is taken daily and this reduces or prevents monthly periods. During cyclic estrogen and progestin therapy, estrogens are taken daily, but progestins are only taken for 10-14 days of the cycle to promote bleeding and monthly cycles. In the last five years, clinical trial data regarding the use of combined estrogen and progestin products in postmenopausal women have identified many disadvantages of this therapy.

There is good evidence that **hormone replacement therapy** increases the risk of heart disease, stroke, breast cancer and blood clots. Disagreement over the significance of new data and how it impacts individual patients has led to controversy in the medical community; however, current guidelines recommend against the routine use of estrogen alone or estrogen and progestin combinations for the prevention of chronic conditions, such as heart disease and cancer in postmenopausal women. Health care providers need to individualize therapy and thoroughly discuss advantages and disadvantages with each patient. When hormonal therapy is used to relieve menopausal symptoms, it is initiated at the lowest effective dose(s) for the shortest possible time in all patients.

Recently, drug manufacturers have developed "designer estrogens" that are pharmacologically classified as **selective estrogen receptor modulators (SERMs)**. This drug class exerts some beneficial effects of estrogen on the body while decreasing many of the harmful effects observed with current estrogen replacement therapy. Raloxifene and tamoxifen are two SERMs that have been shown to improve cholesterol levels and decrease the occurrence of breast cancer. These agents are not currently indicated for the treatment of postmenopausal symptoms; however, raloxifene does decrease the risk of osteoporosis, while tamoxifen is beneficial in breast cancer prevention and treatment.

Phytoestrogens are considered herbal remedies that contain isoflavones and lignans derived from plants that possess estrogen-like biological activity. Common food sources of phytoestrogens include soybeans, flaxseed oil, dates and Mexican yams. Black cohosh and red clover are other plant sources of phytoestrogens. Many of the products that contain these substances are touted to decrease the symptoms of menopause. There is some evidence to support these claims; but, trial results are inconsistent and lack comparisons to prescription drugs. Additionally, ingestion of phytoestrogens has been suggested to lower the risk of breast cancer, improve bone density and decrease cardiovascular disease; however, these claims remain unsubstantiated.

Endometriosis

Endometriosis is an abnormal condition of the **endometrium**, or inner layer of the uterine wall. Endometriosis is a common cause of pelvic pain and infertility in women. The exact prevalence of this condition is unknown because surgical visualization methods are required to make a definitive diagnosis of endometriosis; however, it is generally estimated to occur in 10 percent of women. The cause of endometriosis is unknown; but, factors, such as frequent or heavy menstruation, high estrogen levels and genetic predisposition, seem to be associated with the condition. Symptoms of endometriosis include **dysmenorrhea** (painful menstruation), **dyspareunia** (painful sexual intercourse), chronic pelvic pain, urinary disturbances, low back pain and gastrointestinal disturbances. The drugs of choice in treating endometriosis are nonsteroidal anti-inflammatory drugs (NSAIDs) and oral contraceptives. Other treatments include progestins, gonadotropin-releasing hormone agonists and danazol.

NSAIDs decrease the inflammation involved with endometriosis and, thereby, relieve pelvic pain. The most common side effects of NSAIDs involve the gastrointestinal (GI) tract and include nausea, loss of appetite, stomach upset, abdominal pain and diarrhea. Oral contraceptives are the second drug class of choice in treating endometriosis. These medications are especially useful in adolescents with endometriosis, but are not used in women with a history of thromboembolisms (blood clots) or in smokers over the age of 35 years. Side effects of oral contraceptives are generally mild and include nausea, bloating, headache and **breakthrough bleeding**. Progestin-only agents are also used in the treatment of endometriosis. The most frequent side effects occurring with these medications include breakthrough bleeding, weight gain, fluid retention and mood swings. These agents may not be good for women wanting immediate future fertility because they can cause prolonged **amenorrhea** (abnormal discontinuation of menstruation) and **anovulation** (absence of ovulation). Another option for treating endometriosis is GnRH agonists, such as goserelin (Zoladex®), leuprolide (Lupron®, Viadur® and Eligard®) and nafarelin (Synarel®). The primary limitations in using these agents are the side effects: bone loss, hot flashes, vaginal dryness and insomnia. Finally, danazol, another synthetic hormone agent, is also available as a treatment for endometriosis. This medication was formerly the standard endometriosis treatment, but it has since been replaced by the previously mentioned agents due to its side effect profile. The limitations of this agent include weight gain, acne, hot flashes, decreased breast size, hirsutism and increased cholesterol levels.

Infertility

Infertility is defined as the failure to conceive after one year of frequent contraceptive-free intercourse. The rate of infertility has been rising in the last few decades. Currently, it is estimated that one in 10 couples of reproductive age have some difficulty in conceiving a child. One reason for the increase in infertility rates is that societal trends have led to delaying the start of a family. Often couples do not even think of trying to conceive until they are in their 30s and 40s. Additionally, there are many medical causes of infertility, such as pelvic inflammatory disease, endometriosis and infections of the genitourinary tract. Abnormalities in the normal release of female hormones can inhibit ovulation and, therefore, be a cause of infertility. These abnormalities may be present in the hypothalamus, the pituitary gland and/or the ovaries. Current medications and assisted reproductive techniques have made a significant impact on decreasing infertility due to these hormonal abnormalities.

Females trying to become pregnant are recommended to follow a healthy lifestyle and maintain a nutrient-rich diet, which includes folic acid. Alcohol, smoking and obesity can all adversely effect fertility and need to be avoided. Surgery may be required if the Fallopian tubes are blocked or in cases of severe endometriosis. Females who have difficulty becoming pregnant can often increase their chances by timing intercourse to coincide with ovulation. They can monitor body temperature to help determine when ovulation is occurring and increase sexual activity during that time. Temperatures increase slightly following ovulation and can be accurately measured with basal body thermometers.

Additionally, products that predict ovulation (e.g., Answer Ovulation Kit® and the Clearblue Easy Fertility Monitor®) are available for patients who wish to increase the likelihood of becoming pregnant. These urine tests measure elevations in LH that occur 24-36 hours prior to ovulation. For a follicle in the ovary to develop into an egg and be released, there must be a coordinated effort of the HPO axis. Dysfunction of any part of the HPO axis can result in decreased secretion of the female hormones needed for ovulation. Decreased concentrations of female hormones resulting in infertility can be treated with the administration of selected agents that supplement hormonal concentrations. These ovulation-inducing agents act at specific sites in the axis where the problem is suspected. Gonadorelin mimics the actions of GnRH in the body; GnRH generally stimulates the HPO axis. When there is a problem with the hypothalamus, gonadorelin is administered in a pulsatile manner, intravenously, causing LH and FSH secretion to increase from the pituitary and, thereby, increase the probability of ovulation. Another drug that acts in the hypothalamus by a different mechanism is clomiphene citrate. It binds to estrogen receptors and leads to increases in the release of GnRH, which then stimulates the HPO axis and induces ovulation. Clomiphene is considered a first-line therapy for infertility and is given orally for five days beginning the fifth day of a woman's normal menstrual cycle. Another approach to induce ovulation is to enhance the blood levels of gonadotropins that act on the ovaries to cause egg development and release. As mentioned previously, FSH and LH are naturally occurring gonadotropins that are produced and released from the pituitary into the blood. Drugs have been synthesized that have the same structure as the gonadotropins and are used to supplement hormonal concentrations. Follitropin-alpha and follitropin-beta are man-made versions of FSH, and lutropin alfa is a synthetic form of LH. Gonadotropins are also available from natural sources (e.g., after purification, the urine from postmenopausal women). Urofillitropin has predominately FSH-like activity, while human menopausal gonadotropins (i.e., HMG or menotropins) possess both FSH-like and LH-like activity. If infertility is due to low levels of endogenous FSH or LH and not problems with the ovaries, these agents can greatly enhance the probability of ovulation. Some disadvantages of using the gonadotropins include lack of availability in oral dosage forms, expense and increased likelihood of multiple pregnancies.

In the last few decades, advances in medical techniques have significantly aided in the treatment of infertility. **Assisted reproductive technology (ART)** involves the direct retrieval of eggs from a woman's ovaries and the manipulation of sperm and/or embryos to achieve pregnancy. The most common of these technologies is ***in vitro* fertilization (IVF)**. During IVF, eggs are stimulated to develop inside the ovary following treatment with gonadotropins. These eggs are harvested and physically placed in contact with sperm to become fertilized, often in a test tube outside of the female body. The embryo or embryos are then placed back into the uterus, and gestation can occur naturally. Progesterone supplementation is often administered to sustain the developing fetus. Two classes of drugs that are used in conjunction with ART to alter egg development and release are the GnRH agonists and GnRH antagonists. Both of these classes of drugs are utilized to slow down or halt egg development and release from the ovaries. Nafarelin spray and leuprolide injection are GnRH agonists that mimic the actions of endogenous GnRH in the body. When given in a continuous manner, they delay ovulation. Cetrorelix and ganirelix are GnRH antagonists that inhibit the actions of endogenous GnRH on the pituitary gland, resulting in a delay in ovulation. When an exact time for ovulation is scheduled, the GnRH agonist or antagonist is discontinued and gonadotropins are administered. Ovulation often results, and these techniques allow for many eggs to develop simultaneously and be available for IVF. A disadvantage of utilizing GnRH agonists is hyperstimulation of the ovaries and the development of ovarian cysts.

Sexually Transmitted Diseases

The occurrence of **sexually transmitted diseases (STDs)** is on the rise in the United States. Individuals in their teens and 20s account for most of these cases. A wide variety of different types of

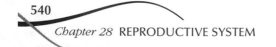

diseases can result from the spread of infectious agents during intimate sexual contact. Classification and treatment of the resulting diseases is usually based on the type of pathogen present and can be classified into one of the following groups: bacterial infections, viral infections, fungal infections, protozoal infections and parasitic infestations. The best way to limit the occurrence of STDs is through monogamous sexual relationships and the use of barrier contraceptive methods, such as male condoms and female condoms. Additionally, vaginal diaphragms and sponges with spermicides can be used for contraception and do provide some degree of protection from a number of STDs. It must also be noted that treatment may need to involve not only the individual first discovered to have an STD but also the individual's recent sexual partner(s). In some cases, treatment of sexual partners is not warranted without testing; however, informing sexual partners that testing may be appropriate could be required by law.

Bacterial Infections

Gonorrhea and **syphilis** are two examples of bacterial infections classified as STDs. Symptoms of these infections can affect the urinary tract and show up as abnormal discharges from the urethra and pain on urination. If left untreated, the bacteria can spread throughout the body and cause organ damage and systemic symptoms. Antibiotics are the main treatment for bacterial infections. Gonorrhea is commonly treated with cephalosporin antibiotics (e.g., ceftriaxone). Alternately, quinolone antibiotics (e.g., ciprofloxacin and ofloxacin) have efficacy against *neisseria gonorrhea* bacteria. Syphilis responds well to intramuscular or intravenous penicillin G. In penicillin-allergic patients, doxycycline may be used.

Viral Infections

Examples of viral STDs are **Human Immunodeficiency Virus / Acquired Immune Deficiency Syndrome (HIV/AIDS), Herpes Simplex Virus (HSV)** and **Human Papillomavirus (HPV)**. Patients with genital herpes show signs of sores and ulcerations on the genitals. The disease is caused by HSV and can be transmitted even when sores are not present. There is no cure for genital herpes, but flare-ups can be controlled and suppressed with oral and topical antiviral medications, such as acyclovir, famciclovir and valacyclovir. Genital warts are caused by HPV and are associated with cervical cancer. Yearly pap smears are used to identify HPV infections. Topically applied products, such as imiquimod cream and podofilox gel, can be used to control symptoms, but, none of these are considered curative.

Fungal Infections

Vaginal candidiasis, also known as a yeast infection, is usually caused by a fungus called *Candida albicans. Candida* normally resides in the gastrointestinal tract where it is not considered pathogenic. Upon exposure to female sexual organs during sex, the fungus can cause itching and irritation, as well as overgrowth of the normal vaginal flora. Sexual contact is not a requirement for developing a yeast infection; but, the male urethra often harbors the fungus and can lead to reinfection after treatment. Intravaginal creams, vaginal suppositories and combination products (e.g., miconazole, clotrimazole, tioconazole) are available over-the-counter to kill *Candida*. Combination products are advantageous because they allow for internal and external relief of symptoms. Terconazole cream or suppositories, and oral antifungals, such as fluconazole, are effective prescription agents used in the treatment of vaginal candidiasis.

Protozoal Infections

Trichomoniasis is an infection that occurs more commonly in women than men and presents with symptoms of pain during urination, vaginal discharge and itch. The protozoan *trichomonas vaginalis* causes this STD and it can be effectively eradicated by the antimicrobial agent metronidazole.

Parasitic Infections

Chlamydia trachomatis is a parasite that causes **chlamydia** infections that commonly affect the genitourinary organs. Most often, the infection does not cause symptoms; but, if present, symptoms can include pain during urination and cloudy urogenital discharge. Chlamydia infections require treatment because persistent infections can lead to pelvic inflammatory disease, ectopic pregnancy and infertility. Successful treatment of chlamydia infections can be achieved with the antibiotic azithromycin or doxycycline. Pubic lice and scabies mites can often be transferred between individuals during intimate sexual contact. In the genital areas, these infestations will often present with redness and intense itching. Preparations of permethrin are available over-the-counter (permethrin 1% creme rinse) and by prescription (permethrin 5% cream) for treatment. Lindane lotion can be applied as an alternative to permethrin, but its use is limited due to the increased potential for toxicity to the nervous system and increased occurrence of seizures. See Table 3 below for a listing of drugs used to treat reproductive and sexual disorders.

Table 3
Drugs Used to Treat Reproductive / Sexual Disorders (Excluding Infectious Diseases)

Drug Class(es)	Generic Name(s)**	Brand Name(s)**	Indication(s)	Available Dose Form(s)
Androgen Hormone Inhibitor	Finasteride	Propecia, Proscar	Enlarging Prostate, Hair Loss	Tablet
Anticholinergic	Oxybutynin	Ditropan, Ditropan XL, Gelnique, Ox	Over-Active Bladder	Extended-Release Tablet, Gel, Patch, Syrup, Topical Gel
Anti-Estrogen	Tamoxifen	Nolvadex	Breast Cancer, Ovulation Stimulation	Tablet
Estrogen Agonist / Antagonist	Raloxifene	Evista	Osteoporosis	Tablet
Gastrointestinal Protectant, Uterine Conractant	Misoprostol	Cytotec, Mifeprex	Gastroesophageal Reflux Disease, Induce Labor, Terminate Pregnancy, Ulcer Prevention	Tablet

Drug Class(es)	Generic Name(s)**	Brand Name(s)**	Indication(s)	Available Dose Form(s)
Hormone	Black Cohosh (Estrogen)	Remifemin	Perimenopausal Symptoms, Post-Menopausal Symptoms	Capsule
Hormone	Cetrorelix	Cetrolide	Ovulation Stimulation	Injectable
Hormone	Clomiphene	Clomid, Serophene	Ovulation Stimulation	Tablet
Hormone	Danazol	Denocrine	Endometriosis	Capsule
Hormone	Estradiol / Levonorgestrel	Climara Pro, Lybrel	Perimenopausal Symptoms, Post-Menopausal Symptoms	Patch, Tablet
Hormone	Estradiol / Norethindrone	Activella, Combi-patch, Mimvey	Perimenopausal Symptoms, Post-Menopausal Symptoms	Patch, Tablet
Hormone	Estradiol Valerate / Dienogestrel	Natazia	Contraception, Endometriosis, Menstrual Cycle Regulation	Tablet
Hormone	Conjugated Estrogens, Estradiol, Estrogen	Alora, Climara, Delestrogen, Depo-Estradiol, Divigel, Elestrin, Esclim, Estrace, Estraderm, Estrasorb, Estratab, Estring, Evamist, Femring, Femtrace, Menostar, Ogen, Ortho-Est, Premarin, Vagifem, Vivelle-Dot	Osteoporosis, Perimenopausal Symptoms, Post-Menopausal Symptoms	Gel, Injectable, Intravaginal Ring, Patch, Tablet, Vaginal Cream, Vaginal Tablet
Hormone	Estrogens and Medroxyprogester-one	Premphase, Prempro	Osteoporosis, Perimenopausal Symptoms, Post-Menopausal Symptoms	Tablet

Table 3 cont.
Drugs Used to Treat Reproductive / Sexual Disorders (Excluding Infectious Diseases)

Drug Class(es)	Generic Name(s)**	Brand Name(s)**	Indication(s)	Available Dose Form(s)
Hormone	Ethinyl Estradiol / Desogestrel	Apri, Azurette, Caziant, Cyclessa, Desogen, Kariva, Mircette, Ortho-cept, Reclipsen, Velivet	Contraception, Endometriosis, Menstrual Cycle Regulation	Tablet
Hormone	Ethinyl Estradiol / Dropirenone	Angeliq, Gianvi, Ocella, Yasmin, Yaz, Zarah	Contraception, Menstrual Cycle Regulation	Tablet
Hormone	Ethinyl Estradiol / Ethynodiol Diacetate	Demulen, Kelnor, Zovia	Contraception, Endometriosis, Menstrual Cycle Regulation	Tablet
Hormone	Ethinyl Estradiol / Etonogestrel	NuvaRing	Contraception, Endometriosis, Menstrual Cycle Regulation	Intravaginal Ring
Hormone	Ethinyl Estradiol / Levonorgestrel	Aviane, Enpresse, Introvale, Jolessa, Lessina, Levora, Loseasonique, Lutera, Nordette, Portia, Quasense, Seasonale, Seasonique, Sronyx, Trivora	Contraception, Endometriosis, Menstrual Cycle Regulation	Tablet
Hormone	Ethinyl Estradiol / Norelgestromin	Ortho-Evra, Ortho Tri-Cyclen	Contraceptive	Patch, Tablet
Hormone	Ethinyl Estradiol / Norethindrone with or without Iron	Aranelle, Balziva, Brevicon, FemHRT, Junel, Leena, Loestrin, Micro-gestin, Modicon, Necon, Norinel, Nortrel, Ortho-Novum, Ovcon, Tri-Norinyl, Zenchent	Birth Control, Endometriosis, Osteoporosis, Perimenopausal Symptoms, Post-Menopausal Symptoms	Chewable Tablet, Patch, Tablet

Drug Class(es)	Generic Name(s)**	Brand Name(s)**	Indication(s)	Available Dose Form(s)
Hormone	Ethinyl Estradiol / Norgestimate	Mononessa, Ortho-Cyclen, Ortho Tri-Cyclen Lo, Previfem, Sprintec, Trinessa, Tri-Previfem, Tri-Sprintec	Contraception, Endometriosis, Menstrual Cycle Regulation	Tablet
Hormone	Ethinyl Estradiol / Norgestrel	Cryselle, Lo/Ovral, Low-Ogestrel, Ogestrel	Contraception, Endometriosis, Menstrual Cycle Regulation	Tablet
Hormone	Follitropin Alpha	Gonal-F	Ovulation Stimulation	Injectable
Hormone	Follitropin Beta	Follistim	Ovulation Stimulation	Injectable
Hormone	Ganirelix	Sanirelex	Ovulation Stimulation	Injectable
Hormone	Gonadorelin	Lutrepulse	Ovulation Stimulation	Injectable
Hormone	Goserelin	Zoladex	Breast Cancer, Endometriosis, Prostate Cancer	Injectable
Hormone	Leuprolide	Eligard, Lupron Depot	Endometriosis, Ovulation Stimulation, Prostate Cancer	Injectable
Hormone	Levonorgestrel	Mirena, Next Choice, Plan B One-Step	Contraception	Intrauterine Device, Tablet
Hormone	Lutropin Alpha	Luveris	Ovulation Stimulation	Injectable
Hormone	Medroxyprogester-one	Depo-Provera, Provera	Birth Control, Perimenopausal Symptoms, Post-Menopausal Symptoms	Injectable, Tablet
Hormone	Megestrol	Megace, Megace ES	Endometriosis, Loss of Appetite	Liquid, Tablet
Hormone	Menotropins	Menopur, Repronex	Ovulation Stimulation	Injectable

Table 3 *cont.*
Drugs Used to Treat Reproductive / Sexual Disorders (Excluding Infectious Diseases)

Drug Class(es)	Generic Name(s)**	Brand Name(s)**	Indication(s)	Available Dose Form(s)
Hormone	Nafarelin	Synarel	Endometriosis	Nasal Spray
Hormone	Norethindrone	Aygestin, Camila, Errin, Heather, Jolivette, Nora BE, Nor-Q-D, Ortho Micronor	Birth Control, Endometriosis, Perimenopausal Symptoms, Post-Menopausal Symptoms	Tablet
Hormone	Norethindrone / Mestranol	Necon	Contraception, Endometriosis, Menstrual Cycle Regulation	Tablet
Hormone	Progesterone	Crinone, Endometrin, Prochieve, Prometrium	Contraception, Menstrual Cycle Regulation	Capsule, Cream, Gel, Injectable, Powder, Tablet, Vaginal Suppository
Hormone	Red Clover (Estrogen)	Promensil, Trinovin	Perimenopausal Symptoms, Post-Menopausal Symptoms	Tablet
Hormone	Soy Isoflavones (Estrogen)	Estroven	Perimenopausal Symptoms, Post-Menopausal Symptoms	Capsule
Hormone	Methyltestosterone, Testosterone	Androderm, Androgel, Android, Delatestryl, Depo-Testosterone, Meth-itest, Testim, Testred, Testopel, Testosterone	Erectile Dysfunction, Low Testosterone	Cream, Gel, Injectable, Lozenge, Patch
Hormone	Urofollitropin	Bravelle	Ovulation Stimulation	Injectable
Phosphodiesterase -5 Inhibitor	Sildenafil	Revatio, Viagra	Erectile Dysfunction, Pulmonary Arterial Hypertension	Injectable, Tablet
Phosphodiesterase -5 Inhibitor	Tadalafil	Adcirca, Cialis	Erectile Dysfunction, Pulmonary Arterial Hypertension	Tablet
Phosphodiesterase -5 Inhibitor	Vardenafil	Levitra	Erectile Dysfunction	Tablet

Drug Class(es)	Generic Name(s)**	Brand Name(s)**	Indication(s)	Available Dose Form(s)
Vasodilator	Alprostadil	Caverject, Edex, Muse, Prostin	Erectile Dysfunction, Patent Ductus Arteriosus	Injectable, Suppository
Vitamin: Water-Soluble	Folic Acid	Folvite	Folic Acid Deficiency, Megaloblastic Anemia, Neural Tube Defect Prevention (Fetal)	Solution, Tablet

**All rights to all brand names and trademarks are held by their respective owners.*

Conclusion

The male and female reproductive systems are very complex, and it is important to comprehend their normal function to understand the disorders caused by genitourinary malfunction. The body produces many hormones that act throughout the body and are important in normal bodily function. Estrogen and progesterone are two of these hormones that play important physiologic roles throughout life. Supplementation or loss of these hormones has profound effects on the body. When health care providers recommend therapies to alter estrogen and progesterone levels, they must treat every patient individually and monitor the therapy for beneficial and/or undesirable effects.

Reproductive disorders, such as endometriosis, infertility, testosterone deficiency and sexually transmitted diseases, can result in decreased quality of life in those who are affected. Combinations of lifestyle changes, nondrug therapies and medication are available to help patients get relief from symptoms of these disorders and to live more productive and eventful lives. Pharmacy technicians must have enough knowledge about common disorders to understand appropriate treatment, including those of the reproductive system. Pharmacists and pharmacy technicians can play a significant role in educating patients about these disorders and helping them get the proper therapy. Disorders of the reproductive system, including sexually transmitted diseases, are based primarily on the type of invading organism identified. Most of these diseases respond well to current drug therapy when the correct diagnosis is determined.

Acknowledgement

The editors wish to acknowledge Dianne E. Miller, R.Ph.; Reta E. Naoum, Pharm.D.; and Gregg S. Potter, Ph.D., R.Ph., for their previous authorship of this chapter, which has been directly updated from the 11th edition of this Manual.

Bibliography

- Centers for Disease Control and Prevention, Sexually Transmitted Diseases, www.cdc.gov/std/, March 9, 2011.

- Dickerson, L., Bucci, K., "Chapter 80, Contraception," Pharmacotherapy: A Pathophysiologic Approach, 5th edition, New York, NY, 2002, pp. 1445-1461.

- Kalantaridou, S.N., Davis, S.R., Calis, K.A., "Hormone Therapy in Women," Pharmacotherapy: A Pathophysiologic Approach, 7th edition, New York, NY, 2008, pp. 1351-1365.

- Knodel, L.C., "Chapter 121, Sexually Transmitted Diseases," Pharmacotherapy: A Pathophysiologic Approach, 7th edition, New York, NY, 2008, pp. 1915-1930.

- Lacy, C.F., Armstrong, L.L., Goldman, M.P., Lance, L.L., Drug Information Handbook, 2010.

- Lee, M., "Chapter 86, Erectile Dysfunction," Pharmacotherapy: A Pathophysiologic Approach, 7th edition, New York, NY, 2008, pp. 1369-1385.

- Mayo Clinic, Male Hypogonadism, www.mayoclinic.com/health/male-hypogonadism/DS00300, March 10, 2011.

- Michigan Pharmacists Association, Pharmacy Certified Technician Training Manual, 11th edition, Lansing, MI, 2008, pp. 367-405.

- National Institutes of Health, www.health.nih.gov/category/WomensHealth, March 9, 2011.

- Natural Medicines Comprehensive Database, http://naturaldatabase.therapeuticresearch.com/nd/Search.aspx?cs=&s=ND&pt=100&id=875&fs=ND&searchid=24671160, Jan. 16, 2011.

- Smith, S., Pfeifer, S., Collins, J., "Diagnosis and Management of Female Infertility," Journal of the American Medical Association, Chicago, IL, Vol. 290, No. 13, pp. 1767-1770, October 2003.

- Snow, K., "Erectile Dysfunction: A Review and Update," Formulary, New York, NY, Vol. 39, pp. 261-268, May 2004.

- Sturpe, D.A., "Chapter 84, Endometriosis," Pharmacotherapy: A Pathophysiologic Approach, 7th edition, New York, NY, 2008, pp. 1345-1350.

- United States Department of Health and Human Services Agency for Healthcare Research and Quality, www.ahrq.gov, March 9, 2011.

- U.S. National Cancer Institute, http://training.seer.cancer.gov/anatomy/reproductive/, March 9, 2011.

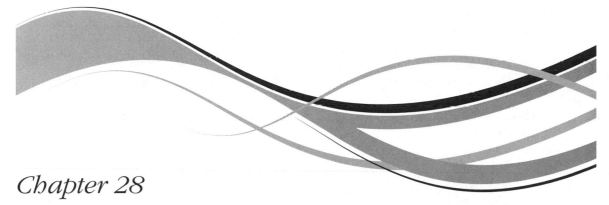

Chapter 28
REVIEW QUESTIONS

1. Which of the following is not a part of the male anatomy?
    a. Epididymus
    b. Flagellum
    c. Vas deferens
    d. Urethra

2. What happens to an egg that has not been fertilized?
    a. It travels to the uterus for implantation
    b. It leaves the body through the urethra
    c. It degenerates in the Fallopian tubes
    d. It is excreted during the menstrual cycle

3. Which of the following connects the uterus with the vagina?
    a. Cervix
    b. Clitoris
    c. Urethra
    d. Vulva

4. Which one of the following classes of drugs is known to cause harm to the developing fetus and must be avoided during pregnancy?
    a. Beta adrenergic antagonists
    b. Calcium channel blockers
    c. Thiazide diuretics
    d. Angiotensin converting enzyme inhibitors

5. Which of the following does the addition of progestins, in the hormonal treatment of postmenopausal women who still have a uterus, decrease the risk of developing?
    a. Breast cancer
    b. Parkinson's Disease
    c. Endometrial cancer
    d. Osteoarthritis

6. Which of the following is not a common symptom of endometriosis?
   a. Dysmenorrhea
   b. Blurred vision
   c. Low back pain
   d. Urinary disturbances

7. Which of the following drugs for erectile dysfunction allows for more flexibility in initiating sexual activity?
   a. Vardenafil
   b. Tadalafil
   c. Sildenafil
   d. Alprostadil

8. Which of the following agents is used in the treatment of infertility and classified as a gonadotropin-releasing hormone agonist?
   a. Estradiol
   b. Nafarelin
   c. Clomiphene citrate
   d. Urofillitropin

9. Which of the following is a common cause of testosterone deficiency?
   a. Undescended testicles
   b. Tuberculosis
   c. Sexual intercourse
   d. Exposure to UV light

10. Which of the following is a parasitic infection that does not usually cause symptoms?
    a. Gonorrhea
    b. Syphilis
    c. Chlamydia
    d. Trichomoniasis

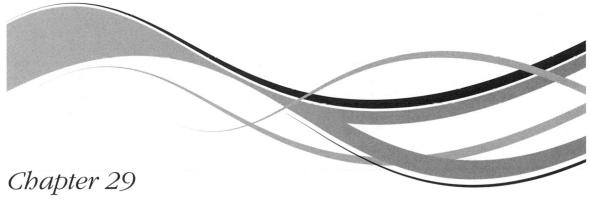

Chapter 29
URINARY SYSTEM

By Andrew E. Britton, MBA, R.Ph.
Gregg S. Potter, Ph.D., R.Ph.

Learning Objectives

This chapter seeks to prepare a pharmacy technician to:

- define and briefly explain benign prostatic hyperplasia (BPH).
- describe the medications used in the treatment of BPH.
- understand the various types of incontinence.
- identify the drugs used in the treatment of incontinence.
- discuss enuresis and its treatment.
- know the causes of urinary tract infections (UTIs).
- identify the most common antibiotics used in the treatment of UTIs.

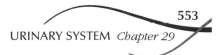

Urinary System

The function of the urinary system is to produce, store, and transport urine. Included in the urinary system are **kidneys, ureters, bladder** and the **urethra**. In the kidneys, urine is produced and then it drains through long tubes called ureters into the bladder. Muscle contraction in the ureters helps to force this urine into the bladder. The bladder stores urine and will contract to expel urine through the urethra and past the urethral sphincter. The movement of urine from the kidneys and through the urethra occurs involuntarily and is controlled by the sympathetic and parasympathetic nervous systems. The **sphincter muscle** at the base of the urethra allows for voluntary control of urination (see Figure 1).

Figure 1
Male and Female Urinary Systems

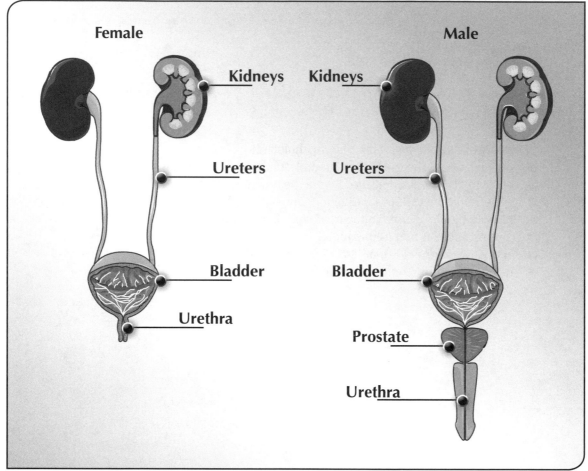

Figure produced using Servier Medical Art, www.servier.com

There are various urological disorders that commonly afflict the U.S. population, including **benign prostatic hyperplasia (BPH)**, **incontinence**, **enuresis** and **urinary tract infections (UTIs)**.

Benign Prostatic Hyperplasia

BPH is an enlargement of the prostate gland in men; however, patients must understand that BPH does not develop into prostate cancer (which causes abnormal growth of the prostate gland and is the second leading cause of cancer death among males). Tests to distinguish between BPH and prostate cancer include a digital rectal exam (the prostate may be felt through the rectum, with a finger, by a trained physician) and an increase in prostate-specific antigen in the blood. BPH is one of the most common medical conditions affecting older men. It is common for the prostate gland to become enlarged as a man matures. As a man ages, the gland goes through two main growth periods. The first occurs early in puberty, when the prostate doubles in size. At approximately age 25, the prostate begins to grow again. This second growth phase frequently results, years later, in BPH. Though the prostate continues to grow during the majority of a man's life, the enlargement doesn't typically cause problems until late in life. According to statistics, BPH affects 50 percent of men age 51-60 years and as many as 90 percent of men over age 80. In patients with BPH, urethra compression becomes excessive and causes difficulty in urination, a weak urine stream and incomplete emptying of the bladder. Many BPH symptoms stem from obstruction of the urethra and gradual loss of bladder function that results in incomplete emptying of the bladder. The symptoms of BPH include changes or problems with urination, such as a hesitant, interrupted, weak stream; urgency and leaking or dribbling of urine; and more frequent urination, particularly at night.

BPH can be treated with drugs, surgery or both. Surgical interventions include **transurethral microwave thermotherapy (TUMT)**, **transurethral needle ablation (TUNA)**, **transurethral resection of the prostate (TURP)** and other procedures. Surgery is considered the gold standard of BPH treatment; but, surgery does carry risks, such as impotence and incontinence, so many patients prefer drug treatment. The start of pharmacologic treatment is often determined by the severity of the symptoms having an impact on the patient's quality of life. The pharmacological management of BPH includes alpha-1 adrenergic antagonists and 5-alpha reductase inhibitors. In some instances, drug therapy includes a combination of one agent from each class. If this is appropriate, there are combination agents available that may be economically beneficial for patients.

Alpha-1 adrenergic antagonists were initially designed for the treatment of hypertension. These drugs cause relaxation of smooth muscles, particularly in the prostate and bladder neck, that improves urine flow and reduces bladder outlet obstruction. Often a decrease in symptoms is observed within days as flow of urine through the urethra is increased. Alpha-1 adrenergic antagonists include both selective and nonselective agents. Nonselective agents include terazosin, doxazosin and prazosin. These agents work in the prostate, but they also reduce smooth muscle tone in the blood vessels. This leads to possible side effects of dizziness and **postural hypotension**. Selective agents include tamsulosin and alfuzosin. These drugs were specifically designed to treat BPH and do not have a significant affect on blood pressure so they have less risk of adverse effects, such as fainting, than the nonselective agents.

5-alpha reductase inhibitors are medications that inhibit production of the hormone dihydrotestosterone (DHT); DHT is involved with prostate enlargement and the stimulation of male reproductive organs. Finasteride and dutasteride are the two 5-alpha reductase inhibitors that are currently available in the United States. The usage of either of these drugs can either prevent progression of prostate growth or actually shrink the prostate in some men. A common side effect associated with these drugs is decreased libido. Another disadvantage of these drugs is that it often takes six to 12 months to observe symptomatic relief. Since this class of drugs directly stops the action of male hormone production, both of these agents are contraindicated in pregnant females and women of childbearing age. Those working in the pharmacy must not handle broken tablets/capsules without protective gloves due to the potential for transdermal absorption and disruption of normal fetal development.

Herbals

Herbal products used for BPH include saw palmetto, stinging nettle and pygeum. Of these, saw palmetto is the most commonly used for BPH, and it has been shown to decrease symptoms in some individuals. Overall, the effectiveness of these herbal agents is still questionable and their use as single agents for BPH is not recommended.

Urinary Incontinence

Control of urination relies on the finely coordinated actions of the smooth muscle tissue of the urethra and bladder, voluntary inhibition and impulses from the nervous system. The body stores urine in the bladder. During urination, muscles in the bladder contract. The contraction forces urine out of the bladder and into the urethra and then out of the body. Simultaneously, muscles surrounding the urethra relax and allow passage of the urine. Spinal nerves control the movement of these muscles. Medications, such as diuretics and some calcium channel blockers, typically cause an increase in urine formation that may worsen symptoms.

Loss of bladder control is called urinary incontinence. There are five different types of urinary incontinence. They are:

- **Stress incontinence:** This is a weakness of the sphincter muscle that pinches off the urethra at the base of the bladder. This causes leakage when abdominal pressure increases (e.g., sneezing, coughing, laughing); it is common during pregnancy.
- **Urge incontinence:** This involves uncontrolled contractions of the bladder.
- **Overflow incontinence:** This is incontinence caused by obstruction of urine flow from the bladder; it is common in elderly men due to prostate enlargement.
- **Functional incontinence:** This is incontinence related to physical or psychological problems that impair the individual's ability to get to the bathroom.
- **Mixed incontinence:** This is a combination of more than one type of incontinence.

Aging itself does not cause incontinence; it can occur for many reasons. For example, urinary tract infections, vaginal irritation and certain medications can cause acute bladder control problems. In certain cases, incontinence lasts longer. This might be attributed to other problems, such as:

- weak bladder muscles.
- overactive bladder muscles.
- blockage from prostate enlargement.
- damage to nerves that control the bladder from diseases (such as multiple sclerosis or Parkinson's Disease).
- disorders, such as arthritis, that make walking to the bathroom painful and slow.

One-third of women older than 65 years have some degree of incontinence and 12 percent have daily incontinence. The disorder is much more prevalent in women than men.

Changes in lifestyle and behavior are initiated before drug therapy. Lifestyle modifications that may alleviate incontinence episodes include weight loss, smoking cessation, decreased consumption of caffeine, decreased alcohol intake, limiting fluid intake after certain hours, maintaining proper hydration throughout the day (but avoiding fluid at night) and exercising. Nondrug treatments of incontinence also include pelvic muscle exercises (also known as **Kegel exercises**) and **biofeedback**. Pelvic muscle exercises work the muscles that are used to stop urination. Strengthening these muscles helps patients hold urine in the bladder for a longer period of time. Biofeedback helps patients become more aware of signals from the body to urinate. Additionally, timed voiding and bladder training can be used to help incontinence sufferers regain proper bladder control.

Drugs that block the effects of the parasympathetic nervous system on the urinary tract are used to treat urinary incontinence. These agents are called muscarinic receptor antagonists and relax the bladder muscle, allowing for increased storage of urine. Commonly used antimuscarinic agents include oxybutynin and tolterodine. Long-acting and extended-release forms of these agents allow for once daily dosing, and a sustained-release oxybutynin transdermal patch is available. Recently-approved antimuscarinics, such as trospium, solifenacin and darifenacin, are expected to have fewer adverse effects (e.g., less dry mouth, less constipation and less blurred vision). Older antimuscarinics, such as propantheline and flavoxate, exhibit more of these effects and, therefore, are only occasionally used for urinary incontinence. Alpha-agonists and estrogens are sometimes used to treat stress incontinence. Antimuscarinic drugs, mentioned previously, are neither appropriate nor effective in treating stress incontinence. Alpha-agonists stimulate urethral closure, and there is a suggested benefit in the treatment of stress incontinence from this action. Pseudoephedrine, which is a nonprescription drug, sometimes is recommended for the treatment of stress incontinence. There are, however, no published studies evaluating pseudoephedrine in the treatment of stress incontinence, and the Food and Drug Administration has not approved this use of the product. Estrogen has been used widely to treat stress incontinence. The rationale for estrogen therapy is its ability to increase urethral blood supply and thickness and to sensitize alpha-receptors in the bladder neck; both of these actions possibly could improve urethral closure. In addition to treatment, bladder control pads (e.g., Attends®, Depends® and Serenity®) are also available to help control unwanted leakage through garments.

Enuresis

Enuresis, or bed-wetting, is an involuntary voiding of urine observed in children. Most children will outgrow this problem with age. In children where symptoms happen frequently, behavioral training, such as fluid restriction before bedtime or moisture sensitive alarms (Potty Pager®, DRISleeper®), can be initiated to decrease occurrences. If these are not successful, medications (e.g., desmopressin and imipramine) may be prescribed, although drug treatment is not recommended for children under six years of age. Desmopressin, which can be given orally or intranasally, acts in the kidneys to decrease the amount of urine formed. Imipramine causes the bladder to relax and be able to hold more urine, decreasing the frequency of urination.

Urinary Tract Infections

UTIs are a serious health problem affecting millions of people annually. Infections involving the urinary tract are common, second only to respiratory infections in occurrence. An estimated 34 percent of adults age 20 or older (61.4 million) self-reported having experienced at least one episode of a urinary tract infection or cystitis. In 2000, there were an estimated 9.1 million physician visits by patients age 20 years, or older, with a urinary tract infection or cystitis listed as a diagnosis. UTIs are most prevalent in sexually active women. This occurs because sexual activity promotes bacteria, specifically the intestinal bacterial Escherichia coli, to move from the gastrointestinal tract to the vagina and surrounding region. The bacteria then colonize that area and continue to migrate up the urethra, the first site of infection of the urinary tract. Although many different bacteria may be responsible for a UTI, *E. coli* is the most common bacterial cause of a UTI. This happens more readily in females than males due to the relatively shorter urethra found in females. If a UTI does occur in a male, the severity of such an infection is much worse and often requires hospitalization to be treated. Although such infections are generally referred to as urinary tract infections, there are specific names for infections that reach the different parts of the urinary tract. **Cystitis** is a broad term referring to inflammation of the bladder that may be caused by multiple sources, one very common source being an infection of the urinary tract (infectious cystitis). If the infection is contained at the urethra, it may be referred to as **infectious urethritis**. If the infection reaches all the way to the kidney(s), it is referred to as **infectious**

pyelonephritis. If the infection is in a male and it reaches the prostate, it may be referred to as **infectious prostatitis**. Further, there are complicated and uncomplicated UTIs. A **complicated UTI** is one that occurs with another condition allowing the urinary tract to be a ready target for bacterial growth. Such a complication could be a kidney stone, prostate enlargement or damage to the nerve controlling the bladder. An **uncomplicated UTI** is one that occurs without any assistance from another condition.

Not everyone with a UTI is symptomatic, but most individuals experience at least some symptoms. Symptoms of a UTI may include a frequent urge to urinate, a painful or burning sensation in portions of the urinary tract or a change in the color or clarity (from clear to cloudy) of the person's urine. Frequently, women feel an uncomfortable pressure above the pubic bone, and some men experience a fullness in the rectum. Commonly, people with a UTI complain that, despite the urge to urinate, only a tiny amount of urine is voided. The urine itself may appear cloudy and even reddish, if blood is present. A fever may indicate that the infection has traveled into the kidneys. Other symptoms of a kidney infection include pain in the back or side below the ribs, nausea and vomiting. Some risk factors that predispose patients to a UTI include incomplete emptying of the bladder, decreased urination frequency or volume (from any cause), BPH, pregnancy and antimuscarinic drugs (e.g., hyoscyamine, ipratropium, oxybutynin and atropine).

Many nondrug therapies are available for the treatment and prevention of a UTI. Drinking plenty of water can dilute the bacterial concentrations in the urine and promote removal of infected urine. Ingestion of cranberry juice increases the natural antibacterial activity of the urine by preventing adherence of bacteria to organ walls within the urinary tract. Pharmacological treatment is antibiotic therapy with antibiotics that are known to kill *E. coli* (or the infecting bacteria when known) and that have high penetration into the urinary tract. The choice of drug and length of treatment depends on the patient's history and the classification of the infection. Generally, oral therapy is appropriate; however, complicated infections or severe infections (especially in men) may require IV antibiotics at the initiation of therapy. In either case, therapy is generally short and may last from three to 14 days depending on the severity of the infection. Many UTIs can be completely cleared with three days of sulfamethoxazole/trimethoprim double-strength taken twice daily. Further, penicillins (e.g., amoxicillin and ampicillin), cephalosporins (e.g., cephalexin) and nitrofurantoin are also commonly used for UTIs. Nitrofurantoin, however, is only recommended for patients with otherwise healthy kidneys due to the need for the kidneys to filter it out from the blood to get it to the urinary tract. In the last decade, quinolone antibiotics, specifically ciprofloxacin and levofloxacin, have become a common choice of physicians for treating a UTI. Quinolones have the advantage of being broad-spectrum, meaning that they kill a wide variety of bacteria that includes gram-positive and gram-negative bacteria; unfortunately, due to their increased use, resistance to these antibiotics is increasing. More narrow-spectrum antibiotics are recommended whenever it is possible to use them. Further, quinolones must be avoided in pregnant women and children due to the potential that they will cause abnormalities in bone and joint development. Fosfomycin is another choice; it comes as a single-dose powder packet that is dissolved in water and drank. Fosfomycin is only used in the treatment of cystitis. In the severest of cases, IV aminoglycosides may be used (e.g., gentamycin and tobramycin) and a combination of drugs may be employed to attempt to prevent the infection from reaching the blood and becoming sepsis (a life-threatening infection of the blood).

Although antibiotics are necessary to eradicate the bacteria, they do not address the immediate symptoms of the patients, including the pain, burning and itching that may come with a UTI. There are many pain relievers and anti-inflammatory drugs that may be helpful; however, phenazopyridine is the drug of choice for urinary discomfort. Phenazopyridine is available both by prescription and over-the-counter (OTC), with the prescription products having a higher strength than the OTC versions. Phenazopyridine is not without its side effects, even though it only works on the urinary tract and generally does not have effects anywhere else in the body. Phenazopyridine causes a patient's secretions (most notably the urine) to turn orange. This orange color can stain fabrics if affected urine comes in contact with the fabric. Further, contact lenses may be discolored, as tears may be affected by this color change. Especially due to its OTC availability, many patients mistakenly believe that the pain relieving effects of phenazopyridine are a cure for a UTI; however, an antibiotic is required in addition to pain relievers to eradicate the infection.

Table 1
Drugs Used to Treat Disorders of the Urinary System

Drug Class(es)	Generic Name(s)**	Brand Name(s)**	Indication(s)	Available Dose Form(s)
5-Alpha Reductase Inhibitor	Dutasteride	Avodart	Enlarging Prostate	Capsule
Antibiotic	Fosfomycin	Monurol	Bacterial Infection	Oral Powder
Antibiotic	Nitrofurantoin Macrocrystals	Furadantin, Microdantin	Bacterial Infection	Capsule, Suspension
Antibiotic	Nitrofurantoin Monohydrate Macrocrystals	Macrobid	Bacterial Infection	Capsule
Antibiotic: Antiprotozoal, Antibiotic: Sulfonamide	Sulfamethoxazole / Trimethoprim	Bactrim, Septra	Bacterial Infection, Pneumocystis Pneumonia Prophylaxis	Injectable, Suspension, Tablet
Antibiotic: Fluoroquinolone	Ciprofloxacin	Cetraxal, Ciloxan, Cipro, Cipro XR, Proquin XR	Bacterial Infection	Injectable, Ophthalmic, Otic, Suspension, Tablet
Antibiotic: Fluoroquinolone	Levofloxacin	Iquix, Levaquin, Quixin	Bacterial Infection	Injectable, Ophthalmic, Tablet
Antibiotic: Fluoroquinolone	Moxifloxacin	Avelox, Moxeza, Vigamox	Bacterial Infection	Injectable, Ophthalmic, Tablet
Antibiotic: Fluoroquinolone	Norfloxacin	Noroxin	Bacterial Infection	Tablet
Antibiotic: Penicillin	Amoxicillin	Amoxil	Bacterial Infection	Capsule, Chewable Tablet, Powder (for Suspension)
Antibiotic: Penicillin	Amoxicillin / Potassium Clavulanate	Augmentin	Bacterial Infection	Extended-Release Tablet, Powder (for Suspension), Tablet
Antibiotic: Penicillin	Ampicillin	Omnipen, Polycillin, Principen	Bacterial Infection	Capsule, Injectable, Powder, Suspension

Table 1 *cont.*
Drugs Used to Treat Disorders of the Urinary System

Drug Class(es)	Generic Name(s)**	Brand Name(s)**	Indication(s)	Available Dose Form(s)
Anticholinergic	Darifenacin	Darifenacin	Over-Active Bladder	Extended-Release Tablet
Anticholinergic	Fesoterodine	Toviaz	Over-Active Bladder	Extended-Release Tablet
Anticholinergic	Flavoxate	Urispas	Over-Active Bladder	Tablet
Anticholinergic	Oxybutynin	Ditropan, Ditropan XL, Gelnique, Oxytrol	Over-Active Bladder	Extended-Release Tablet, Gel, Patch, Syrup, Tablet
Anticholinergic	Solifenacin	Vesicare	Over-Active Bladder	Tablet
Anticholinergic	Tolterodine	Detrol, Detrol LA	Over-Active Bladder	Extended-Release Tablet, Tablet
Anticholinergic	Trospium	Sanctura, Sanctura XR	Over-Active Bladder	Extended-Release Tablet, Tablet
Antidepressant: Tricyclic	Imipramine	Tofranil, Tofranil-PM	Attention Deficit Hyperactivity Disorder, Bed Wetting, Depression, Pain, Panic Disorder	Capsule, Tablet
Antihypertensive: Alpha-Blocker	Doxazosin	Cardura	High Blood Pressure	Extended-Release Tablet, Tablet
Antihypertensive: Alpha-Blocker	Prazosin	Minipress	High Blood Pressure	Capsule, Tablet
Antihypertensive: Alpha-Blocker	Terazosin	Hytrin	High Blood Pressure	Capsule
Hormone	Desmopressin Acetate	DDAVP	Bed Wetting	Injectable, Nasal Spray, Tablet
Pain Reliever	Phenazopyridine	AZO, Pyridium	Urinary Pain	Tablet

Drug Class(es)	Generic Name(s)**	Brand Name(s)**	Indication(s)	Available Dose Form(s)
Selective Alpha-1 Blocker	Tamsulosin	Flomax	Enlarging Prostate, Urethral Constriction, Urethral Obstruction	Capsule

*All rights to all brand names and trademarks are held by their respective owners.

Conclusion

Urological disorders affect a significant number of people in the United States each year. Some urological disorders are transient, some are permanent and some build over time. BPH, which is a noncancerous enlargement of the prostate gland, primarily affects elderly men. A UTI, a bacterial infection of the urinary tract, primarily affects young, sexually-active women. Incontinence is another urological disorder that is more prevalent in women than in men. Nondrug treatments for incontinence, such as bladder training, can be very useful in helping patients to regain bladder control. Enuresis occurs mainly in children and can be treated with both pharmacological and behavioral therapies. Infections of the urinary tract account for millions of physician visits each year. Although treatment choices for each of these conditions will be made by physicians in collaboration with pharmacists, a pharmacy technician would do very well to be familiar with the myriad of disorders associated with the urinary tract.

Acknowledgement

The editors wish to acknowledge Andrew E. Britton, MBA, R.Ph., and Gregg S. Potter, Ph.D., R.Ph., for their previous authorship of this chapter, which was directly updated from the 11th edition of this Manual.

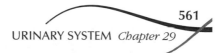

Bibliography

- Cole, E., Prince, R., "Chapter 114, Urinary Tract Infections and Prostatitis," Pharmacotherapy: A Pathophysiologic Approach, 5th edition, New York, NY, 2002, pp. 1981-1996.
- Cotran, R.S., et. al., Robbins' Pathologic Basis of Disease, 6th edition, Philadelphia, PA, 1999.
- Dorland, N.W., Novak, P.D., Dorland's Pocket Medical Dictionary, 26th edition, Philadelphia, PA, 2001.
- Douglass, M., Lin, J., "Update on the Treatment of Benign Prostatic Hyperplasia," *Formulary*, New York, NY, Vol. 40, pp. 50-64, February 2005.
- Fantl, J.A., Cardozo, L., McClish, D.K., "Estrogen Therapy in the Management of Urinary Incontinence in Postmenopausal Women: A Meta-Analysis. First Report of the Hormones and Urogenital Therapy Committee," *Obstetrics & Gynecology*, Vol. 83, pp. 12-18, January 1994.
- Lacy, C., Armstrong, L., Goldman, M., Lance, L., Drug Information Handbook, Ohio, 2005.
- Lee, M., "Chapter 85, Management of Benign Prostatic Hyperplasia," Pharmacotherapy: A Pathophy-siologic Approach, 5th edition, New York, NY, 2002, pp. 1533-1542.
- McConnell, J.D., "Epidemiology, Etiology, Pathophysiology, and Diagnosis of Benign Prostatic Hyperplasia," *Campbell's Urology*, Philadelphia, PA, Vol. 2. No. 7, pp. 1429-1452, 1998.
- Michigan Pharmacists Association, Pharmacy Certified Technician Training Manual, 9th edition, Lansing, MI, 2004, pp. 281-289.
- Ouslander, J., "Management of Overactive Bladder," *New England Journal of Medicine*, Waltham, MA, Vol. 350, No. 8, pp. 786-797, February 2004.
- Rover, E., Wyman, J., Lackner, T., Guay, D., "Chapter 86, Urinary Incontinence," Pharmacotherapy: A Pathophysiologic Approach, 5th edition, New York, NY, 2002, pp. 1543-1556.
- Stewart, S., McGhan, W., Offerdahl, T., Corey, R., "Overactive Bladder Patients and the Role of the Pharmacist," *Journal of the American Pharmaceutical Association*, Washington, D.C., Vol. 42, No. 3, pp. 469-476, May/June 2002.
- Thiedke, C., "Nocturnal Enuresis," *American Family Physician*, Kansas, Vol. 67, No. 7, pp. 1499-1506, April 2003.
- Thom, D., "Variation in Estimates of Urinary Incontinence Prevalence in the Community: Effects of Differences in Definition, Population Characteristics, and Study Type," *Journal of American Geriatrics Society*, Malden, MA, Vol. 46, pp. 473-480, 1998.

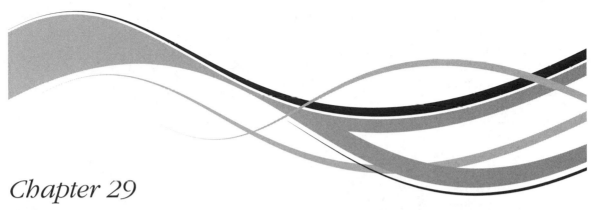

Chapter 29

REVIEW QUESTIONS

1. Which group does BPH most commonly affect?
    a. Older men
    b. Sexually-active women
    c. Boys in puberty
    d. Men and women equally

2. Which of the following is an example of a selective agent specifically designed to treat BPH?
    a. Terazosin (Hytrin®)
    b. Alfuzosin (Uroxatral®)
    c. Doxazosin (Cardura®)
    d. Prazosin (Minipress®)

3. Which of the following is a common side effect associated with 5-alpha reductase inhibitors?
    a. Dizziness
    b. Postural hypotension
    c. Decreased libido
    d. Photosensitivity

4. Which herbal supplement has been shown to decrease symptoms of BPH in certain individuals?
    a. Saw palmetto
    b. Ginseng
    c. Stinging nettle
    d. Pygeum

5. Which of the following is not a type of incontinence?
    a. Urge
    b. Overflow
    c. Gastric
    d. Stress

6.   Which of the following has been widely used to treat stress incontinence?
      a. Estrogen
      b. Tolterodine
      c. Oxybutynin
      d. Tamulosin

7.   Which of the following treatments for enuresis causes the bladder to relax and be able to hold more urine?
      a. Desmopression
      b. Imipramine
      c. Terazosin
      d. Ciprofloxacin

8.   Which drug is available both orally and intranasally for the treatment of enuresis?
      a. Sildenafil
      b. Desmopressin
      c. Metronidazole
      d. Indinavir

9.   Phenazopyridine has which of the following unique effects?
      a. Turning the urine orange
      b. Dry mouth
      c. Turning the urine cloudy
      d. Causing the bladder to hold more urine before causing the urge to void

10.   Which of the following antibiotics for a UTI is only recommended for patients with otherwise healthy kidneys?
      a. Ampicillin
      b. Amoxicillin
      c. Trimethoprim/sulfamethoxazole
      d. Nitrofurantoin

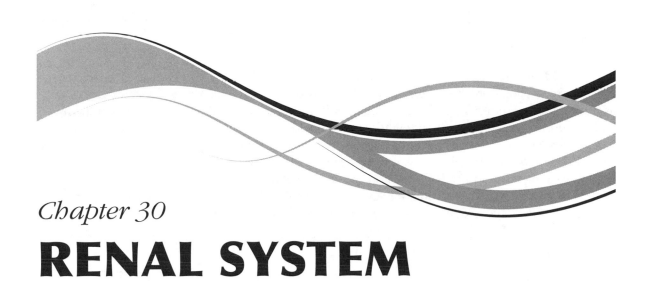

Chapter 30

RENAL SYSTEM

By Jessica M. Bessner, Pharm.D.

Learning Objectives

This chapter seeks to prepare a pharmacy technician to:

- understand the major functions of the kidney.
- understand the ways to measure kidney function.
- compare and contrast acute renal failure and chronic kidney disease.
- understand the management of acute renal failure and chronic kidney disease.
- describe the complications of chronic kidney disease.

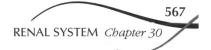

Introduction

The **kidneys** are two, dark-red, bean-shaped organs located toward the middle of the back receiving some protection from the lower two ribs. These organs function primarily to filter substances, such as waste products, drugs, metabolites of drugs and waste products, and excess fluid, out of the blood and into urine. Additional functions of the kidneys include secretion of substances and reabsorption of electrolytes back into the body. This helps maintain blood pressure and electrolyte balance. Because some drugs and their metabolites are eliminated here, kidney function becomes important when dosing these medications. Kidney function can decline abruptly, which is called **acute renal failure (ARF),** or gradually, called **chronic kidney disease (CKD)**. This chapter briefly covers the multiple functions of the kidneys, kidney disease and treatments for kidney disease.

Figure 1
Anatomy and Physiology

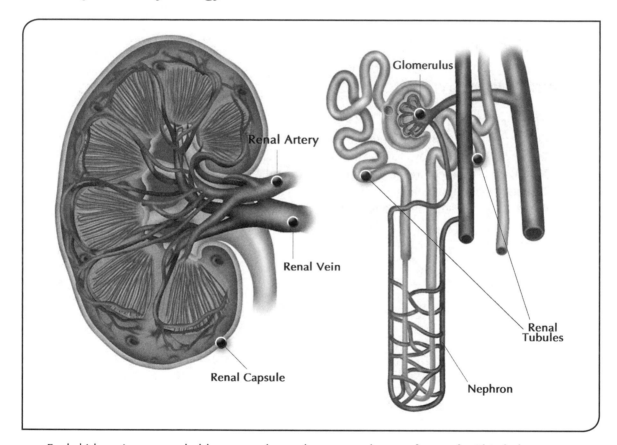

Each kidney is surrounded by a membrane known as the **renal capsule**. This helps to protect against trauma and infections. Each kidney contains approximately one million nephrons. A **nephron** is a microscopic tubule that filters wastes out of the blood. Each nephron consists of the glomerulus and the renal tubule. The **glomerulus** is a group of capillaries that functions as the main component in the filtration process. The **renal tubule** is a long, tube-like structure that collects urine. Each day, many liters of blood flow through the **renal artery** to enter the kidney. Blood is cleaned and urine is formed through the following three mechanisms: filtration, reabsorption and secretion. As blood flows through the renal artery, fluid and electrolytes leave the blood and are filtered across a membrane to the nephrons. Nutrients, water and other necessary substances are reabsorbed back into the blood. Finally, any additional waste products that are left in the blood after the first two processes are actively secreted back into the tubule. After these three processes, the purified blood will flow through the **renal vein** to exit the kidney and flow back to the heart. What is left in the tubule will be excreted, or eliminated, as it flows from the ureter to the bladder. This process is how many drugs are removed from the body unchanged or after they are metabolized elsewhere.[1] The kidneys also function to secrete substances such as renin, erythropoietin and vitamin D. **Renin** is an enzyme that works to regulate blood pressure; **erythropoietin** is a necessary protein in the production of red blood cells by the bone marrow. Finally, vitamin D_3 is activated by the kidney, which is important in bone formation and the absorption of calcium.[2]

Kidney Function

Any alteration to kidney function is associated with a change in the **glomerular filtration rate (GFR)**. The GFR is a measurement that determines the extent of a patient's kidney function. This is not usually measured directly because that is difficult and costly; however, it can be estimated by calculating a patient's **creatinine clearance (CrCl)**. **Creatinine** is produced by muscle breakdown and is eliminated by glomerular filtration. As kidney function declines, less creatinine is eliminated in the urine and more creatinine can be found in the blood. A creatinine level can be measured either by a 24-hour urine collection or, more commonly, by determining a serum (blood) level, otherwise known as the serum creatinine (SCr) level. The most common method to estimate CrCl is by using an equation known as the **Cockcroft-Gault equation**.[2] The **Modification of Diet in Renal Disease (MDRD)** four-factor equation (there is also a six-factor equation that is used even less often) is gaining ground as being the preferred equation in some hospitals. Some hospitals only use the MDRD equation for patients with established kidney disease and use the Cockcroft-Gault equation for all other patients. These are not the only ways to estimate GFR, and other methods may be used by a particular pharmacy, hospital or institution.

Cockcroft-Gault Equation for CrCl:

$$CrCl = \frac{(140-age) \times weight}{72 \times SCr} \times 0.85 \text{ if female}$$

CrCl = Creatinine clearance
Age = Measured in whole years
Weight = Body weight measured in kg
SCr = Measured serum (blood) creatinine (mg/dL)

A correction factor is applied (multiplying by 0.85) when the equation is used to estimate the CrCl for a woman.

MDRD Four-Factor Equation:

$$eGFR = 186 \times SCr^{-1.154} \times Age^{-0.203} \times (1.210 \text{ if black}) \times (0.742 \text{ if female}) \times (0.94 \text{ if lab is IDMS-calibrated})$$

eGFR = Estimated Glomerular Filtration Rate
SCr = Measured serum (blood) creatinine (mg/dL)
Age = Measured in whole years
IDMS = Isotope Dilution Mass Spectroscopy

A correction factor is applied (multiplying by 1.210) when the equation is used to estimate the GFR for a patient of African decent. Another correction factor is applied (multiplying by 0.742) if the patient is female. Finally, if the lab that processes the SCr measurement uses machines that are IDMS-calibrated, then a final correction factor (multiplying by 0.94) is applied.

Acute Renal Failure

Acute renal failure (ARF) is commonly characterized by an abrupt increase in serum creatinine by more than 50 percent over a 24- to 48-hour period.[3] Urine production decreases, serum creatinine increases and **blood urea nitrogen (BUN)** increases. The causes of ARF are classified into three groups: pre-renal failure, intrinsic renal failure and post-renal obstruction. **Pre-renal failure** is so called because it is due to a decline in blood flow to the kidney, which is a failure of the systems before the kidney, rather than due to a failure of the kidneys. Examples of conditions that may cause this are liver failure, congestive heart failure, dehydration and hemorrhage. **Intrinsic renal failure** results from structural damage to the kidney, usually from a blood clot in the kidney or as an adverse effect from a medication. **Post-renal obstruction** is due to a blockage of urine flow from the kidney out of the body. The treatment for ARF is driven by the cause of the renal failure.

Treatment of Acute Renal Failure

The ultimate goal in treating ARF is that the patient survives the incident; renal failure is a life-threatening condition and so any failure of the kidneys, regardless of how acute, must be taken seriously to prevent permanent damage to the kidneys and to hopefully allow the patient to regain life-sustaining kidney function. Treatment, as mentioned, is based on the cause of the ARF; however, three treatment modalities exist that may be used in combination or alone to treat ARF. First, the offending agent or situation may be withdrawn or reversed (e.g., the drug causing the problem is stopped, the patient is rehydrated if dehydration is the issue). Second, there are drugs that can help protect the kidneys that may be employed when the situation calls for them. Third, a machine can be used to substitute for the kidneys while the kidneys attempt to repair themselves; this is called dialysis. In addition to the treatment appropriate for the situation, fluid buildup and serum electrolyte buildup needs to be avoided. Medications, such as diuretics, can remove excess fluid while other medications (such as calcium, glucose, insulin and kayexalate) may be used to help control an increase in serum potassium levels.[3]

Prevention of Acute Renal Failure

Because ARF is sometimes caused by an avoidable factor, efforts to prevent ARF in high-risk patients can be worthwhile. Some high-risk patients include those who have prior kidney or liver damage, patients with diabetes, the elderly and those who are already being treated with a **nephrotoxic agent** (a medication that is known to cause damage to the kidneys). Prevention can be accomplished by avoiding nephrotoxic agents altogether or administering a renal-protective therapy (e.g., hydration or N-acetylcysteine) prior to the administration of these damaging agents.

Chronic Kidney Disease

Chronic kidney disease (CKD) is a result of gradual damage to the kidneys caused by diseases, such as diabetes or hypertension. Often, there is not an early marked increase in serum creatinine, as in acute renal failure.[4] Protein found in the urine on several occurrences is often an early sign of CKD. CKD is staged by degree of kidney function (see Table 1). Stage 1 represents mild damage, while stage 5 represents **end-stage renal disease (ESRD)** and is characterized by minimal kidney function.

Table 1
Stages of Chronic Kidney Disease[4]

GFR (mL/min)	CKD Stage
≥ 90 (with kidney damage)	1
60-89 (with kidney damage)	2
30-59	3
15-29	4
< 15	5

Treatment of Chronic Kidney Disease

Treatment of CKD is predominantly focused around managing the causative disease and preventing further damage to the kidneys. Aggressive management of diabetes or hypertension is necessary to preserve the function of the kidneys. One method of protection is by treating patients with diabetes, or hypertension, with angiotensin-converting enzyme (ACE) inhibitors or angiotensin II receptor blockers (ARB).[5] These agents reduce the blood pressure, which will slow progression of CKD, and they help to decrease the amount of protein excreted in the urine.

End-Stage Renal Disease

ESRD occurs when the kidneys lose a majority of function and can no longer clear waste products, or toxins, from the body. Survival in ESRD depends on one of two options: the patient must receive dialysis, or the patient must receive a kidney transplant.

There are many types of dialysis and it is a complicated process well beyond the scope of this chapter. Further, there are serious risks and potential complications that can come from undergoing a kidney transplant. This is a decision that must be carefully made in collaboration between the patient's physicians, the patient and the patient's family.

Treatment of End-Stage Renal Disease

Dialysis is a technique to remove wastes from the blood using a method other than a kidney. In dialysis, a semi-permeable membrane functions like an artificial kidney to filter waste products and excess fluid out of the body. There are two types of dialysis: hemodialysis and peritoneal dialysis. **Hemodialysis** is a process by which a patient's blood is run through an external machine while **peritoneal dialysis** is a process that is performed inside the patient's body. Dialysis is a process that needs to be maintained for the life of the patient or until a kidney transplant can be performed. A **kidney transplant** is a process by which a single, healthy kidney is taken from a donor and placed into a recipient to replace the nonfunctioning kidneys, which are usually left in place.[5] The recipient must take immunosuppressive drugs (drugs that suppress the immune system) for life in order to prevent a rejection of the new kidney.

Anemia of Chronic Kidney Disease

Anemia is one of the severe complications of CKD. It is a reduced production of red blood cells that carry oxygen throughout the body. This occurs due to the inability of the kidneys to produce erythropoietin. Healthy kidneys synthesize approximately 90 percent of circulating erythropoietin, which is a hormone necessary for red blood cell production.[4,5] A damaged kidney simply cannot meet this quota. Some symptoms that result from the reduced oxygen delivery include fatigue, headache and some cardiac complications.[4] Anemia may also be due to an iron deficiency. Iron replacement therapy is relatively inexpensive and may be accomplished through oral, or IV, supplementation. Oral iron is preferably taken on an empty stomach for maximum absorption, but many patients cannot tolerate iron on an empty stomach and so most patients take iron with food. Many dialysis patients require intravenous supplementation because oral doses are not effective enough to achieve the desired levels of iron. Treatment of anemia due to CKD includes supplementation with an erythropoietin-stimulating agent (ESA). These agents are either administered subcutaneously or intravenously once or three times each week depending on the agent and the need of the patient. Patients may experience cardiovascular adverse events, such as hypertension, and are at an increased risk for blood clots while using an ESA. Additional complications of CKD, as well as treatments for CKD, are listed in Table 2.

Table 2
Treatment for Chronic Kidney Disease and Other Kidney Disorders

Drug Class(es)	Generic Name(s)**	Brand Name(s)**	Indication(s)	Available Dose Form(s)
Anti-Anemia: Hematopoietic	Darbepoetin Alfa	Aranesp	Anemia from: Chronic Renal Failure or Nonmyeloid Cancer	Injectable
Anti-Anemia: Hematopoietic	Epoetin Alfa	Epogen, Procrit	Anemia from: Chemotheraphy, Chronic Renal Failure or Zidovudine	Injectable
Antihypertensive: Angiotensin-Converting Enzyme Inhibitor	Benazepril	Lotensin	Acute Coronary Syndrome, Heart Failure, High Blood Pressure	Tablet
Antihypertensive: Angiotensin-Converting Enzyme Inhibitor	Captopril	Capoten	Acute Coronary Syndrome, Heart Failure, High Blood Pressure	Tablet
Antihypertensive: Angiotensin-Converting Enzyme Inhibitor	Enalapril	Vasotec	Acute Coronary Syndrome, Heart Failure, High Blood Pressure	Tablet
Antihypertensive: Angiotensin-Convertin Enzyme Inhibitor	Fosinopril	Monopril	Acute Coronary Syndrome, Heart Failure, High Blood Pressure	Tablet

Drug Class(es)	Generic Name(s)**	Brand Name(s)**	Indication(s)	Available Dose Form(s)
Antihypertensive: Angiotensin-Converting Enzyme Inhibitor	Lisinopril	Prinivil, Zestril	Acute Coronary Syndrome, Heart Failure, High Blood Pressure	Tablet
Antihypertensive: Angiotensin-Converting Enzyme Inhibitor	Moexipril	Univasc	Acute Coronary Syndrome, Heart Failure, High Blood Pressure	Tablet
Antihypertensive: Angiotensin-Converting Enzyme Inhibitor	Perindopril	Aceon	Acute Coronary Syndrome, Heart Failure, High Blood Pressure	Tablet
Antihypertensive: Angiotensin-Converting Enzyme Inhiitor	Quinapril	Accupril	Acute Coronary Syndrome, Heart Failure, High Blood Pressure	Tablet
Antihypertensive: Angiotensin-Converting Enzyme Inhibitor	Ramipril	Altace	Acute Coronary Syndrome, Heart Failure, High Blood Pressure	Tablet
Antihypertensive: Angiotensin-Converting Enzyme Inhibitor	Trandolapril	Mavix	Acute Coronary Syndrome, Heart Failure, High Blood Pressure	Tablet
Antihypertensive: Angiotensin-Converting Enzyme Inhibitor; Diuretic: Thiazide / Thiazide-Like	Lisinopril / Hydrochlorothiazide	Prinzide, Zestoretic	High Blood Pressure	Tablet
Antihypertensive: Angiotensin Receptor Blocker	Candesartan	Atacand	Heart Failure, High Blood Pressure	Tablet
Antihypertensive: Angiotensin Receptor Blocker	Eprosartan	Tevetan	Heart Failure, High Blood Pressure	Tablet
Antihypertensive: Angiotensin Receptor Blocker	Irbesartan	Avapro	Heart Failure, High Blood Pressure	Tablet

Table 2 cont.
Treatment for Chronic Kidney Disease and Other Kidney Disorders

Drug Class(es)	Generic Name(s)**	Brand Name(s)**	Indication(s)	Available Dose Form(s)
Antihypertensive: Angiotensin Receptor Blocker	Losartan	Cozaar	Heart Failure, High Blood Pressure	Tablet
Antihypertensive: Angiotensin Receptor Blocker	Olmesartan	Benicar	Heart Failure, High Blood Pressure	Tablet
Antihypertensive: Angiotensin Receptor Blocker	Telmisartan	Micardis	Heart Failure, High Blood Pressure	Tablet
Antihypertensive: Angiotensin Receptor Blocker	Valsartan	Diovan	Heart Failure, High Blood Pressure	Tablet
Antihypertensive: Direct Renin Inhibitor	Aliskiren	Tekturna	High Blood Pressure	Tablet
Biguanide	Metformin	Glucophage, Glucophage XR	Diabetes	Extended-Release Tablet, Tablet
Biguanide / Sulfonylurea	Glyburide / Metformin	Glucovance	Diabetes	Tablet
Calcimemetic	Cinacalcet	Sensipar	High Blood Calcium	Tablet
Diuretic: Aldosterone Antagonist, Potassium-Sparing	Eplerenone	Inspra	High Blood Pressure	Tablet
Diuretic: Aldosterone Antagonist, Potassium-Sparing	Spironolactone	Aldactone	High Blood Pressure	Tablet
Diuretic: Loop Diuretic	Bumetanide	Bumex	Edema, Heart Failure, High Blood Pressure	Injectable, Tablet
Diuretic: Loop Diuretic	Ethacrynic Acid	Edecrin	Edema, Heart Failure, High Blood Pressure	Injectable, Solution, Tablet

Drug Class(es)	Generic Name(s)**	Brand Name(s)**	Indication(s)	Available Dose Form(s)
Diuretic: Loop Diuretic	Furosemide	Lasix	Edema, Fluid Retention, Heart Failure, High Blood Pressure	Injectable, Solution, Tablet
Diuretic: Loop Diuretic	Toresmide	Demadex	Heart Failure, High Blood Pressure	Injectable, Tablet
Diuretic: Potassium-Sparing	Amiloride	Midamor	High Blood Pressure	Tablet
Diuretic: Potassium-Sparing	Triamterene	Dyrenium	High Blood Pressure	Capsule
Diuretic: Potassium-Sparing Diuretic: Thiazide / Thiazide-Like	Hydrochlorothiazide / Triamterene	Dyazide, Maxzide	High Blood Pressure	Capsule, Tablet
Diuretic: Thiazide / Thiazide-Like	Chlorothiazide	Diuril	High Blood Pressure	Liquid, Tablet
Diuretic: Thiazide / Thiazide-Like	Chlorthalidone	Hygroton, Thalitone	High Blood Pressure	Tablet
Diuretic: Thiazide / Thiazide-Like	Hydro-chlorothiazide	Esidrix, HydroDIURIL, Microzide, Oretic	High Blood Pressure	Liquid, Tablet
Diuretic: Thiazide / Thiazide-Like	Indapamide	Lozol	High Blood Pressure	Tablet
Diuretic: Thiazide / Thiazide-Like	Methylclothiazide	Enduron	High Blood Pressure	Tablet
Diuretic: Thiazide / Thiazide-Like	Metolazone	Mykrox, Zaroxolyn	High Blood Pressure	Tablet

Table 2 *cont.*
Treatment for Chronic Kidney Disease and Other Kidney Disorders

Drug Class(es)	Generic Name(s)**	Brand Name(s)**	Indication(s)	Available Dose Form(s)
Mineral	Calcium Acetate	Calphron, Eliphos, Phoslo	High Blood Phosphorus, Kidney Failure	Capsule, Tablet
Mineral	Potassium Chloride	K-Dur, Klor-Con	Low Potassium	Capsule, Effervescent Powder, Extended-Release Capsule, Extended-Release Tablet, Injectable, Powder
Nonsteroidal Anti-Inflammatory Drug: Nonselective	Ibuprofen	Advil, Motrin	Gout, Osteoarthritis, Rheumatoid Arthritis	Capsule, Chewable Tablet, Liquid, Tablet
Potassium-Removing Resin	Sodium Polystyrene Sulfonate	Kayexalate	High Potassium	Powder, Suspension
Systemic Alkalizer	Sodium Bicarbonate	Neut	Antacid, Systemic or Urinary Inappropriate Acidity	Tablet
Trace Element	Carbonyl Iron	FeoSol, IronChews	Iron Deficiency	Chewable Tablet, Suspension, Tablet
Trace Element	Ferric Gluconate	Ferrlecit	Iron Deficiency	Injectable
Trace Element	Ferrous Aspartate	FE Aspartate	Iron Deficiency	Tablet
Trace Element	Ferrous Fumerate	Ferro-Sequels, Hemocyte	Iron Deficiency	Extended-Release Tablet, Tablet
Trace Element	Ferrous Gluconate	Fergon	Iron Deficiency	Tablet
Trace Element	Ferrous Sulfate	Feosol, Fer-Gen-Sol	Iron Deficiency	Elixir, Solution, Syrup, Tablet
Trace Element	Ferrous Sulfate / Ascorbic Acid	Fero Grad 500	Iron Deficiency	Extended-Release Tablet
Trace Element	Ferrous Sulfate Exsiccated (Dried)	Feosol, Feratab, Slow FE	Iron Deficiency	Extended Release Tablet

Drug Class(es)	Generic Name(s)**	Brand Name(s)**	Indication(s)	Available Dose Form(s)
Trace Element	Ferumoxytol	Feraheme	Iron Deficiency	Injectable
Trace Element	Iron Dextran	DexFerrum, InFeD	Iron Deficiency	Injectable
Trace Element	Iron Sucrose	Venofer	Iron Deficiency	Injectable
Trace Element	Polysaccharide Iron	Ferrex 150, Niferex	Iron Deficiency	Capsule, Elixir
Trace Element	Polysaccharide Iron / Ascorbic Acid	Niferex-150	Iron Deficiency	Capsule
Trace Element	Sodium Ferric Gluconate Complex	Ferrlecit	Iron Deficiency	Solution
Urinary Alkalizer	Potassium Citrate	Urocit-K	Kidney Stones	Extended-Release Tablet
Vitamin D Analog	Calcitriol	Rocatrol	Low Bone Density	Capsule
Vitamin D Analog	Doxercalciferol	Hectorol	Hyperpara-thyroidism	Capsule, Injectable
Vitamin D Analog	Ergocalciferol	Calciferol, Drisdol	Osteomalacia	Capsule, Liquid
Vitamin D Analog	Paricalcitol	Zemplar	Hyperpara-thyroidism	Capsule, Injectable
Vitamin Fat-Soluble	Cholicalciferol (Vitamin D), Ergocalciferol	Drisdol	Low Calcium Absorption, Osteomalacia, Osteoporosis	Capsule, Tablet

**All rights to brand names and trademarks are held by their respective owners. There may be additional brand names for some of the products listed.*

Conclusion

The kidneys are very important for many life functions, including filtering the blood and maintaining fluid and electrolyte balances in the body. It is therefore important for health care professionals to understand how to monitor kidney function and to understand the management of both acute renal failure and chronic kidney disease. This can help prevent initial or further damage to the kidneys. Pharmacy technicians may be called upon to help perform calculations relating to CrCl or GFR and may assist in flagging drugs that can be harmful to the kidneys to ensure that only the right patients receive those drugs.

References

1. Marieb, E.N., Mallart, J., "The urinary system," Human Anatomy, 3rd edition, Update, San Fransisco, Benjamin Cummings, 2003, pp. 676-686.
2. Comstock, T.J., "Chapter 42, Quantification of renal function," Pharmacotherapy; A Pathophysiologic Approach, 5th edition, McGraw-Hill, 2002, pp. 753-769.
3. Mueller, B.A., "Chapter 43, Acute renal failure," Pharmacotherapy; A Pathophysiologic Approach, 5th edition, McGraw-Hill, 2002, pp. 771-795.
4. National Kidney Foundation, www.kidney.org, Sept. 9, 2010.
5. Lewis, M.J., St. Peter, W.L., Kasiske, B.L., "Chapter 44, Pathophysiology and therapeutics of progressive renal disease," Pharmacotherapy; A Pathophysiologic Approach, 5th edition, McGraw-Hill, 2002, pp. 797-842.
6. National Kidney Disease Education Program, www.nkdep.nih.gov, Nov. 30, 2010.

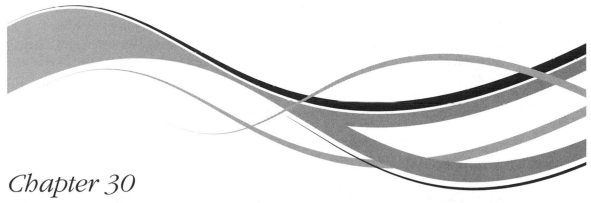

Chapter 30

REVIEW QUESTIONS

1. Through which structure does blood enter into the kidney?
    a. Renal vein
    b. Nephron
    c. Renal tubule
    d. Renal artery

2. Which of the following is not a mechanism by which blood is cleaned in the nephrons?
    a. Filtration
    b. Secretion
    c. Reabsorption
    d. Emission

3. Which enzyme is secreted by the kidneys to regulate blood pressure?
    a. Erythropoietin
    b. Calcium
    c. Renin
    d. Aldosterone

4. As kidney function declines, more creatinine can be found in the blood.
    a. True
    b. False

5. Acute renal failure is characterized by a decrease of serum creatinine by more than 50 percent over a 24- to 48-hour period.
    a. True
    b. False

6. Which of the following is not a condition that may cause pre-renal failure?
   a. Dehydration
   b. Blood clot in the kidney
   c. Hemorrhage
   d. Liver failure

7. Stage 5 chronic kidney disease is characterized by an elevated GFR and usually requires dialysis.
   a. True
   b. False

8. Which of the following medication classes aids in protecting kidney function?
   a. ESA
   b. Beta blockers
   c. ACE inhibitors
   d. Beta agonists

9. Peritoneal dialysis is a process that is performed inside the patient's body.
   a. True
   b. False

10. Which of the following medications is not a treatment for anemia?
    a. ESA
    b. Phosphate binders
    c. INFeD®
    d. Iron sucrose

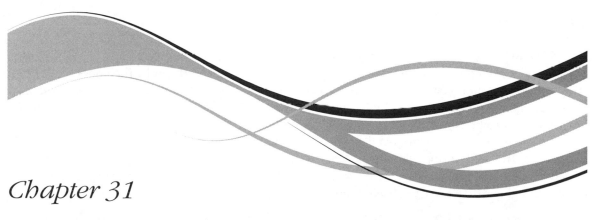

Chapter 31

ENDOCRINE SYSTEM

By Joan M. Rider, Pharm.D., CDE, BC-ADM

Learning Objectives

This chapter seeks to prepare a pharmacy technician to:

- list the glands that make up the endocrine system.
- describe the mechanism of hormone/receptor binding.
- explain what is meant by a "negative feedback system" used by the endocrine system.
- determine why the pituitary gland is often referred to as the "master gland" of the endocrine system.
- depict the proposed roles of each hormone in the endocrine system and consider the types of medication therapy that may be used to treat disorders in each category.

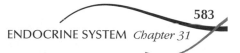

Introduction

The endocrine system consists of several types of **glands**. Each gland secretes or releases a different type of hormone into the blood stream to normalize or regulate the body. The endocrine system is a major information system just like the central nervous system (CNS). **Hormones** help to regulate many functions of an animal (including humans), such as mood, growth and development, tissue function and metabolism.[1,2] The term hormone is derived from the Greek word *horme* meaning "to set into motion." Hormones are produced either in small bursts at regular intervals or due to some outside stimulus.[1,2] The field of study that deals with disorders of endocrine glands is called **endocrinology**, a branch of internal medicine, and the physicians in this branch of medicine are called **endocrinologists**.[1,2] The glands that are commonly thought to make up the endocrine system are as follows (see Figure 1)[1]:

- Adrenal glands
- Pancreas
- Parathyroid gland
- Pituitary gland
- Thyroid gland
- Testes (males) / ovaries (females)

Figure 1
Endocrine System

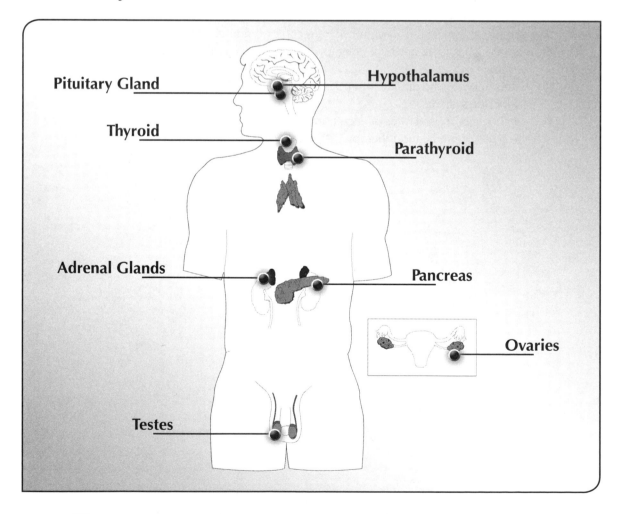

Hormone release is dependent on the body's natural feedback mechanisms. The main feedback system involved in the regulation of many of the endocrine hormones is the **hypothalamic-pituitary axis (HPA)**. This system is controlled by a **negative feedback loop** that helps maintain hormone levels in a narrow therapeutic range to maintain **homeostasis** (balance).[1] What is meant by calling this system a negative feedback loop is best understood through a real example of how it works. If blood sugar is too low, the body uses cortisol to increase blood sugar (through the release of sugar stored in the liver).[3] The hypothalamus secretes a hormone called corticotropin-releasing hormone. Corticotropin-releasing hormone tells the pituitary gland to secrete Adrenocorticotropic Hormone (ACTH). ACTH goes to the adrenal glands and stimulates the production of cortisol. Cortisol not only increases blood sugar, but it also stops the hypothalamus from making corticotropin-releasing hormone and it stops the pituitary gland from secreting ACTH. Once enough cortisol reaches these other glands, they will stop producing corticotropin-releasing hormone and ACTH until the blood sugar returns to being too low. In this way, from the perspective of the hypothalamus, the feedback it gets from taking the action of producing corticotropin-releasing hormone is a negative response (stop making this hormone) from the target of the corticotropin-releasing hormone. This interrelatedness of hormones makes endocrinology very difficult because information must be collected not just on the hormone or gland in question, but every hormone or gland that has a connecting hormone relationship, because the root cause of a symptom may not be the gland that directly has effects to cause that symptom. As in the previous example, if a patient was having a problem with high cortisol levels, then it could be the adrenal glands overproducing cortisol, but it could also be the pituitary overproducing ACTH leading to an overproduction of cortisol. Or, it could be the hypothalamus overproducing corticotropin-releasing hormone leading to high cortisol production. Further, it could be that the hypothalamus or the pituitary have been damaged in such a way as to not understand the message to stop making their hormones when cortisol is present. As shown, it can become very complicated! This chapter seeks to provide a basic understanding of how this interwoven system of glands and hormones regulates the body, what disorders are commonly seen when this system breaks down in some way and what drugs are available to attempt to address these breakdowns.

Pituitary Gland

The **pituitary gland**, or **hypophysis**, is one of the smallest endocrine glands. About the size of a pea, it weighs about five grams and is located at the base of the brain below the hypothalamus. The pituitary gland is somewhat protected in a bony cavity known as the **sella turcica** and is covered by a "fold" called the **diaphragm sellae**. The pituitary gland is mostly controlled through hormones released by the hypothalamus. The hypothalamus regulates many functions through the body; however, one of its main functions is to control the release of hormones from the pituitary gland.[4-6] The pituitary gland is separated from the upper parts of the brain by a membrane that does not allow cerebrospinal fluid surrounding the brain to reach the pituitary gland. This helps to ensure that the hormones constantly going in and out of the pituitary do not have effects on the rest of the brain; further, since the pituitary needs access to chemicals in the blood that are normally filtered out before blood reaches the brain, the pituitary must be separate to avoid contamination of the brain but still allow the brain to receive signals from the pituitary, based on the levels of chemicals in the blood that affect the pituitary gland. The pituitary gland is divided into two distinct regions: the **anterior lobe** and the **posterior lobe**. The posterior pituitary secretes two main hormones: oxytocin and vasopressin. **Oxytocin** is released in large amounts after the dilation of the cervix and vagina during labor and after stimulation of the nipples, facilitating birth and breastfeeding. Studies have begun to investigate oxytocin's role in various behaviors, including orgasm, social recognition, pair bonding, anxiety and maternal behaviors.[4-6] **Vasopressin**, also known as argipressin or antidiuretic hormone (ADH), controls which molecules are filtered into the urine by the kidneys and which molecules stay in the blood. This regulation of kidney filtration plays a large role in how much water (fluid) the body holds back and how much it allows to go into the production of urine. As part of this fluid-regulation ability, vasopressin also has the ability to increase blood pressure.[4-6] The anterior pituitary secretes different hormones than the posterior pituitary. Some of the many hormones produced in the anterior pituitary are **growth hormones** (GH or somatotropin), ACTH and thyroid-stimulating hormone (TSH). **Somatotropes** are cells that secrete growth hormone; somatotropes comprise one-third to one-half of the anterior pituitary. GH secretion is increased when growth-hormone-releasing hormone (GHRH) is released from the hypothalamus. ACTH, vasopressin, GH releasing peptide, sleep, exercise, stress and certain medications activate this system. The release of GH is inhibited by somatostatin. Other things that may inhibit the release of GH include high blood sugar after meals, increased free fatty acids in the blood, elevated insulin-like growth factor (ILGF), progesterone and some medications.[4,5] GH decreases the use of glucose by the body, increases the breakdown of the body's lipids (cholesterol) and increases muscle mass. It also increases the hepatic (liver) release of glucose, impairs the body's ability to use insulin and impairs the tissue's ability to use glucose. It is secreted in a pulsating fashion, with most of the bursts occurring at night. GH has a half-life of 30 minutes, so levels during waking hours are usually not detectable. If GH is released during the day, it is most likely to occur after meals, during exercise or with stress. Secretion of GH is the lowest in infants; it then increases to a peak during adolescence. Levels begin to decline again through the middle-age years.[4-6]

Pituitary Gland Disorders

When GH secretion is not regulated properly, the result can be **acromegaly** or **gigantism**. Both conditions occur when GH occurs in excess. Acromegaly affects only about 50-70 adults per million, and gigantism is even rarer. The difference between the two conditions is when they occur in life. Acromegaly is when GH excess occurs in adulthood. Gigantism is when GH excess occurs before the bones of an affected child have not yet stopped growing. The most common cause of both conditions is a GH-secreting pituitary tumor.[4-6] Surgical removal of the pituitary tumor is the treatment of choice for most cases of gigantism and acromegaly. If the tumor cannot be completely removed with surgery, medication is used to control the effects of GH on the body. Somatostatin analogs inhibit the release of GH. Dopamine agonist treatments have also been used, but these are generally less effective than the somatostatin analogs. Radiation therapy is effective but used as a last resort.[4-6]

Adrenal Glands

The human body has two **adrenal glands** that are located directly on top of each kidney. Each gland is 4-6 cm in length, 2-3 cm in width and weighs approximately 4 g. Each adrenal gland is divided into two major parts: the **adrenal medulla** and the **adrenal cortex**. The adrenal medulla makes up 10 percent of the total gland and secretes catecholamines (e.g., norepinephrine and epinephrine). The adrenal cortex makes up the other 90 percent; however, the cortex is further divided into three zones. The **zona glomerulosa** secretes **aldosterone** (a mineralocorticoid); aldosterone is part of the body's system for retaining or releasing water and electrolytes. Further, aldosterone is a component of the **renin-angiotensin-aldosterone system (RAAS)** that has an effect on blood pressure and controls the body's electrolyte and water balance by altering potassium and magnesium secretion and kidney reabsorption of sodium. It is 15 percent of the adrenal cortex. The **zona fasiculta** is in the middle and accounts for 60 percent of the cortex. This zone is high in cholesterol and secretes the **glucocorticoids** (steroids). Glucocorticoids help regulate the metabolism of food, as well as reduce the body's inflammatory response. Cortisol, mentioned earlier, is the main steroid produced by this area of the adrenal cortex. The last zone is the **zona reticularis** that produces sex hormones (e.g., testosterone, estrogens).[7,8] As with all aspects of the endocrine system, the interrelationship between the adrenal glands and other areas of the body is extensive.

Adrenal Gland Disorders

Cushing's syndrome occurs when the adrenal gland is functioning excessively. The symptoms of Cushing's syndrome are due to the higher than normal levels of glucocorticoids being released by the adrenal glands. Cushing's syndrome may be induced by administering steroids in high doses, or it may result from a dysfunction of the endocrine system. About 70 percent of Cushing's syndrome cases are due to the pituitary gland overproducing ACTH, leading to an overstimulation of the adrenal glands. Tumors that secrete ACTH, or tumors in the hypothalamus that secrete corticotropin-releasing hormone, make up about 12 percent of the cases. Of all cases of Cushing's syndrome, 18 percent are due to ACTH-independent tumors that occur in the adrenal glands.[7-9] Treatment of Cushing's syndrome is based on the root cause of the overproduction of glucocorticoids when possible; however, drugs exist that directly suppress glucocorticoid production. Mitotane is successful at suppressing glucocorticoid production in 30-40 percent of patients with Cushing's syndrome. Ketoconazole (Nizoral®), an antifungal drug, can also be used alone or in combination to control the production of excess glucocorticoids. When a tumor is responsible for the presentation of Cushing's syndrome, the most widely-used treatment is surgical removal of the tumor.

Addison's disease is the opposite of Cushing's syndrome; it occurs when there is abnormally low function of the adrenal gland. With Addison's disease, the actual tissue of the adrenal cortex is usually damaged (this can be part of the cause or can be the effect). This destruction leads to deficiencies in all of the hormones produced by the adrenal cortex (not just the glucocorticoids). Unless Addison's disease occurs because a patient is taking a steroid medication that suppresses the adrenal glands, the cause of Addison's disease is still unknown. The chronic use of certain steroid medications can lead to the body shutting off its natural production of steroids. This shutdown in natural steroid production can lead to Addison's disease when the pituitary gland, hypothalamus and adrenal glands actually break down and stop producing hormones naturally. In this case, the patient becomes completely dependent on hormone supplementation and cannot survive without taking hormone medications. It takes a significant amount of destruction, however, to get to this point; it requires 90 percent of the adrenal glands to be affected to begin experiencing noticeable symptoms.[7,8,10] Treatment of Addison's disease involves replacing the hormones that the adrenal glands are not making. The two hormones that generally must be replaced are cortisol and aldosterone; the other hormones produced by the adrenal glands can be produced elsewhere in the body and do not, generally, need to be supplemented. Cortisol can be replaced orally with hydrocortisone (Cortef®) tablets. Aldosterone can be replaced orally with fludrocortisone (Florinef®) tablets.

Thyroid Gland

The **thyroid gland** is shaped like a butterfly and sits over the trachea but behind the Adam's apple. The gland is divided equally to either side of the trachea by a thin connective tissue known as the **isthmus**.[11-13] The thyroid gland mainly absorbs iodine and produces thyroid hormone; **thyroid hormone** is generally responsible for controlling metabolism by helping cells use oxygen and carbon-based molecules in the process of creating and using energy. The hypothalamus in the brain releases thyrotropin-releasing hormone (TRH). The release of TRH tells the pituitary gland to release thyroid-stimulating hormone (TSH). This TSH, circulating in the blood stream, is what tells the thyroid to make thyroid hormones. Low levels of circulating thyroid hormone trigger the hypothalamus to begin this process; high levels of circulating thyroid hormone stop the hypothalamus from releasing TRH. Thyroid hormone is actually a mixture of molecules with liothyronine (or Triiodothyronine) and thyroxine being the most prevalent. Thyroxine is actually a mixture of two molecules that are mirror images of each other; only the "left-handed" version (levothyroxine) is effective in the body. Further, levothyroxine has to be converted into liothyronine to be used by cells. Levothyroxine is also called T4 because it is a tyrosine (an amino acid) with four iodines attached to it. Liothyronine is also called

T3 because it is a tyrosine with three iodines attached to it. The thyroid can directly make T4 much more efficiently than it can produce T3, so most of the T3 found in the body starts as T4 and is then converted into T3 as cells need it. Although it is not necessary for a pharmacy technician to be familiar with the chemistry behind this conversion process, these molecules are included here to help provide a visual representation of what the thyroid is doing to make T4 and convert it to T3; note the four "I" atoms on the T4 and the three "I" atoms on the T3 (see Figure 2).[11-13]

Figure 2
Thyroid Conversion of T4 to T3

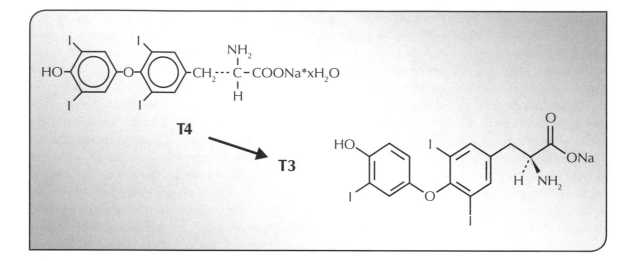

Thyroid Gland Disorders

It is estimated that 40 million people in the United States have a thyroid disease; however, only half of those with thyroid disease have been diagnosed. Women are at the greatest risk of developing a thyroid disorder. One out of eight women will likely develop thyroid problems during her lifetime, and that risk increases with age and family history.[14] Thyroid disorders are either a problem with over-production of thyroid tissue or an imbalance in the thyroid, or thyroid-stimulating hormones. Thyroid disorders can be caused by a myriad of factors; however, those exposed to radiation, those with a high dietary intake of isoflavones (e.g., soy), those taking lithium or amiodarone, tobacco smokers, those exposed to perchlorate, those exposed to high levels of fluoride and those with an imbalance in their dietary iodine intake are at higher risk for developing a thyroid disorder. Further, those individuals with a family history of thyroid disorders, those with another endocrine disorder, those with an autoimmune disease, those with a family history of autoimmune diseases, those with chronic fatigue syndrome, those with fibromyalgia, women and those over 60 years of age are all at a higher risk of developing a thyroid disorder.

A **thyroid goiter** is an enlargement of the thyroid gland. Goiters are often removed for cosmetic reasons or, more commonly, because they compress the trachea and the esophagus, making breathing and swallowing difficult.[11-13] If a goiter is small, doesn't appear to cause problems and is functioning appropriately, it may just be kept under observation. Thyroid hormone replacement with levothyroxine may slow the release of TSH from the pituitary gland and can decrease the size of a goiter. If inflammation of the thyroid gland is causing the thyroid to swell, aspirin (or prednisone) may be used to treat the inflammation. Surgical removal of all, or part, of the thyroid gland (called a **thyroidectomy**) may be an option if the goiter is large (and uncomfortable) or causes difficulty breathing or swallowing. Thyroid hormone supplementation may be used alone or in combination with surgery. In some cases, radioactive iodine can be used to treat an overactive thyroid gland. Because the thyroid is the only part of the body that takes up and stores iodine, radioactive iodine can be delivered to the thyroid where it kills off thyroid cells (in the same way radiation kills off cancer cells) but leaves other tissues unaffected. Destruction, by radioactivity or surgical removal, of thyroid tissue often leads to an underproduction of thyroid hormones that requires supplementation with thyroid hormone drugs.[11-13]

Females are more likely to have thyroid cancer than men at a rate of three to one. It occurs in the United States at a rate of approximately 37,000 new cases diagnosed each year. It can occur in any age group; however, it is most commonly diagnosed after 30 years of age. The older a patient is at diagnosis, the more likely the cancer will be aggressive and difficult to treat. There are four known types of thyroid cancer: papillary and/or mixed papillary/follicular cancer accounts for 78 percent of cases, follicular and/or hurthle-cell accounts for 17 percent of cases; medullary accounts for 4 percent and anaplastic accounts for only 1 percent.[15] The vast majority of those diagnosed with thyroid cancer have excellent long-term survival (papillary and follicular cancers have more than a 97 percent cure rate if treated appropriately). Most patients present with a nodule on their thyroid that typically does not cause symptoms. Although as much as 75 percent of the U.S. population will have a thyroid nodule at some point in their lives, the vast majority are benign and cause no symptoms. The chance of developing a nodule increases with age, with 90 percent of those 80 years and older having had (or having) at least one benign nodule present on the thyroid. Thyroid cancer is generally treated with surgery followed by treatment with radioactive iodine.[15]

Hyperthyroidism occurs when too much thyroid hormone is produced. Current methods used for treating a patient with hyperthyroidism are radioactive iodine, anti-thyroid drugs or thyroidectomy. Each method has advantages and disadvantages and is selected for individual patients based on individual needs at the given time.[9-11] Two anti-thyroid drug treatments commonly used to treat hyperthyroidism are methimazole (Tapazole®) and propylthiouracil. **Hypothyroidism** occurs when too little thyroid hormone is produced. Current methods used for treating a patient with hypothyroidism are supplementation with T4, supplementation with T3 and supplementation with a mixture of T3 and T4.[11-13]

Diabetes

Diabetes mellitus, or simply diabetes, is a group of diseases characterized by high blood glucose levels that result from defects in the body's ability to produce and/or use insulin.[16-19] **Insulin** is a hormone made in the pancreas that helps the body convert sugar, protein and fat into energy.[3,16-18] Diabetes is generally divided into four main categories: type 1, type 2, gestational and other.[16-18] The average age of onset for **type 1 diabetes** is around 10 years old; however, it can affect people of any age. It results from destruction of the insulin-producing cells of the pancreas (pancreatic beta-cells). Once destroyed, these cells can no longer produce insulin (or other chemicals like amylin that are important for metabolism), and, therefore, patients must receive insulin supplementation to live. The cause of this destruction is not fully known; however, it is believed that a combination of genetic predisposition and environmental factors are responsible. One possible environmental factor is a viral infection in a susceptible individual; more diagnoses of type 1 diabetes occur in the fall and spring than in the winter and summer, and this may be attributable to rates of viral infections.[16-20]

Type 2 diabetes results from a progressive problem secreting insulin, as well as a development of a resistance to insulin throughout the body. Type 2 diabetes represents 90-95 percent of all diabetes cases in the United States.[21] It is highly genetic; however, environmental factors play a large role in determining whether or not it develops during a person's lifetime. Genetically at-risk children may be acquiring the disease earlier because of the increased insulin resistance associated with early obesity resulting from poor eating habits.[22,23] Healthy habits, including eating a balanced diet and regularly exercising, can help children avoid or reverse developing type 2 diabetes.

Pregnant women who have never had diabetes before, but who have high blood sugar levels during pregnancy, are said to have **gestational diabetes**. Gestational diabetes affects 135,000 pregnant women in the United States each year.[24] Gestational diabetes generally onsets in late pregnancy (26-28 weeks). Untreated or poorly controlled diabetes can cause birth defects to occur. Newborns may have very low blood glucose levels at birth, are at a higher risk for breathing problems, may have larger than usual organs that lead to complications and are at a higher risk for developing type 2 diabetes later in life. Although a woman who develops gestational diabetes may return to normal blood glucose levels after the pregnancy, such women are 66 percent more likely to have gestational diabetes on future pregnancies than they were going into their first pregnancy.[16-19,24,25]

The values listed in Table 1 are used for diagnosing diabetes; however, different values may be used to monitor a patient's diabetes once it is diagnosed. The diagnosis of diabetes, or pre-diabetes, is generally based on a repeated measure of a **fasting blood glucose (FBG)** or on an **oral glucose tolerance test (OGTT)**. A FBG is obtained by a blood draw after fasting for at least eight hours prior to the sample being taken. At least two FBG tests, done apart from one another, are required to diagnose a patient with diabetes or pre-diabetes. An OGTT is a test done in a physician's office. It involves having the patient fast for eight to 12 hours before beginning the test. A FBG level is taken before the test begins. The patient then consumes a specific amount of sugar. Another blood glucose level is taken two hours after the sugar is ingested. If the patient's blood glucose at fasting and at two hours is higher than the limits, then a diagnosis of diabetes or pre-diabetes is made. A diagnosis of diabetes is a serious change to a patient's life. Patients with diabetes have significant effects from their diabetes on many different organ systems (see Table 2).

Table 1
Normal, Pre-diabetes and Diabetes Diagnostic Tests[16,17,26]

	HbA1c	FBG	OGTT
Normal Range	< 5.7 percent	< 100 mg/dL	< 140 mg/dL
Prediabetes	5.7 percent to 6.4 percent	100 mg/dL to 126 mg/dL	140 mg/dL to 200 mg/dL
Diabetes	> 6.4 percent	> 126 mg/dL	> 200 mg/dL

Patients may test their blood sugar using home blood glucose monitors. Generally, patients not using insulin will test no more than two times daily (once while fasting and once two hours after a meal). Patients using insulin may test as often as eight times daily if they are struggling to keep their blood sugar under control. Although the targets for fasting and postprandial blood glucose (two hours after a meal) are individualized for each patient, the general target for fasting blood sugar is between 70 mg/dL and 110 mg/dL. The target for postprandial blood sugar is generally less than 140 mg/dL. Further tests may be done to monitor a patient's blood sugar control. A **hemoglobin A1c** (HbA1c or A1c) measures an average blood glucose over the previous 60-90 days. Nondiabetic patients range from 4.0-6.2 percent on an A1c test; the target for patients with diabetes is an A1c of less than 7 percent with lower results corresponding to better long-term control and prevention of the harmful effects of diabetes. It is recommended that an A1c be drawn every three to six months and no less often than annually for every patient with diabetes.

Table 2
Chronic Complications of Diabetes[16,17,27]

Type of Complication	Prevention of Complication
Heart Disease, Hypertension, Stroke	Keep blood pressure at or below goal (< 130/80 mmHg) and blood sugar at goal; maintain a healthy lifestyle
Kidney Disease	Keep blood pressure at or below goal; maintain a healthy lifestyle
Foot Complications (Skin Changes, Calluses, Foot Ulcers, Poor Circulation, Amputation)	Inspect feet daily for sores and seek medical treatment if sores appear or changes occur
Nerve Damage (Diabetic Neuropathy)	Keep blood sugar at or below goal
Sleep Apnea	Maintain a healthy lifestyle; keep a healthy weight
Blindness, Glaucoma, Cataracts	Keep blood sugar and blood pressure at or below goal
Tooth and Gum Disease	Brush and floss teeth twice daily; see a dentist every six months

Although maintaining a healthy lifestyle that includes a balanced diet and 23-30 minutes of exercise at least three times per week is important for everyone, especially those with diabetes, sometimes this is not enough to keep blood sugar levels under control. Many treatment options exist to help patients maintain a healthy blood sugar level. There are many classes of oral medications that can be used to lower blood sugar. Further, there are injectable options that either supplement insulin or work on pathways related to the body's use of sugar. Sulfonylureas were the only class of oral diabetic medicine available from 1950 to 1995. Sulfonylureas help the body release more insulin from the pancreas. They may also make it easier for insulin to work. Sulfonylureas are usually taken before meals. If food is consumed shorlty after taking a sulfonylurea, the patient's blood sugar will drop significantly; therefore, sulfonylureas are only taken if food is going to be consumed. A sulfonylurea may be used alone, along with another oral medication or in combination with insulin. All sulfonylureas may cause the blood sugar levels to drop below normal levels (they may cause **hypoglycemia**). Symptoms of hypoglycemia can include nervousness, dizziness, sweating, weakness and a pounding heart.

There is only one biguanide currently available in the United States, metformin, and it is considered the first-line agent for most patients with type 2 diabetes. Metformin causes the liver to release stored sugar into the blood more slowly making it easier for insulin to work. Also, metformin may change how fat and sugar are absorbed through the intestines, leading to a more even blood sugar level after a meal. Metformin alone will not cause hypoglycemia. The most common side effect of metformin is an upset of the gastrointestinal (GI) tract (e.g., gas/bloating, diarrhea or constipation, nausea and abdominal pain). Metformin is not recommended for patients with poorly-functioning kidneys and must be stopped if a patient will be receiving another drug that will reduce kidney function (such as radiocontrast dye used during some CT scans). Metformin is generally started at a small dose, 500 mg/day, and then the dose is slowly increased until the goal of 2,000 mg/day is reached. Unless extreme circumstances exists, patients must reach 2,000 mg/day to get the maximum benefit from metformin; the increase in dose from 500 mg/day to 2,000 mg/day is not done in response to blood glucose targets but is done, regardless of blood glucose levels, to achieve the maximum benefits.

The alpha-glucosidase inhibitors slow down the digestion of carbohydrates after a meal. This means postprandial blood sugar levels don't rise so sharply. Alpha-glucosidase inhibitors must be taken with the first bite of each meal. An alpha-glucosidase inhibitor may be taken alone or in combination with other oral anti-diabetes drugs. Alpha-glucosidase inhibitors themselves do not cause hypoglycemia or **hyperinsulinemia** (too much insulin in the blood). Thiazolidinediones (TZDs) work by making the body's cells more responsive to insulin. Sometimes TZDs are called insulin sensitizers. TZDs are taken once daily. A TZD alone will not cause hypoglycemia. TZDs may be combined with other anti-diabetes medications. Recently, this class of medications, specifically rosiglitazone, has come under suspicion of causing serious negatives effects on the heart, so the use of TZDs in patients not already taking a TZD is less likely. Meglitinides help the body release more insulin from the pancreas similarly to the sulfonylureas. Meglitinides respond to the body's blood sugar level by signaling the pancreas to put out more insulin when the blood glucose level is high. Meglitinides may be used alone or with other drugs, but not at the same time as a sulfonylurea. Meglitinides are taken before meals and only work if food is present (unlike the sulfonylureas that work even in the absence of food). Meglitinides can cause hypoglycemia, but the risk of this is less than with the sulfonylureas.

All patients with type 1 diabetes, and some patients with type 2 diabetes, need insulin supplementation (see Table 3).

Table 3
Activity of Different Types of Insulin

Type of Insulin	Example**	Onset	Peak	Duration
Ultra Short-Acting Insulin	Humalog, Novolog, Apidra	5 minutes	1 hour	2-4 hours
Short-Acting Insulin	Humulin R	30 minutes	2-4 hours	6-8 hours
Intermediate-Acting Insulin	Humulin N	2-4 hours	6-12 hours	18-24 hours
Long-Acting Insulin	Lantus, Levemir	Continuous duration; no pronounced peak		

**All rights to all brand names and trademarks are held by their respective owners.

A physician will collaborate with the patient and sometimes a pharmacist (especially a certified diabetes educator) to prescribe the type(s) of insulin that is best for the patient. Insulin can be provided to the patient in vials so that doses may be drawn from those vials with a needle and syringe. Insulin also comes in prefilled devices that resemble a pen that can be used to inject insulin after a pen-needle is added. A pharmacist will train patients on how to use insulin; a pharmacy technician can assist in this process by ensuring that all of the necessary demonstration supplies are available to a pharmacist going into a training session. Some general principles that hold true for all of the currently available insulin products include the following:

- Insulin products not currently in use must be refrigerated
- Insulin products currently in use may be stored at room temperature (the duration of room temperature storage allowed for each product varies, but 28 days is the most common length of time that a vial or pen may be stored outside the refrigerator)

- Cold insulin hurts to inject, so it is recommended to allow products to warm to room temperature before first use
- Insulin must never be frozen
- Solid floating particles are not acceptable if insulin is to be injected (although some insulin is cloudy and some is clear, there is not to be any solid chunks floating in the insulin)
- Reusing needles hurts more because the needle becomes dull after just one use
- Insulin is injected subcutaneously or intravenously but not intramuscularly except under the most extreme conditions

Ketoacidosis

Ketoacidosis (also called diabetic ketoacidosis or DKA) happens when there is no insulin in the blood and glucose can't be used by the body's cells. This occurs more commonly in people with type 1 diabetes. The body starts using stored fat for energy instead of carbohydrates (sugars). When fat is broken down to its most base components, **ketones** are formed. Although this is usually going in small quantities, the body cannot handle large amounts of ketones. The symptoms of ketoacidosis include extreme thirst, loss of appetite, abdominal pain, nausea, vomiting, flushed skin, fever, frequent urination, drowsiness, alcohol breath and rapid breathing. If the person is not given fluids and insulin right away, ketoacidosis can lead to coma and death. Generally, the liver processes the small amounts of ketones produced from normal fat breakdown. If the liver reaches its capacity to process ketones, the excess will filter through the kidneys into the urine. This is the level where ketoacidosis is becoming serious and intervention must be made; diagnostic strips that are dipped into a patient's urine to determine if ketones are present are available to help patients experiencing the possible symptoms of ketoacidosis to determine what course of action to take. Uncontrolled diabetes can lead to ketoacidosis; however, poorly-controlled diabetes can also have many consequences. Damage to the nerves, eyes, feet, kidneys and heart are the most common long-term complications from poorly-controlled diabetes. Many of these complications are also related to high blood pressure, so patients with diabetes are typically on blood pressure medication to protect these organs.[28] See Table 4 for a list of drugs commonly used to treat endocrine system disorders.

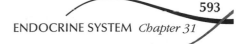

Table 4
Drugs Used to Treat Endocrine System Disorders

Drug Class(es)	Generic Name(s)**	Brand Name(s)**	Indication(s)	Available Dose Form(s)
Alpha-Glucosidase Inhibitor	Acarbose	Precose	Diabetes	Tablet
Alpha-Glucosidase Inhibitor	Miglitol	Glyset	Diabetes	Tablet
Amylin Analog	Pramlintide	Symlin	Diabetes	Injectable
Anabolic Steroid	Fluoxymester-one	Androxy	Low Testosterone	Tablet
Anabolic Steroid	Oxandrolone (Schedule 3)	Oxandrin	Bone Pain, Weight Gain	Tablet
Anabolic Steroid	Oxymetholone (Schedule 3)	Anadrol-50	Anemia	Tablet
Anabolic Steroid / Estrogen	Esterified Estrogens / Methyltestoster-one	Covaryx, Covaryx HS, Estratest, Estratest HS	Menopausal Symptoms (e.g., Hot Flashes)	Tablet
Antibiotic: Antifungal	Ketoconazole	Nizoral	Cushing's Syndrome, Fungal Infection, Psoriasis	Cream, Foam, Gel, Shampoo, Tablet
Anti-Cancer	Mitotane	Lysodren	Cushing's Syndrome	Tablet
Anti-Diarrhea: Anti-Secretory; Somatostatin Analog	Octreotide	Sandostatin	Acromegaly, Diarrhea, Variceal Bleeding	Injectable
Anti-Osteoporosis: Bisphosphonate	Alendronate	Fosamax, Fosamax Plus D	Osteoporosis	Liquid, Tablet
Anti-Osteoporosis: Bisphosphonate	Etidronate	Didronel	Osteoporosis	Tablet
Anti-Osteoporosis: Bisphosphonate	Ibandronate	Boniva	Osteoporosis	Injectable, Tablet
Anti-Osteoporosis: Bisphosphonate	Pamidronate	Aredia	Osteoporosis	Injectable

Drug Class(es)	Generic Name(s)**	Brand Name(s)**	Indication(s)	Available Dose Form(s)
Anti-Osteoporosis: Bisphosphonate	Risedronate	Actonel	Osteoporosis	Tablet
Anti-Osteoporosis: Bisphosphonate	Zoledronic Acid	Reclast, Zometa	Osteoporosis	Injectable
Anti-Thyroid	Methimazole	Tapazole	Hyperthyroidism	Tablet
Anti-Thyroid	Propylthiouracil	Not Available	Hyperthyroidism	Tablet
Anti-Thyroid	Sodium Iodide (I 131)	Hicon	Hyperthyroidism	Capsule, Liquid
Blood Sugar Elevator	Glucagon	Glucagen	Low Blood Sugar	Injectable
Calcimimetic	Cinacalcet	Sensipar	High Blood Calcium	Tablet
Dipeptidyl Peptidase-4 Inhibitor	Saxagliptin	Onglyza	Diabetes	Tablet
Dipeptidyl Peptidase-4 Inhibitor	Sitagliptin	Januvia	Diabetes	Tablet
Dipeptidyl Peptidase-4 Inhibitor / Biguanide	Saxagliptin / Metformin	Kombiglyze XR	Diabetes	Extended-Release Tablet
Dipeptidyl Peptidase-4 Inhibitor / Biguanide	Sitagliptin / Metformin	Janumet	Diabetes	Tablet
Dopamine Receptor Agonist	Bromocriptine	Cycloset, Parlodel	Acromegaly, Diabetes (Type 2), Parkinson's Disease	Capsule, Tablet
Glucagon-Like Peptide 1 Receptor Agonist	Exenatide	Byetta	Diabetes	Injectable
Glucagon-Like Peptide 1 Receptor Agonist	Liraglutide	Victoza	Diabetes	Injectable

Table 4 *cont.*
Drugs Used to Treat Endocrine System Disorders

Drug Class(es)	Generic Name(s)**	Brand Name(s)**	Indication(s)	Available Dose Form(s)
Growth Hormone	Mecasermin	Increlex	Growth Failure	Injectable
Growth Hormone	Somatropin	Genotropin, Humatrope, Norditropin, Omnitrope, Saizen, Serostim, Tev-Tropin, Zorbtive	Growth Failure	Injectable
Growth Hormone Releasing Factor	Tesamorelin	Egrifta	Lipodystrophy (HIV/AIDS-Infected Patients)	Injectable
Hormone	Calcitonin	Fortical, Miacalcin	Osteoporosis	Injectable, Nasal Spray
Hormone	Desmopressin Acetate	DDAVP	Bedwetting, Urinary Incontinence	Injectable, Nasal Spray, Tablet
Insulin: Intermediate-Acting	Insulin Isophane (NPH)	Humulin N, Novolin N	Diabetes	Injectable (Store Refrigerated; Use at Room Temperature)
Insulin: Intermediate-Acting / Regular	Insulin Isophane (NPH) / Insulin Regular	Humulin 50/50, Humulin 70/30, Novolin 70/30	Diabetes	Injectable (Store Refrigerated; Use at Room Temperature)
Insulin: Intermediate-Acting / Very Fast-Acting	Insulin Aspart / Insulin Aspart Protamine	Novolog Mix 70/30	Diabetes	Injectable (Store Refrigerated; Use at Room Temperature)
Insulin: Intermediate-Acting / Very Fast-Acting	Insulin Lispro / Insulin Isophane	Humalog Mix 50/50, Humalog Mix 75/25	Diabetes	Injectable (Store Refrigerated; Use at Room Temperature)
Insulin: Long-Acting	Insulin Detemir	Levemir	Diabetes	Injectable (Store Refrigerated; Use at Room Temperature)
Insulin: Long-Acting	Insulin Glargine	Lantus	Diabetes	Injectable (Store Refrigerated; Use at Room Temperature)

Drug Class(es)	Generic Name(s)**	Brand Name(s)**	Indication(s)	Available Dose Form(s)
Insulin: Regular	Insulin Regular	Humulin R, Novolin R	Diabetes	Injectable (Store Refrigerated; Use at Room Temperature)
Insulin: Very Fast-Acting	Insulin Aspart	Novolog	Diabetes	Injectable (Store Refrigerated; Use at Room Temperature)
Insulin: Very Fast-Acting	Insulin Glulisine	Apidra	Diabetes	Injectable (Store Refrigerated; Use at Room Temperature)
Insulin: Very Fast-Acting	Insulin Lispro	Humalog	Diabetes	Injectable (Store Refrigerated; Use at Room Temperature)
Meglitinide	Nateglinide	Starlix	Diabetes	Tablet
Meglitinide	Repaglinide	Prandin	Diabetes	Tablet
Meglitinide / Biguanide	Repaglinide / Metformin	Prandimet	Diabetes	Tablet
Mineralocorti-coid	Fludrocortisone	Florinef	Addison's Disease	Tablet
Phenylalanine Hydroxylase Cofactor	Sapropterin	Kuvan	Phenylketonuria	Tablet
Somatostatin Analog	Lanreotide	Somatuline	Acromegaly	Injectable
Sulfonylurea	Chlorpropamide	Not Available	Diabetes	Tablet
Sulfonylurea	Glimepiride	Amaryl	Diabetes	Tablet
Sulfonylurea	Glipizide	Glucotrol, Glucotrol XL	Diabetes	Extended-Release Tablet, Tablet
Sulfonylurea	Glyburide	Diabeta, Glynase, Micronase	Diabetes	Tablet
Sulfonylurea	Tolazamide	Tolinase	Diabetes	Tablet
Sulfonylurea	Tolbutamide	Orinase, Tol-Tab	Diabetes	Tablet
Sulfonylurea / Biguanide	Glipizide / Metformin	Metaglip	Diabetes	Tablet

Table 4 *cont.*
Drugs Used to Treat Endocrine System Disorders

Drug Class(es)	Generic Name(s)**	Brand Name(s)**	Indication(s)	Available Dose Form(s)
Sulfonylurea / Biguanide	Glyburide / Metformin	Glucovance	Diabetes	Tablet
Sulfonylurea / Thiazolidin-edione	Glimepiride / Pioglitazone	DuetAct	Diabetes	Tablet
Sulfonylurea / Thiazolidin-edione	Glimepiride / Rosiglitazone	Avandaryl	Diabetes	Tablet
Thiazolidin-edione	Pioglitazone	Actos	Diabetes	Tablet
Thiazolidin-edione	Rosiglitazone	Avandia	Diabetes	Tablet
Thiazolidin-edione / Biguanide	Pioglitazone / Metformin	ActoPlus Met, ActoPlus Met XR	Diabetes	Extended-Release Tablet, Tablet
Thiazolidin-edione / Biguanide	Rosiglitazone / Metformin	Avandamet	Diabetes	Tablet
Thyroid Hormone	Liothyronine	Cytomel	Hypothyroidism	Injectable, Tablet
Thyroid Hormone	Liothyronine / Levothyroxine, Liotrix	Armour Thyroid, Thyrolar	Hypothyroidism	Tablet
Vasopressin Receptor Antagonist	Conivaptan	Vaprisol	Low Blood Sodium	Injectable
Vasopressin Receptor Antagonist	Tolvaptan	Samsca	Low Blood Sodium	Tablet

**All rights to all brand names and trademarks are held by their respective owners.

Conclusion

The endocrine system is a highly complex system. The interrelatedness of the glands and hormones with all other functions of the body means that nearly all other diseases must be thought of in the context of how they affect the endocrine system and how the endocrine system affects the progression of those other diseases. Nearly every American will either be affected by a thyroid condition or diabetes either personally or in contact with a family member or friend. It is absolutely essential that every pharmacy technician be able to assist pharmacists with the complex task of helping patients manage these complex disease that often require many different drugs from many different classes.

Acknowledgement

The author wishes to acknowledge Kimberly K. Daugherty, Pharm.D., BCPS, and Stephen H. Freed, R.Ph., CDE, for their previous authorship of certain sections of this chapter, which were directly updated from the 11th edition of the Manual.

References

1. Melmed, S., Jameson, J.L., "Chapter 332, Principles of Endocrinology," Harrison's Principles of Internal Medicine, 17th edition, New York, NY, 2008, pp. 2187-2194.
2. Your Adrenal Glands, www.endocrineweb.com/endocrinology/your-adrenal-glands, Nov. 9, 2010.
3. What is Insulin, www.endocrineweb.com/conditions/diabetes/diabetes-what-insulin, Nov. 9, 2010.
4. Melmed, S., Jameson, J.L., "Chapter 328, Disorders of the Anterior Pituitary and Hypothalamus," Harrison's Principles of Internal Medicine, 15th edition, New York, NY, 2008, pp. 2195-2216.
5. Chen, J.T., Dang, D.K., Pucino, F., Calis, K.A., "Chapter 43, Pituitary Gland Disorders," Pharmacotherapy Principles and Practice, 1st edition, New York, NY, 2008, pp. 701-720.
6. Parker, K.L., Schimmer, B.P., "Pituitary Hormones and Their Hypothalamic Releasing Factors," Goodman and Gilman's The Pharmacological Basis of Therapeutics, 11th edition, York, NY, 2006, pp. 1541-1562.
7. Williams, G.H., Dluhy, R.G., "Chapter 336, Disorders of the Adrenal Cortex," Harrison's Principles of Internal Medicine, 17th edition, New York, NY, 2008, pp. 2247-2268.
8. Dang, D.K., Chen, J.T., Pucino, F., Calis, K.A., "Chapter 42, Adrenal Gland Disorders," Pharmacotherapy Principles and Practice, 1st edition, New York, NY, 2008, pp. 685-700.
9. Cushing's syndrome, www.mayoclinic.com/health/cushings-syndrome/DS00470, Aug. 26, 2010.
10. Adrenal Insufficiency and Addison's disease, http://endocrine.niddk.nih.gov/pubs/addison/addison.htm, Aug. 26, 2010.
11. Katz, M.D., "Chapter 41, Thyroid Disorders," Pharmacotherapy Principles & Practice, 1st edition, New York, NY, 2008, pp. 667-684.
12. Jameson, J.L., Weetman A.P., "Chapter 335, Disorders of the Thyroid Gland," Harrison's Principles of Internal Medicine, 17th edition, New York, NY, 2008, pp. 2224-2246.
13. Your Thyroid Gland, www.endocrineweb.com/conditions/thyroid/your-thyroid-gland, Nov. 8, 2010.
14. Statistics About Thyroid Disorders, www.wrongdiagnosis.com/t/thyroid/stats.htm, Aug. 28, 2010.
15. Thyroid Cancer, www.endocrineweb.com/thyroidca.html, Aug. 28, 2010.

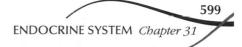

16. Cook, C.L., Johnson, J.T., Wade, W.E., "Chapter 40, Diabetes," Pharmacotherapy Principles and Practice, 1st edition, New York, NY, 2008, pp. 643-666.

17. Powers, A.C., "Chapter 338, Diabetes Mellitus," Harrison's Principles of Internal Medicine, 17th edition, York, NY, 2008, pp. 2275-2304.

18. American Diabetes Association (ADA), Diabetes Basics, www.diabetes.org/diabetes-basics/?utm_source=WWW&utm_medium=GlobalNavDB&utm_campaign=CON, Nov. 8, 2010.

19. American Diabetes Association, Symptoms, www.diabetes.org/diabetes-basics/symptoms/, Nov. 10, 2010.

20. American Diabetes Association. Standards of the American Diabetes Association - 2010, Position Statement, http://care.diabetesjournals.org/content/33/Supplement_1/S11.full.pdf, Nov. 16, 2010.

21. American Diabetes Association, Diabetes Statistics, www.diabetes.org/diabetes-basics/diabetes statistics, Nov. 9, 2010.

22. Centers for Disease Control and Prevention, National Diabetes Fact Sheet, 2007: General Information, www.cdc.gov/diabetes/pubs/pdf/ndfs_2007.pdf, Nov. 10, 2010.

23. American Diabetes Association, Facts about Type 2, www.diabetes.org/diabetes-basics/type-2/facts-about-type-2.html, Nov. 9, 2010.

24. Everyday Health, You Can Help Children Avoid Type 2 Diabetes, www.everydayhealth.com/type-2-diabetes/helping-kids-avoid-diabetes.aspx, Nov. 9, 2010.

25. American Diabetes Association, What is Gestational Diabetes?, www.diabetes.org/diabetes-basics/gestational/what-is-gestational-diabetes.html, Nov. 10, 2010.

26. American Diabetes Association, Summary of Revisions for the 2010, http://care.diabetesjournals.org/content/33/Supplement_1/S3.full.pdf, Nov. 16, 2010.

27. American Diabetes Association, Symptoms, www.diabetes.org/diabetes-basics/symptoms/?utm_source=WWW&utm_medium=DropDownDB&utm_content=Symptoms&utm_campaign=CON, Nov. 10, 2010.

28. American Diabetes Association, Ketoacidosis (DKA), www.diabetes.org/living-with-diabetes/complications/ketoacidosis-dka.html, Nov. 10, 2010.

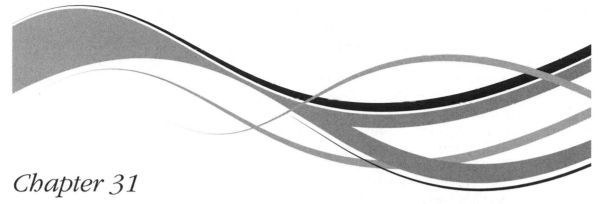

Chapter 31
REVIEW QUESTIONS

1. What is the main function of a gland?
    a. To regulate the many functions of the pituitary
    b. To secrete hormones
    c. To suppress cortisol release
    d. To cause thyroid-stimulating hormone to be released
    e. None of the above

2. Which of the following are glands in the endocrine system?
    a. Adrenal glands, pancreas, pituitary gland and hypothalamus
    b. Pancreas, parathyroid gland and thyroid gland
    c. Adrenal glands, parathyroid gland and pituitary gland
    d. Parathyroid gland, pituitary gland and thyroid gland
    e. All of the above

3. TSH exerts its effect on which gland?
    a. Parathyroid gland
    b. Pancreas
    c. Pituitary gland
    d. Thyroid gland
    e. Adrenal glands

4. Which of the following disorders is an excess of GH in adults and is properly paired with one of its treatments?
    a. Acromegaly; Fludrocortisone
    b. Acromegaly; Octreotide
    c. Gigantism; Cabergoline
    d. Cushing's Syndrome; Octreotide
    e. Cushing's Syndrome; Lanreotide

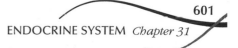

5. Which thyroid cancer is the most common and has the best prognosis?
   a. Papillary and/or mixed papillary/follicular
   b. Follicular and/or Hurthle cell
   c. Medullary
   d. Anaplastic
   e. All have a similar incidence and prognosis

6. Which type of diabetes is caused by a destruction of pancreatic beta cells?
   a. Type 1 diabetes
   b. Type 2 diabetes
   c. Gestational diabetes
   d. Maturity onset
   e. Chemical-induced diabetes

7. Which type of diabetes is the most common form of diabetes?
   a. Type 1 diabetes
   b. Type 2 diabetes
   c. Gestational diabetes
   d. Drug-induced diabetes
   e. B and C

8. Which of the following is not a long-term complication from diabetes?
   a. Eye damage
   b. Nerve damage
   c. Ketoacidosis
   d. Kidney damage

9. Which of the following is true of an HbA1c test?
   a. It represents a two- to three-month average of a patient's blood sugar
   b. The goal A1c is less than 7 percent
   c. It is recommended that all patients with diabetes receive this test at least annually and preferably every three to six months
   d. All of the above are true

10. What condition results when there is enough insulin in the body but the body isn't able to use it properly to reduce blood glucose?
    a. Insulin resistance
    b. Gestational diabetes
    c. Type 1 diabetes
    d. Hypoglycemia

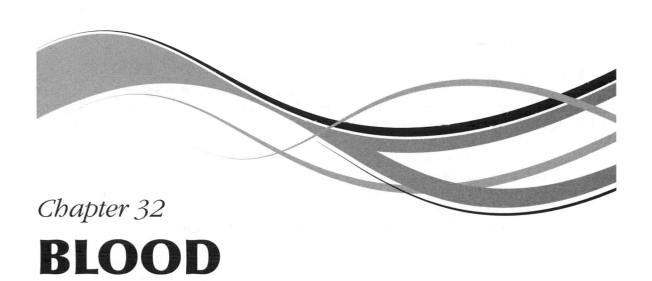

Chapter 32

BLOOD

By Renee R. Koski, Pharm.D., CACP

Learning Objectives

This chapter seeks to prepare a pharmacy technician to:

- describe erythrocytes, leukocytes and platelets, specifically focusing on where they are produced, their function and what happens if their levels are abnormal.
- explain what microcytic and macrocytic anemias are and how they are treated.
- describe how blood clots form and how they are treated.
- discuss sickle cell anemia and how it is treated.
- discuss hemophilia and how it is treated.

Introduction

An average 70 kg patient is made up of seven percent blood by volume (or 5 L). The blood is made up of cells and plasma. White blood cells (WBCs or **leukocytes**) and **platelets** make up less than two percent of the cells in blood. The rest of the blood cell composition is red blood cells (RBCs or erythrocytes). WBCs, RBCs and platelets are produced in the bone marrow. All blood cells come from stem cells, which undergo differentiation in the bone marrow. This process of formation and development of blood cells is called **hematopoiesis**. There are several substances (certain proteins, called **hematopoietins**, and colony stimulating factors) that stimulate hematopoiesis.[1] Disorders of the blood include anemia, hemophilia and blood clots, and they can occur in anyone from infants to the elderly. Many medications are currently available to help treat and prevent these problems. This chapter will review characteristics and disorders of blood cells, including their treatment.

Blood Cells

■ Erythrocytes

Erythrocytes are the simplest structured cells in the body. Their main function is to transport **hemoglobin**, a protein that carries oxygen from the lungs to the tissues. **Erythropoiesis** is the normal production of RBCs. **Erythropoietin**, a circulating hormone, is the main factor that stimulates RBC production. A lack of oxygen (**hypoxia**) in the body stimulates the production of erythropoietin by the kidney. Erythropoietin stimulates the bone marrow to produce immature RBCs (called **reticulocytes**) until the hypoxia is relieved. After the reticulocytes are released into the blood, they circulate for one to two days before maturing into erythrocytes. Erythrocytes circulate for 120 days before being destroyed by the **reticuloendothelial system** (a system in the body that destroys unwanted substances).[1,2]

Several substances are necessary for the development of erythrocytes, including iron, vitamin B_{12} (cyanocobalamin) and folic acid. Iron is required for hemoglobin production in RBCs. Vitamin B_{12} and folic acid are essential for DNA synthesis. Normally, these nutrients are found in a well-balanced diet.[1,2]

There are several laboratory tests that physicians use to assess a patient's erythrocyte population, including an RBC count (of a sample of known size), hemoglobin level, hematocrit, reticulocyte count and some erythrocyte indices (see Table 1). If the RBC count, hemoglobin and/or hematocrit are low, a patient is said to have anemia. The erythrocyte indices could be high or low, depending on what type of anemia is present. The reticulocyte count increases with acute blood loss due to the patient's bone marrow trying to compensate for the low number of erythrocytes circulating.[3]

Table 1
Erythrocyte Blood Tests[3]

Blood Test	Adult Normal Range	Measure of
Red Blood Cell Count (RBC)	Men: 4.5-5.9 x 10⁶ cells/µL Women: 4.1-5.1 x 10⁶ cells/µL	Number of erythrocytes per unit volume
Hemoglobin (HGB)	Men: 14-17.5 g/dL Women: 12.3-15.3 g/dL	Concentration of hemoglobin per unit volume
Hematocrit (HCT)	Men: 42-50 percent Women: 36-45 percent	Total volume of erythrocytes relative to total volume of whole blood in a sample
Reticulocyte Count	0.5-2.5 percent of RBCs	Indirect measure of recent RBC production
Erythrocyte Indices		
Mean Corpuscular Volume (MCV)	80-96 femtoliters/cell	Average cell volume $MCV = HCT \div RBC$
Mean Corpuscular Hemoglobin (MCH)	27.5-33.2 picograms/cell	Average mass of hemoglobin in the RBC $MCH = HGB \div RBC$
Mean Corpuscular Hemoglobin Concentration (MCHC)	33.4-35.5 g/dL	Average concentration of hemoglobin in the RBC $MCHC = HGB \div HCT$

■ Leukocytes

Leukocytes have a somewhat complex classification system (see Figure 1). There are two main types of leukocytes: phagocytes and lymphocytes. **Phagocytes** consist of granulocytes (neutrophils, eosinophils and basophils) and monocyte macrophages. **Lymphocytes** consist of T-cells and B-cells. B-cells are converted into plasma cells, which produce **immunoglobulins** (Ig). The main functions of phagocytes are to engulf and digest other cells and pathogens. The main functions of lymphocytes are to recognize and destroy foreign proteins. Leukocyte production in the bone marrow is stimulated by granulocyte-macrophage colony stimulating factors and a protein called interleukin-2 (IL-2).[3,4]

Figure 1

Leukocyte Classification[3,4]

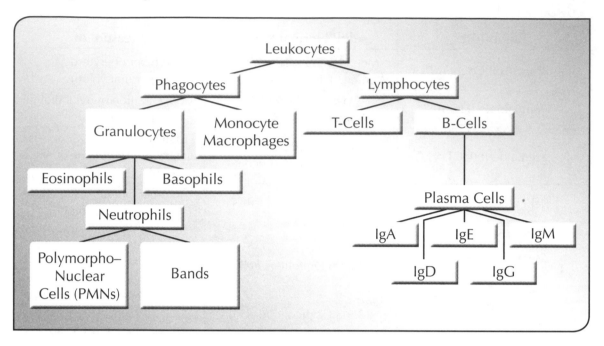

- ■ **Phagocytes**
  - • **Granulocytes** defend the body against infecting organisms (e.g., bacteria). After being released into the blood from the bone marrow, mature granulocytes circulate for one day before they migrate into the tissues. They live for two to three days in the tissues before being destroyed during defense activities or by the body because they have aged.[3,4]
  - • **Neutrophils** are the most prevalent circulating white cells. They are subdivided into **polymorphonuclear leukocytes** (mature cells, a.k.a. segs) and **band leukocytes** (immature cells, a.k.a. bands or stabs). They are produced in response to acute stress (e.g., a bacterial infection, heart attack or trauma). When called to a site of injury, they digest (**phagocytize**) invaders and usually kill themselves in the process.[3,4]
  - • **Eosinophils** are present in the intestinal mucosa and the lungs where foreign proteins enter the body. Eosinophils can phagocytize bacteria, yeast and parasites. They are also involved in hypersensitivity (allergic) reactions.[3,4]
  - • **Basophils** produce histamine and heparin, and they are increased in chronic inflammation.[3,4]
  - • **Monocyte macrophages** remove foreign substances from the body. They enter the circulation from the bone marrow in an immature form. In 16-36 hours, they enter the tissues where they mature. They are present in multiple organs (e.g., lymph nodes, lungs, liver and spleen). They help destroy old RBCs, proteins and lipids (fats). They are increased in tuberculosis, **endocarditis** (an infection of the heart) and other types of infections.[3,4]

- ■ **Lymphocytes**
  Lymphocytes recognize and destroy foreign proteins. They give the body's defense system memory against foreign invaders. Lymphocytes are made up of T-lymphocytes (T-cells) and B-lymphocytes (B-cells). T-cells are involved in hypersensitivity reactions, defense against fungal and viral infections, and prevention of neoplastic cancerous growth. With the help of

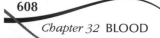

T-cells, B-cells are converted into plasma cells. Plasma cells produce antibodies, also called Ig (immunoglobulin). Antibodies give our body the memory to recognize and prevent certain infections. There are five classes of immunoglobulins: Immunoglobulin-G (IgG), Immuno-globulin-M (IgM), Immunoglobulin-A (IgA), Immunoglobulin-E (IgE) and Immunoglobulin-D (IgD). They all have different roles in the body.[3,4]

There are several laboratory tests that physicians use to assess a patient's leukocyte popula-tion. These include a WBC count, with or without differential. A differential includes count-ing the segmented and band neutrophils, lymphocytes, monocyte macrophages, eosinophils and basophils. The normal range for the WBC count is 4,300-10,800 mm[3] (see Table 2).[3]

Table 2
Leukocyte Blood Tests – Adult Normal Values[3]

Leukocyte	Percent Differential
Band Neutrophils	3-5
Basophils	0 1
Eosinophils	0-4
Lymphocytes	20-40
Monocytes	2-8
Segmented Neutrophils	45-73
White Blood Cells (WBC)	100

Leukocytes can increase in **leukemia**, a form of cancer affiliated with an excess production of leukocytes. The lymphocyte population can increase or decrease in **lymphoma**, cancer of lymphoid tissue. Table 3 lists other typical reasons for patients to have high or low values for the various types of leukocytes.[3]

Table 3
Disorders of Leukocytes[3]

Leukocyte	Increased Levels Name of Disorder and a Common Cause	Decreased Levels – Name of Disorder and a Common Cause
Basophils	Basophilia: Chronic Inflammation	Not Applicable
Eosinophils	Eosinophilia: Allergic Disorders	Eosinopenia: Acute Infection
Lymphocytes	Lymphocytosis: Viral Infection	Lymphopenia: Human Immunodeficiency Virus (HIV)
Monocytes	Monocytosis: Tuberculosis	Not Applicable
Neutrophils	Neutrophilia: Bacterial Infection	Neutropenia: Antineoplastic Agents

■ Platelets

Platelets are "cell-like" but do not have nuclei and cannot reproduce. Platelet production in the bone marrow is stimulated by a protein, called **thrombopoietin**, and colony stimulating factors, called **megakaryocytes**. The normal concentration of platelets in the blood is 150,000 to 450,000 cells/microliter. The main function of **platelets** is to promote blood clotting during bleeding.[5,6]

Platelet cytoplasm contains substances that are similar to those found in muscle cells. These substances store calcium ions and synthesize enzymes, prostaglandins (substances involved in vasodilation and vasoconstriction), adenosine triphosphate (ATP) (energy molecule), adenosine diphosphate (ADP) (energy molecule) and molecules that repair damaged vascular walls.[5] Platelet membranes contain substances that play a role in heart attacks, strokes and blood clots. These substances avoid adherence to normal endothelium but adhere to injured areas of the vessel wall, contributing to heart attacks and strokes. They are also involved in blood clotting, which is important to stop bleeding but can also be an adverse condition.[5]

A high platelet count, called **thrombocythemia**, is associated with a splenectomy (removal of spleen), infection and other disorders. A low platelet count, called **thrombocytopenia**, is caused by certain drugs (antineoplastic agents, heparin, etc.), as well as by some clotting disorders such as **thrombotic thrombocytopenic purpura** (**TTP**). A low platelet count puts a patient at risk for bleeding. A low or high platelet count can occur in leukemia.[6]

In a person without a clotting disorder, **coagulation** (formation of a blood clot) is initiated within seconds after an injury occurs to the blood vessel **endothelium**, a layer of thin, flat cells that lines the interior surface of blood vessels. This process of forming the initial blood clot is called **primary hemostasis**. It occurs as a result of platelets adhering to the damaged area and to each other (aggregation) to form a hemostatic plug (which stops blood flow) at the site of the injury. **Secondary hemostasis** then follows; this is when clotting factors from the plasma respond in a complex cascade (see Figure 2) to form fibrin strands which strengthen the platelet plug. Clotting factors are generally indicated by Roman numerals with a lowercase "a" appended to indicate an active form. The coagulation cascade of secondary hemostasis has two pathways: the Contact Activation Pathway (formally known as the Intrinsic Pathway) and the Tissue Factor Pathway (formally known as the Extrinsic Pathway) that lead to fibrin formation.[7,8]

Figure 2
The Coagulation Cascade[8]

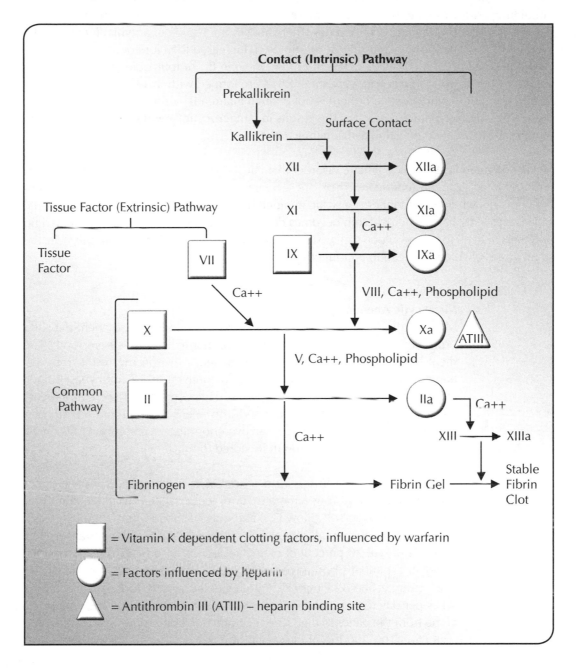

Blood Disorders

■ **Anemia** is defined as a reduction in the amount of hemoglobin, or the number of RBCs, circulating. It is associated with certain nutritional deficiencies, acute and chronic diseases, genetic disorders and taking certain drugs. There are several causes of anemia, including decreased RBC production, increased RBC destruction, increased RBC loss or abnormal hemoglobin production. If the body is deficient of iron, vitamin B_{12} or folic acid, anemia can also result. If there is not enough iron, very small RBCs are formed with insufficient hemoglobin, resulting in microcytic anemia. If there is not enough vitamin B_{12} or folic acid present in the body, RBCs do not mature correctly. This results in a **macrocytic anemia**, where large-sized, abnormal RBCs called **megaloblastic anemia** are formed.[9]

Sickle cell anemia (SCA) is a genetic disorder that causes abnormal hemoglobin production. It mostly affects African Americans. There are several variants of sickle cell disease, but it generally occurs when a child inherits a sickle hemoglobin trait from each parent. The abnormal sickle (crescent-shaped) hemoglobin becomes deoxygenated (loses its oxygen), forming rigid polymers that deform red blood cells. This can cause vaso-occlusion (constriction) in the small vessels, which can lead to painful crises.[10]

- **Treatment of Anemia**
  - ■ **Microcytic Anemia**

    Most iron in the body is present in hemoglobin in RBCs, so anemia is the most prominent feature of iron deficiency. Iron normally comes from foods, such as meat, eggs, greens and dried fruit. Deficiency of iron my result from inadedequate ingestion, decresed absorption (including from gastric bybass surgery) or utilization, blood loss (including menstruation) or increased requirements (infants and adolescents have increased iron needs during rapid growth periods. Iron deficiency anemia is diagnosed by performing seceral blood tests, including levels or iron and ferritin (iron in its stored form).[3,9,11]

    Iron therapy is given in the form of iron salts or complexes. Iron producs are available orally as ferrous fumerate (Ferro-Sequels®), ferrous gluconate (Fergon®), ferrous sulfate (Feo-sol®, Slow FE®) and polysaccharide-iron complex (Niferex®). The amount of elemental iron in each product differs based on its absorption. For example, about 20 percent of elemental iron is absorbed from a ferrous sulfate tablet. If a patient's body needs 200 mg/day of elemental iron, he/she would need to take one 325 mg (65 mg elemental iron) ferrous sulfate tablet three times per day to get a total daily dose of 195 mg (the other 5 mg would need to come from the patient's diet). The recommended dose of iron for iron-deficiency anemia is 100-200 mg of elemental iron per day depending on the severity of the anemia. The average length of iron therapy for anemia is six months. To help absorb more oral iron form the gastrointestinal (GI) tract, ascorbic acid (vitamin C) may be administered concurrently with the iron. A product that contains iron and ascorbic acid is Fero-Grad 500®. Adverse effects of oral iron preparations include constipation, diarrhea, dark stools, nausea and occasional GI pain. Iron in large amounts is toxic. Poisoning is usually due to accidental overdose. To reduce the risk of pediatric poisoning, iron should be kept out of the reach of children. Antacids (e.g., Tums®, calcium carbonate) coffee, tea and milk decrease iron absorption. Iron may interfere with the absorption of tetracycline, levothyroxine and some other drugs. Oral iron should be given between meals and at

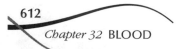

least two hours before an antacid. Liquid iron preparations may be taken through a straw to prevent staining of the teeth. Oral iron products are available without a prescription in the United States.[9,12,13]

Paternal (injectable) iron is used to treat iron deficiency when oral iron preparations are inneffective or cannot be used. It is also used for iron deficiency anemia in patients with chronic kidney disease. Fatal **anaphylactic reactions** (an allergic hypersensitivity reaction of the body to a foreign protein or drug) have occured with parenteral iron, so it should be reserved for patients in whom a clearly established indication exists.[9,13]

- **Macrocytic Anemia**
  Vitamin B_{12} and folic acid are chemically unrelated essenial vitamins (required and not produced by the body). Deficiencies lead to impaired DNA synthesis, inhibited cell **mitosis** (division), and abnormal maturing and functioning of cells. These problems are most often seen in cells that undergo rapid cell division (e.g., in the GI tract and bone marrow). Deficiencies in either vitamin B_{12} or folic acid can lead to anemia. Severe B_{12} deficiency can also lead to neurological damage.[9]

  Since the body stores vitamin B_{12}, it takes years to become deficient if supplements are not taken. Most vitamin B_{12} comes from animal products, so strict vegetarians may need to take vitamin B_{12} supplements. The cause of vitamin B_{12} deficiency is ususally impaired oral absorption. Oral vitamin B_{12} is considered an extrinsic factor that must combine with an intrinsic factor, found in the GI tract, for absorption. The intrinsic factor is a **glycoprotein** (compound consisting of a carbohydrate and protein) that is normally present in the gastric juice. Certain people can experience a deficiency of an intrinsic factor (including patients undergoing gastric bypass surgery), leading to impaired vitamin B_{12} absorption. The vitamin B_{12} intrinsic factor complex is absorbed through the ileum (lower portion of the small intestine) by a transport system. Vitamin B_{12} is transported to many tissues in need of it, with any extra being stored in the liver. Vitamin B_{12} given by intramuscular or subcutaneous injection avoids absorption problems and can be given daily at first to replenish body stores, and then once a month for maintenance. There is no evidence that vitamin B_{12} injections have any benefit in persons who do not have a deficiency. Oral vitamin B_{12} is available withou a prescription as a dietary supplement. Vitamin B_{12} deficiency is diagosed by checking a patient's blood level.[9,11,13]

  Folic acid is found in fresh green vegetables, meat and eggs. Folic acid is given orally to treat a deficiency or to prevent deficiencies in patients who have liver failure, alcoholism, skin diseases, renal failure or have undergone gastric bypass surgery. In addition, folic acid may be administered to pregnant women (or those women seeking to become pregnant), who are folic acid deficient, to prevent neural tube defects in the fetus. Products containing less than 1 mg/tablet of folic acid d not require a prescription in the United States; products containing 1 mg/tablet or more of folic acid require a prescription in the United States. Folic acid deficiency is diagnosed by checking a blood level of folic acid. Folic acid should never be administered at doses greater than 0.4 mg/day unless vitamin B_{12} deficiency is ruled out because folic acid supplementation can mask the neurological symptoms of vitamin B_{12} deficiency. This could result in the progression of the neurological consequences associated with vitamin B_{12} deficiency.[9,11,13]

Parenteral folic acid is usually reserved for reversing the effects of certain cancer chemotherapy. Folinic acid (Leucovorin®) is an active form of folic acid that is available orally and by injection, and is used as an adjunct to cancer chemotherapy. It is not routinely used to correct folic acid deficiency because it is more expensive, and oral folic acid is just as effective.[9,13]

- **Anemia Associated with Other Diseases**
  For treatment of patients with chronic anemia, such as seen with kidney disease, erythropoietin is available for parenteral administration to stimulate RBC production. In addition, erythropoietin may be used for the treatment of anemia in cancer patients who are receiving chemotherapy, HIV patients who are experiencing zidovudine-induced anemia and premature infants who are experiencing anemia. Erythropoietin can be administered by subcutaneous or intravenous injection. The commonly available erythropoietins are: epoetin alpha (Epogen®, Procrit®) and darbepoetin alfa (Aranesp®). The most common adverse effects include **hypertension** (high blood pressure) and **thrombosis** (blood clots).[9,13]

- **Sickle Cell Anemia (SCA)**
  Analgesics, such as acetaminophen, nonsteroidal anti-inflammatory drugs (NSAIDs), and opioids are used to treat the pain associated with SCA. Hydroxyurea (Droxia®, Hydrea®), a cancer drug, can decrease the frequency of sickle cell crises. It increases the production of fetal hemoglobin, which, in turn, decreases the sickling of RBC. A side effect of hydroxyurea is bone marrow suppression so treatment with hydroxyurea must be carefully monitored by prescribers, pharmacists and patients. Patients with SCA are prone to infections, so it is very important that they receive all appropriate immunizations. Further, they are sometimes given prophylactic penicillin. They also have an increased need for folic acid requiring daily supplementation.[10,14]

■ **Hemophilia**
Hemophilia is a collection of conditions characterized by deficiencies in certain blood clotting factors (i.e., Factors VIII and IX) that prevent blood from clotting, which leads to bleeding. Bleeding can occur anywhere, but it occurs mostly in the joints, muscles and GI tract. The disease is classified as mild, moderate or severe, depending on how much of the involved clotting factors patients have in their blood.[7]

- **Treatment of Hemophilia**
  Clotting factors from normal human plasma are donated and available to prevent and limit existing bleeding in hemophilia patients. Patients with Hemophilia A have a deficiency in Factor VIII so they can be treated with Factor VIII complex infusions. Patients with Hemophilia B (Christmas disease) have a Factor IX deficiency in their blood, so they can be treated with Factor IX complex infusions. Sometimes, patients can develop antibodies to their clotting factors. They can be treated with Factor VIIa complex (NovoSeven RT®) or an anti-inhibitory coagulant complex (Feiba VH® or Feiba NF®). The choice of clotting factor product depends on the type of hemophilia and the safety, purity and cost of the products. The downfall of human-derived products is the fear of spreading viral diseases (e.g., viral hepatitis, HIV/AIDS). Virus-inactivating techniques and protein purification to produce high purity products were introduced in the 1980s and 1990s to produce safer human-derived products (Factor VIII: Monoclate P®, Factor IX: Mononine®). Recombinant factor replacement products are also now available (Factor VIII: Recombinate®, Factor IX: Benefix®).[7,13]

■ **Blood Clots**

Blood clots can occur in arteries or veins. Cholesterol, red blood cells, platelets, fibrin and other substances adhere to injured endothelium in the arteries forming a clot (thrombus). Patients who have this buildup of substances in the arteries are said to have **atherosclerotic** heart disease. If this occurs in the heart, it may block blood flow. This can lead to damage and a painful lack of oxygen to part of the heart. Acute heart problems related to this plaque buildup include unstable angina (evolving heart attack) and myocardial infarction (heart attack). These acute heart disorders are collectively known as acute coronary syndromes (ACS). If such a thrombus occurs in the brain, it can cause a cerebral vascular accident (CVA, stroke). Heart attacks and strokes are often fatal. High cholesterol, high blood pressure, diabetes, smoking and family history are among the most common contributing factors to heart attacks and strokes.[15]

Clots can also occur in veins (usually deep veins within the legs). This is generally referred to as **deep vein thrombosis (DVT)**. A patient experiencing a DVT usually has a painful, swollen and red extremity. If part of the clot breaks off and travels through the blood stream it is called an **embolus**. Clots from the legs usually embolize to the lungs and cause what is called a **pulmonary embolism (PE)**. A PE is usually painful and can be fatal. If a clot starts in the heart, it can embolize to the brain and cause a stroke.[8]

A clot in the legs can occur as a result of several processes. Damage to the vessel wall due to pooled blood or trauma can cause platelets to aggregate at the damaged site and activate the clotting cascade. The clotting cascade can also be turned on if the patient is deficient of proteins that normally keep the clotting cascade in check. Atrial fibrillation (an irregular heart rhythm) and prosthetic heart valves can increase the risk of developing a clot in the heart. Pregnancy, prolonged immobility (airplane rides, being bedridden), orthopedic surgery, certain malignancies and estrogen use can all increase the risk of developing a clot in the veins.[8]

• **Prevention and Treatment of Blood Clots**

If a patient has clots or is prone to repeated clots, medications are given to prevent the clot formation or to counteract the coagulation process. These medications include antiplatelets, anticoagulants and thrombolytics.[8,15]

■ **Antiplatelet Drugs**

Antiplatelet medications interfere with platelet aggregation (the initial step in blood clot formation). Oral antiplatelet drugs include aspirin, dipyridamole (Persantine®), ticlopidine (Ticlid®), clopidogrel (Plavix®), prasugrel (Effient®) and NSAIDs, such as ibuprofen (Advil®, Motrin®). The parenteral antiplatelet drugs include the glycoprotein IIb/IIIa receptor antagonists, including abciximab (Reopro®), eptifibatide (Integrilin®) and tirofiban (Aggrastat®). Aspirin binds to platelets irreversibly, while the other antiplatelet drugs bind reversibly.[13,15]

Aspirin is the prototype for all current antiplatelet drugs. In a low dose (81 mg-325 mg), it has been shown to prevent heart attacks. It may also reduce the risk of other vascular events, like a stroke or **transient ischemic attack** (temporary interference of blood supply to the brain). It is recommended at the first sign of an acute myocardial infarction for patients to chew and swallow one 325 mg nonenteric-coated aspirin as soon as possible. Then, a dose of aspirin should be repeated daily (indefinitely). Taking aspirin can increase the risk of bleeding; this is especially true if aspirin is used in combination with other drugs that increase the risk of bleeding (NSAIDs, anticoagulants). It can cause stomach upset when taken daily, so patients can take it with food, milk or antacids to diminish this side effect. Also, enteric-coated aspirin will not dissolve until it gets to the small intestine (reducing stomach discomfort). Hypersensitivity reactions to aspirin may occur; a hypersensitivity reaction can appear as rash, asthma-like broncho-spasm and even anaphylaxis.[13,15,16]

Aspirin is the preferred antiplatelet drug in most cases, but, ticlopidine, clopido-grel or prasugrel can be used in patients who are allergic to aspirin. Ticlopidine has been associated with causing **neutropenia** (low number of white blood cells; this puts patients at risk of infections) and thrombotic thrombocytopenic purpura (a disorder that causes patients to develop clots despite having a low number of platelets). Aspirin is combined with clopidogrel, or one of the other oral an-tiplatelet drugs, for patients undergoing a percutaneous coronary intervention (PCI) (e.g., a stent placement).[13,15]

Dipyridamole is not usually used alone and is available in combination with aspirin in a capsule called Aggrenox®, which is indicated to prevent recurrent strokes. NSAIDs are not used for antiplatelet purposes. They are used for their anti-inflammatory and antipyretic, fever-reducing properties. The IIb/IIIa-recep-tor antagonists are used in conjunction with anticoagulants and/or thrombolytics in the hospital, during PCI and for the treatment of ACS.[13,15]

- **Anticoagulants**
  Anticoagulant medications stop or slow the clotting process. Heparin is an an-ticoagulant that slows the clotting process by binding to and accelerating the ef-fects of **antithrombin III**. Antithrombin III is an enzyme that inhibits the clotting cascade by inactivating Factor Xa. Heparin also prevents the conversion of pro-thrombin (Factor II) to thrombin (Factor IIa) to prevent further formation of a clot (see Figure 2). Heparin itself cannot dissolve clots. The body's own process must do this over time. The anticoagulant effect of heparin is monitored with a blood test called a **partial thromboplastin time (PTT)**. Heparin is given subcutaneously or by continuous intravenous (IV) infusion. The main side effect of heparin is bleeding. If bleeding occurs, heparin's effect can be neutralized by protamine sulfate given IV. Another serious side effect that sometimes occurs with heparin is thrombocytopenia (a decrease in the number of platelets). Thrombocytopenia requires heparin therapy to be discontinued.[8,17]

Low molecular weight (LMW) fractions of heparin, such as enoxaparin (Lo-venox®), dalteparin (Fragmin®) and tinzaparin (Innohep®), have been approved for subcutaneous administration to treat blood clots and also to prevent clots when patients are at risk (e.g., after hip or knee replacement surgery). The LMW heparins, when compared to regular heparin, have similar effects, similar bleed-ing rates, less frequent dosing (once or twice daily) and no routine laboratory testing required. They bind to antithrombin III to inactivate Factor Xa but they do not have a direct effect on Factor II. The most common side effect of LMW hepa-rins is bruising at the injection site. If someone develops thrombocytopenia from heparin, they could also get it from LMW heparins. Anticoagulants that can be used in patients with heparin induced thrombocytopenia (HIT) include lepirudin (Refludan®) and argatroban. These drugs are direct thrombin (Factor II) inhibi-tors and are administered by IV. Fondaparinux (Arixtra®) is a Factor Xa inhibitor

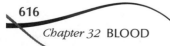

administered subcutaneously. It is used to treat and prevent blood clots and can also be used in patients with HIT.[8,13,17]

In addition to the injectable anticoagulants discussed, two oral anticoagulants are available. **Warfarin** (Coumadin®) is an oral anticoagulant that is used to treat and prevent blood clots. It prevents the activation of clotting factors that require vitamin K. Vitamin K is involved in activating Factors II, VII, IX and X (see Figure 2). The anticoagulant effects occur when circulating clotting factors become depleted. The full anticoagulation effects from warfarin are not seen for at least five days after commencing therapy. The warfarin dose is then adjusted based on a blood test called the international normalized ratio (INR). Warfarin is the preferred medication for long-term prevention of clots in patients with DVT, prosthetic heart valves and chronic atrial fibrillation. The duration of warfarin therapy can be as short as one month (for atrial fibrillation converted to normal sinus rhythm) or as long as the patient remains alive (for chronic atrial fibrillation, recurrent blood clots or prosthetic heart valve replacement).[8,13,17]

Warfarin is not given to pregnant patients because it can cross the placenta and damage the fetus. Heparin does not cross the placenta and may be used in pregnancy. Warfarin is known to interact with many medications (e.g., antibiotics, aspirin), causing an increased bleeding risk. Careful monitoring of the patient's INR is necessary when medications interacting with warfarin are added or discontinued. Diet also plays a role in warfarin therapy; vitamin K or vitamin K-rich foods (green leafy vegetables) may interfere with the effects of warfarin. A vitamin K consistent diet is recommended for patients who are taking warfarin therapy. Elevated INR due to overanticoagulation with warfarin can be reversed by administering vitamin K. Vitamin K is available orally and by injection.[8,13,17]

A second oral anticoagulant was approved for use in 2010. Dabigatran etexilate (PRADAXA®), 75 mg and 150 mg capsules, are available to reduce the risk of stroke and systemic embolism in patients with nonvalvular atrial fibrillation. Dabigatran works in the blood by blocking the action of thrombin, which inhibits the clot-making process.

Although dabigatran and warfarin are both anticoagulants, there are significant differences between the medications. Dabigatran is currently approved in the U.S. for individuals with nonvalvular atrial fibrillation, warfarin treats other clotting disease. In addition, warfarin has more interactions with other medications.

A research study comparing the efficacy and safety of dabigatran and warfarin in patients with nonvalvular atrial fibrillation found that patients taking dabigatran 150 mg twice daily had a 34 percent reduced risk of stroke compared with patients taking warfarin, with similar rates of major bleeding. Patients taking dabigatran 150 mg twice daily had more stomach upset and stopped taking their medication more often than patients taking warfarin.

The Food and Drug Administration (FDA) issued a safety alert in December 2011, and revised the label for dabigatran, due to post-marketing reports of serious bleeding events in patients taking the medication. The FDA recommended that patients using dabigatran continue to do so as directed and not stop taking if without consulting with a health care professional.[18,19]

- **Thrombolytics**

    To dissolve a newly-formed clot, such as in a heart attack or stroke, a thrombolytic can be administered. Examples of thrombolytics include alteplase (Activase®), reteplase (Retavase®) and tenecteplase (TNKase®). They exert their action through the activation of plasminogen to plasmin in the clotting cascade. Plasmin, in turn, breaks down fibrin in the thrombus. These medications can also be used to dissolve clots that block off an IV catheter. Thrombolytic agents interact with anticoagulants, antiplatelet drugs and NSAIDs, causing an increased risk of bleeding.[13,15] See Table 4 for a comprehensive list of products used to treat blood disorders.

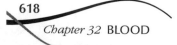

Table 4
Drugs Used to Treat Blood Disorders[4]

Drug Class(es)	Generic Name(s)**	Brand Name(s)**	Indication(s)	Available Dose Form(s)
Anti-Anemia: Hematopoietic	Darbepoetin Alfa	Aranesp	Anemia from Chronic Renal Failure or Nonmyeloid Cancer	Injectable
Anti-Anemia: Hematopoietic	Epoetin Alfa	Epogen, Procrit	Anemia from Chemotherapy, Chronic Renal Failure or Zidovudine	Injectable
Anticoagulant: Antithrombin III Inhibitor	Heparin (Unfractionated)	Not Available	Acute Coronary Syndrome, Deep Vein Thrombosis, Pulmonary Embolism	Injectable
Anticoagulant: Factor Xa Inhibitor	Fondaparinux	Arixtra	Deep Vein Thrombosis, Pulmonary Embolism	Injectable
Anticoagulant: Low Molecular Weight Heparin	Dalteparin	Fragmin	Acute Coronary Syndrome, Deep Vein Thrombosis	Injectable
Anticoagulant: Low Molecular Weight Heparin	Enoxaparin	Lovenox	Acute Coronary Syndrome, Deep Vein Thrombosis, Pulmonary Embolism	Injectable
Anticoagulant: Low Molecular Weight Heparin	Tinzaparin	Innohep	Deep Vein Thrombosis, Pulmonary Embolism	Injectable
Anticoagulant: Thrombin Inhibitor	Argatroban	Not Available	Anticoagulation in Heparin-Induced Thrombocytopenia	Injectable
Anticoagulant: Thrombin Inhibitor	Bivalirudin	Angiomax	Acute Coronary Syndrome, Percutaneous Coronary Intervention	Injectable
Anticoagulant: Thrombin inhibitor	Dabigatran Extelate Mesylate	PRADAXA	Nonvalvular Atrial Fibrillation	Capsule

Table 4 *cont.*
Drugs Used to Treat Blood Disorders[4]

Drug Class(es)	Generic Name(s)**	Brand Name(s)**	Indication(s)	Available Dose Form(s)
Anticoagulant: Thrombin Inhibitor	Desirudin	Iprivask	Deep Vein Thrombosis, Pulmonary Embolism	Injectable
Anticoagulant: Thrombin Inhibitor	Lepirudin	Refludan	Anticoagulation in Heparin-Induced Thrombocytopenia	Powder (for Injection)
Anticoagulant: Vitamin K Epoxide Reductase Inhibitor	Warfarin	Coumadin, Jantoven	Deep Vein Thrombosis, Pulmonary Embolism	Solution, Tablet
Antihemophilic	Anti-Inhibitor Coagulant Complex	Feiba NF, Feiba VH	Hemophilia A and B with Inhibitors	Injectable
Antihemophilic	Coagulation Factor VIIa (Recombinant)	NotoSeven RT	Hemophilia A and B with Inhibitors	Injectable
Antihemophilic	Factor IX Complex	Bebulin VH, Profilnine SD	Hemophilia B	Injectable
Antihemophilic	Factor IX (Human)	AlphaNine SD, Mononine	Hemophilia B	Injectable
Antihemophilic	Factor IX (Recombinant)	Benefix	Hemophilia B	Injectable
Antihemophilic	Factor VIII (Human)	Alphanate, Hemofil M, Koate-DVI, Monoclate-P	Hemophilia A	Injectable
Antihemophilic	Factor VIII (Recombinant)	Advate, Helixate FS, Kogenate FS, Recombinate, ReFacto, Xyntha	Hemophilia A	Injectable
Antihyperlipidemic	Omega-3 Fish Oil	Lovaza	High Triglycerides	Capsule
Antihyperlipidemic: Bile Acid Sequestrant	Cholestyramine	Questran	High Cholesterol	Powder
Antihyperlipidemic: Bile Acid Sequestrant	Colesevelam	WelChol	High Cholesterol	Tablet

Drug Class(es)	Generic Name(s)**	Brand Name(s)**	Indication(s)	Available Dose Form(s)
Antihyperlipidemic: Bile Acid Sequestrant	Colestipol	Colestid	High Cholesterol	Granules, Tablet
Antihyperlipidemic: Fibrate	Fenofibrate	Antara, Fenoglide, Lipofen, Lofibra, Tricor, Triglide, Trilipix	High Triglycerides	Capsule, Tablet
Antihyperlipidemic: Fibrate	Gemifibrozil	Lopid	High Triglycerides	Tablet
Antihyperlipidemic: HMC-CoA Reductase Inhibitor (Statin)	Atorvastatin	Lipitor	Acute Coronary Syndrome, Hyperlipidemia	Tablet
Antihyperlipidemic: HMC-CoA Reductase Inhibitor (Statin)	Fluvastatin	Lescol, Lescol XL	Acute Coronary Syndrome, High Cholesterol	Capsule, Extended-Release Tablet
Antihyperlipidemic: HMC-CoA Reductase Inhibitor (Statin)	Lovastatin	Altoprev, Mevacor	Acute Coronary Syndrome, High Cholesterol	Extended-Release Tablet, Tablet
Antihyperlipidemic: HMC-CoA Reductase Inhibitor (Statin)	Pravastatin	Pravachol	Acute Coronary Syndrome, Hyperlipidemia	Tablet
Antihyperlipidemic: HMC-CoA Reductase Inhibitor (Statin)	Rosuvastatin	Crestor	Acute Coronary Syndrome, High Cholesterol	Tablet
Antihyperlipidemic: HMC-CoA Reductase Inhibitor (Statin)	Simvastatin	Zocor	Acute Coronary Syndrome, High Cholesterol	Tablet
Antiplatelet	Aspirin / Dipyridamole	Aggrenox	Stroke Prevention	Capsule
Antiplatelet	Cilostazol	Pletal	Pain with Walking	Tablet

Table 4 *cont.*
Drugs Used to Treat Blood Disorders[4]

Drug Class(es)	Generic Name(s)**	Brand Name(s)**	Indication(s)	Available Dose Form(s)
Antiplatelet	Dipyridamole	Persantine	Deep Vein Thrombosis Prevention, Pulmonary Embolism Prevention	Tablet
Antiplatelet	Ticlopidine	Ticlid	Stroke	Tablet
Antiplatelet: Adenoside Diphosphate Receptor Antagonist	Clopidogrel	Plavix	Acute Coronary Syndrome, Heart Attack Prevention, Stroke Prevention	Tablet
Antiplatelet: Adenoside Diphosphate Receptor Antagonist	Prasugrel	Effient	Acute Coronary Syndrome	Tablet
Antiplatelet: Glycoprotein IIb / IIa Receptor Antagonist	Abciximab	ReoPro	Acute Coronary Syndrome, Percutaneous Coronary Intervention	Injectable
Antiplatelet: Glycoprotein IIb / IIa Receptor Antagonist	Eptifibatide	Integrilin	Acute Coronary Syndrome, Percutaneous Coronary Intervention	Injectable
Antiplatelet: Glycoprotein IIb / IIa Receptor Antagonist	Integrilin	Eptifibatide	Acute Coronary Syndrome	Injectable
Antiplatelet: Glycoprotein IIb / IIa Receptor Antagonist	Tirofiban	Aggrastat	Acute Coronary Syndrome	Injectable
Heparin Antagonist	Protamine Sulfate	Not Available	Heparin Overdose	Injectable
Plasma Volume Expander	Albumin	Albuminar-5, Albuminar-25, Buminate, Flexbumin 25%	Low Plasma Volume	Injectable

Drug Class(es)	Generic Name(s)**	Brand Name(s)**	Indication(s)	Available Dose Form(s)
Potassium-Removing Resin	Sodium Polystyrene Sulfonate	Kayexelate	High Potassium	Powder, Suspension
Systemic Alkalizer	Sodium Bicarbonate	Neut	Antacid, Systemic or Urinary Inappropriate Acidity	Tablet
Thrombolytic: Thrombolytic Enzyme	Urokinase	Abbokinase	Acute Pulmonary Embolism, Catheter Clearance, Heart Attack	Injectable
Thrombolytic: Tissue Plasminogen Activator	Alteplase (Recombinant)	Activase, Cathflo Activase	Acute Coronary Syndrome, Catheter Clearance, Pulmonary Embolism	Injectable
Thrombolytic: Tissue Plasminogen Activator	Reteplase	Retevase	Acute Coronary Syndrome	Injectable
Thrombolytic: Tissue Plasminogen Activator	Streptokinase	Kabikinase	Acute Coronary Syndrome	Injectable
Thrombolytic: Tissue Plasminogen Activator	Tenecteplase	TNKase	Acute Coronary Syndrome	Injectable
Trace Element	Carbonyl Iron	FeoSol, IronChews	Iron Deficiency	Chewable Tablet, Suspension, Tablet
Trace Element	Ferric Gluconate	Ferrlecit	Iron Deficiency	Injectable
Trace Element	Ferrous Aspartate	FE Aspartate	Iron Deficiency	Tablet
Trace Element	Ferrous Fumerate	Ferro-Sequels, Hemocyte	Iron Deficiency	Extended-Release Tablet, Tablet
Trace Element	Ferrous Gluconate	Fergon	Iron Deficiency	Tablet
Trace Element	Ferrous Sulfate	FeoSol, Fer-Gen-Sol	Iron Deficiency	Elixir, Solution, Syrup, Tablet
Trace Element	Ferrous Sulfate / Ascorbic Acid	Fero Grad 500	Iron Deficiency	Extended-Release Tablet

Table 4 cont.
Drugs Used to Treat Blood Disorders[4]

Drug Class(es)	Generic Name(s)**	Brand Name(s)**	Indication(s)	Available Dose Form(s)
Trace Element	Ferrous Sulfate Exsiccated (Dried)	Feosol, Feratab, Slow FE	Iron Deficiency	Extended-Release Tablet
Trace Element	Ferumoxytol	Feraheme	Iron Deficiency	Injectable
Trace Element	Iron Dextran	DexFerrum, InFeD	Iron Deficiency	Injectable
Trace Element	Iron Sucrose	Venofer	Iron Deficiency	Injectable
Trace Element	Polysaccharide Iron	Ferrex 150, Niferex	Iron Deficiency	Capsule, Elixir
Trace Element	Polysaccharide Iron / Ascorbic Acid	Niferex-150	Iron Deficiency	Capsule
Trace Element	Sodium Ferric Gluconate Complex	Ferrlecit	Iron Deficiency	Solution
Vitamin D Analog	Calcitriol	Rocaltrol	Low Bone Density	Capsule
Vitamin D Analog	Doxercalciferol	Hectorol	Hyperparathyroidism	Capsule, Injectable
Vitamin D Analog	Ergocalciferol	Calciferol, Drisdol	Osteomalacia	Capsule, Liquid
Vitamin D Analog	Paricalcitol	Zemplar	Hyperparathyroidism	Capsule, Injectable
Vitamin: Fat-Soluble	Choliclciferol (Vitamin D), Ergocalciferol	Drisdol	Low Calcium Absorption, Osteomalacia, Osteoporosis	Capsules, Tablets
Vitamin: Fat-Soluble, Warfarin Antagonist	Phytonadione (Vitamin K)	Mephyton	Coagulation Disorders, Warfarin Overdose	Injectable, Solution, Tablet
Vitamin: Water-Soluble	Cyanocobalamin (Vitamin B_{12})	Nascobal	Vitamin B_{12} Deficiency	Extended-Release Tablet, Injectable, Lozenge, Nasal Spray, Solution, Sublingual Tablet, Tablet

Drug Class(es)	Generic Name(s)**	Brand Name(s)**	Indication(s)	Available Dose Form(s)
Vitamin: Water-Soluble	Folic Acid	Folvite	Folic Acid Deficiency, Megaloblastic Anemia , Neural Tube Defect Prevention (Fetal)	Solution, Tablet

*All rights to all brand names and trademarks are held by their respective owners. There may be additional brand names for the products listed.

Conclusion

The three main types of cells in the blood are erythrocytes, leukocytes and platelets. The main function of erythrocytes is to carry oxygen to the tissues. The classification of leukocytes is complex, and their main function is to get rid of foreign substances in the body. An important function of platelets is to promote clotting in order to stop bleeding. There are several disorders of the blood, including anemia, hemophilia and blood clots. There are many types of anemia, and treatment depends on what type of anemia a patient has. Microcytic anemia is usually caused by iron deficiency and is treated with iron replacement. Macrocytic anemia is usually caused by folic acid or vitamin B_{12} deficiency and is treated with the respective replacement. Sickle cell anemia cannot be reversed and it is painful. It is treated with hydroxyurea, which decreases the painful episodes, and with analgesics. Hemophilia is treated by replacing the patient's deficient clotting factors. Blood clots can be prevented with antiplatelet drugs or anticoagulants. Blood clots are treated with heparin or LMW heparins, warfarin, fondaparinux and sometimes thrombolytics. Understanding various blood disorders and how agents inhibit or activate the coagulation cascade can provide pharmacy technicians with key information needed to suport pharmacists and adequately care for patients.

References

1. Uthman, E., Blood Cells and the CBC, http://web2.airmail.net/uthman/blood_cells.html, June 28, 2010.

2. Guyton, A.C., "Chapter 32, Red Blood Cells, Anemia, and Polycythemia," Textbook of Medical Physiology, 8th edition, Philadelphia, PA, 1991, pp. 356-364.

3. Hutson P.R., "Chapter 14, Hematology: Red and White Blood Cell Tests," Basic Skills in Interpreting Laboratory Data, 4th edition, Bethesda, MD, 2009, pp. 339-362.

4. Guyton, A.C., "Chapter 33, Resistance of the Body to Infection: I. Leukocytes, Granulocytes, the Monocyte-Macrophage System, and Inflammation," Textbook of Medical Physiology, 8th edition, Philadelphia, PA, 1991, pp. 365-373.

5. Guyton, A.C., "Chapter 36, Hemostasis and Blood Coagulation," Textbook of Medical Physiology, 8th edition, Philadelphia, PA, 1991, pp. 390-399.

6. Allen, S.M., dela Pena, L.E., "Chapter 15, Hematology: Blood Coagulation Tests," Basic Skills in Interpreting Laboratory Data, 4th edition, Bethesda, MD, pp. 363-390.

7. Bickert, B., Kwiatkowski, J.L., "Chapter 110, Coagulation Disorders," Pharmacotherapy: A Pathophysiologic Approach, 6th edition, New York, NY, 2005, pp. 1833-1854.

8. Haines, S.T., Zeolla, M., Witt, D.M., "Chapter 26, Venous Thromboembolism," Pharmacotherapy: A Pathophysiologic Approach, 6th edition, New York, NY, 2005, pp. 373-414.

9. Ineck, B., Mason, B.J., Thompson, E.G. "Chapter 109, Anemias," Pharmacotherapy: A Pathophysiologic Approach, 6th edition, New York, NY, 2005, pp. 1805-1832.

10. Chan, C.Y.J., Moore, R., "Chapter 111, Sickle Cell Disease," Pharmacotherapy: A Pathophysiologic Approach, 6th edition, New York, NY, 2005, pp. 1855-1874.

11. Miller, A.D., Smith, K.M., "Medication and Nutrient Administration Considerations After Bariatric Surgery," American Journal of Health-System Pharmacists, Vol. 63, pp. 1852-1857, Oct. 1, 2006.

12. Alleyne, M., Horne, M.K., Miler, J.L., "Individualized Treatment For Iron Deficiency Anemia In Adults," American Journal of Medicine, Vol. 121, pp. 943-48, November 2008.

13. Kastrup, E.K., Drug Facts and Comparisons, St. Louis, MO, 2010.

14. Field, J.J., DeBraun, M.R., Vichinsky, E.P., "Overview of the Management of Sickle Cell Disease," www.uptodate.com/contents/overview-of-the-management-of-sickle-cell-disease, MA, 2010.

15. Talbert, R.L., "Chapter 23, Ischemic Heart Disease," Pharmacotherapy: A Pathophysiologic Approach, 6th edition, New York, NY, 2005, pp. 261-290.

16. Bhatt, D.L., Topol, E.J., "Antiplatelet and Anticoagulant Drugs," Treatment Guidelines from the Medical Letter, Vol. 6, pp. 29-36, May 2008.

17. Du Breuil, A.L., Umland, E.M., "Outpatient Management of Anticoagulation Therapy," American Family Physician, Vol. 75, pp. 1031-1042, April 1, 2007.

18. Spinler, S.A., "A Patient's Guide to Taking Dabigatran Etexilate," Circulation, American Heart Association, 2011.

19. Food and Drug Administration, www.fda.gov/Safety/MedWatch/SafetyInformation/SafetyAlertsforHumanMedicalProducts/ucm282820.html, Jan. 26, 2012.

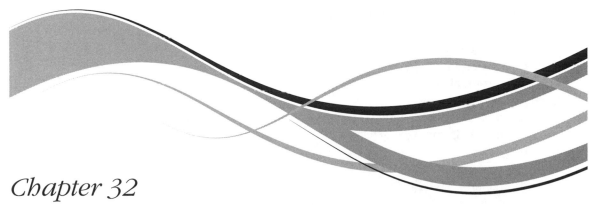

Chapter 32
REVIEW QUESTIONS

1. Which of the following types of cells in the blood carry oxygen to the tissues?
   a. Erythrocytes
   b. Leukocytes
   c. Platelets
   d. Basophils

2. Which of the following types of granulocytes increase in the presence of an acute bacterial infection?
   a. Eosinophils
   b. Basophils
   c. Neutrophils
   d. Lymphocytes

3. Which of the following is the main function of platelets?
   a. Fight infections
   b. Stop bleeding
   c. Carry oxygen to tissues
   d. Prevent allergic reactions

4. Microcytic anemia is the result of:
   a. vitamin B_{12} deficiency.
   b. folic acid deficiency.
   c. iron deficiency.
   d. vitamin B_6 deficiency.

5. Macrocytic anemia is the result of:
   a. vitamin B_{12} or folic acid deficiency.
   b. iron or vitamin C deficiency.
   c. vitamin K or folic acid deficiency.
   d. vitamin B_6 or vitamin C deficiency.

6. The effect of aspirin on blood cells is best described as:
    a. antiplatelet.
    b. anticoagulant.
    c. hemostatic.
    d. thrombolytic.

7. An injectable anticoagulant that accelerates the process of antithrombin III is:
    a. tissue plasminogen activator.
    b. dextran.
    c. warfarin.
    d. heparin.

8. The long-term anticoagulant of choice for preventing clots in patients with chronic atrial fibrillation or DVT is:
    a. tissue plasminogen activator.
    b. warfarin.
    c. heparin.
    d. enoxaparin.

9. Which of the following drugs is used to prevent painful crises in patients with sickle cell anemia?
    a. Aminocaproic acid
    b. Human Factor IX complex
    c. Pyridoxine
    d. Hydroxyurea

10. Giving which of the following factors would be an appropriate treatment for someone with Hemophilia A?
    a. Factor VII
    b. Factor VIII
    c. Factor IX
    d. Factor X

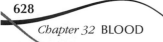

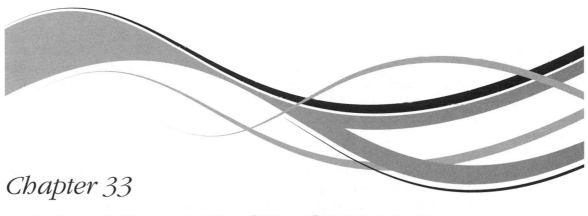

Chapter 33
IMMUNE SYSTEM

By Dean A. Van Loo, Pharm.D.

Learning Objectives

This chapter seeks to prepare a pharmacy technician to:

- describe the function of the immune system.
- differentiate between innate and adaptive immunity.
- differentiate between cellular and humoral immunity.
- list the different types of white blood cells and their functions.
- list the components of the combination antiretrovirals.
- classify the antiretrovirals by class (nucleoside reverse transcriptase inhibitors, non-nucleoside reverse transcriptase inhibitors, protease inhibitors, fusion inhibitors, integrase inhibitors, receptor blockers) and list the common adverse effects of each class.
- recognize the drugs used for prophylaxis of pneumocystis pneumonia and mycobacterium avium complex (MAC) and the most common adverse effect for each.
- explain how the medications used for preventing rejection of transplanted organs work and the common complications of that immune suppression.

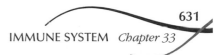

Introduction

The immune system is a complex and intricate system that usually works well to protect us. It is designed to defend the body against foreign substances (e.g., microorganisms, parasites, cancer cells and transplanted organs and tissues). Using its network of organs and cells, the immune system protects the body from disease and illness through **adaptive immunity** and **innate immunity**. Innate, or nonspecific, immunity is a basic resistance to disease that the body possesses from the moment of creation. This type of immunity consists mostly of barriers used as defense. These barriers, such as skin, chemicals in the blood and mucous membranes, help deter invading **pathogens** (biological agents that cause disease or illness to a host). Another type of immunity, adaptive, or acquired, immunity comes into play when innate immunity is breached. Adaptive immunity is more complex than innate immunity and involves an immune response to the foreign invader. A response usually consists of sending certain types of cells to destroy the threat. Adaptive immunity has the ability, as its name implies, to "remember" pathogens it has encountered previously and tailor its response to be more efficient.

Immune System Components

Components of the immune system include: barriers, immune cells, **immune globulin** (**antibodies**), immune complement, cytokines and other inflammatory mediators. The barriers of the body include the skin and mucous membranes; these barriers are the first line of defense for keeping pathogens from getting into the body. When these barriers are disrupted through injuries (such as burns), the potential for infection increases dramatically. If a pathogen gets beyond these barriers, the immune system will send white blood cells, among other things, to destroy the pathogen. There are many types of white blood cells involved in immunity, including **neutrophils**, **lymphocytes**, **monocytes**, **eosinophils**, and **basophils**. Although eosinophils and basophils are important, few medications target this part of the immune system; thus, this chapter will not discuss this portion of the immune system any further. Neutrophils and monocytes are the predominant cells often called "**phagocytes.**" They function predominantly as part of the innate, or non-specific, immunity. Lymphocytes are principally responsible for functions related to adaptive immunity. Lymphocytes are divided into T-cells and B-cells. **B-cells** are responsible for making antibodies (immune globulin) and **T-cells** work with antibodies to eliminate an invading pathogen. The **soluble mediators**, the parts of the immune system that are not cells and dissolved into blood or plasma, make up the majority of the humoral immunity and are immune globulin, immune complement (or complement) and inflammatory mediators. Immune globulin specifically binds with certain parts of the pathogen to make it more difficult for the pathogen to function; further, this tags the pathogen for destruction by specific white blood cells. Complement performs similar functions to immune globulin, but in a non-specific way. The inflammatory mediators, such as cytokines, recruit and direct the white blood cells to where they need to go.

Human Immunodeficiency Virus

Human immunodeficiency virus (HIV) infection attacks a specific type of T-lymphocyte called a CD4 cell. As the disease progresses, the elimination of the CD4 cells results in a profound immune deficiency, leading to multiple opportunistic infections, such as pneumocystis pneumonia (PCP) and mycobacterium avium complex (MAC). HIV infection can be transmitted in one of three modes: parenteral (e.g., blood transfusions, sharing of needles, needle sticks), sexual or perinatal (during pregnancy, birth or breastfeeding). Sexual contact is the most common route of infection in adults; whereas, perinatal transmission is the most common route of transmission in infants and children. Drugs used to treat any infectious agent must target biological features or processes unique to the infecting organism to prevent adverse effects to the host. The life cycle of HIV has several unique processes which have been identified for therapeutic intervention (see Figure 1). HIV initially adheres to a CD4 cell at the CCR5 or CXCR4 receptor; the CCR5 receptor is a target for the CCR5 receptor blocker maraviroc. The virus then fuses with the cell and injects its **ribonucleic acid (RNA)** into the cell; this fusion step is the next target and is where the fusion inhibitor enfuvirtide works. The genetic information of HIV is contained on single-strand RNA and must be transcribed onto **deoxyribonucleic acid (DNA)** for replication inside the human cell. HIV possesses a unique enzyme to force this process to occur, called **reverse transcriptase**. This enzyme is the prime target for drug therapy and where the classes nucleoside reverse transcriptase inhibitors (NRTI) and non-nucleoside reverse transcriptase inhibitors (NNRTI) work. Once the genetic information of HIV is replicated, it must be inserted into the cellular genome in order to exert its effect. The enzyme responsible for this integration is called integrase and is the target of the integrase inhibitor raltegravir. Once the viral genetic protein has taken over the cell, it starts to produce the components of new **virons**. The large proteins within the new virons must be "cut" into functional pieces to produce a virus capable of causing infection. This is accomplished with another unique enzyme called protease, which is the final current target of HIV therapies, where the protease inhibitors (PI) exert their activity.

Figure 1
HIV Life-Cycle

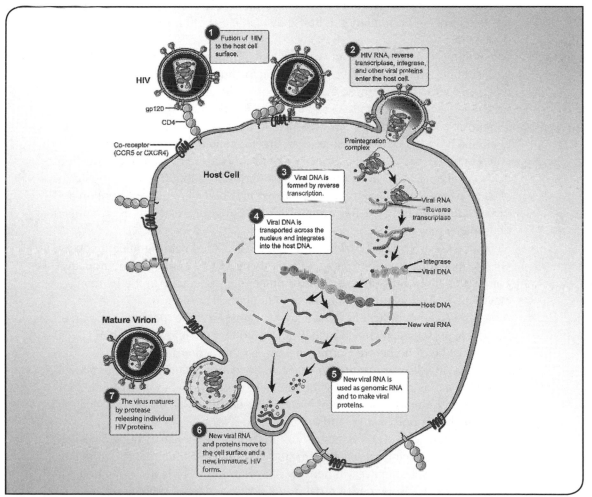

Courtesy of the National Institute of Allergy and Infectious Diseases, www.niaid.nih.gov/topics/ HIVAIDS/Understanding/Biology/pages/hivreplicationcycle.aspx

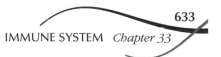

Drugs Used to Treat HIV

Food and Drug Administration (FDA) approved drugs to treat HIV infection are included in Table 1. Many of these drugs have been given abbreviations (e.g., Zidovudine is also known as AZT); these abbreviations can be found in the text below. Although these abbreviations can be helpful in remembering the many drugs available to manage HIV infection, these are not recommended for use on prescriptions due to possible confusion with other drugs that could lead to medication errors.

■ **Nucleoside Reverse Transcriptase Inhibitors**
Nucleoside reverse transcriptase inhibitors (NRTIs) inhibit the enzyme reverse transcriptase by mimicking the **nucleosides** that are being incorporated into the DNA being transcribed from the viral RNA. The most serious adverse effect from taking any drug in this class is **lactic acidosis** (a buildup of lactic acid in the bloodstream at a faster rate than the body can eliminate it) that often occurs with liver damage.

- Zidovudine (Retrovir®, AZT) was the first antiretroviral agent to be used clinically. Intolerance, which is common, and some rare, but serious, effects including bone marrow suppression such as anemia, leukopenia and thrombocytopenia; peripheral neuropathy; and **lipodystrophy** (fat loss in the face and extremities and fat accumulation in the abdomen and back) made the need to find new agents imperative. Zidovudine is the only antiretroviral available as an intravenously-injectable formulation; this IV formulation is used exclusively for HIV positive mothers during labor. It is also available as both a solid and liquid oral dose form.
- Lamivudine (Epivir®, 3TC) and emtricitabine (Emtriva™) are the best tolerated NRTIs. Although they still have the potential to cause lactic acidosis and peripheral neuropathy, both of these events are extremely rare. Lamivudine and emtricitabine are available as both a solid and liquid oral dose form.
- Didanosine (Videx®, ddi) is very sensitive to acid, it must be taken on an empty stomach and is only available in an enteric-coated formulation. As with all enteric-coated capsules, the capsule cannot be crushed or emptied; but, ddi is also available in an oral solution. It is a useful drug, but it is well-known for causing pancreatitis. Due to the relationship between alcohol consumption and pancreatitis, alcohol must be avoided while taking this medication. Peripheral neuropathy may also occur.
- Stavudine (Zerit®, d4T) is a useful drug but is associated with significant adverse effects (including lipodystrophy and potentially severe peripheral neuropathy). The neuropathy results in weakness or numbness, especially in the extremities. Stavudine is available in both a solid and liquid oral dose form.
- Abacavir (Ziagen®, ABC) has great activity against HIV. The most serious side effect is a hypersensitivity reaction that can be life-threatening. A test called HLA-B 5701 must be done before starting therapy, and if it comes back positive or if a patient has an allergic reaction to abacavir, they must never receive the medication. Abacavir is metabolized by the same enzyme that metabolizes alcohol (alcohol dehydrogenase), so alcohol must be avoided when taking this medication. It is available in both a solid and liquid oral dose form.
- Tenofovir (Viread™, TDF) is actually a nucleotide (rather than nucleoside) reverse transcriptase inhibitor, which means it has a slightly different structure than the other NRTIs, but in every other way is similar. Tenofovir is well-tolerated, but it may cause rare instances of renal insufficiency and bone problems (osteomalacia). It is available only as a solid oral dose form.

■ Protease Inhibitors

As described earlier, **protease inhibitors (PIs)** act by inhibiting the enzyme protease, resulting in a newly replicated immature virus incapable of infecting new CD4 cells. All of the protease inhibitors are metabolized by the liver, which has major implications for drug interactions. The package insert must be consulted whenever beginning any protease inhibitor therapy and every time a new drug is prescribed for the patient to avoid serious drug interactions. Patients must be advised to strictly adhere to their dosing schedule when taking PIs to prevent the development of resistance. Most PIs are very poorly absorbed and are immediately metabolized by the liver. For this reason, one PI will be given with ritonavir to inhibit the metabolism of the PI and result in a "boosting" of the levels; ritonavir will block the metabolism of other PIs so that they stay in the system longer and have their effect prolonged. Common adverse effects reported with PI include hyperglycemia, increased bleeding episodes in hemophiliac patients and fat redistribution (lipodystrophy) with or without lipid abnormalities.

- Saquinavir (Invirase®, SQV) was the first FDA-approved protease inhibitor. Due to significant problems with bioavailability, saquinavir must always be used with ritonavir to increase levels and must be taken within two hours after a meal. It is available only as a solid oral dose form.

- Indinavir (Crixivan®, IDV) is very susceptible to moisture and will degrade quickly if exposed to moist conditions. For this reason, the medication must be left in the original container that includes a **desiccant** (drying agent). The drug is only stable for three days out of the original container. For optimal absorption, patients must be advised to take indinavir one hour before, or two hours after, a meal. An unusual adverse effect associated with indinavir is the formation of kidney stones due to the insolubility of indinavir and its metabolites in the urine. Therefore, patients must drink 48 ounces of noncaffeinated fluids every day while taking indinavir. It is available only as a solid oral dose form.

- Ritonavir (Norvir®, RTV) has the most adverse effects and drug interactions of all the PIs. The most frequent side effects include weakness, gastrointestinal (GI) intolerance, diarrhea, anorexia, abdominal pain, change in sense of taste, numbness in the lips and **paresthesia** (tingling sensations). The package insert must be consulted with every new prescribed drug to avoid drug interactions. Ritonavir is taken with meals and one hour after antacids. The capsule form must be stored in the refrigerator, but it is stable for 30 days at room temperature; the oral solution must be stored at room temperature. The taste of ritonavir oral solution may be improved by mixing it with chocolate milk or another flavored dietary supplement within one hour of dosing.

- Nelfinavir (Viracept®, NFV) is associated with mild-to-moderate diarrhea that may be relieved with the over-the-counter loperamide (Immodium®). Nelfinavir is best absorbed with a small meal. It is also available as powder for suspension that is taken orally after reconstitution.

- Fosamprenavir (Lexiva™, FPV) is a prodrug of amprenavir and most commonly causes a rash, but can also rarely result in kidney stones. It is available as both a solid and liquid oral dose form.

- Lopinavir/ritonavir (Kaletra®, LPVr) is a combination of two protease inhibitors. The ritonavir increases the lopinavir concentrations. The adverse effects are similar to those of ritonavir. It is available as both a solid and liquid oral dose form. The oral solution contains 42 percent alcohol (by volume) and must be taken with food.

- Atazanavir (Reyataz™, ATV) may have less of the metabolic class effects (e.g., hyperglycemia, hyperlipidemia and fat redistribution) than the other PIs. One important drug interaction: any drug that decreases stomach acid will also reduce the absorption of atazanavir. If the patient is on an H_2 antagonist (such as famotidine), the atazanavir must be given before the H_2 antagonist or at least 10 hours after it. Proton pump inhibitors must be avoided when using atazanavir; but, if they must be used together, the atazanavir must be boosted by using ritonavir. Atazanavir may also result in the increase of bilirubin levels. Atazanavir is available only as a solid oral dose form and must be taken with food.

- Darunavir (Prezista™, DRV) is a very effective PI that is fairly well-tolerated. The most serious adverse effect is a skin rash that may, at times, be very severe. Darunavir may also cause liver toxicity. It is available only as a solid oral dose form, and it must always be boosted with ritonavir. Darunavir must be taken with food.
- Tipranavir (Aptivus®, TPV) is another PI that must always be boosted with ritonavir. It has a sulfonamide moiety in its structure, so it must be avoided in patients with a serious sulfa allergy. It has a rare, but serious, adverse effect of intracranial hemorrhage, and it may also cause liver toxicity. The capsules must be refrigerated but are stable at room temperature for up to 60 days; the oral solution must not be refrigerated.

■ **Nonnucleoside Reverse Transcriptase Inhibitors**

Nonnucleoside reverse transcriptase inhibitors (NNRTIs) exert their antiretroviral effects as noncompetitive inhibitors of reverse transcriptase. Common adverse effects include the development of a rash and an increase in liver enzyme levels (transaminases), as well as drug interactions.

- Nevirapine (Viramune®, NVP) was the first FDA-approved NNRTI. Nevirapine has many drug interactions since it induces the liver to metabolize faster. It actually induces its own metabolism, which is why it is dosed daily for two weeks and then it is dosed twice daily. Nevirapine also causes liver toxicity, especially in women with a CD4 count greater than 250 cells/mm^3 or men with a CD4 count greater than 400 cells/mm^3, and must not be used in these populations. It is available as both a solid and liquid oral dose form.
- Delavirdine (Rescriptor®, DLV) is a rarely used medication due to its three times per day dosing and relatively poor activity. It has the standard adverse effects of rash and liver toxicity. It comes only as a solid oral dose form that can be dispersed in water if needed.
- Efavirenz (Sustiva®, EFV) is currently the most commonly used medication in this class. It is relatively well-tolerated; although, the class effects of rash and liver toxicity may occur. The most common adverse effects are confusion and other central nervous system effects. For this reason, the drug is usually given at bedtime usually resulting in vivid dreams. Efavirenz is available as a solid oral dose form that is taken on an empty stomach to slow absorption and reduce adverse effects.
- Etravirine (Intelence™, ETR) is a newer NNRTI and can be used when there is HIV resistance to the other NNRTI. The main adverse effects of etravirine are the standard class adverse effects.

■ **Fusion Inhibitors**

Enfuvirtide (Fuzeon®, T20) is the only available fusion inhibitor. It is only available as an injectable and is given subcutaneously like insulin. It can be very difficult to prepare the injection due to difficulty in solubilizing the powder. Once reconstituted, the solution must be refrigerated if it is not used immediately and is stable for only 24 hours. The most common adverse effects are redness and hard lumps at the injection sites.

CCR5 Receptor Antagonists

CCR5 receptor antagonists are a class of small molecules that antagonize the CCR5 receptor. The C-C motif chemokine receptor CCR5 is involved in the HIV entry process. Maraviroc (Selzentry™, MVC) is a rarely used medication (block the CCR5 receptor on the CD4 cell preventing HIV from being able to enter certain cells). In order to use this agent, a test to ensure that the patient's specific strain of HIV is dependent on the CCR5 receptor must be performed. The most common adverse effects are abdominal pain and musculoskeletal pain. Many other HIV drugs interact with this medication. Maraviroc is only available in a solid oral dose form.

Integrase Inhibitors

Raltegravir (Isentress™, RAL) is currently the only available integrase inhibitor. Raltegravir is a very well-tolerated and easy-to-use medication. It targets integrase, an HIV enzyme that integrates the viral genetic material into human chromosomes, a critical step in the pathogenesis of HIV. Raltegravir is only available as a solid oral dose form.

Combination Products

In order to adequately treat HIV, the use of combinations of different antiretrovirals must be used. The most effective of these regimens are called **highly active antiretroviral therapy (HAART)**. Because adherence is such an important issue in HIV therapy, combination products are often used so it is important to be familiar with the different products available. Table 1 contains a list of the various combination products available. The most up-to-date recommendations are available at www.aidsinfo.nih.gov.

Occupational Exposure to HIV

Health care workers are at risk of contracting HIV from exposure to the virus through significant mucous membrane exposure or accidental needle sticks. The Centers for Disease Control and Prevention (CDC) has published guidelines for **postexposure prophylaxis (PEP)** for HIV infection. It is recommended to administer, within one to two hours of exposure, a combination of two NRTIs or a full HAART regimen, depending on the extent of the exposure. If the exposure is deemed significant, therapy is continued for four weeks.

Opportunistic Infection Prophylaxis Regimens

Drugs used as prophylaxis against PCP and MAC are listed in Table 1.

Pneumocystis Pneumonia

Pneumonia caused by *Pneumocystis jiroveci* is the most common, life-threatening infection in HIV patients. *Pneumocystis jiroveci* is widespread in the environment and up to 80 percent of the population has been exposed. Infection does not occur unless a patient has a suppressed immune system. HIV patients with CD4 counts less than 200 cells/mm³ must receive prophylaxis for PCP. Sulfamethoxazole and trimethoprim in combination is the current drug of choice. For patients who cannot tolerate sulfamethoxazole/trimethoprim, dapsone is an alternative. Adverse effects of sulfamethoxazole/trimethoprim include rash, nausea and anemia. Both sulfamethoxazole/trimethoprim and dapsone regimens may provide additional prophylaxis against the disease toxoplasmosis. Pentamidine by nebulization (administration of a fine spray) once each month is another option. This treatment can be associated with bronchospasm. Atovaquone is an option for patients who cannot receive either sulfamethoxazole/trimethoprim or pentamidine. The most common adverse effects are headache, nausea and diarrhea.

■ Mycobacterium Avium Complex Infection

Mycobacterium avium complex infection (MAC) is a nontuberculosis organism commonly found in water and soil. Systemic MAC infection is considered an end-stage **acquired immune deficiency syndrome (AIDS)** complication, consisting of high fevers, diarrhea, night sweats, malaise, weight loss, anemia and neutropenia. Patients with CD4 counts less than 50 cells/mm³ must receive prophylaxis for MAC. Azithromycin once weekly or clarithromycin daily are the current drugs of choice. Adverse effects are minimal but may include GI upset. Patients unable to tolerate azithromycin or clarithromycin may be prescribed rifabutin. Adverse effects of rifabutin include rash, GI intolerance, **uveitis** (inflammation of the iris, ciliary body or the layer of blood vessels and connective tissue between the white of the eye and the retina of the eye), hepatitis and orange-brown coloring of bodily secretions (tears, sweat, sputum, urine and feces) and skin. Patients must be warned that soft contacts may be permanently stained if worn while taking rifabutin. There are also multiple drug interactions with rifabutin.

Organ Transplant

There are more than 100,000 people on the United Network for Organ Sharing list awaiting transplantation of a solid organ in the United States. This list includes patients who are candidates for a transplanted kidney, pancreas, liver, heart, lung or intestines. Depending on the organ that the patient is waiting for, and how sick the patient is, the wait can range from hours to years after being placed on the waiting list. The decision to transplant an organ is not taken lightly, and once the decision is made and the transplant complete, a lifetime of taking immunosuppressant drugs is required to prevent rejection.

Immunosuppression

There are three main types of transplant organ rejection: hyper acute, acute and chronic. **Hyperacute organ rejection** is caused by preformed cytotoxic antibodies that are directed against donor organ markers. An example of hyperacute rejection would be if the blood type of the organ donor and of the organ recipient do not match. If there is a mismatch, hyperacute rejection would occur. This can happen within minutes of sewing the organ in and usually requires removal of the organ. **Acute organ rejection**, or cellular organ rejection (T-cell mediated), occurs when the host immune system has a reaction to the markers on the donor organ (immediately recognizes it as foreign). This can happen at any time after the transplant but occurs more frequently in the early period (between seven and 21 days after transplantation). **Chronic organ rejection**, or humoral organ rejection (B-cell mediated), is when the host body forms antibodies against the donor organ. Again, this can happen at any time after the transplant; however, it generally occurs later (three months or more after transplantation). Diagnosing graft rejection can be challenging, and clinical scenarios must be closely matched with laboratory and **histological** findings. In kidney transplant patients, signs that the patient may be experiencing organ rejection include an increase in serum creatinine, a decrease in urine output, and pain or tenderness over the transplanted kidney. It would also be expected that the liver enzymes would be elevated in the blood if a liver transplant patient is experiencing rejection. Heart and lung transplant patients may experience shortness of breath, and heart transplant patients may experience edema. The only way to absolutely confirm the diagnosis of organ rejection is with an organ biopsy.

When patients are evaluated for transplant, the specific markers on the organs are matched as closely as possible in an attempt to decrease the risk of the patient's body "rejecting" the new organ.

Even if all of the organ markers are matched perfectly, the transplant recipient will be on immunosuppressive medications for the rest of his or her life. In the period immediately after the transplant operation, the patients will receive an immunosuppressive that is for "induction therapy." This is given in hopes of eliminating all preformed antibodies against the new organ. Medications used for induction include antithymocyte globulins (ATG or Atgam® and RATG or Thymoglobulin®), muomonab-CD-3 (OKT3®) and anti-interleukin-2 (IL-2) receptor monoclonal antibodies, such as daclizumab (Zenepax®) and basiliximab (Simulect®). These agents are listed in Table 1.

The exact way that the antithymocyte globulins work is very complex. They are a mix of different types of antibodies (polyclonal) that ultimately act to suppress the cellular portion (T-cells) of the immune system. They can be used as induction therapy or to reverse acute rejection episodes. They have many adverse reactions (including fever, chills, dizziness and headaches) that can be minimized by slowing the infusion rate and by pre-medicating with acetaminophen (Tylenol®) and diphenhydramine (Benadryl®). Patients on these medications also may experience **thrombocytopenia** (decreased platelet count) and **leukopenia** (decreased white blood cell count). The doses of these medications must be decreased if the patient experiences thrombocytopenia or leukopenia. Patients on these medications are also at an increased risk for infections. Prophylactic medications must be added against common infectious agents when these medications are taken; this is done in similar ways to those discussed for patients with HIV-AIDS.

The IL-2 receptor antagonists are a single type of antibody (monoclonal) and are utilized only as induction therapy. They are not as immune suppressive as the antithymocyte globulins, but they are very effective as induction therapies. Activated T-cells have an IL-receptor on their surface. These medications bind to this receptor and inactivate the T-cell. Daclizumab and basiliximab are both very well-tolerated and do not cause thrombocytopenia or leukopenia like Atgam® and Thymoglobulin®.

Muromonab-CD3 (OKT3®) is a monoclonal antibody that is a very potent immunosuppressant. It is usually reserved as induction therapy for high-risk patients or to reverse steroid-resistant, acute cellular rejection episodes. It is very immunosuppressive and has a complex mechanism of action. It has many severe adverse effects, including **flash pulmonary edema** (fluid in the lungs) and **anaphylaxis** (allergic reaction to the first dose). Pre-medicating with acetaminophen, diphenhydramine and corticosteroids may help minimize some of these adverse effects. Patients must be carefully examined prior to receiving this medication to rule out fluid overload. This can be done by obtaining a chest x-ray within 24 hours of planned administration and checking for a greater than three percent weight gain within the week prior to the planned administration.

Maintenance Immunosuppression

There are many immunosuppressive drug regimens utilized in transplantation. Most commonly, a three-drug combination is used. Multiple medications are used because they each have unique mechanisms of action without overlapping toxicities. This allows maximal suppression of the immune system while limiting the adverse effects of each of the medications. These medications are listed in Table 1.

The first group of medications that is used to prevent graft rejection in solid organ transplant patients includes cyclosporine (Sandimmune®, Neoral®) and tacrolimus (Prograf®). These medications work by suppressing the production of T-cells (preventing T-cell mediated rejection). The doses are patient specific and are determined based on blood levels that are drawn immediately prior to the morning dose of the medication (this is referred to as a "trough blood level"). Some of the adverse effects that may occur in patients who are on these medications include acute and chronic kidney toxicities, hypertension (usually when blood levels are elevated) and elevated cholesterol levels. Cyclosporine can also cause hair growth on the face, the trunk of the body and the arms and legs, as well as **gingival hyperplasia** (thickening of the gums). These medications are metabolized by a common enzyme in the liver so drug interactions are common; and, all other medications that the patient is on must be evaluated for the possibility of interacting with either cyclosporine or tacrolimus. The two forms of cyclosporine (Sandimmune® and Neoral®) have different dosing, so care must be taken in dispensing to ensure the correct product is used.

Corticosteroids (primarily methylprednisolone and prednisone) are used to both prevent graft rejection and to reverse acute rejection episodes. They also inhibit the production of T-cells (preventing or reversing cellular rejection). Initially, after the transplant procedure, the corticosteroid doses are high and then are tapered down to a maintenance dose over the first few days. These medications have many significant adverse effects, including insomnia, elevated blood glucose, elevated cholesterol, weakening of the bones (osteoporosis), mental status changes and stomach irritation. They are always taken with food, and the patient must take precautions when in the sunlight (e.g., sunscreen use, minimizing exposed skin, etc.)

Azathioprine (Imuran®) and mycophenolate (Cellcept®, Myfortic®) belong to the third group of medications commonly used to prevent organ rejection. These medications have a unique mechanism of action that involves the suppression of the T-cells (prevents cellular rejection) and some B-cells (prevents humoral rejection). Of these two medications, mycophenolate is more frequently used and tends to have more favorable outcomes. The main adverse effects with these medications are a decrease in the white blood cell count (more common with azathioprine) and stomach upset (more common with mycophenolate). Cellcept® can be toxic to touch, so care must be used when handling it. Myfortic® is an enteric coated form of mycophenolate, which decreases stomach upset and toxicity while handling the tablet compared to Cellcept®. Dosing is different between the two forms, so care must be used to ensure the correct form is dispensed. Neither form should ever be crushed, and the capsules must never be opened without using appropriate precautions (wearing gloves, gowns and a face mask). Sirolimus (Rapamune®) is an immunosuppressant with a unique mechanism of action. It was approved by the FDA in 1999 for the prophylaxis of organ rejection in renal transplant patients, in combination with cyclosporine and prednisone. It is a macrolide antibiotic with immunosuppressive properties that inhibits the development of cells in the growth cycle. It is dosed once daily and must be separated from cyclosporine by at least four hours. The side effect profile for sirolimus includes an increase in serum cholesterol and triglycerides and an increased risk of fluid collection around the kidney (**lymphocele**). It is metabolized by the same common enzyme system as cyclosporine and tacrolimus, so all concurrent medications must be checked for possible drug interactions.

There are risks to suppressing a patient's immune system. These include, but are not limited to, increasing the risk of infections and increasing the risk of certain types of cancers. Many of the infections are similar to those seen in patients with AIDS, but one of the most troubling is **cytomegalovirus (CMV)** infection. This is a common herpes virus that, in patients with a normal immune system, is generally not of concern; however, when a patient is immunosuppressed, it can be devastating. Ganciclovir (Cytovene®) or valganciclovir (Valcyte®) are medications that post-transplant patients are generally placed on to prevent them from acquiring an active disease from this virus. These medications are generally continued for the first three months after the transplant, the duration may vary depending on the risk for the transplant patient of acquiring the virus. Valganciclovir is a prodrug of ganciclovir to improve absorption of the orally-administered drug. The most troubling adverse effect of these drugs is a dose-dependent (i.e., the higher the dose, the more the effect is seen) bone marrow suppression most often observed as leukopenia.

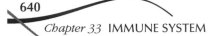

Table 1

Drugs Used to Treat Immune System Disorders

Drug Class(es)	Generic Name(s)**	Brand Name(s)**	Indication(s)	Available Dose Form(s)
Anti-Rejection: Immune Globulin	Antithymocyte Globulin, Lymphocyte Globulin	Thymoglobulin	Organ Transplant Rejection	Injectable
Anti-Rejection: Immune Globulin	Antithymocyte Globulin / Lymphocyte Globulin	Atgam	Organ Transplant Rejection Prevention	Injectable
Anti-Rejection: Immunosuppressive	Basilizimab	Simulect	Immunosuppression, Organ Transplant Rejection Prevention	Injectable
Anti-Rejection: Immunosuppressive	Daclizumab	Zenapax	Immunosuppression, Organ Transplant Rejection Prevention	Injectable
Anti-Rejection: Immunosuppressive	Mycophenolate Mofetil	CellCept, Myfortic	Immunosuppression, Organ Transplant Rejection Prevention	Capsule, Suspension, Tablet
Anti-Rejection: Immunosuppressive	Sirolimus	Rapamune	Immunosuppression, Organ Transplant Rejection Prevention	Solution, Tablet
Anti-Rejection: Immunosuppressive	Tacrolimus	Prograf	Immunosuppression, Organ Transplant Rejection Prevention	Capsule, Injectable
Anti-Rejection: Immunosuppressive, Anti-Rheumatic Drug	Cyclosporine	Gengraf, Neoral, Restasis, Sandimmune	Organ Transplant Rejection Prevention, Psoriasis, Rheumatoid Arthritis, Tear Prevention	Capsule, Injectable, Ophthalmic, Solution
Anti-Rejection: Monoclonal Antibody	Muromonab-CD3	OKT3	Organ Transplant Rejection Prevention	Injectable
Anti-Rheumatic: Disease-Modifying Anti-Rheumatic Drug, Immunosuppressive	Azathioprine	Azasan, Imuran	Immunosuppression, Rheumatoid Arthritis	Injectable, Tablet
Antiviral	Acyclovir	Zovirax	Herpes Viral Infection, Varicella Virus Infection	Capsule, Injectable, Solution, Tablet

Table 1 *cont.*
Drugs Used to Treat Immune System Disorders

Drug Class(es)	Generic Name(s)**	Brand Name(s)**	Indication(s)	Available Dose Form(s)
Antiviral	Adefovir	Hepsera	Hepatitis B Infection	Tablet
Antiviral	Entecavir	Baraclude	Hepatitis B Infection	Solution, Tablet
Antiviral	Famciclovir	Famvir	Herpes Infection	Tablet
Antiviral	Ganciclovir	Cytovene	Cytomegalovirus Prophylaxis	Capsule, Injectable
Antiviral	Ribavirin	Copegus, Rebetol, Virazole	Hepatitis C Infection	Capsule, Solution, Solution for Inhalation, Tablet
Antiviral	Valacyclovir	Valtrex	Herpes Infection	Tablet
Antiviral	Valganciclovir	Valcyte	Cytomegalovirus Prophylaxis	Tablet
Antiviral: Chemokine Receptor 5 Antagonist	Maraviroc	Selzentry	Human Immunodeficiency Virus / Acquired Immune Deficiency Syndrome	Tablet
Antiviral: Combination	Abacavir / Lamivudine	Epzicom	Human Immunodeficiency Virus / Acquired Immune Deficiency Syndrome	Tablet
Antiviral: Combination	Abacavir / Lamivudine / Zidovudine	Trizivir	Human Immunodeficiency Virus / Acquired Immune Deficiency Syndrome	Tablet
Antiviral: Combination	Efavirenz / Emtricitabine / Tenofovir	Atripla	Human Immunodeficiency Virus / Acquired Immune Deficiency Syndrome	Tablet
Antiviral: Combination	Emtricitabine / Tenofovir	Truvada	Human Immunodeficiency Virus / Acquired Immune Deficiency Syndrome	Tablet

Drug Class(es)	Generic Name(s)**	Brand Name(s)**	Indication(s)	Available Dose Form(s)
Antiviral: Combination	Lamivudine / Zidovudine	Combivir	Human Immunodeficiency Virus / Acquired Immune Deficiency Syndrome	Tablet
Antiviral: Fusion Inhibitor	Enfuvirtide	Fuzeon	Human Immunodeficiency Virus / Acquired Immune Deficiency Syndrome	Powder for Injection
Antiviral: Integrase Inhibitor	Raltegravir	Isentress	Human Immunodeficiency Virus / Acquired Immune Deficiency Syndrome	Tablet
Antiviral: Neuraminidase Inhibitor	Oseltamivir	Tamiflu	Influenza	Capsule, Liquid
Antiviral: Neuraminidase Inhibitor	Zanamivir	Relenza	Influenza	Powder for Inhalation
Antiviral: Nonnucleoside Reverse Transcriptase Inhibitor	Abacavir	Ziagen	Human Immunodeficiency Virus / Acquired Immune Deficiency Syndrome	Solution, Tablet
Antiviral: Nonnucleoside Reverse Transcriptase Inhibitor	Delavirdine	Rescriptor	Human Immunodeficiency Virus / Acquired Immune Deficiency Syndrome	Tablet
Antiviral: Nonnucleoside Reverse Transcriptase Inhibitor	Didanosine	Videx	Human Immunodeficiency Virus / Acquired Immune Deficiency Syndrome	Solution, Tablet
Antiviral: Nonnucleoside Reverse Transcriptase Inhibitor	Efavirenz	Sustiva	Human Immunodeficiency Virus / Acquired Immune Deficiency Syndrome	Capsule, Tablet

Table 1 *cont.*
Drugs Used to Treat Immune System Disorders

Drug Class(es)	Generic Name(s)**	Brand Name(s)**	Indication(s)	Available Dose Form(s)
Antiviral: Nonnucleoside Reverse Transcriptase Inhibitor	Emtricitabine	Emtriva	Human Immunodeficiency Virus / Acquired Immune Deficiency Syndrome	Capsule
Antiviral: Nonnucleoside Reverse Transcriptase Inhibitor	Etravirine	Intelence	Human Immunodeficiency Virus / Acquired Immune Deficiency Syndrome	Tablet
Antiviral: Nonnucleoside Reverse Transcriptase Inhibitor	Lamivudine	Epivir	Human Immunodeficiency Virus / Acquired Immune Deficiency Syndrome	Solution, Tablet
Antiviral: Nonnucleoside Reverse Transcriptase Inhibitor	Neviraprine	Viramune	Human Immunodeficiency Virus / Acquired Immune Deficiency Syndrome	Suspension, Tablet
Antiviral: Nonnucleoside Reverse Transcriptase Inhibitor	Stavudine	Zerit	Human Immunodeficiency Virus / Acquired Immune Deficiency Syndrome	Capsule, Solution
Antiviral: Nonnucleoside Reverse Transcriptase Inhibitor	Telbivudine	Tyzeka	Hepatitis B Infection	Solution, Tablet
Antiviral: Nonnucleoside Reverse Transcriptase Inhibitor	Tenofovir	Viread	Human Immunodeficiency Virus / Acquired Immune Deficiency Syndrome	Tablet
Antiviral: Nonnucleoside Reverse Transcriptase Inhibitor	Zidovudine	Retrovir	Human Immunodeficiency Virus / Acquired Immune Deficiency Syndrome	Capsule, Injectable, Solution, Tablet

Drug Class(es)	Generic Name(s)**	Brand Name(s)**	Indication(s)	Available Dose Form(s)
Antiviral: Protease Inhibitor	Atazanavir	Reyataz	Human Immunodeficiency Virus / Acquired Immune Deficiency Syndrome	Capsule
Antiviral: Protease Inhibitor	Darunavir	Prezista	Human Immunodeficiency Virus / Acquired Immune Deficiency Syndrome	Tablet
Antiviral: Protease Inhibitor	Fosamprenavir	Lexiva	Human Immunodeficiency Virus / Acquired Immune Deficiency Syndrome	Suspension, Tablet
Antiviral: Protease Inhibitor	Indinavir	Crixivan	Human Immunodeficiency Virus / Acquired Immune Deficiency Syndrome	Capsule
Antiviral: Protease Inhibitor	Lopinavir / Ritonavir	Kaletra	Human Immunodeficiency Virus / Acquired Immune Deficiency Syndrome	Solution, Tablet
Antiviral: Protease Inhibitor	Nelfinavir	Viracept	Human Immunodeficiency Virus / Acquired Immune Deficiency Syndrome	Powder, Tablet
Antiviral: Protease Inhibitor	Ritonavir	Norvir	Human Immunodeficiency Virus / Acquired Immune Deficiency Syndrome	Capsule, Solution
Antiviral: Protease Inhibitor	Saquinavir	Invirase	Human Immunodeficiency Virus / Acquired Immune Deficiency Syndrome	Capsule, Tablet

Table 1 *cont.*
Drugs Used to Treat Immune System Disorders

Drug Class(es)	Generic Name(s)**	Brand Name(s)**	Indication(s)	Available Dose Form(s)
Antiviral: Protease Inhibitor	Tipranavir	Aptivus	Human Immunodeficiency Virus / Acquired Immune Deficiency Syndrome	Capsule, Solution
Corticosteroid	Methylprednisolone	Depo-Medrol, Medrol, Medrol Dosepak, Solu-Medrol	Acute Asthma Exacerbation, Gout, Osteoarthritis, Rheumatoid Arthritis, Severe Asthma, Skin Inflammation	Capsule, Solution
Corticosteroid	Prednisolone	Prelone	Acute Asthma Exacerbation, Severe Allergic Reaction, Severe Asthma	Liquid, Syrup, Tablet
Corticosteroid	Prednisone	Deltasone, Stelapred	Acute Asthma Exacerbation, Gout, Rheumatoid Arthritis, Severe Allergic Reaction, Severe Asthma	Liquid, Tablet
Hormone	Levothyroxine	Levothroid, Levoxyl, Synthroid, Tirosint, Unithroid	Hypothyroidism	Injectable, Tablet
Immunodilator	Interferon Alfa-2b	Intron-A	Chronic Hepatitis B, Chronic Hepatitis C, Human Immunodeficiency Virus-Related Kaposi's Sarcoma	Injectable
Immunodilator	Peginterferon Alfa-2a	Pegasys	Hepatitis B Infection, Hepatitis C Infection	Injectable
Pain Reliever, Topical Irritant	Capsaicin	Capzasin, Capzasin-HP, Zostrix	Osteoarthritis	Cream, Gel, Liquid

**All rights to all brand names and trademarks are held by their respective owners. There may be additional brand names for some of the products listed.

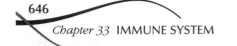

Conclusion

The immune system is an important defense mechanism for the body; however, when the immune system malfunctions, patients are at risk for a number of infections. Drugs used to treat HIV, drugs used to prevent transplanted organ rejection and the antibiotics to treat the opportunistic infections of concern in these patients may be seen quite rarely. Therefore, it is imperative that a pharmacy technician remain updated and knowledgeable about the medications used to treat these conditions for such an occasion as a patient presenting to a pharmacy in need of one or more of these special drugs.

Bibliography

- National Institute of Allergy and Infectious Diseases, www.niaid.nih.gov/topics/immuneSystem/Pages/default.aspx, Aug. 16, 2010.
- National Institute of Allergy and Infectious Diseases, www.niaid.nih.gov/topics/HIVAIDS/Understanding/Biology/pages/hivreplicationcycle.aspx, Aug. 16, 2010.
- Panel on Antiretroviral Guidelines for Adults and Adolescents, Guidelines for the use of antiretroviral agents in HIV 1 infected adults and adolescents, Department of Health and Human Services, Dec. 1, 2009, pp. 1-161, available at www.aidsinfo.nih.gov/ContentFiles/AdultandAdolescentGL.pdf, Aug. 16, 2010.
- Centers for Disease Control and Prevention, Updated U.S. Public Health Service guidelines for the management of occupational exposures to HIV and recommendations for Postexposure Prophylaxis, MMWR 2005, Vol. 54 (No. RR-9), pp. 1-24.
- Centers for Disease Control and Prevention, Guidelines for Prevention and Treatment of Opportunistic Infections in HIV-Infected Adults and Adolescents, MMWR 2009, Vol. 58 (RR-4), pp. 1-216.
- United Network for Organ Sharing, www.unos.org, Aug. 16, 2010.

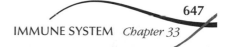

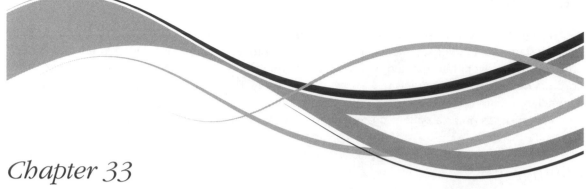

REVIEW QUESTIONS

1.   What is the primary function of the immune system?
     a.   To induce a febrile response
     b.   To protect the body from pathogens (foreign substances)
     c.   To regulate the hormones in the body
     d.   To control the heart rate

2.   Which of the following is a part of the adaptive immunity system?
     a.   Lymphocytes
     b.   Neutrophils
     c.   Skin
     d.   Mucous membranes

3.   Which of the following is a part of the humoral immunity system?
     a.   Neutrophils
     b.   Immune Globulin
     c.   Eosinophils
     d.   Skin

4.   Which of the following cells would be the best example of a "phagocyte?"
     a.   Eosinophils
     b.   Basophils
     c.   Neutrophils
     d.   Punxsutawneyphil

5.   Which of the following combination of antiretrovirals is in Atripla®?
     a.   Zidovudine and lamivudine
     b.   Zidovudine, lamivudine and abacavir
     c.   Tenofovir and emtricitabine
     d.   Tenofovir, emtricitabine and efavirenz

6. Which of the following agents is an example of a protease inhibitor?
   a. Abacavir
   b. Combivir
   c. Atazanavir
   d. Retrovir

7. Which of the following agents is the most likely to result in the adverse effect of lipodystrophy?
   a. Tenofovir
   b. Efavirenz
   c. Raltegravir
   d. Ritonavir

8. Which of the following drugs will be most effective for the prophylaxis of PCP?
   a. Azithromycin
   b. Trimethoprim/Sulfamethoxazole
   c. Rifabutin
   d. Ganciclovir

9. Which of the following is the most likely adverse effect associated with inhaled pentamidine?
   a. Orange-brown body fluid discoloration
   b. GI upset
   c. Bronchospasm
   d. Liver toxicity

10. Which of the following infections is most troubling in patients receiving immunosuppressant drugs following organ transplantation?
    a. CMV
    b. RSV
    c. VZV
    d. HIV

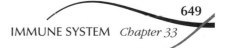

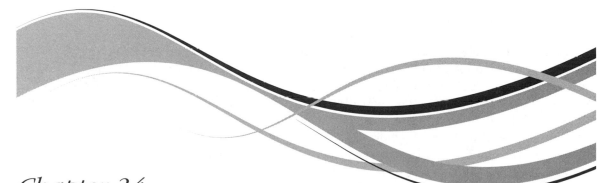

Chapter 34

MUSCULOSKELETAL SYSTEM

By   Claire T. Lee, Pharm.D.

Learning Objectives

This chapter seeks to prepare a pharmacy technician to:

■ describe the major components of the musculoskeletal system.

■ explain how the various components of the musculoskeletal system work together to allow movement.

■ understand the differences between the various types of bones, joints and muscles.

■ explain factors that may contribute to the development of osteoporosis.

■ list treatment options for osteoporosis.

■ understand the most common cause of osteomalacia

■ name the most common cause of osteoarthritis.

■ list and describe the various treatments available for osteoarthritis.

■ differentiate rheumatoid arthritis from osteoarthritis.

■ list common side effects associated with corticosteroid use.

■ explain the various treatment options used for gout.

■ describe the options available for the treatment of fibromyalgia.

Introduction

The **musculoskeletal system** is a highly complex structure composed of bones, ligaments, tendons, joints and muscles. While each of these structures is separate and distinct, they must work together in a controlled way to enable the body to move and perform tasks. Disorders of the musculoskeletal system are not uncommon. These disorders can have a significant impact on a person's quality of life and ability to perform activities of daily living.

This chapter will discuss the individual parts of the musculoskeletal system. It will also provide an overview of common conditions that affect this system and common treatments used for the management of these disorders.

Bones

The bones of the body serve a variety of functions. They provide support and protection for the body's more delicate internal structures. Bones also work with muscles and other soft tissues to enable the body to move. The bones additionally serve as production sites for blood cells and storage sites for mineral and energy reserves.[1]

The composition of any given bone in the human body is not constant. **Bone metabolism** is a process that occurs continuously and at variable rates in bones throughout the body. This process, often referred to as **bone remodeling**, depends on the balanced interplay of two types of bone cells: osteoblasts and osteoclasts. **Osteoblasts** are responsible for the production of new bone through the maturation of **osteocytes**, or mature bone cells. **Osteoclasts**, on the other hand, cause bone resorption. **Bone resorption** results in the removal of bone matrix or the breakdown of bone. For bone remodeling to occur, at the appropriate rate for maintenance of bone health, osteoblast and osteoclast activity must remain balanced.[1]

The process of bone remodeling is highly susceptible to the effects of hormones and vitamins. Growth hormone, thyroid hormone, calcitonin and parathyroid hormone are just some of the hormones that can affect the rate of bone resorption. The activity of some of these hormones depends on the levels of calcium and phosphorus in the blood. Calcium and phosphorous are the main mineral components of bone and their presence, or absence, in the blood can cause hormones to react. Reaction of these hormones results in the return of calcium and phosphorus levels to normal in most cases. Vitamins A, C and D are a few of the vitamins that can have an effect on bone remodeling. Constant dietary intake of vitamins is necessary for proper bone health.[1]

Bones are classified according to shape and size. **Long bones**, as their name implies, are greater in length than width. Examples of long bones include bones in the thigh, forearm and fingers. **Short bones** are approximately as long as they are wide. The small bones in the wrist and feet are examples of short bones. The kneecap is another example. **Flat bones** are another type of bone and include the sternum (breastbone) and the bones that form the roof of the skull. The final classification is **irregular bones** that have complex shapes. The bones that make up the spinal column fit into this category.[1] See Figure 1 for a visual overview of the human skeletal structure.

Figure 1
Human Skeleton

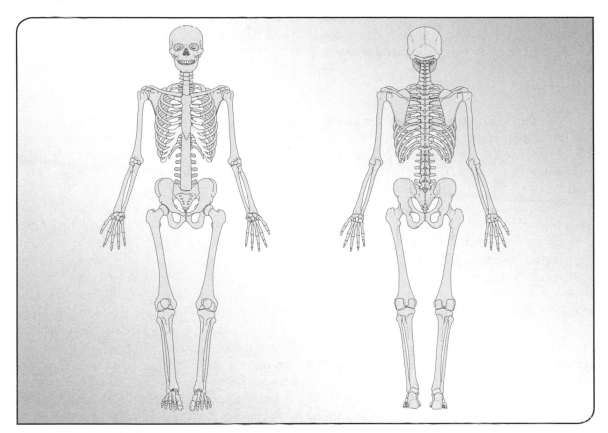

Joints

Joints, which are also referred to as articulations, are places in the body where two bones come together. Joints allow variable degrees of freedom of movement for the bones to which they attach. For example, the shoulder is a freely moving joint, while the joints in the skull are stationary and allow little to no movement at all.[1] Joints are classified based on the type of connective tissue that binds the surfaces of the bones. The three types of joints are: fibrous joints, cartilaginous joints and synovial joints.[1] **Fibrous joints** attach bones via dense regular connective tissue and are immovable or only slightly movable. Examples of fibrous joints include those that connect the skull bones to one another and those that join the ulna and radius together in the forearm.[1] **Cartilaginous joints** connect bones together via cartilage. **Cartilage** is a type of supporting connective tissue that adds stability to joints. An example is the cartilage that joins the ribs to the sternum in the chest. While these joints are immovable, not all cartilaginous joints function this way. An example of a slightly movable cartilaginous joint is the cartilage between the vertebra in the spine.[1] The final type of joint is the **synovial joint**. This joint classification is unique in that these joints are freely movable and the bones are separated by a joint cavity or space. Examples of synovial joints include the shoulder, knee, elbow and hip.[1]

Ligaments and Tendons

Both ligaments and tendons are composed of dense, regular, connective tissue. This connective tissue is mostly made up of collagen fibers. **Collagen** is a protein that is strong, flexible and resistant to stretching. Ligaments and tendons help to strengthen and stabilize joints in the body. **Ligaments** connect bones to one another, while **tendons** are responsible for binding muscle to bone.[1]

Muscles

The muscle tissues in the human body are unique and are responsible for a variety of activities that the body performs on a daily basis. Some of these activities are voluntary, such as waving to a friend, while others occur constantly without any conscious effort. Examples of involuntary muscle movements include the constriction of the pupil when the eye is exposed to light or the digestion of food.[1]

Three different classifications of muscles exist in the human body. Since each of these muscle types performs a unique, but wide, range of tasks, muscles are able to carry out a wide variety of functions. These muscle types include: skeletal muscle, cardiac muscle and smooth muscle.[1]

Skeletal muscle, along with the other components of the musculoskeletal system, facilitates movement. Skeletal muscle also helps to keep the body in an erect position by maintaining posture. Temperature regulation, storage and movement of materials, and support are other important functions of the skeletal muscles. Skeletal muscles require large amounts of energy to do their job. The fibers of skeletal muscle are **striated**, meaning that they run parallel, or next to, one another. Movements of the skeletal muscles in the human body are voluntary and require input from the voluntary nervous system in order to function.[1] **Cardiac muscle** is striated (similar to skeletal muscle); however, unlike skeletal muscle, cardiac muscle has the ability to generate nerve impulses without nervous system stimulation. This means that cardiac muscle fibers are autorhythmic and do not require a signal from outside the cardiac muscle cell to contract. Although the generation of an impulse is not mediated by the nervous system, the rate of the contraction of cardiac muscle, or the heart beat, is controlled by the nervous system.[1] **Smooth muscle** is under involuntary control. Contraction of smooth muscle is slow, sustained for an extended period of time and resistant to fatigue. Energy requirements for smooth muscle fibers are much less than that for skeletal and cardiac muscles. An example of something that occurs as a result of smooth muscle contraction is the movement of food and waste products through the gastrointestinal tract.[1] See Figure 2 below for a visual overview of the human muscular structure.

Figure 2
Human Muscular Structure

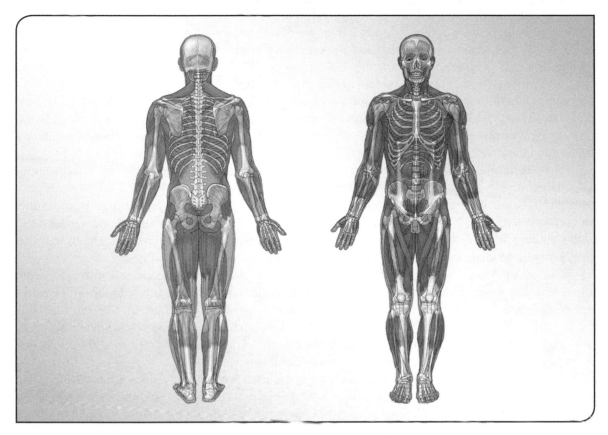

Diseases of the Musculoskeletal System

Musculoskeletal system diseases, disorders and syndromes are numerous. Patients with dysfunction of their musculoskeletal system experience a reduced ability to move around, symptoms that may affect their ability to think clearly and, very often, extreme pain. The conditions to be discussed in this chapter include osteoporosis, osteomalacia, osteoarthritis, rheumatoid arthritis, gout and fibromyalgia. See Table 1 following an overview of each of these conditions for a list of the most common medications used to treat musculoskeletal disorders.

Osteoporosis

Osteoporosis is the most common bone disease in humans. The National Osteoporosis Foundation estimates that 10 million Americans currently have osteoporosis and that this number could double or even triple by the year 2040. Falls and fractures associated with osteoporosis can cause significant morbidity and mortality problems for affected individuals.[2] Osteoporosis develops when bone removal by osteoclasts occurs at a faster rate than bone formation by osteoblasts. This imbalance can be partially attributed to menopause in women and aging in older patients of either gender. Osteoporosis can also develop if bone mineralization does not occur appropriately. In this case, osteoblast and osteoclast activity are balanced but, due to a vitamin or mineral deficiency, the bones that are formed are weak.[2]

Many factors have been associated with an increased risk of osteoporosis-related fractures. Lifestyle factors, such as low calcium intake or excessive smoking and alcohol intake, can contribute to the risk for the development of osteoporosis. Genetic factors, endocrine disorders, gastrointestinal disorders, several other conditions and certain forms of medication therapy can also contribute to osteoporosis development.[2] Because osteoporosis often results from easily identifiable risk factors, the National Osteoporosis Foundation recommends routine screening for high-risk individuals, including all women age 65 years and older and all men ages 70 years and older. Screening assessments can help identify individuals who are eligible for prevention therapy and those who may already be experiencing symptoms in need of treatment.[2]

Current Food and Drug Administration (FDA)-approved pharmacologic options for osteoporosis prevention and/or treatment include: bisphosphonates, calcitonin, estrogens and/or hormone therapy, parathyroid hormone and estrogen agonist/antagonist therapy. A variety of conditions can lead to the development of osteoporosis. For this reason, a full patient assessment is necessary before beginning medication therapy for osteoporosis.[2]

The bisphosphonates are indicated for the prevention and treatment of post-menopausal osteoporosis. They work by inhibiting bone resorption by osteoclasts. By blocking this bone removal process, osteoclasts indirectly increase bone mass. Medications in the bisphosphonate drug class include: alendronate (Fosamax®, Fosamax® Plus D), ibandronate (Boniva®), risendronate (Actonel®, Actonel® with Calcium) and zoledronic acid (Reclast®). Bisphosphonates are generally well-tolerated; but, side effects can include: gastrointestinal upset, inflammation of the esophagus and gastric ulcer.[2]

Calcitonin (Miacalcin®, Fortical®) is indicated for the treatment of osteoporosis in women who are at least five years post-menopausal. Calcitonin is a hormone that is naturally found in the body. It is responsible for directly inhibiting bone resorption by osteoclasts. Calcitonin, administered as a medication, acts through the same mechanism. Calcitonin can be administered via an intranasal spray or given by subcutaneous injection. Side effects are rare; but, some patients experience **rhinitis** (runny nose) or **epistaxis** (nose bleed) when using the intranasal spray.[3,4]

Estrogens and/or hormonal therapy are sometimes used for the prevention of the development of osteoporosis; however, some of these therapies have been associated with increased serious adverse effects. Therefore, use is limited to low doses for short periods of time. Medications in this class include: Climara®, Estrace®, Estraderm®, Estratab®, Ogen®, Ortho-Est®, Premarin®, Vivelle®, Activella®, Femhrt®, Premphase® and Prempro®.[2]

Raloxifene (Evista®) is an estrogen agonist/antagonist indicated for the prevention and treatment of osteoporosis in post-menopausal women. Raloxifene works in the bone to prevent bone resorption and in the breast to reduce the risk of invasive breast cancer. Side effects of raloxifene include hot flashes and a slightly increased risk of deep vein thrombosis.[2]

Teriparatide (Forteo®) is a recombinant form of parathyroid hormone indicated for the treatment of osteoporosis in several high-risk patient populations. Parathyroid hormone, like calcitonin, is naturally found in the body. Parathyroid hormone stimulates osteoblast function, which is how teriparatide works to increase bone mass. Teriparatide is given via subcutaneous injection and has been associated with leg cramps and dizziness.[2,4]

In addition to prescription-only medications indicated for the prevention and treatment of osteoporosis, calcium and vitamin D can be obtained over-the-counter and taken on a daily basis to improve bone health. The National Osteoporosis Foundation recommends at least 1,200 mg of calcium each day and 800-1,000 IU of vitamin D each day for individuals age 50 years and older.[2]

Osteomalacia

Osteomalacia, which is another bone disorder, is relatively rare in the United States. Osteomalacia is characterized by inadequate and delayed mineralization of mature bone that most commonly results from severe vitamin D deficiency.[5] Many foods in the United States are fortified with vitamin D, so deficiency due to insufficient dietary intake is rare. Secondary causes of vitamin D deficiency are more common and include disorders of the small bowel, liver, gall bladder and pancreas.[5] Vitamin D deficiency indirectly causes osteomalacia. Vitamin D normally regulates and enhances the absorption of calcium from the intestine. When vitamin D levels are low, calcium is not absorbed appropriately and calcium is unable to work in concert with phosphate to properly mineralize the bones. This results in abnormalities in bone density.[5] Unlike osteoporosis, which is often referred to as a "silent disease" because of its lack of obvious symptoms, osteomalacia can cause varying degrees of skeletal pain and tenderness. Pain may initially manifest in the lower back, but it could eventually spread to the feet, ribs, spine and other sites.[5] Since vitamin D deficiency is the most common cause of osteomalacia, correction of the deficiency is the most common treatment. High doses of vitamin D are administered in oral drops or capsules of ergocalciferol (Calciferol®, Drisdol®).[3]

Arthritis

Arthritis is the term commonly used to describe a group of diseases collectively referred to as inflammatory joint diseases. Arthritis can be categorized as inflammatory or non-inflammatory and infectious or noninfectious. The two most common types of arthritis are osteoarthritis and rheumatoid arthritis, which are classified as inflammatory and noninfectious.[5]

Osteoarthritis

Osteoarthritis is most commonly found in load-bearing synovial joints. It typically occurs as a result of trauma, excessive joint loading or instability of the joint that results in excessive joint loading. The most common cause of osteoarthritis is obesity. The excessive weight put on the joint sets into motion a series of events that result in the breakdown of cartilage in synovial joints. This breakdown causes increased friction in the joint, further destruction of articular cartilage, bone changes, joint space narrowing and eventually results in inflamed, painful and deformed joints.[6] Osteoarthritis typically does not occur until after 50 years of age, and the disease becomes progressively worse with advancing age. The pain associated with osteoarthritis can be significant and can occur with motion or at rest.[6]

Treatment of osteoarthritis is tailored specifically to each individual patient based on the number of joints affected by the disease, the patient's perceived level of pain and disability, other medical conditions of the patient and the medications the patient is taking. The first treatment option for osteoarthritis is typically a nonmedication therapy. For example, since obesity is the most common cause of osteoarthritis and also a major predictor of disease progression, diet modification is recommended in order to encourage weight loss. Physical therapy may also be an option for certain patients.[6] Medication therapy for osteoarthritis is aimed at relieving pain associated with the disease. It is important to remember that nonmedication therapies must be continued even after medication therapy is initiated.[6] The first-line therapy for osteoarthritis pain is acetaminophen (Tylenol®). Acetaminophen works by inhibiting the formation of prostaglandins that are responsible for the pain sensations felt in the inflamed joint. Side effects of acetaminophen include liver toxicity that can occur if more than the recommended amount of acetaminophen is taken.[6] If acetaminophen does not sufficiently reduce the pain associated with a patient's osteoarthritis, then the patient may try nonsteroidal anti-inflammatory drugs (NSAIDs). NSAIDs work by inhibiting prostaglandin formation and act to reduce pain at lower doses and reduce inflammation at higher doses. NSAIDs available to treat osteoarthritis include ibuprofen (Motrin®, Advil®), aspirin (Bayer®, Ecotrin®), naproxen (Aleve®, Anaprox®, Naprosyn®), sulindac (Clinoril®), diclofenac (Voltaren®, Pennsaid®), indomethacin (Indocin®), meloxicam (Mobic®), piroxicam (Feldene®) and celecoxib (Celebrex®). NSAIDs can cause gastrointestinal upset, fluid retention (bloating) and tinnitus (ringing in the ears).[4,6]

Topical therapies may be used in combination with oral acetaminophen, or NSAIDs, in order to improve pain control. Capsaicin cream and topical diclofenac (Pennsaid®, Voltaren® Gel) are two topical therapies that decrease inflammation at the site of application. Capsaicin may cause local side effects including stinging, redness and burning.[6] There are a variety of other agents available for patients who do not experience sufficient pain relief with the use of acetaminophen, NSAIDs or topical therapies. Options include glucosamine and chondroitin, corticosteroid injections (Aristospan®, Depo-Medrol®), hyalurate injections (Hyalgan®, Supartz®, Synvisc®, Orthovisc®), opioid analgesics (e.g., Oxycontin®, OxyIR®), tramadol (Ultram®) and a variety of novel new medications that are being investigated. The most important thing to remember is that each patient will experience different levels of pain relief with each therapy, so medication choice is made based on patient specific factors and the patient's response to therapy.[4,6]

Rheumatoid Arthritis

The second type of arthritis, rheumatoid arthritis, is a **systemic autoimmune disorder**. This means that the body's immune system cannot differentiate self from nonself tissues. The immune system, therefore, attacks synovial tissue and other connective tissues in the joint space. The inflammation caused by this attack of the immune system is variable. Rheumatoid arthritis commonly manifests symmetrically. For example, if the right knee were affected by rheumatoid arthritis, it is highly likely that the left knee would also be affected.[7] **Rheumatoid arthritis** differs significantly from osteoarthritis in that it is a **systemic disease**. When a disease is systemic, it affects the body as a whole. The skin, lungs, eyes, heart and lymph nodes are all examples of other body parts or systems that can be affected by rheumatoid arthritis. Because rheumatoid arthritis has the potential to impact so many body systems, the symptoms are not confined to pain. Patients with rheumatoid arthritis can also experience fatigue, weakness, low-grade fever, loss of appetite, muscle pain, etc. Joint deformity is also commonly seen late in the disease's progression.[7] Similarly to osteoarthritis, rheumatoid arthritis patients can benefit significantly from non-medication therapy. Rest, in moderation, can help alleviate pain and stress on joints; however, excessive rest can lead to decreases in range of motion and eventual muscle wasting. Weight reduction and physical therapy are other non-medication therapy options.[7]

The medications available to treat rheumatoid arthritis include: NSAIDs, corticosteroids, **disease-modifying anti-rheumatic drugs (DMARDs)**, and biologic response modifiers.[7] NSAIDs must not be used alone, but rather in combination therapy with DMARDs or biologic response modifiers. NSAIDs do not slow disease progression. Corticosteroids are used in rheumatoid arthritis patients because they interfere with the inflammatory and autoimmune processes. Long-term and/or high dose corticosteroid use is not recommended due to the potential for adverse effects. These adverse effects include, but are not limited to, increased blood pressure, impaired wound healing, hormonal imbalances, increased blood sugar, increased risk of stomach ulcer formation and increased risk of infection.[4,7] DMARDs modify the clinical course of rheumatoid arthritis. This means that they slow the progression of the disease and help patients gain remission status leading to significant improvements in the patient's quality of life. DMARDs must be initiated within three months of disease diagnosis. Medications in this class include: methotrexate (Rheumatrex®, Trexall®), hydroxychloroquine (Plaquenil®), sulfasalazine (Azulfidine®), leflunomide (Arava®), azathioprine (Azasan®, Imuran®), D-penicillamine (Cuprimine®, Depen®), gold sodium thiomalate (Myochrysine®), minocycline (Minocin®), cyclosporine (Gengraf®, Neoral®, Sandimmune®) and cyclophosphamide. Side effects include liver dysfunction, kidney dysfunction and decreases in blood cell formation.[4,7]

Biological response modifiers include: etanercept (Enbrel®), infliximab (Remicade®), adalimumab (Humira®), anakinra (Kineret®), abatacept (Orencia®) and rituximab (Rituxin®). These agents block or interfere with various steps of the inflammatory process. Because biological response modifiers have disease modifying activity, these medications are sometimes included in the DMARDs category. They are sometimes used when other DMARDs fail to achieve the desired effects but are significantly more expensive than other medications used to treat rheumatoid arthritis. Side effects associated with biologic response modifiers include increased risk of tuberculosis infection, allergic reactions and cardiac problems.[4,7]

Gout

Gout is another disease that affects the joints of the body. For this reason, it is commonly referred to as "gouty arthritis." Gout typically only affects one joint at a time (most frequently the great, or big, toe). Other joints commonly affected by gout include the insteps of the feet, the ankles, heels, knees, wrists, fingers and elbows. Gout is a disease characterized by periods of acute "gout attacks" that can be extremely painful. These attacks typically last one week.[8]

Although patients with gout often have similar symptoms to those with osteoarthritis or rheumatoid arthritis, the causes and treatments of these diseases are very different. The inflammation and pain associated with gout occurs through a separate process than that associated with osteoarthritis and rheumatoid arthritis. Gout is most commonly caused by an elevation of serum urate (uric acid). Serum urate is a substance naturally found in the body; however, increased production of urate or decreased excretion from the body can result in elevated concentrations in the serum. When the concentration of urate in the serum exceeds a certain level, urate crystals form and deposit in the joints. This sets the inflammatory process into motion.[8]

Gout attacks can be treated with NSAIDs, colchicine (Colocrys®), corticosteroids (Sterapred®, Medrol®) and various forms of nonmedication therapy.[4,8] NSAIDs are first choice medications for the treatment of gout. Therapy begins as soon as possible. Ideally, therapy begins immediately at the onset of an attack. Indomethacin (Indocin®) is the most commonly used NSAID for gout attacks; but, naproxen (Aleve®, Anaprox®, Naprosyn®), sulindac (Clinoril®), ibuprofen (Advil®, Motrin®) and piroxicam (Feldene®) are all also routinely used. Side effects, as stated above, include primarily gastrointestinal upset.[8]

Colchicine is an extremely effective medication used for the treatment of gout attacks. It works by interfering with the inflammatory process and is most effective when initiated within 24 hours of the onset of a gout attack. Although colchicine is an extremely effective treatment option, the high rate of side effects limits its use. Side effects include gastrointestinal problems in up to 80 percent of patients.[8] Corticosteroids can also be used in gout attacks; however, their use is limited by side effects that include increased blood sugar, increased risk of osteoporosis and muscle weakness.[8]

In addition to medications, several nonmedication therapies can be used to improve the symptoms of gout attacks. These include dietary reduction of saturated fat intake, weight loss, restriction of alcohol consumption and joint exercises.[8]

Fibromyalgia

Fibromyalgia is a disease characterized by widespread generalized musculoskeletal pain. Patients with fibromyalgia also commonly experience sleep disturbances, headache, morning stiffness, anxiety, memory problems and episodes of lightheadedness.[9] The diagnosis of fibromyalgia is difficult because its symptoms are nonspecific and often overlap with other diseases; however, patients with fibromyalgia experience a painful response at some of 18 specific pressure points covering the body. Painful response at 11 of the 18 sites indicates that the patient most likely has fibromyalgia.[9]

Three medications are currently approved by the Food and Drug Administration (FDA) for the treatment of fibromyalgia: pregabalin (Lyrica®), duloxetine (Cymbalta®) and milnacipran (Savella®). Anti-depressants are also commonly used to offset the symptoms of fibromyalgia.[10]

Pregabalin was the first medication approved by FDA for the treatment of fibromyalgia. It has some pain relieving activity and works by blocking nervous system stimulation. Side effects include swelling of the arms and legs, dizziness, headache, blurred vision and weight gain.[10]

Anti-depressants are commonly used in fibromyalgia treatment. Duloxetine and milnacipran are currently the only two antidepressants with FDA approval for the treatment of fibromyalgia. They work by improving pain, sleep quality and general quality of life. Other antidepressants commonly used for the treatment of fibromyalgia include amitriptyline (Elavil®) and fluoxetine (Prozac®).[9,10]

Nonmedication therapy is also important in the treatment of fibromyalgia. Because fibromyalgia is a disease that frequently occurs in patients who also suffer from anxiety and/or depression, cognitive behavioral strategies (such as counseling) are common methods of therapy. Exercise is also an option, and patient education is crucial.[9]

Table 1
Medications Used to Treat Musculoskeletal Disorders

Drug Class(es)	Generic Name(s)**	Brand Name(s)**	Indication(s)	Available Dose Form(s)
Analgesic	Acetaminophen	Tylenol	Osteoarthritis	Capsule, Chewable Tablet, Drops, Gel Cap, Gel Tab, Liquid, Suppository, Tablet
Anticonvulsant	Pregabalin	Lyrica	Fibromyalgia	Capsule
Antidepressant	Amitriptyline	Elavil	Fibromyalgia	Tablet
Antidepressant	Duloxetine	Cymbalta	Fibromyalgia	Capsule
Antidepressant	Fluoxetine	Prozac, Sarafem	Fibromyalgia	Capsule, Tablet
Antidepressant	Milnacipran	Savella	Fibromyalgia	Tablet
Anti-Inflammatory	Colchicine	Colcrys	Gout	Tablet
Anti-Rheumatic	Hyaluronate Injection	Hyalgan, Orthovisc, Supartz, Synvisc	Osteoarthritis	Injection
Biologic Response Modifier	Abatacept	Orencia	Rheumatoid Arthritis	Injection
Biologic Response Modifier	Adalimumab	Humira	Rheumatoid Arthritis	Injection
Biologic Response Modifier	Anakinra	Kineret	Rheumatoid Arthritis	Injection
Biologic Response Modifier	Etanercept	Enbrel	Rheumatoid Arthritis	Injection
Biologic Response Modifier	Infliximab	Remicade	Rheumatoid Arthritis	Injection
Biologic Response Modifier	Rituximab	Rituxan	Rheumatoid Arthritis	Injection
Bisphosphonate	Alendronate	Fosamax, Fosamax Plus D	Osteoporosis	Liquid, Tablet
Bisphosphonate	Ibandronate	Boniva	Osteoporosis	Injection, Tablet
Bisphosphonate	Risedronate	Actonel	Osteoporosis	Tablet
Bisphosphonate	Zoledronic Acid	Reclast	Osteoporosis	Infusion
Corticosteroid	Corticotrophin	H.P. Acthar	Gout	Injection
Corticosteroid	Triamcinolone Acetonide	Kenalog	Gout	Cream, Injection, Ointment

Drug Class(es)	Generic Name(s)**	Brand Name(s)**	Indication(s)	Available Dose Form(s)
Corticosteroid	Triamcinolone Hexacetonide	Aristospan	Osteoarthritis	Injection
Corticosteroid	Methylprednisol-one	Medrol, Medrol Dosepak	Gout, Rheumatoid Arthritis	Oral
Corticosteroid	Methylprednisol-one Acetate	Depo-Medrol	Osteoarthritis	Injection
Corticosteroid	Prednisone	Deltasone, Sterapred	Gout, Rheumatoid Arthritis	Oral
DMARD	Azathioprine	Azasan, Imuran	Rheumatoid Arthritis	Injection, Tablet
DMARD	Cyclophosphamide	Not Available	Rheumatoid Arthritis	Injectable, Tablet
DMARD	Cyclosporine	Gengraf, Neoral, Sandimmune	Rheumatoid Arthritis	Capsule, Liquid
DMARD	D-penicillamine	Cuprimine, Depen	Rheumatoid Arthritis	Capsule, Tablet
DMARD	Gold Sodium Thiomalate	Myochrysine	Rheumatoid Arthritis	Injection
DMARD	Hydroxychloro-quine	Plaquenil	Rheumatoid Arthritis	Tablet
DMARD	Leflunomide	Arava	Rheumatoid Arthritis	Tablet
DMARD	Methotrexate	Rheumatrex, Trexall	Rheumatoid Arthritis	Tablet
DMARD	Minocycline	Minocin	Rheumatoid Arthritis	Capsule, Tablet
DMARD	Sulfasalazine	Azulfidine	Rheumatoid Arthritis	Tablet
Estrogen Agonist / Antagonist	Raloxifene	Evista	Osteoporosis	Tablet
Hormone	Calcitonin	Fortical, Miacalcin	Osteoporosis	Injection, Intranasal Solution
Hormone	Estradiol, Norethindrone	Activella	Osteoporosis	Tablet
Hormone	Estrogen	Climara, Estrace, Estraderm, Estratab, Ogen, Ortho-Est, Premarin, Vivelle	Osteoporosis	Patch, Tablet, Vaginal Cream

Table 1 *cont.*
Medications Used to Treat Musculoskeletal Disorders

Drug Class(es)	Generic Name(s)**	Brand Name(s)**	Indication(s)	Available Dose Form(s)
Hormone	Estrogens / Medroxy-progesterone	Premphase, Prempro	Osteoporosis	Tablet
Hormone	Ethinyl Estradiol, Norethindrone	Femhrt	Osteoporosis	Tablet
Natural Product	Capsaicin	Capzasin, Capzasin-HP, Zostrix	Osteoarthritis	Cream, Gel, Liquid
Natural Product	Glucosamine / Chondroitin	Not Available	Osteoarthritis	Capsule, Tablet
NSAID	Aspirin	Bayer, Ecotrin	Osteoarthritis, Rheumatoid Arthritis	Capsule, Tablet
NSAID	Celecoxib	Celebrex	Osteoarthritis, Rheumatoid Arthritis	Capsule
NSAID	Diclofenac	Flector, Pennsaid, Voltaren	Osteoarthritis, Rheumatoid Arthritis	Capsule, Gel, Patch, Solution, Tablet
NSAID	Ibuprofen	Advil, Motrin	Gout, Osteoarthritis, Rheumatoid Arthritis	Capsule, Chewable Tablet, Liquid, Tablet
NSAID	Indomethacin	Indocin	Gout, Osteoarthritis, Rheumatoid Arthritis	Capsule, Liquid
NSAID	Meloxicam	Mobic	Osteoarthritis, Rheumatoid Arthritis	Liquid, Tablet
NSAID	Naproxen	Aleve, Anaprox, Naprosyn	Gout, Osteoarthritis, Rheumatoid Arthritis	Capsule, Liquid, Tablet
NSAID	Piroxicam	Feldene	Gout, Osteoarthritis, Rheumatoid Arthritis	Capsule
NSAID	Sulindac	Clinoril	Gout, Osteoarthritis, Rheumatoid Arthritis	Tablet
Opioid Analgesic	Oxycodone	OxyContin, OxyIR	Osteoarthritis	Capsule, Tablet
Opioid Analgesic	Tramadol	Ultram	Osteoarthritis	Tablet

Drug Class(es)	Generic Name(s)**	Brand Name(s)**	Indication(s)	Available Dose Form(s)
Parathyroid Hormone Analog	Teriparatide	Forteo	Osteoporosis	Injection
Vitamin	Calcium Carbonate	Maalox, Oyst-Cal 500, Rolaids, Tums	Osteomalacia, Osteoporosis	Chewable Tablet, Tablet
Vitamin	Calcium Carbonate, Vitamin D	Caltrate, Oyst-Cal-D, Viactiv	Osteomalacia, Osteoporosis	Chewable Tablet, Tablet
Vitamin	Calcium Citrate	Cal-Citrate, Citracal	Osteomalacia, Osteoporosis	Tablet
Vitamin	Vitamin D	Not Available	Osteomalacia, Osteoporosis	Various
Vitamin D Analog	Ergocalciferol	Calciferol, Drisdol	Osteomalacia	Capsule, Drops

Conclusion

The bones, joints, ligaments, tendons and muscles of the musculoskeletal system all work together to allow the body to move. Disorders of the musculoskeletal system have the potential to have a profound impact on the quality of life of the affected individual. It is important for a pharmacy technician to understand these disorders and their treatments.

References

1. O'Loughlin, V.D., McKinley, M., Human Anatomy, New York: McGraw Hill, 2006, pp. 147-398.

2. National Osteoporosis Foundation, www.nof.org, July 14, 2010.

3. O'Connell, M.B., Vondracek, S.F., "Chapter 93, Osteoporosis and Other Metabolic Bone Diseases," Pharmacotherapy: A Pathophysiologic Approach, 7th edition, New York, NY, 2008, pp. 1483-1504.

4. Lexi-Comp, Inc., Lexi-Comp Drug Information, PDA Software.

5. McCance, K.L., Huether, S.E., Pathophysiology: The Biologic Basis for Disease in Adults and Children, 5th edition, St. Louis: Elsevier-Mosby, 2006, pp. 1471-1572.

6. Buys, L.M., Elliot, M.E., "Chapter 95, Osteoarthritis," Pharmacotherapy: A Pathophysiologic Approach, 7th edition, New York: New York, 2008, pp. 1519-1537.

7. Schuna, A.A., "Chapter 94, Rheumatoid Arthritis," Pharmacotherapy: A Pathophysiologic Approach, 7th Edition, New York: New York, 2008, pp. 1505-1517.

8. Ernst, M.E., Clark, E.C., Hawkins, D.W., "Chapter 96, Gout and Hyperuricemia," Pharmacotherapy: A Pathophysiologic Approach, 7th edition, New York: New York, 2008, pp. 1539-1550.

9. Chakrabarty, S., Zoorob, R., Fibromyalgia, *American Family Physician*, 2007, Vol. 76, No. 2, pp. 248-254.

10. U.S. Food and Drug Administration, www.fda.gov/downloads/AboutFDA/CentersOffices/CDER/UCM192786.pdf, July 13, 2010.

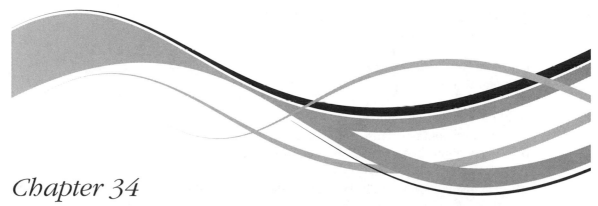

Chapter 34
REVIEW QUESTIONS

1. Which type of cell is responsible for the formation of bone?
    a. Osteocyte
    b. Osteoclast
    c. Osteoblast
    d. None of the above

2. The knee is an example of a _____.
    a. fibrous joint.
    b. synovial joint.
    c. cartilaginous joint.
    d. long joint.

3. Skeletal muscle has the ability to perform which of the following functions?
    a. Facilitate movement
    b. Regulate temperature
    c. Support the body
    d. All of the above

4. Which of the following statements is false?
    a. Collagen fibers are the major component of the connective tissue in ligaments and tendons.
    b. Ligaments and tendons help to stabilize joints.
    c. Ligaments connect bones to one another.
    d. Tendons connect bones to one another.

5. Which of the following is not recommended for the prevention and/or treatment of osteoporosis?
    a. Bisphosphonates
    b. Nonsteroidal anti-inflammatory drugs (NSAIDs)
    c. Raloxifene
    d. Calcium 1,200 mg + vitamin D 800-1,000 IU

6. What is the most common cause of osteomalacia?
   a. Vitamin D deficiency
   b. Obesity
   c. Inadequate calcium intake
   d. Vitamin C deficiency

7. Which of the following statements is false?
   a. The most common cause of osteoarthritis is obesity.
   b. Osteoarthritis becomes worse with advancing age.
   c. Osteoarthritis is a curable disease.
   d. Treatment of osteoarthritis is aimed at improving the individual patient's quality of life.

8. Which of the following is/are adverse effects associated with the use of corticosteroids?
   a. Impaired wound healing
   b. Increased blood sugar
   c. Increased risk of stomach ulcer formation
   d. All of the above

9. Of the medications used to treat gout, which of the following is usually considered first-line therapy?
   a. Nonsteroidal anti-inflammatory drugs (NSAIDs)
   b. Colchicine
   c. Corticosteroids
   d. None of the above

10. Which of the following medications is not currently approved by the FDA for treatment of fibro-myalgia?
    a. Duloxetine (Cymbalta®)
    b. Tramadol (Ultram®)
    c. Milnacipran (Savella®)
    d. Pregabalin (Lyrica®)

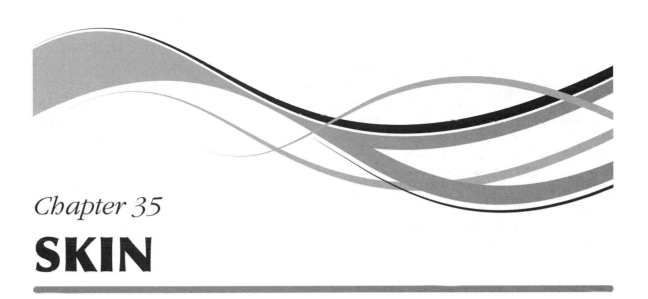

Chapter 35
SKIN

By Jodie L. Elder, Pharm.D., BCPS

Learning Objectives

This chapter seeks to prepare a pharmacy technician to:
- describe the anatomy and function of the skin.
- discuss acne and how it is treated.
- discuss the pathology and treatment of eczema.
- describe appropriate prevention and treatment for sunburn.
- discuss pathology and treatment of psoriasis.

Introduction

The skin is one of the largest organs of the body and performs several important functions. In addition to providing a protective barrier and assisting in temperature control, the skin is also involved in vitamin synthesis. The skin is composed of three main layers: the epidermis, dermis and hypodermis. The **epidermis** is the outermost layer of skin and serves to control the skin's water content (and drug absorption to lower layers of the skin). The **dermis** is the middle layer and contains hair follicles, nerve endings, blood vessels and **melanin** (pigment) cells. The **hypodermis** is the deepest layer and serves to cushion the skin.[1,2] See Figure 1 for a visual representation of the skin's layers. There are many disorders of the skin, including acne, eczema, psoriasis and sunburn. This chapter will review common characteristics of these disorders, including the actions that prevent these diseases, the lesions that accompany these maladies and the therapies that treat these conditions. Descriptions of the types of skin lesions discussed in this chapter are listed in Table 1.

Figure 1
Layers and Structure of the Skin

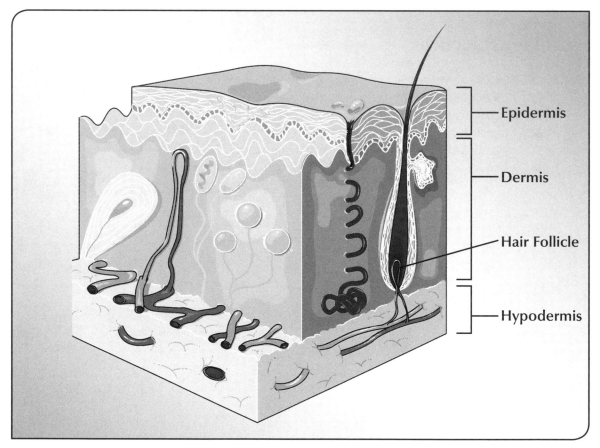

Epidermis

Dermis

Hair Follicle

Hypodermis

Figure was produced using Servier Medical Art, www.servier.com

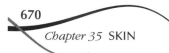

Table 1
Types of Skin Lesions[1]

Type	Description
Bullae	Blisters (fluid-filled) larger than 0.5 cm in size
Macules	Flat lesions of any shape or size that differ from surrounding skin because of their color
Nodule	Solid, round or oval-shaped lesions with varying depth of involvement into the skin
Papules	Small, solid, elevated lesions that are less than 1 cm in diameter
Plaque	A flat, raised area with a relatively large surface area in comparison with its height above the surrounding skin
Vesicle	Blisters (fluid-filled) less than 0.5 cm in size
Wheal	Rounded or flat-topped papules or plaques that characteristically disappear within hours, and usually itch

Acne

It is estimated that 40-50 million people in the United States are affected by **acne**, making it the most common skin disorder. Although it is most common in adolescents and young adults, up to five percent of adults suffer from the condition. There are four primary factors involved in the pathology of acne:

- abnormal **keratinization** of skin cells in the follicular canal;
- androgen-responsive excess **sebum** production;
- **colonization** with *Propionibacterium acnes (P. acnes)*; and
- inflammation.

At puberty, abnormal cohesion occurs between the epithelial cells that cover the unit, called keratinization, which decreases outflow of sebum through the follicular canal. **Androgens** cause the sebaceous glands to become multilobular, which results in an increased sebum output. *P. acnes* usually is found in skin; but, the combination of abnormally **desquamated** cells and excessive levels of sebum in the follicle produce an environment that promotes the growth of *P. acnes*. As sebum accumulates behind the keratotic plug, dilation distorts the normal follicular structure, forming a **microcomedone**, which may become a **closed comedone** (also known as a white head).

Contrary to popular belief, diet has not been proven to contribute significantly to the development of acne. Medications (including lithium, barbiturates and corticosteroids) and physical factors (including friction and cosmetics) may cause or worsen the condition. Acne can be described as noninflammatory and/or inflammatory. **Noninflammatory acne** consists of microcomedones that develop into open (blackheads) and closed (whiteheads) comedones with minimal colonization by *P. acnes*. With inflammatory acne, *P. acnes* thrive in the sebum and release **lipase**, which causes inflammation. As inflammation progresses, the risk of scarring increases. Inflammatory lesions consist of papules, pustules and nodules. A **papule** is a red, raised lesion of less than 5 mm in size that occurs in the epidermis. **Pustules** occur when the follicle ruptures in the outer layers of the skin, allowing pus to be visible in the center of the lesion. If the inflammation is severe and deep in the dermis, nodules or painful cysts may develop.

Acne is usually classified based on the number, type and location of lesions. Two classification systems are commonly used and are based on severity. The most commonly used classification system describes mild as noninflammatory papules or pustules; moderate as inflammatory papules and pustules; and severe as many inflammatory papules and pustules with frequent scarring present. The type and location of lesions are more important to dictate treatment rather than the number of lesions. Goals of treatment include relieving patient discomfort, preventing pitting or scarring, and limiting psychosocial distress.

Topical Treatment of Acne

Benzoyl peroxide has a long history of safety and efficacy in the topical treatment of mild to moderate acne and is used in combination therapy for moderate to severe acne. The primary mechanism of action for benzoyl peroxide is antibacterial. Benzoyl peroxide is available over-the-counter (OTC) and by prescription in a variety of dosage forms and concentrations ranging from 2.5-10 percent, and is generally applied sparingly once or twice daily to the affected areas. Benzoyl peroxide is commonly used in combination with other topical antibiotics to improve efficacy and decrease antibiotic resistance. Improvements are seen with both noninflammatory and inflammatory lesions in approximately three weeks with maximal benefit, defined a 50-75 percent reduction in the number of lesions seen between eight and 12 weeks after initiating therapy. Common side effects are local and include dryness, irritation, redness and photosensitivity. Side effects can be reduced by starting with the lowest dose of benzoyl peroxide (2.5 percent), by using water-based formulations (e.g., creams and lotions) and by applying the products once daily at first. Allergic contact dermatitis, characterized by inflammation and pruritus (itching), can, rarely, result from the use of benzoyl peroxide; however, this reaction resolves soon after discontinuing therapy. Patients must be made aware that benzoyl peroxide may bleach hair and fabric (including towels, sheets, pillow cases and clothing). Clinical data have shown higher concentrations (greater than 10 percent) are no more effective than 2.5-5 percent formulations in reducing the number of lesions and may cause significantly more irritation, which may impact patient adherence to therapy. Recent microsphere formulations of benzoyl peroxide have shown fewer side effects and similar efficacy to traditional products; but, these newer formulations are significantly more expensive than older formulations. Benzoyl peroxide is available in both prescription and OTC products; unlike some products where prescriptions are similarly formulated but with a higher dose, note that benzoyl peroxide's highest available dose, 10 percent, is available without a prescription.

Topical retinoids are commonly used to treat all types of acne. Tretinoin, adapalene and tazarotene have all been shown to be effective in mild to severe acne and are available as cream, gel and microsphere gel. Retinoids help stimulate skin-cell turnover, which restores normal keratinization, and they decrease *P. acnes* colonization by decreasing sebum production to resolve and prevent both noninflammatory and inflammatory acne. They also decrease inflammation by inhibiting neutrophil and monocyte chemotaxis (white blood cell movement). Recent evidence indicates that topical retinoids reduce the expression of a protein called toll-like receptor 2 (TLR-2) that is part of the immune system; a reduction of TLR-2 expression reduces the ability of *P. acnes* to trigger the body's normal inflammatory response. Tretinoin is the only pure topical retinoid available; both tazarotene and adapalene are chemically changed retinoid. Since all three drugs act in the same way, they are all considered retinoids. All of these products require a prescription. Retinoids decrease the thickness of the stratum corneum and may appear to worsen acne in the first few weeks of treatment. Reduction of lesions can be seen as early as four weeks after treatment initiation; but, maximum benefit may not be seen for up to 12 weeks after starting retinoid therapy. The most common adverse effects are all local reactions and include redness, dryness, irritation, peeling and photosensitivity. Exposure to both sunlight and a retinoid can significantly worsen the retinoid's irritation to the skin. It is recommended that patients avoid tanning beds and use a broad-spectrum sunscreen with a sun protection factor (SPF) of at least

15 on all areas exposed to the retinoid. Retinoids are usually applied once daily (in the evening) 10 -30 minutes after cleansing the face; this is done to minimize the irritation caused by application of the drug. Microsphere formulations may help to minimize the irritation compared to nonmicrosphere formulations. When used in combination with other topical therapies, retinoids may increase absorption of the other agents; patients initiating a retinoid while still using other topical therapies on the same areas must be made aware of the potential effects of absorbing the other drug into the body.

Topical antibiotics may be used for mild to moderate acne to decrease the number of *P. acnes* bacteria present on the skin and to potentially reduce inflammation directly. Antibiotics do not resolve existing lesions; however, they do prevent future lesions from forming. Commonly used topical antibiotics include: clindamycin, erythromycin, sodium sulfacetamide (sulfa) and (less frequently) tetracycline. Due to the chance for increased bacterial resistance, it is recommended that topical antibiotics be used in combination with benzoyl peroxide or topical retinoids to ensure that bacteria exposed to the antibiotic are killed off. Generally, these topical antibiotics are applied up to twice daily to the affected area(s). Another topical antibiotic that can be used is azelaic acid, a naturally-occurring dicarboxylic acid commonly found in grains like wheat and barley. Azelaic acid helps to restore normal keratinization, has an antimicrobial effect in acne, and is commercially available as a 20 percent cream or a 15 percent gel. Although only the 20 percent cream is Food and Drug Administration (FDA) approved for acne treatment, clinical studies have shown that 15 percent azelaic acid gel may be effective for the treatment of comedonal and mild-to-moderate inflammatory acne. Azelaic acid may cause less irritation than either retinoids or benzoyl peroxide and may be used for patients who cannot tolerate side effects of other topical medications. All of the topical antibiotics mentioned in this section require a prescription.

Salicylic acid, resorcinol and sulfur have mild **keratolytic** and anti-inflammatory effects in the treatment of mild acne. Combination formulations with resorcinol and sulfur have been shown to reduce the numbers of acne lesions present on a patient's skin. Salicylic acid may improve the absorption of other topical medications and must be combined with caution. Although many different formulations of salicylic acid exist, the most commonly used preparations are pre-soaked pads and face/body washes. These are used one to three times daily on the areas affected by the acne. These ingredients are available in both over-the-counter and prescription preparations. Dapsone five percent aqueous gel is approved for acne treatment in patients 12 years of age and older. Dapsone has antibacterial and anti-inflammatory properties. Adverse effects with topical dapsone are minimal, but include dryness and redness. Although the maximum benefits of using dapsone are reached approximately 10 weeks after initiating therapy, results can be seen in as little as two weeks. See Table 2 for more topical treatments for acne.

Table 2
Selected Topical Treatments for Acne

Drug Class(es)	Generic Name(s)**	Brand Name(s)**	Indication(s)	Available Dose Form(s)
Anti-Acne: Antibiotic	Azelaic Acid	Azelex, Finacea	Acne	Cream, Gel
Anti-Acne: Antibiotic	Benxoyl Peroxide	Benzac, Benziq, Brevoxyl, Clearasil, Micro, NeoBenz, Pan-Oxyl, Triaz, Zoderm	Acne	Cleanser, Cream, Foam, Gel, Liquid, Lotion, Pre-Soaked Cloths, Soap

Table 2 *cont.*
Selected Topical Treatments for Acne

Drug Class(es)	Generic Name(s)**	Brand Name(s)**	Indication(s)	Available Dose Form(s)
Anti-Acne: Antibiotic	Clindamycin	Cleocin T, Clindagel, Clindamax, Evoclin Foam	Acne, Bacterial Infection	Capsule, Foam, Gel, Lotion, Pre-Soaked Pads, Solution
Anti-Acne: Antibiotic	Clindamycin / Benzoyl Peroxide	Acanya, Benzaclin, Duac	Acne	Gel
Anti-Acne: Antibiotic	Erythromycin	Akne-Mycin, Ery-Tab	Bacterial Infection	Gel, Ointment, Pre-Soaked Pads, Solution, Powder for Suspension, Suspension, Tablet
Anti-Acne: Antibiotic	Erythromycin / Benzoyl Peroxide	Benzamycin	Acne	Gel
Anti-Acne: Antibiotic	Sulfacetamide with or without Sulfur	Klaron, Plexion, Rosac, Rosula	Acne	Cream, Emulsion, Foam, Gel, Lotion, Pre-Soaked Pads, Soap, Suspension, Wash
Anti-Acne: Antibiotic / Retinoid	Adapalene / Benzoyl Peroxide	Epiduo	Acne	Gel
Anti-Acne: Antibiotic, Antibiotic: Tetracyclin Anti-Rheumatic: Disease-Modifying Anti-Rheumatic Drug	Minocycline	Arestin, Dynacin, Minocin, Solodyn	Acne, Bacterial Infection, Rheumatoid Arthritis	Capsule, Extended-Release Tablet, Injectable, Tablet
Anti-Acne: Antibiotic / Retinoid	Clindamycin / Tretinoin	Veltin, Ziana	Acne	Gel
Anti-Acne: Retinoid	Adapalene	Differin	Acne	Cream, Gel, Lotion
Anti-Acne: Retinoid	Amnesteem, Claravis, Isoretinoin, Sotret	Accutane	Severe Acne	Capsule

Drug Class(es)	Generic Name(s)**	Brand Name(s)**	Indication(s)	Available Dose Form(s)
Anti-Acne: Retinoid	Tazaroene	Tazorac	Acne	Cream, Gel
Anti-Acne: Retinoid	Tretinoin	Atralin, Avita, Retin-A, Tretin-X	Acne	Topical: Cream, Gel, Micro Gel

**All rights to all brand names and trademarks are held by their respective owners. There may be additional brand names for some of the products listed.*

Oral Medications for Acne

Oral antibiotics are the first-line therapy for moderate to severe inflammatory acne and are often used in combination with topical medications. They are also used for patients with mild to moderate inflammatory acne who do not respond to topical treatments, or patients with acne on the chest or back. Antibiotics work by decreasing the number of bacteria on the skin that are thought to stimulate the inflammation involved in acne. Improvement in the visible signs of acne can be seen in as little as two weeks; however, maximum improvement usually takes three to four months. Tetracycline, minocycline, doxycycline, erythromycin, azithromycin and trimethoprim-sulfamethoxazole have all been used for the treatment of acne. Doxycycline is associated with increased photosensitivity; other antibiotics may have undesirable gastrointestinal effects or cause vaginal yeast infections in women. Trimethoprim-sulfamethoxazole is reserved for severe cases of acne that do not respond to other antibiotics because of its usefulness in treating other common infections. Exposing a patient to these antibiotics on a routine basis can cause bacteria in places other than the skin to become resistant to these antibiotics. Potential side effects of trimethoprim-sulfamethoxazole include rash, photosensitivity, dizziness and (extremely rarely) **Steven-Johnson's syndrome**. Dermatologists generally recommend limiting treatment with systemic antibiotics to no more than three months per treatment; however, many patients will need to repeat the treatment since acne is a chronic disorder.

Another option is isotretinoin, which is a synthetic 13-cis-isomer of tretinoin and the only oral medication that targets all four factors that contribute to acne. Due to the severe adverse effects, use is limited to severe acne that does not respond to other medications. Isotretinoin is administered at doses of 0.5 mg/kg/day to 1.0 mg/kg/day for approximately five months (as tolerated by the patient and as needed to control the signs of acne). Adverse effects include dry lips, dry skin, skin peeling, itching, decreased night vision and mild muscle symptoms. These adverse effects go away once therapy is discontinued. Due to the known risk of birth defects with isotretinoin, prescribers, pharmacies and patients must fully participate in the **iPLEDGE program** in order to prescribe, dispense and receive isotretinoin. In the iPLEDGE program, treatment with isotretinoin requires two negative pregnancy tests, the use of two forms of birth control beginning the month prior to therapy until one month after therapy is discontinued, cholesterol and liver function monitoring (blood work), and patients must answer a series of questions about their lifestyle. Only one month of the medication may be dispensed at each fill to ensure that the required pregnancy tests are performed and are negative. Prescriptions of isotretinoin may not have refills. Cholesterol and liver enzyme blood work is needed since isotretinoin may increase cholesterol levels. Increased thoughts of suicide in teenagers treated with the medication is a concern; providers are required to monitor psychiatric symptoms and provide patients with counseling options. Remission of acne occurs in 90 percent of patients; repeat cycles may be prescribed if acne recurs.

The hormone boost found in birth control (contraceptives) is an effective treatment option for women with moderate to severe acne or menstrual flares that require hormone-based contraceptives for gynecological purposes. Premenstrual worsening of acne is very common. Seven in 10 women frequently experience flare-ups of acne two to seven days before the onset of menses, with gradual improvement at the beginning of the next menstrual cycle. Fluctuation in hormone levels is thought to increase sebum production; so, oral contraceptives may help by decreasing the hormones released by the ovaries. Patients must be made aware that it may take three to six months before any acne benefit is seen from taking hormone-based contraceptives. Several oral contraceptives have been approved by the FDA for the treatment of acne; however, any estrogen-containing oral contraceptive may improve acne symptoms. The androgen-receptor blocker spironolactone and the antiandrogen cyproterone acetate have also been used in the treatment of acne and may be most beneficial when **hirsutism** is present. Spironolactone alone, or in combination with oral contraceptives, has resulted in significant improvement in 85 percent of women with acne in some studies. Doses between 50 mg and 200 mg have been studied, with most patients starting on 100 mg daily. Significant adverse effects with spironolactone use include menstrual irregularities, breast tenderness and serum potassium level elevations. Spironolactone is contraindicated during pregnancy due to the risk of female characteristics developing in a male fetus.

Nondrug Options for Acne

Although drugs play a significant role in the treatment of acne, all patients can benefit from some general skin-care principles. It is recommended that patients wash their face twice daily with a gentle cleanser and avoid abrasives or irritating products (such as scrubs or toners that contain alcohol). Patients must be informed of the characteristics of the formulations for topical products. Gels usually have a high alcohol content; alcohol allows for better absorption of the target drug. Gels also may be more drying and, therefore, best for oily skin. A cream or an ointment may be better tolerated than a gel in patients with dry or sensitive skin. For best results, the entire susceptible area, not just the lesions, must be treated. Temperature and humidity also may play roles in acne development. Hot, humid weather stimulates sweating, which leads to swelling and narrowing of the follicle opening, resulting in duct obstruction. Showering after athletic activity may remove excess sweat to minimize this swelling. Sunlight or ultraviolet light may temporarily improve the appearance of acne by drying and peeling the skin, but can aggravate the condition and mask symptoms. Broad-spectrum sunscreen with SPF 30 can be used to prevent this aggravation.

Acne is a common skin disorder, which may be chronic. Treatment is usually based on the severity and type of lesions. Mild acne may be treated with topical treatments alone. Moderate to severe acne often requires a combination of oral treatments and topical therapies. Isotretinoin is usually only used for acne that does not respond to oral antibiotics and other treatments. Patient compliance with treatment regimens is necessary for the best treatment outcomes.

Eczema

Eczema (also known as atopic dermatitis), is the most common skin disorder in children. Eczema is commonly seen in children with asthma and allergies and may persist into adulthood. Common symptoms include itching, redness and swelling. Oozing vesicles may or may not be present. Eczema is commonly seen in infants on the face and scalp. In children, it may be seen on the neck, wrists and ankles. In adults, eczema is most common on the upper arms, back and wrists. Several triggers may worsen eczema, including allergens, irritants, humidity, dry skin, infection and stress. Prevention of eczema involves minimizing exposure to allergens or skin irritants and drinking water to stay hydrated. To control symptoms and lesions, patients with eczema benefit by bathing daily with a mild nonsoap cleanser in warm water, being careful not to scrub or rub the skin. Bath oils and moisturizers

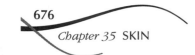

may help to hydrate and lubricate the skin, helping to decrease irritation. It is recommended that patients also wear loose-fitting clothes and keep their fingernails short to prevent scratching of the skin that may lead to infection.

Topical treatment with corticosteroids (e.g., hydrocortisone) are recommended for the treatment of eczema and may help to decrease itching and inflammation. Corticosteroid formulations vary in potency but must always be used sparingly. Corticosteroids are generally applied to the affected areas up to four times daily, depending on the severity of the lesions. Topical steroids are not applied around the eyes or to infected skin. Long-term use of corticosteroids may lead to chronic irritation of the area and thinning of the skin. Table 3 lists some commonly used topical corticosteroids.

Table 3
Commonly Used Topical Corticosteroids

Drug Class(es)	Generic Name(s)**	Brand Name(s)**	Indication(s)	Available Dose Form(s)
Corticosteroid	Alclometasone	Alclovate	Skin Inflammation	Cream, Ointment
Corticosteroid	Amcinonide	Not Available	Skin Inflammation	Cream, Lotion, Ointment
Corticosteroid	Betamethasone	Beta-Val, Celestone, Diprolene, Diprosone, Luxiq, Valisone	High Blood Calcium, Skin Inflammation	Cream, Foam, Lotion, Ointment, Solution
Corticosteroid	Clobetasol	Clobex, Cormax, Olux, Temovate, Temovate E	Skin Inflammation	Cream, Lotion, Ointment, Shampoo, Solution, Spray
Corticosteroid	Clocortolone	Cloderm	Skin Inflammation	Cream
Corticosteroid	Desonide	Desonate, Desonil, DesOwen, LoKara, Verdeso	Skin Inflammation	Cream, Foam, Gel, Lotion, Ointment
Corticosteroid	Desoximetasone	Topicort	Skin Inflammation	Cream, Gel, Ointment
Corticosteroid	Diflorasone	Apexicon	Skin Inflammation	Cream, Ointment
Corticosteroid	Fluocinolone	Capex, Derma-Smoothe FS, DermOtic, Retisert	Skin Inflammation	Cream, Ointment, Ophthalmic Implant, Otic Oil, Shampoo, Solution

Table 3 *cont.*
Commonly Used Topical Corticosteroids

Drug Class(es)	Generic Name(s)**	Brand Name(s)**	Indication(s)	Available Dose Form(s)
Corticosteroid	Fluocinonide	Vanos	Skin Inflammation	Cream, Gel, Ointment, Solution
Corticosteroid	Flurandrenolide	Cordran	Skin Inflammation	Cream, Lotion, Tape
Corticosteroid	Fluticasone	Cutivate, Flonase, Flovent Diskus, Flovent HFA, Veramyst	Allergies, Asthma	Aerosol, Cream, Lotion, Nasal Spray, Ointment, Powder for Inhalation
Corticosteroid	Halcinonide	Halog	Skin Inflammation	Cream, Ointment
Corticosteroid	Halobetasol	Ultravate	Skin Inflammation	Cream, Ointment
Corticosteroid	Hydrocortisone	Cortef	Inflammation	Cream, Foam, Gel, Injectable, Lotion, Ointment, Rectal Suppository
Corticosteroid	Mometasone	Asmanex Twisthaler, Elocon Nasonex	Allergies, Asthma, Skin Inflammation	Cream, Lotion, Nasal Spray, Ointment, Powder for Inhalation, Solution
Corticosteroid	Prednicarbate	Dermatop	Skin Inflammation	Cream, Ointment
Corticosteroid	Triamcinolone	Aristopan, Kenalog, Nasacort AQ	Allergies, Inflammation, Osteroarthritis	Cream, Dental Paste, Injectable, Nasal Spray, Ointment

Oral antihistamines (e.g., diphenhydramine) block histamine release and may, therefore, block the itching response. Oral diphenhydramine may be used to decrease itching; however, it is associated with significant drowsiness, which limits its use. Topical preparations are available, but diphenhydramine may not properly absorb through the skin to the root cause of the itching. Therefore, the topical products may not be as effective as the oral options. Using a newer antihistamine (e.g., cetirizine, loratadine or fexofenadine) can provide the same relief from itching as diphenhydramine but generally does not produce the excessive drowsiness seen with diphenhydramine. Further, the new antihistamines are generally taken only once daily, whereas diphenhydramine must be taken every four to six hours to provide coverage throughout the day.

If patients with eczema develop oozing lesions, astringents and antibiotics may be used. Astringents containing aluminum acetate decrease oozing and may be used to soak the affected area two to four times each day. Topical antibiotics may be used if the skin becomes infected (usually indicated by yellow crusting) to decrease the presence of bacteria on the skin and heal the affected area. Ointments are not generally recommended if the patient has oozing lesions.

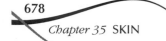

Prescription treatments that are used for eczema include topical tacrolimus and pimecrolimus. These medications work by decreasing the immune response that contributes to the inflammation in eczema. Advantages to tacrolimus and pimecrolimus are that they can be used on the face and eyelid area and are approved for use in patients as young as two years of age. The biggest disadvantage to these two medications is that they are costly. Side effects are generally local and may include mild burning or stinging. More seriously, tacrolimus and pimecrolimus have been linked to a risk of developing certain cancers and must, therefore, be avoided in patients with a history or higher risk of certain cancers.

Atopic dermatitis is a common skin disorder characterized by redness and itching. Nondrug therapies such as avoidance of allergens/irritants and moisturizers are essential to treatment. Treatment may require topical corticosteroids that help to decrease inflammation and itching. Tacrolimus and pimecrolimus are alternative topical medications for the treatment of eczema but are reserved for more severe cases due to their potentially serious risks.

Sunburn

Excessive sun exposure and ultraviolet (UV) radiation have been linked to cancer, premature wrinkles, sunburn and cataracts. It may worsen many skin disorders, including acne and herpes simplex infection (cold sores). Some medications may increase patient sensitivity to the sun (photosensitivity), including some antibiotics and some seizure medications (see Table 4). Sunburn is characterized by redness, tenderness, swelling and sometimes itching. More severe sunburn may lead to vesicles, **bullae**, fever and chills.

Table 4
Select Medications that Cause Photosensitivity

Carbamazepine	Glyburide	Ketoconazole	Sulfamethoxazole
Doxycycline	Hydrochlorothiazide	Lamotrigine	Tetracycline
Furosemide	Isotretinoin	Minocycline	Trimethoprim

Sunburn may be prevented by minimizing exposure to ultraviolet radiation from the sun, wearing sunglasses with UV protection and wearing protective clothing. Broad spectrum (protecting against both types of UV light: UVA and UVB) with a sun protection factor (SPF) of at least 15 is recommended. The SPF is an indication of how well UVB is filtered by the product (e.g., SPF 15 filters 94 percent of UVB rays, while SPF 30 filters 97 percent of UVB rays). For UVA rays, a four-star rating scale is used (the stars indicate: low, medium, high and highest). Patients must be advised that the term "water resistant" indicates that a product maintains the listed SPF for at least 40 minutes while sweating or swimming. Products claiming to be "very water resistant" maintain the listed SPF for at least 80 minutes when swimming or sweating. Many sunscreen products contain more than one ingredient, so it is important to use a product with appropriate UV protection for the circumstance (see Table 5 for a list of sunscreen active ingredients). Products must be applied generously (approximately one ounce covers the entire body surface) at least 15-30 minutes prior to exposure and be reapplied every two to three hours.

Treatment of Sunburn

Nondrug treatments for sunburn include applying cool compresses, soaking the skin in cool tap water for 15-30 minutes, and drinking water to stay hydrated. Protectants (e.g., aloe, cocoa butter and moisturizers) may help to rehydrate the skin and prevent rubbing or irritation. If vesicles or bullae are present, patients can use cool tap water soaks three to six times daily to help hydrate the skin and cool the burn. Topical antibiotics (as discussed in eczema treatment) may be used if the sunburn is oozing. Antibiotic ointments may be used if the skin is intact; if the skin is oozing, creams must be used. Topical anesthetics (e.g., benzocaine or lidocaine) may be used to relieve pain and itching associated with a sunburn; but, they may only be used over small body areas with intact skin. If there is broken skin or blisters, lower strengths of anesthetics may be considered. Anesthetics may be applied three to four times daily for up to seven days. If pain persists beyond seven days, if the burn is severe or if the burn covers greater than two percent of the body surface area, then the patient will need to see a physician for treatment options. Oral anti-inflammatory medications (e.g., aspirin, naproxen and ibuprofen) inhibit **prostaglandin** (necessary part of the body's inflammatory response). These medications may be useful to decrease the swelling and redness associated with sunburn.

Sunburn is a preventable skin disorder; by minimizing UV exposure, including with the use of broad spectrum sunscreen, patients can avoid the pain and irritation that comes with sunburn. Patients on medications that cause photosensitivity must be made aware of their increased risk for sunburn. Treatment of sunburn typically involves cooling the skin and using protectants. Topical anesthetics and oral anti-inflammatory medications may help reduce the discomfort associated with sunburn.

Table 5
Sunscreen Active Ingredients

Ingredient	Protection from UV	Comments
Avobnzone	A	Protection for entire UVA range
Menthyl Anthranilate	A	Mostly UVA absorption; used in combination
Para-Aminobenzoic Acid (PABA)	A	May cause skin reactions; penetrates deep into skin; stains clothing
Terephthalyidene Dicampor Sulphonic Acid	A	Mid-range UVA protection
Trolamin Salicylate	A	Weak sunscreen; does not adhere well
Cinoxate	B	Does not adhere well
Homosalate	B	Weak sunscreen; does not adhere well
Octyl Methoxycinnamate	B	Does not adhere well
Octyl Salicylate	B	Weak sunscreen; does not adhere well
Padimate O	B	PABA derivative; does not stain clothing
Phenyl Benzimidazole	B	UVB absorption only
Sulisobenzone	B	Mostly UVB absorption; may cause skin reactions
Dioxybenzone	A & B	Mostly UVB absorption; can asorb into UVA range; may cause skin reactions
Octocrylene	A & B	Does not adhere well; can also absorb some UVA
Oxybenzone	A & B	Mostly UVB absorption; can absorb into UVA range; found in cosmetics; may cause skin reactions
Titanium Dioxide	A & B	Reflects light; a thick layer is required; may discolor clothing; occlusive
Zinc Dioxide	A & B	Reflects light; a thick layer is required; may discolor clothing; occlusive

Psoriasis

Psoriasis is a common, chronic skin disorder that occurs when the body produces skin cells too quickly. Instead of taking weeks to produce skin cells, the immune system sends a signal to produce skin cells in days. This increase in skin cells leads to the formation of plaques that may be itchy or painful. The plaques may appear dry, scaly, red or silvery. The most commonly affected areas are the elbows, the knees, the wrists and the scalp. The most common type of psoriasis is plaque psoriasis. Psoriasis may occur at any age, but most patients with psoriasis first see symptoms appear between 15-30 years of age. Typically, psoriasis waxes and wanes with certain seasons of the year or periods of time that are often associated with the wax and wane of the seasons.

Treatment of Psoriasis

Topical corticosteroids are the most commonly used medications for the treatment of psoriasis. Steroids are available in a variety of vehicles, including creams, ointments, gels, lotions, foams, shampoos and sprays. As mentioned previously, adverse effects of corticosteroids include thinning of the skin and changes in skin appearance.

Calcipotriene is a form of vitamin D that is used topically to treat psoriasis. It slows skin cell growth. It is available as a cream or solution, and common side effects may include local burning or stinging. Calcipotriene is also available combined with betamethasone, a steroid, in both an ointment applied to the body and a suspension applied to the scalp.

For more severe psoriasis, or psoriasis that does not respond to topical treatment, oral medications are used (e.g., methotrexate, cyclosporine and acitretin). Methotrexate is an **immunosuppressant** (decreases the body's immune response) and is very effective. However, it is associated with serious side effects, including liver toxicity and birth defects. More common side effects with methotrexate include nausea and blood disorders. Cyclosporine is also an immunosuppressant that has been effective in treating severe psoriasis, but it may damage the kidneys and has many drug interactions. Acitretin is an oral retinoid used for severe psoriasis. Side effects of acitretin include dry skin, hair loss, peeling of the skin, increased liver enzymes and increased cholesterol levels. Acitretin has the same severe birth defects as istretinoin, but the effects of acitretin last much longer. Patients on acitretin must avoid pregnancy and blood donation for at least three years after taking the medication.

The newest medications to treat psoriasis, T-cell inhibitors and tumor necrosis factor (TNF) inhibitors, inhibit the immune response involved in psoriasis. These medications are used for more severe psoriasis covering large areas of the body and are given by injection or intravenously. These injectable medications are significantly more expensive than the other medications used to treat psoriasis. T-cell inhibitors (e.g., alefacept and efalizumab) are associated with "flu-like" symptoms, some blood abnormalities and an increased risk of infection. TNF inhibitors (e.g., etanercept, infliximab and adalimumab) are associated with a higher than usual risk of contracting serious infections. Infliximab is only available as an intravenous infusion. Medication storage is important, as many of these medications require refrigeration to maintain drug stability and potency. Ustekinumab is a human monoclonal antibody that has shown benefit in psoriasis, but it, too, has been associated with serious side effects.

Psoriasis is a common skin disorder involving an abnormal immune response and an increased production of skin cells. Mild psoriasis over small areas may be treated with topical treatments including corticosteroids, calcipotriene or topical retinoids, such as tazerotene. Severe psoriasis covering large body areas may necessitate treatment with oral or injectable therapies that are associated with significant side effects. Severity of disease, side effect potential and cost must all be considered when selecting treatments for psoriasis. See Table 6 for a list of systemic medications used to treat psoriasis. In addition, Table 7 provides other common medications used to treat skin-related conditions.

Table 6
Systemic Medications for Psoriasis

Drug Class(es)	Generic Name(s)**	Brand Name(s)**	Indication(s)	Available Dose Form(s)
Anti-Cancer: Antimetabolite, Anti-Rejection: Immunosuppressive, Disease-Modifying Anti-Rheumatic Drug	Methotrexate	Folex, Rheumatrex, Trexall	Multiple Cancers, Psoriasis, Rheumatoid Arthritis	Injectable, Tablet
Anti-Rejection: Immunosuppressive, Anti-Rheumatic: Disease-Modifying Anti-Rheumatic Drug	Cyclosporine	Gengraf, Neoral, Restasis, Sandimmune	Organ Transplant Rejection Prevention, Psoriasis, Rheumatoid Arthritis, Tear Production	Capsule, Injectable, Ophthalmic Solution, Solution
Anti-Rheumatic: Biologic Response Modifier	Efalizumab	Raptiva	Psoriasis	Injectable
Anti-Rheumatic: Biologic Response Modifier, T-Cell Inhibitor	Alefacept	Amevive	Psoriasis	Injectable
Anti-Rheumatic: Biologic Response Modifier, T-Cell Inhibitor, TNF Inhibitor	Etanercept	Enbrel	Psoriasis, Rheumatoid Arthritis	Injectable
Anti-Rheumatic: Biologic Response Modifier, TNF Inhibitor	Adalimumab	Humira	Psoriasis, Rheumatoid Arthritis	Injectable
Monoclonal Antibody	Ustekinumab	Stelara	Psoriasis	Injectable
Retinoid	Acitretin	Soriatane	Psoriasis	Capsule
TNF Inhibitor	Infliximab	Remicade	Crohn's Disease, Inflammatory Conditions, Psoriasis, Rheumatoid Arthritis	Injectable

**All rights to brand names and trademarks are held by their respective owners.*

Table 7
Other Common Medications Used to Treat Skin-related Conditions

Drug Class(es)	Generic Name(s)**	Brand Name(s)**	Indication(s)	Available Dose Form(s)
Antihistamine	Hydroxyzine	Atarax, Vistaril	Allergies, Anxiety, Insomnia, Itching	Capsule, Injectable, Suspension, Syrup, Tablet
Antihistamine, Anti-Nausea	Diphenhydramine	Benadryl, Unisom	Insomnia, Motion Sickness (Nausea), Skin Allergies, Vomiting	Aerosol, Capsule, Cream, Dissolving Strip, Elixir, Gel, Gel Cap, Injectable, Solution, Syrup, Tablet
Corticosteroid	Triamcinolone	Aristopan, Kenalog, Nasacort AQ	Allergies, Inflammation, Osteoarthritis	Cream, Dental Paste, Injectable, Nasal Spray, Ointment

**All rights to all brand names and trademarks are held by their respective owners.

Bibliography

- Cheigh, N., Dermatologic drug reactions, self-treatable skin disorders, and skin cancer, Pharmacotherapy: a Pathophysiologic Approach, 7th edition, New York, 2005, pp. 1741-1753.

- Scott, S., Martin, R.I., Atopic dermatitis and dry skin, Handbook of Nonprescription Drugs; Washington D.C., American Pharmacists Association, 2006, pp. 711-728.

- West, D.P., Loyd, A., Bauer, K.A., West, L.E., Scuderi, L., Micali, G., "Chapter 100, Acne Vulgaris," Pharmacotherapy: A Pathophysiologic Approach, 7th edition, http://0-www.ac-cesspharmacy.com.libcat.ferris.edu/content.aspx?aID=3212082.

- Cheigh, N.H, "Chapter 102, Atopic Dermatitis," Pharmacotherapy: A Pathophysiologic Approach, 7th edition, http://0-www.accesspharmacy.com.libcat.ferris.edu/content.aspx?aID=3212748.

- Wasserbauer, N., Ballow, M., "Atopic Dermatitis," *The American Journal of Medicine*, 2009, Vol. 122, pp. 121-125.

- Ference, J.D., Last, A.R., "Choosing topical corticosteroids," *American Family Physician*, 2009, Vol. 79, No. 2, pp. 135-140.

- Carroll, D., Crosby, K., "Prevention of sun-induced skin disorders," Handbook of Nonprescription Drugs, Washington, D.C., American Pharmacists Association, 2006, pp. 817-837.

- Bowman, J., "Minor burns and sunburn," Handbook of Nonprescription Drugs, Washington, D.C., American Pharmacists Association, 2006, pp. 852-868.

- Land, V., Small, L., "The evidence on how to best treat sunburn in children: a common treatment dilemma," *Pediatric Nursing*, 2008, Vol. 34, pp. 343-348.

- Baron, E., Kirkland, E., Santo Domingo, D., "Advances in photoprotection," *Dermatology Nursing*, 2008, Vol. 20, pp. 265-273.

- Hexsel, C., Bangert, S., Hebert, A., Lim, H., "Current sunscreen issues: 2007 food and drug administration sunscreen labeling recommendations and combination sunscreen/insect repellent products," *Journal of the American Academy of Dermatology*, 2008, Vol. 59, pp. 316-323.

- West, D.P., Loyd, A., West, L.E., Bauer, K.A., Musumeci, M.L., Micali, G., "Chapter 101, Psoriasis," Pharmacotherapy: A Pathophysiologic Approach, 7th edition, http://0-www.ac-cesspharmacy.com.libcat.ferris.edu/content.aspx?aID=3212393.

- Mentor, A., Korman, N.J., Elmets, C.A., Feldman, S.R., et al., "Guidelines of care for the management of psoriasis and psoriatic arthritis: Section 3, Guidelines of care for the management of psoriasis with topical therapies," *Journal of the American Academy of Dermatology*, 2009, Vol. 60, pp. 643-659.

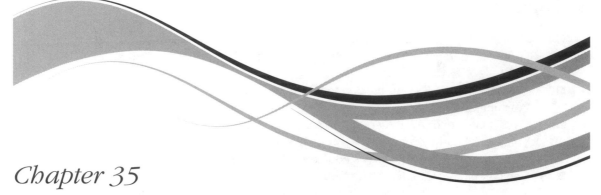

Chapter 35
REVIEW QUESTIONS

1. Which of the following is not a side effect of benzoyl peroxide?
    a. Redness
    b. Dryness
    c. Photosensitivity
    d. Thinning of skin

2. The primary mechanism of action of tretinoin is:
    a. antibacterial.
    b. to stimulate cell turnover.
    c. astringent.
    d. immunosuppressive.

3. Which of the following is a side effect of topical tretinoin?
    a. Liver toxicity
    b. Decreased night vision
    c. Peeling skin
    d. Bleaching of the skin and fabrics

4. Patients with eczema must be warned to:
    a. avoid allergens that worsen eczema.
    b. bathe in hot water twice daily.
    c. use topical antibiotics to prevent eczema.
    d. apply ointment to broken skin.

5. Which of the following is a side effect of long-term hydrocortisone cream use?
    a. Thinning of skin
    b. Peeling
    c. Darkening of skin
    d. Itching

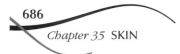

6. All of the following medications may cause photosensitivity except:
    a. doxycycline.
    b. sulfamethoxazole.
    c. metformin.
    d. isotretinoin.

7. Which of the following sunscreen ingredients filters UVA and UVB rays?
    a. Titanium dioxide
    b. Para-Aminobenzoic Acid (PABA)
    c. Homosalate
    d. Cinoxate

8. Which of the following is a local anesthetic used to treat pain associated with sunburn?
    a. Aloe vera
    b. Hydrocortisone
    c. Benzocaine
    d. Naproxen

9. All of the following are potential side effects of methotrexate except:
    a. liver toxicity.
    b. hair loss.
    c. nausea.
    d. birth defects.

10. Which of the following is an injectable medication to treat severe psoriasis?
    a. Methotrexate
    b. Tazaroterene
    c. Adalimumab
    d. Hydrocortisone

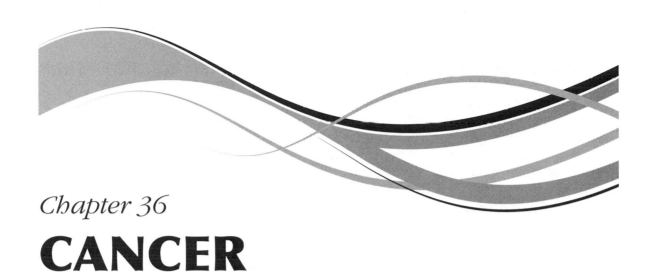

Chapter 36
CANCER

By   Claire E. Saadeh, Pharm.D., BCOP
     Kari L. Vavra, Pharm.D.

Learning Objectives

This chapter seeks to prepare a pharmacy technician to:

- compare and contrast therapeutic modalities utilized in the treatment of cancer.
- describe the mechanism of action of common chemotherapy agents, targeted therapies, endocrine therapies and biologic response modifiers utilized in the treatment of cancer.
- identify common side effects associated with all of the pharmacologic agents.
- discuss safe handling techniques and medication error prevention strategies that should be used in preparing and dispensing chemotherapy.
- identify supportive care issues that may be encountered in the oncology patient.
- discuss the important role that pharmacists and pharmacy technicians serve as members of the health care team in caring for patients with cancer.

Introduction

Cancer, a group of diseases characterized by uncontrolled growth and spread of abnormal cells, may result in serious illness and possibly death. An estimated 1.6 million new cases of cancer will be diagnosed in the United States in 2011, and more than 570,000 Americans are expected to die of cancer-related causes. Approximately 25 percent of all deaths in the United States are due to cancer, making it the second leading cause of death behind heart disease. More than 100 different types of cancer are known to exist. Currently, prostate (in men), breast (in women), lung and colorectal cancer are the most common cancers in the United States.

Cancer Overview

■ Origins of Cancer

Differences exist between normal and cancer cell growth. With normal cells, growth mechanisms in the body produce cells as needed to sustain life. When cells become too old to function properly, or become damaged, the body tries to repair these cells. If repair is not possible, then cells are programmed to die and are replaced with new cells. Thus, there is a balance between cell growth and death. With cancer, however, there is a lack of balance between cell growth and death. Normal cells may become cancer cells if they are exposed to a **carcinogen** (a cancer-causing substance) that damages the cells. These damaged cells cannot be repaired and continue to grow. Eventually, the cells form a mass called a **tumor**. If the tumor mass becomes large enough, it has the ability to invade neighboring tissues. Cancer cells can also break away and spread, or **metastasize**, to other parts of the body, such as the liver, lung, brain and bone.

■ Causes of Cancer

In many cases, it is difficult to determine the cause of cancer. In general, cancer may be inherited, caused by exposure to something in the environment, caused by exposure to a carcinogenic substance, or caused by a combination of these factors. Examples of environmental cancer risks include exposure to excessive amounts of ionizing radiation, ultraviolet radiation and/or secondhand smoke. Carcinogenic substances that have been linked to cancer include tobacco (ingestion by smoking, chewing, etc.), asbestos, pesticides and many other chemicals. Certain viruses and bacteria have also been associated with cancer, such as human papillomavirus (HPV) causing cervical cancer, Epstein-Barr virus causing lymphoma and hepatitis B virus causing liver cancer.

Occasionally, medications used for beneficial or healing purposes may also cause cancer. Selected drugs and hormones known to cause cancer include the following: agents that suppress the immune system (e.g., azathioprine, cyclosporine), antiestrogens (e.g., tamoxifen), chemotherapy agents (e.g., alkylating agents) and estrogens (e.g., hormone replacement therapy).

Other factors that may have an association with, or contribute to, cancer development include poor diet, excessive consumption of alcohol, chewing tobacco, lack of physical activity and obesity. To reduce cancer risk, the following recommendations are encouraged by the American Cancer Society (ACS): eat a healthy diet (choose healthy portion sizes, eat less processed/red meats, eat more whole grains and eat five or more servings of fruits and vegetables per day); limit intake of alcoholic beverages (no more than two drinks per day for men and one drink per day for women); avoid chewing tobacco; increase physical activity (at least 30 minutes of moderate to vigorous physical activity five or more days per week); and maintain a healthy weight.

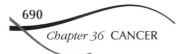

■ Cancer Prevention

Although genetics and family history are unavoidable, lifestyle changes, cancer screening and chemoprevention may help reduce the risk of developing cancer. Harmful behaviors, such as tobacco use, ultraviolet radiation exposure, poor diet, lack of physical activity and being overweight should be avoided. Likewise, secondhand smoke and chemical exposure should be limited.

Chemoprevention is the use of substances, such as drugs, vitamins or vaccines, to decrease the risk of, prolong the development of, or stop the recurrence of cancer in patients at high risk. Chemoprevention strategies to reduce the risk of developing cancer have been studied in clinical trials for many years. Examples include drugs, such as the selective estrogen receptor modulators (SERMS) (e.g., tamoxifen and raloxifene) for breast cancer; 5-alpha-reductase inhibitors (e.g., finasteride) for prostate cancer; the HPV vaccine for cervical cancer; and aspirin, nonaspirin, nonsteroidal anti-inflammatory drugs (NSAIDs), and cyclooxygenase-2 (COX-2) inhibitors (e.g., celecoxib) for colorectal cancer. Despite being extensively studied for cancer prevention, the use of 5-alpha-reductase inhibitors and aspirin/NSAIDs/COX-2 inhibitors is not currently recommended for use by the general population at this time. SERMS and the HPV vaccine, on the other hand, are currently recommended for cancer risk reduction in certain patients.

■ Screening and Early Detection

Screening for cancer involves using different kinds of tests, such as physical exams, imaging procedures (x-rays), laboratory tests and genetic tests, to look for cancer at an early stage (before symptoms appear). Finding cancer early, before it has time to grow and spread, improves the chances of successful treatment, survival and cure. Several organizations, including the ACS, have published screening guidelines for the early detection of cancer. ACS guidelines are available for breast, cervical, colorectal, endometrial and prostate cancer. To view the complete ACS Screening Guidelines for the Early Detection of Cancer, please refer to the document *Cancer Facts and Figures 2012* available online at www.cancer.org.

■ Clinical Presentation

General signs and symptoms of cancer may include unexplained weight loss, fever, fatigue, pain or skin changes. Many different diseases other than cancer may cause these, so signs and symptoms of cancer are not always obvious. The following warning signs, however, are more suggestive of cancer and should be noted:

Change in bowel habits or bladder function
A sore that does not heal
Unusual bleeding or discharge
Thickening or lump in the breast or other parts of the body
Indigestion or trouble swallowing
Obvious change in a wart or mole or any new skin change
Nagging cough or hoarseness

For many reasons, people may not tell their physician about these signs or symptoms. Fear or anxiety about being diagnosed with cancer may prevent people from seeking help. People may think that the symptoms aren't important or that the symptoms will go away without treatment; however, all of these signs and symptoms are important, even if a person doesn't have cancer, and they should be discussed with a physician.

■ Diagnosis, Staging and Performance Status

To make a diagnosis of cancer, several tests and procedures may be utilized, including laboratory tests, imaging procedures (x-rays) to look inside the body and/or a biopsy to remove a sample of the suspected cancerous cells or tissue.

Once a diagnosis has been made, staging is the next step. Staging involves determining the size of the tumor and whether or not the cancer has spread to other parts of the body. This will help in choosing a therapy protocol and estimating the likely outcome. The TNM classification is one of the most common staging systems and is based on the size and/or extent of the tumor (T), the extent of spread to the lymph nodes (N) and the extent of spread to other parts of the body (metastasis) (M). After classifying T, N and M, a numerical stage of I through IV is assigned, with stage I representing early disease (no spread to other organs) and stage IV representing late disease (spread to other organs).

Also at the time of diagnosis, it is important to determine a patient's performance status. Performance status scales, such as the Eastern Cooperative Oncology Group (ECOG) scale, are used to indicate how well a patient will tolerate chemotherapy and what effect chemotherapy will have on patient activity and quality of life. The ECOG scale ranges from zero to four, with zero representing a fully active patient and four representing a bedridden, disabled patient. The lower the number the better the treatment prognosis, or outcome; therefore, patients with a performance status of three or four generally will not receive treatment with chemotherapy.

Treatment

In general, treatment for cancer may be different for every patient and depends on the type of cancer, cancer stage and overall health and performance status of the patient. More than one doctor may be involved in the treatment plan. Treatment options may include surgery, radiation therapy and/or pharmacologic therapy (chemotherapy, targeted therapy, endocrine therapy or biological response modifiers). Any of these treatment options may be used alone or in combination.

■ Surgery

Some patients may undergo surgery as part of their diagnostic work-up to determine the primary location of the tumor, to obtain a tissue sample (biopsy) or to determine the extent of cancer involvement as part of the staging process. In most situations, surgery is used to remove a known tumor mass (and possibly surrounding tissues and/or lymph nodes) for those with early stage disease in which a cure is possible. For those with advanced stage cancer, surgery is not indicated unless it is needed for **palliation** to control symptoms (e.g., pain, blocked airways in the lungs, bowel obstruction, bleeding) that are distressing to the patient.

■ Radiation Therapy

Radiation therapy is a form of localized cancer treatment that uses an external beam of high-energy rays (or particles) to destroy cancer cells. Internal radiation therapy (or **brachytherapy**) is another type of radiation therapy in which radioactive materials are placed at or near the site of the cancer. Radiation therapy may be a primary treatment option for patients who are unable to undergo surgery or it may be used after surgery with or without chemotherapy. In some cases, radiation therapy may be used for those with advanced stage cancer for palliation and symptom control.

■ Pharmacologic Therapy

Surgery and radiation are considered localized treatments and if used alone may not completely eliminate the cancer for those with early stage disease. Systemic, pharmacologic treatment, therefore, is often a necessary addition to the treatment plan. For those patients presenting with advanced stage disease at diagnosis, localized therapies are ineffective and systemic pharmacologic therapy alone is required (depending on the tumor type). Hematological cancers, such as leukemia and lymphoma, require systemic pharmacologic treatment as well.

The goal of pharmacologic treatment varies depending on the type of cancer and the cancer stage. **Neoadjuvant therapy** is chemotherapy (with or without radiation therapy) given prior to surgery to help reduce the tumor size. This makes it easier, and possibly safer, to reach and surgically remove the tumor. **Adjuvant therapy** is chemotherapy (with or without radiation therapy) administered after surgery to ensure that any potentially remaining cancer cells do not survive. Both neoadjuvant and adjuvant therapies are utilized in early stage cancer when the cancer is considered curable. **Palliative therapies** are used in the setting of advanced cancer that is not possible to cure. Treatment in the palliative setting may prolong the life expectancy of the patient, prevent further spread of the cancer or, most importantly, help alleviate some of the cancer-related symptoms experienced by the patient. **Salvage therapy** is treatment given after failure of any of the primary treatments.

A variety of pharmacologic treatment options are currently available. Traditional chemotherapy agents target rapidly dividing cells. Unfortunately, these effects are not specific to cancer cells. Fast-growing cells that normally are found within the body include: bone marrow and the gastrointestinal tract. A major side effect that can result from chemotherapy treatments is bone marrow suppression (**myelosuppression**), which includes **neutropenia** (decline in white blood cell counts), **anemia** (decline in red blood cell counts) and/or **thrombocytopenia** (decline in platelet counts). Nausea and vomiting, **mucositis** (painful ulcers in the mouth and/or esophagus) and diarrhea are common gastrointestinal side effects. Recent advances in new drug development have focused on targeted anticancer therapies which specifically inhibit one or several processes required for tumor-cell growth. Most of these targeted agents do not significantly affect the normal cells within the body; therefore, they have a better side effect profile compared to traditional chemotherapy. Some of these newer agents may be combined with traditional chemotherapy. **Endocrine therapies** are used for tumors that depend on hormones for growth and survival (e.g., breast and prostate cancer). Endocrine therapies are usually not combined with chemotherapy. Instead, such therapies are used sequentially, either before or after chemotherapy administration, depending on the stage of cancer and whether the tumor has spread after primary treatment. Biological response modifiers (or biologic agents) are agents that boost the immune system and are often used in the treatment of melanoma or kidney cancer.

■ Chemotherapy

A variety of chemotherapy agents are used to treat cancer. In most cases, these agents are used in combination and are given on a monthly basis (every 21 or 28 days) for a certain number of months or until the patient's tumor no longer responds to treatment (disease progression). Each chemotherapy agent is categorized primarily by its mechanism of action. Some chemotherapy agents may have several indications (types of cancer treated by the drug) approved by the Food and Drug Administration (FDA); however, a clinician may use FDA-approved drugs for many non-FDA-approved indications.

- **Alkylating Agents**
  The **alkylating agents** work by stopping deoxyribonucleic acid (DNA) and protein synthesis within the cancer cell nucleus, preventing the cancer cell from dividing.

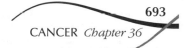

As a class, these agents can cause significant myelosuppression, nausea and vomiting, sterility and infertility. Some of these agents have been known to cause cancer (leukemia), appearing anywhere from one to 20 years after administration. Cyclophosphamide, cisplatin and carboplatin are the most commonly used alkylating agents and appear in many different cancer chemotherapy regimens. Of all the chemotherapy agents, cisplatin causes the most nausea and vomiting, not only during administration but also for up to seven days after administration.

- **Antimetabolites**

  Some of the **antimetabolites** (methotrexate and pemetrexed) work by affecting proteins or enzymes that are necessary for growth and survival within cells. Others work by disrupting DNA and/or ribonucleic acid (RNA) synthesis within the cell nucleus. As a class, these agents can cause a great deal of myelosuppression, nausea and vomiting, and mucositis. Methotrexate, at doses greater than 1,000 mg/m², requires additional supportive care measures to reduce the risk of or to prevent myelosuppression and mucositis from occurring. Patients will receive a nonchemotherapy agent called leucovorin (folinic acid) to rescue the body's normal cells from depletion of proteins necessary for growth and survival. Note that folinic acid and folic acid are not the same; pay close attention to these two drugs to avoid confusion. The amount of leucovorin given differs depending on the cancer type and the chemotherapy regimen; the dose of leucovorin is usually based upon a patient's methotrexate blood level.

- **Antimicrotubules**

  These agents work by stopping **microtubules** (structures within the cell responsible for cell division) from assembling properly. Ultimately, this causes DNA damage leading to cells that are no longer able to divide and grow. All of the agents within this class (except for vincristine) cause significant myelosuppression. **Peripheral neuropathy** (tingling or pain that occurs in the toes and/or fingers) is also a very common side effect associated with this class. Docetaxel, ixabepilone and paclitaxel require a medication regimen prior to administration to reduce the risk of allergic-type reactions. Paclitaxel-albumin is a newer formulation of paclitaxel with a significantly lower risk of allergic-type reactions. This agent is not interchangeable with paclitaxel and should not be substituted for the standard formulation. In general, the antimicrotubules cause the least amount of nausea and vomiting of all the chemotherapy agents.

- **Enzyme Inhibitors**

  These agents work by affecting enzymes within the cell, responsible for specific DNA function and repair mechanisms. Daunorubicin, doxorubicin, epirubicin, idarubicin and mitoxantrone are also classified as anthracycline antitumor antibiotics and are all known to cause damage to the heart (**cardiac toxicity**). This side effect is usually seen after a patient has received multiple cycles; therefore, it is very important to document and to total the administered doses over the entire time that the patient receives chemotherapy (including courses given in the past). Most of the anthracyclines have a suggested, maximum, lifetime dose that must not be exceeded. The solutions of daunorubicin, doxorubicin and idarubicin are orange/red in color; when eliminated from the body through urination, these may cause the urine to change from a yellow to a pink/red or orange color. This is a harmless effect and should not be confused with blood in the urine. Mitoxantrone solution is blue and may cause the urine to look green/blue in color. Daunorubicin and doxorubicin

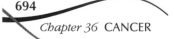

are also available as liposomal formulations and cannot be interchanged with each other or with their standard formulation. Irinotecan, another enzyme inhibitor, can cause significant diarrhea that may be life-threatening if not managed properly. All patients need to take loperamide (Imodium®) immediately at the onset of any diarrheal episodes. All of the enzyme inhibitors can cause myelosuppression, nausea and vomiting, and mucositis.

- **Miscellaneous Chemotherapy Agents**

  A few agents cannot be classified into one of the above chemotherapy categories. Bleomycin is a chemotherapy agent that has been associated with a significant risk of lung toxicity, especially at higher doses; therefore, the lifetime dose of bleomycin is monitored closely.

■ Targeted Therapy

Recent research in **oncology** (the study of cancer) has led to the discovery of specific targets, located primarily on or within cancer cells, that can be attacked by anti-cancer drugs. These agents are generally known as "targeted therapies." These agents work on or target the outside surface of the cancer cell, or they target a specific enzyme or substance within the cancer cell that is needed to produce cell signals. Those agents that target the outside cell surface are known as monoclonal antibodies, and those that work inside the cancer cell are known as kinase inhibitors. If either of these pathways is blocked, cancer cells cannot grow and survive.

- **Monoclonal Antibodies**

  These agents can be used alone, or in combination with chemotherapy, for a variety of cancer types. All of the monoclonal antibodies are administered by intravenous (IV) infusion. One of the most common side effects associated with the monoclonal antibodies is an infusion reaction that can occur during administration of the drug. Symptoms usually include fever, chills, decreased blood pressure and trouble breathing. Infusion reactions can be prevented by pre-medicating with acetaminophen (Tylenol®) and diphenhydramine (Benadryl®) and by slowing the infusion rate.

- **Kinase Inhibitors**

  To date, all of the FDA-approved kinase inhibitors are administered orally and, unlike the monoclonal antibodies, are not combined with chemotherapy. A unique side effect associated with the kinase inhibitors is dry skin and/or an acne like rash that occurs on the face, neck or upper chest. This rash can be mild to severe depending on the patient. Corticosteroid creams and ointments should not be used for treatment. Instead, topical or systemic antibiotics for managing acne may be prescribed and are generally more effective.

■ Endocrine Therapy

Endocrine therapy (hormone therapy) may be used to treat hormone-dependent cancers. These agents work by counteracting the effect of the body's own hormones that may make a certain cancer grow. Examples of hormone-dependent cancers include breast and prostate cancer. For patients diagnosed with breast cancer, tests are conducted on a biopsy sample to determine if the cells are hormone-dependent. If positive, the patient may receive treatment with an antiestrogen or an aromatase inhibitor. Many breast cancer patients receive chemotherapy as part of their treatment course; this is sometimes followed by antiestrogen or aromatase inhibitor therapy after the completion of all chemotherapy cycles. The currently available antiestrogens include fulvestrant (Faslodex®), tamoxifen (Nolvadex®) and toremifene (Fareston®). The currently available aromatase inhibitors include anastrozole (Arimidex®), exemestane (Aromasin®) and letrozole (Femara®). Side effects include hot flashes and clotting in the legs, or deep vein thrombosis (DVT).

For men diagnosed with prostate cancer, initial endocrine treatment includes a luteinizing hormone releasing hormone (LH-RH) agonist such as goserelin (Zoladex®), histrelin (Vantas®), leuprolide (Eligard®) or triptorelin (Trelstar®). Side effects of LH-RH agonists include breast enlargement, decrease in sexual drive, impotence and hot flashes. Often, when an LH-RH agonist is started, symptoms such as those associated with prostate cancer (increased frequency to urinate, decreased amount of urine, painful urination, others) may occur. This is known as tumor flare. These symptoms are not a sign of the cancer growing or worsening; rather, they are an extension of the LH-RH agonist's mechanism of action and the lag time needed for the drug to take effect. Sometimes antiandrogens are given to help prevent or reduce the symptoms associated with tumor flare. Examples of antiandrogens include bicalutamide (Casodex®), flutamide (Eulexin®) and nilutamide (Nilandron®). Degarelix (Firmagon®), an LH-RH antagonist, and abiraterone (Zytiga®), an antiandrogen, are recent FDA-approved agents used in treating advanced-stage prostate cancer.

■ Biological Response Modifiers

Biological response modifiers are typically used for a limited number of cancers that may have occurred as a result of disruption to the immune system. Aldesleukin (Proleukin®) is an agent used to treat kidney cancer and melanoma. Interferon-alpha (Roferon®, Intron-A®) is used in the treatment of kidney cancer and leukemia. Denileukin diftitox (Ontak®) is used to treat one type of lymphoma. In general, these drugs are very hard for patients to handle. Severe chills, fevers, flu-like symptoms and infusion reactions are some of the most common and significant side effects associated with this class of drugs.

Sipuleucel-T (Provenge®) is an immunotherapy agent recently FDA-approved for the management of prostate cancer no longer responding to endocrine therapy. Although its exact mechanism of action is unclear, it is thought to cause the body's own immune system to target a certain protein (antigen) that is found in most prostate cancers. Common side effects include infusion reactions, back pain and chills.

Chemotherapy Administration

■ Dosing and Administration

Prior to processing and preparing chemotherapy, it is necessary to ensure that it is safe to administer. Many clinical and laboratory values need to be considered. The blood components (hemoglobin, white blood cells and platelets) are the most important pre-treatment laboratory values requiring review and assessment by the pharmacist or pharmacy technician before preparing chemotherapy. In general, the following levels are usually required for safe administration:

- a hemoglobin level of 10 g/dL
- a white blood cell count of 3,000/mm^3 or an absolute neutrophil count of 1,500/mm^3
- a platelet count of 100,000/mm^3.

If one or more of these "threshold" values is not achieved, then chemotherapy administration may be held or delayed until the value(s) improve. In addition to the blood components, it is necessary to review and assess a patient's kidney and liver function since one or both of these organs are

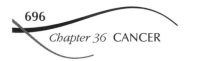

responsible for eliminating chemotherapy from the body. If the renal or hepatic function is lower than normal, doses should be adjusted accordingly. Finally, depending on patient factors (age, nutritional status), treatment factors (previous chemotherapy) and co-existing medical conditions (heart disease), further dosage reductions may be needed.

Several calculation methods may be used to determine a patient's dose of chemotherapy. The most common way to calculate the dose is based on the patient's body surface area (BSA). BSA is a measured indication of the surface of the body based on the patient's weight and height. Since the patient's weight may change throughout the course of treatment, it is important to not only monitor the patient's weight, but also adjust the chemotherapy calculations using the new weight from one month (or cycle) to another. An average BSA is 1.74 mg/m²; however, for patients with a BSA greater than 2 mg/m², a strong collaboration between the prescriber (the oncologist) and a pharmacist is essential to ensuring proper dosing. Many of the targeted therapies are dosed based on a patient's weight (in mg/kg) or as a fixed dose (in mg) irrespective of a patient's weight. When reviewing, processing and dispensing chemotherapy, it is very important to pay special attention to these different dosing strategies. Some drugs, such as carboplatin, have their own formula for determining the total dose. Dosing for this agent is based on the Calvert equation; the Calvert equation takes into account a patient's kidney function. Regardless of the calculation, it is important that dosages are calculated correctly and always verified (double checked) by another pharmacist and/or pharmacy technician based on the pharmacy's protocol. Administration of the wrong drug, dose, route and/or frequency can result in severe toxicity, impairment and/or death.

■ **Safety and Handling Issues**
In handling chemotherapy agents, special precautions should be observed to prevent health care worker exposure to these hazardous substances. Exposure may occur through various mechanisms (e.g., absorption into the skin, inhalation into the lungs and/or ingestion into the gastrointestinal tract) during drug preparation, transfer, storage or administration. Given the hazardous nature of these substances, and the potential risk to health care workers, the American Society of Health-System Pharmacists (ASHP) has published guidelines on handling these agents. Recommendations involve safety programs, labeling and packaging, the work environment, ventilation controls, personal protective equipment, work practices and hazardous waste containment and disposal.

Chemotherapy agents being prepared for IV administration should be prepared in a vertical (vs. horizontal) laminar flow hood. Personal protective equipment, including gloves, gowns, shoe coverings and hair coverings, are essential. During any contact with chemotherapy agents, high-quality, powder-free, gloves must be worn and doubled-up for maximum protection. Gloves may be worn for a maximum of 30 minutes, unless damaged or contaminated, before being replaced. Protective gowns must be made of a lint-free, low-permeability, fabric with a closed front, long sleeves and tight-fitting elastic or knit cuffs. All personal protective equipment must be worn once and discarded appropriately after use. Any health care worker responsible for preparing chemotherapy agents must be properly trained in aseptic technique, with routine assessment of competency. Policies and procedures for handling hazardous substances must be established for the pharmacy, nursing and any other departments where staff may have contact with these agents.

■ **Guidelines for Preventing Errors**
Medication errors involving chemotherapy, more so than with other drugs, may be deadly. Therefore, it is essential to verify all drugs, doses, routes and frequencies very carefully. Safe handling techniques must be used at all steps during the preparation and administration process. Policies and procedures must also be in place to manage medication errors if/when they occur.

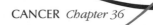

Administering a larger chemotherapy dose, or administering a drug sooner than prescribed, may result in severe side effects, organ damage, permanent injury and/or death. Under-dosing is also considered a medication error and may compromise treatment outcomes. Guidelines on preventing medication errors with chemotherapy agents are available from ASHP. A summary of these recommendations are found in Table 1.

Table 1
ASHP Guidelines on Preventing Medication Errors with Chemotherapy Agents

Prescribing	• Since oral chemotherapy orders eliminate the opportunity for another health care worker to verify the order, they should not be allowed. • "STAT" orders for chemotherapy agents should be avoided. Orders for chemotherapy should only be placed when there is enough staff present to properly perform all safety checks. • Standardized chemotherapy order forms are recommended. Essential components include the dosafe form, patient-specific data (weight), drug dosage, calculations, route, rate, vehicle solution, vehicle volume, administration schedule, duration of treatment, and the date and time of administration. Additionally, the generic drug name, rather than the brand name, is preferred; abbreviations and acronyms are discouraged as well. • Order forms should include pre-treatment medications (hydration) and supportive care agents to ensure comprehensive care.
Preparing	• All information on the original chemotherapy order form should be verified with the treatment protocol, product package labeling, etc. • When preparing two or more agents, only one medication should be compounded at a time. • Chemotherapy agents administered by a route other than intravenously should be clearly labeled and easy to distinguish. • Standardized chemotherapy labels are recommended and should be applied as soon as the agent is prepared. • A second health care worker, such as a pharmacist, should check for errors in order entry and drug admixture.
Dispensing	• During the distribution process, the chemotherapy should be inspected by the receiver, with special attention on the appearance (color).
Administering	• Prior to administering chemotherapy, the patient's name and another unique identifiers should be cross-checked with the drug label. • The final product should be verified one last time with the original order. • After administration, the patient name, chemotherapy name, dose, route, rate, starting date and time, completion date and time (or duration of administration), and any side effects should be documented.

Supportive Care

Medications used along with the chemotherapy regimen are necessary to help prevent or reduce the severity of many of the side effects associated with cancer chemotherapy. The most common supportive care measures and medications are discussed here, while Table 2 provides an overview of other supportive care issues encountered in the oncology patient.

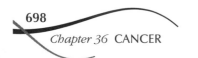

Table 2
Supportive Care Issues Often Encountered in the Oncology Patient

Side Effect / Supportive Care Issue	Description / Definition
Alopecia	Hair loss anywhere on the body, including the head, face, arms, legs, underarms or pubic region
Anxiety	A feeling of nervousness, apprehension, fear or worry
Constipation	Bowel movements that come less often than normal, are painful and/or are hard, dry or difficult to pass
Depression	An ongoing feeling of sadness, worthlessness or hopelessness; may be accompanied by loss of energy, interest or pleasure and/or thoughts of death or suicide
Diarrhea	Bowel movements that come more often than normal and/or are soft, loose or watery
Extravasation	Leakage of chemotherapy from the vein into the surrounding tissue during intravenous administration; may result in redness, pain, irritation and/or tissue damage
Fatigue	A mild to extreme feeling of weakness and/or tiredness
Hypercalcemia	A high blood calcium level; a complication of cancer (commonly breast and lung cancer)
Hypersensitivity Reactions	An immune-mediated reaction to chemotherapy that may result in hives, swelling, itching, flushing, a skin rash and/or difficulty breathing
Infertility / Sterility	Inability to produce (conceive) a child; a woman may not be able to get pregnant or a man may not be able to get a woman pregnant
Loss of Appetite / Weight Loss	Loss of the desire to eat; may result from cancer or cancer treatment side effects (nausea, vomiting, diarrhea, mouth sores, pain, depression, etc.)
Mucositis	Painful ulcers in the mouth and/or esophagus
Pain	Often described as a dull or aching type of pain, pain in the bones or sharp, tingling-type pain (peripheral neuropathy); may affect any part of the body, at or away from the tumor site
Tumor Lysis Syndrome	A complication of chemotherapy occurring from rapid destruction of a large number of cancer cells; the following may result: a high blood uric acid level, a high blood potassium level, a high blood phosphorus level and/or a low blood calcium level

Nausea and vomiting are the most feared side effects from a patient's perspective. Approximately 70-80 percent of patients will experience nausea and/or vomiting during treatment. The **emetogenic potential**, or likelihood of causing nausea and vomiting, for a particular therapy or regimen varies depending on both the patient and the agent; further, nausea and vomiting may be increased when agents are used in combination. For most chemotherapy regimens, a typical antiemetic regimen will consist of the following: a selective serotonin antagonist [ondansetron (Zofran®), granisetron (Kytril®), dolasetron (Anzemet®) or palonosetron (Aloxi®)] and a neurokinin-1 antagonist [aprepitant (Emend®)] and a corticosteroid [dexamethasone (Decadron®)]. Since these agents each work differently to block vomiting pathways, prevention of nausea and vomiting is more successful when all of these agents are given together.

With the potential for bone marrow suppression, anemia may result. The role of red blood cells in the body is to carry oxygen to all tissues. In patients with anemia, the tissues don't receive enough oxygen, and, therefore, fatigue or tiredness (more so than usual) may result. This can significantly impact the patient's ability to function on a daily basis. Treatment of anemia may involve replacement of the lost red blood cells with blood transfusions or medications to boost red blood cell production. Erythropoiesis-stimulating agents (ESAs), such as epoetin alfa (Epogen®, Procrit®) or darbepoetin alfa (Aranesp®), are prescription medications that stimulate the bone marrow to make more red blood cells. These agents are used to decrease transfusion requirements and potentially improve a patient's quality of life. ESAs are only to be used to treat chemotherapy-related anemia if the patient is currently receiving chemotherapy (for noncurative purposes only) and if the hemoglobin level is less than 10 g/dL. Epoetin alfa is commonly administered subcutaneously (SQ) once per week, while darbepoetin alfa may be given SQ once per week or every three weeks. Using the lowest dose possible and discontinuing treatment at the end of the chemotherapy course is very important.

Neutropenia is a common side effect of cancer chemotherapy. The role of white blood cells in the body is to fight infection. In patients with neutropenia (especially prolonged or severe neutropenia), there is an increased risk for infection that can be life threatening. Once infection occurs, patients need to be hospitalized and treated with antibiotics. Preventing neutropenia is important and possible with prescription medications. Colony-stimulating factors (CSFs), such as filgrastim (Neupogen®), pegfilgrastim (Neulasta®) and sargramostim (Leukine®), are prescription medications that enhance white blood cell production and reduce the incidence, severity and duration of neutropenia, potentially decreasing the risk of infection. In general, patients receiving a chemotherapy regimen with a high risk of neutropenia are recommended to receive a CSF. All CSFs are administered by SQ injection 24-72 hours after chemotherapy. Pegfilgrastim is given only once per chemotherapy cycle, whereas filgrastim and sargramostim are given once daily until the absolute neutrophil count returns to a safe level (generally 2,000-3,000/mm^3).

Platelets are another blood component that may be harmed with cancer chemotherapy, resulting in thrombocytopenia. The role of platelets in the body is to control clotting and to stop bleeding. In patients with thrombocytopenia, easy bruising and bleeding may occur. Treatment of thrombocytopenia usually involves platelet transfusions.

Role of the Pharmacist

In caring for patients with cancer, a pharmacist is an essential member of the health care team. Pharmacists provide care beyond chemotherapy dosage calculation, verification and preparation. Providing drug information to other health care professionals and educating patients, family members and other caregivers is a critical role for pharmacists. Drug information may include discussions about chemotherapy agents, potential side effects and their management, or other concerns in groups small or large; written information on drug use or new drugs; or training staff on the safe handling and use of chemotherapy agents. Another important role that pharmacists perform is the routine monitoring of laboratory parameters to ensure safe chemotherapy administration (e.g., pharmacists monitor kidney and liver function and adjust doses, or change therapy, based on organ function.) Side effects and drug interactions must be monitored as well to ensure that patients experience minimal toxicity, which is another role for pharmacists. Pharmacists also provide a vital role in making recommendations for the prevention and management of supportive care issues that may be encountered during treatment with a given chemotherapy regimen. Finally, it is important for pharmacists to stay current with new treatment options, supportive care measures and evidence-based guidelines as they emerge. As an essential member of the health care team, pharmacists fulfill many roles and have a valuable impact on patient care.

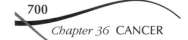

Role of the Pharmacy Technician

One of the most important roles that pharmacy technicians provide is preparation and dispensing of chemotherapy. Technicians are responsible for handling chemotherapy agents in a safe manner (wearing protective clothing), preparing chemotherapy agents appropriately and having a thorough knowledge of pharmacy calculations and training in IV admixture. As part of the chemotherapy preparation process, pharmacy technicians are also responsible for maintaining the vertical laminar airflow hood, such as cleaning up spills, disinfecting the hood, etc. In some institutions, pharmacy technicians are responsible for maintaining drug and supply inventories, ordering supplies and restocking the chemotherapy drug storage area. Having the necessary chemotherapy agents available for each patient is crucial. Responsibilities may also include assisting other members of the health care team (e.g., verifying dosages and calculations by double-checking a pharmacist or another technician, delivering chemotherapy, determining administration time, disposing of chemotherapy waste, etc.). Pharmacy technicians, together with pharmacists, help to ensure the quality of all chemotherapy services used in the care of patients with cancer.

Conclusion

Cancer is a major health problem with absolutely no limitations. Every age, sex, ethnic group, region and economic level may be affected. In the United States, more than 11 million people alive today have received a diagnosis of cancer, are undergoing treatment for cancer, or have survived cancer. With the ever-increasing number of new cancer diagnoses each year, new therapies are being discovered, researched and marketed at a faster pace than ever before. Therefore, it is vital for pharmacists and pharmacy technicians to stay current on new treatments, research and clinical trials as they come to the forefront. Although treatment often takes center stage, it's certainly not the only area of focus for pharmacists and pharmacy technicians. From the patient with cancer to the patient's family members and friends, cancer causes tremendous emotional and physical turmoil. During this distressing time, support and encouragement are more important than ever. Pharmacists and pharmacy technicians in all practice settings must be well-equipped to provide this support and encouragement.

Table 3
Drugs Used to Treat Cancer

Drug Class(es)	Generic Name(s)**	Brand Name(s)**	Indication(s)	Available Dose Form(s)
Anti-Cancer	Bleomycin	Blenoxane	Multiple Cancers	Injectable
Anti-Cancer	Bortezomib	Velcade	Lymphoma, Multiple Myeloma	Injectable
Anti-Cancer	Hydroxyurea	Droxia, Hydrea	Multiple Cancers, Sickle Cell Anemia	Capsule
Anti-Cancer	Romidepsin	Istodax	Lymphoma	Injectable
Anti-Cancer	Vorinostat	Zolinza	Lymphoma	Capsule
Anti-Cancer: Alkylating Agent	Bendamustine	Treanda	Leukemia	Injectable
Anti-Cancer: Alkylating Agent	Carboplatin	Paraplatin	Ovarian Cancer	Injectable
Anti-Cancer: Alkylating Agent	Cisplatin	Platinol	Bladder Cancer, Ovarian Cancer, Testicular Cancer	Injectable
Anti-Cancer: Alkylating Agent	Ifosfamide	Ifex	Testicular Cancer	Injectable
Anti-Cancer: Alkylating Agent	Oxaliplatin	Eloxatin	Colon Cancer	Injectable
Anti-Cancer: Alkylating Agent	Temozolomide	Temodar	Brain Cancer	Capsule, Injectable
Anti-Cancer: Alkylating Agent, Anti-Rheumatic: Disease-Modifying Anti-Rheumatic Drug	Cyclophosphamide	Cytoxan	Multiple Cancers, Rheumatoid Arthritis	Injectable, Tablet
Anti-Cancer: Antimetabolite	Capecitabine	Xeloda	Breast Cancer, Colon Cancer	Tablet
Anti-Cancer: Antimetabolite	Cytarabine	ARA-C, Cytosar	Leukemia	Injectable
Anti-Cancer: Antimetabolite	Fludarabine	Fludara, Oforta	Leukemia	Injectable, Tablet
Anti-Cancer: Antimetabolite	Fluorouracil	5-FU, Adrucil, Carac, Efudex	Multiple Cancers	Cream, Injectable, Topical Solution
Anti-Cancer: Antimetabolite	Gemcitabine	Gemzar	Multiple Cancers	Injectable

Drug Class(es)	Generic Name(s)**	Brand Name(s)**	Indication(s)	Available Dose Form(s)
Anti-Cancer: Antimetabolite	Nelarabine	Arranon	Leukemia, Lymphoma	Injectable
Anti-Cancer: Antimetabolite	Pemetrexed	Alimta	Lung Cancer	Injectable
Anti-Cancer: Antimetabolite	Pralatrexate	Folotyn	Lymphoma	Injectable
Anti-Cancer: Antimetabolite, Anti-Rheumatic: Disease-Modifying Anti-Rheumatic Drug	Methotrexate	Folex, Rheumatrex, Trexall	Multiple Cancers, Psoriasis, Rheumatoid Arthritis	Injectable, Tablet
Anti-Cancer: Antimicrotubule	Cabazitaxel	Jevtana	Prostate Cancer	Injectable
Anti-Cancer: Antimicrotubule	Docetaxel	Taxotere	Multiple Cancers	Injectable
Anti-Cancer: Antimicrotubule	Ixabepilone	Ixempra	Breast Cancer	Injectable
Anti-Cancer: Antimicrotubule	Paclitaxel	Taxol	Multiple Cancers	Injectable
Anti-Cancer: Antimicrotubule	Paclitaxel-Albumin	Abraxane	Breast Cancer	Injectable
Anti-Cancer: Antimicrotubule	Vincristine	Oncovin	Leukemia, Lymphoma	Injectable
Anti-Cancer: Antimicrotubule	Vinorelbine	Navelbine	Lung Cancer	Injectable
Anti-Cancer: DNA Demethylation Agent	Azacitidine	Vidaza	Myelodysplastic Syndrome	Injectable
Anti-Cancer: DNA Demethylation Agent	Decitabine	DACOGEN	Myelodysplastic Syndrome	Injectable
Anti-Cancer: Enyzme Inhibitor	Daunorubicin / Daunorubicin Lipsomal	Cerubidine, DaunoXome	HIV-Associated Kaposi's Sarcoma, Leukemia	Injectable
Anti-Cancer: Enzyme Inhibitor	Doxorubicin / Doxorubicin Liposomal	Adriamycin, Doxil	HIV-Associated Kaposi's Sarcoma, Multiple Cancers, Multiple Myeloma	Injectable

Table 3 *cont.*
Drugs Used to Treat Cancer

Drug Class(es)	Generic Name(s)**	Brand Name(s)**	Indication(s)	Available Dose Form(s)
Anti-Cancer: Enzyme Inhibitor	Epirubicin	Ellence	Breast Cancer	Injectable
Anti-Cancer: Enzyme Inhibitor	Etoposide	Etopophos, Toposar, VePesid	Lung Cancer, Testicular Cancer	Capsule, Injectable
Anti-Cancer: Enzyme Inhibitor	Idarubicin	Idamycin	Leukemia	Injectable
Anti-Cancer: Enzyme Inhibitor	Irinotecan	Camptosar	Colon Cancer	Injectable
Anti-Cancer: Enzyme Inhibitor	Mitoxantrone	Novantrone	Leukemia, Prostate Cancer	Injectable
Anti-Cancer: Immunomodulator	Lenalidomide	Revlimid	Multiple Myeloma, Myelodysplastic Syndrome	Capsule
Anti-Cancer: Kinase Inhibitor	Dasatinib	Sprycel	Leukemia	Injectable
Anti-Cancer: Kinase Inhibitor	Erlotinib	Tarceva	Lung Cancer, Pancreatic Cancer	Tablet
Anti-Cancer: Kinase Inhibitor	Everolimus	Afinitor	Kidney Cancer	Tablet
Anti-Cancer: Kinase Inhibitor	Imatinib	Gleevec	Leukemia, Myelodysplastic Syndrome	Tablet
Anti-Cancer: Kinase Inhibitor	Lapatinib	Tykerb	Breast Cancer	Tablet
Anti-Cancer: Kinase Inhibitor	Nilotinib	Tasigna	Leukemia	Capsule
Anti-Cancer: Kinase Inhibitor	Pazopanib	Votrient	Kidney Cancer	Tablet
Anti-Cancer: Kinase Inhibitor	Sorafenib	Nexavar	Kidney Cancer, Liver Cancer	Tablet
Anti-Cancer: Kinase Inhibitor	Sunitinib	Sutent	Kidney Cancer, Stomach Cancer	Capsule
Anti-Cancer: Kinase Inhibitor	Temsirolimus	Torisel	Kidney Cancer	Injectable
Anti-Cancer: Kinase Inhibitor	Vanditahib	Caprelsa	Thyroid Cancer	Tablet
Anti-Cancer: Monoclonal Antibody	Alemtuzumab	Campath	Leukemia	Injectable

Drug Class(es)	Generic Name(s)**	Brand Name(s)**	Indication(s)	Available Dose Form(s)
Anti-Cancer: Monoclonal Antibody	Bevacizumab	Avastin	Multiple Cancers	Injectable
Anti-Cancer: Monoclonal Antibody	Cetuximab	Erbitux	Colon Cancer, Head and Neck Cancer	Injectable
Anti-Cancer: Monoclonal Antibody	Ipiluminab	Yervoy	Melanoma	Injectable
Anti-Cancer: Monoclonal Antibody	Ofatumumab	Arzerra	Leukemia	Injectable
Anti-Cancer: Monoclonal Antibody	Panitumumab	Vectibix	Colon Cancer	Injectable
Anti-Cancer: Monoclonal Antibody	Trastuzumab	Herceptin	Breast Cancer	Injectable
Anti-Cancer: Monoclonal Antibody, Anti-Rheumatic: Biologic Response Modifier	Rituximab	Rituxan	Lymphoma, Rheumatoid Arthritis	Injectable
Anti-Estrogen	Tamoxifen	Nolvadex	Breast Cancer, Ovulation Stimulation	Tablet
Hormone	Goserelin	Zoladex	Breast Cancer, Endometriosis, Prostate Cancer	Injectable
Hormone	Leuprolide	Eligard, Lupron Depot	Endometriosis, Ovulation Stimulation, Prostate Cancer	Injectable
Hormone	Megestrol	Megace, Megace ES	Endometriosis, Loss of Appetite	Liquid, Suspension, Tablet
Immunodilator	Thalidomide	Thalomid	GI Bleeding, Multiple Myeloma, Nausea, Vomiting	Capsule

*** All rights to all brand names and trademarks are held by their respective owners. There may be additional brand names for some of the products listed.*

Bibliography

- "Cancer Facts and Figures 2011," American Cancer Society, Atlanta, GA, pp. 1-60, 2011.
- Medina, P.J., Fausel, C., "Chapter 130, Cancer Treatment and Chemotherapy," Pharmacotherapy: A Pathophysiologic Approach, 7th edition, New York, NY, 2008.
- American Cancer Society, www.cancer.org, Aug. 10, 2010.
- National Cancer Institute, www.cancer.gov, Aug. 10, 2010.
- Ettinger, D.S., Armstrong, D.K., Barbour, S., Berger, M.J., Bierman, P.J., Bradbury, B., et al., "NCCN Clinical Practice Guidelines in Oncology: Antiemesis, Version 2.2010," National Comprehensive Cancer Network, Fort Washington, PA, pp. 1-36, 2010.
- "ASHP guidelines on handling hazardous drugs," *American Journal of Health-System Pharmacy*, Vol. 63, pp. 1172-1793, 2006.
- "ASHP guidelines on preventing medication errors with antineoplastic agents," *American Journal of Health-System Pharmacy*, Vol. 59, pp. 1648-1668, 2002.

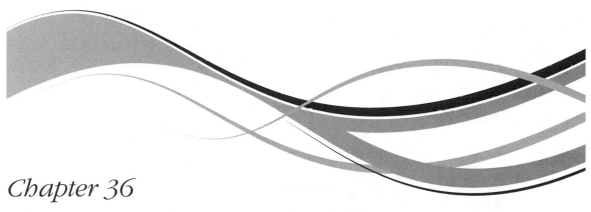

Chapter 36

REVIEW QUESTIONS

1. Which of the following is true regarding radiation therapy?
   a. Radiation therapy cannot be used in combination with chemotherapy
   b. Radiation therapy is not effective for controlling symptoms associated with cancer
   c. Radiation therapy is considered a form of localized therapy
   d. Radiation therapy is more effective than chemotherapy in eliminating cancer from the body

2. KS is a 60-year-old woman who will be starting chemotherapy for early stage (curable) breast cancer. She has already had surgery (removal of her left breast) and radiation therapy. Which of the following terms best describes her chemotherapy?
   a. Neoadjuvant therapy
   b. Adjuvant therapy
   c. Palliative therapy
   d. Salvage therapy

3. AM is a 56-year-old man who will be receiving chemotherapy with idarubicin and cytarabine. Which of the following best describes the mechanism of action of cytarabine?
   a. Stops microtubules within the cell from assembling
   b. Stops enzymes within the cell from repairing themselves
   c. Stops signals within the cell from communicating
   d. Stops DNA or RNA synthesis within the cell

4. TS is a 65-year-old woman receiving therapy with trastuzumab. Which of the following best describes the mechanism of action for this drug?
   a. Targets the outside of the cancer cell, thereby blocking cancer cells from growing
   b. Targets a hormone produced by the body, thereby blocking cancer cells from dividing
   c. Stimulates the immune system, thereby causing cancer cells to be attacked
   d. Stops DNA and/or RNA synthesis, thereby causing cancer cell death

5. MP is a 70-year-old man who received chemotherapy this morning in the clinic. He calls you in the pharmacy complaining of nausea and vomiting. Which of the following pharmacologic therapies would you expect to cause a significant amount of nausea and vomiting?
    a. Rituximab
    b. Erlotinib
    c. Cisplatin
    d. Tamoxifen

6. JT is a 66-year-old woman who comes into the pharmacy to show you a rash and very dry skin on her face. She mentions to you that she started a new drug for her cancer about one or two weeks ago. Which of the following agents would you expect to cause this side effect?
    a. Bevacizumab
    b. Erlotinib
    c. Bleomycin
    d. Interferon-alpha

7. You receive the following order in the pharmacy today:
    Docetaxel 75 mg/m^2 IV, total dose = 142.5 mg
    Cyclophosphamide 600 mg/m^2 IV, total dose = 1,400 mg
    Patient's BSA = 1.9 m^2

    Which of the following actions is most appropriate?
    a. Discuss with the pharmacist; the dose of docetaxel is not calculated properly
    b. Discuss with the pharmacist; the dose of cyclophosphamide is not calculated properly
    c. Discuss with the pharmacist; both doses of chemotherapy are not calculated properly
    d. Proceed with processing the order; calculations are appropriate

8. Where must IV chemotherapy be prepared?
    a. In the chemotherapy clinic, at a dedicated desktop for IV preparation
    b. In the patient's room, to ensure fast drug delivery
    c. In the pharmacy, in a vertical laminar flow hood
    d. In the pharmacy, in a horizontal laminar flow hood

9. Which of the following supportive care regimens is appropriate for the prevention of chemotherapy-induced nausea and vomiting?
    a. Ondansetron, dexamethasone and aprepitant
    b. Acetaminophen, diphenhydramine and granisetron
    c. Diphenhydramine, dexamethasone and aprepitant
    d. Vitamin B$_{12}$, folinic acid and palonosetron

10. Which of the following statements is true regarding the use of filgrastim?
    a. This agent is used to prevent neutropenia in patients at high-risk
    b. This agent stimulates the immune system to produce red blood cells, white blood cells and platelets
    c. This agent is used as a rescue therapy for high dose methotrexate
    d. This agent is used in conjunction with a biologic response modifier

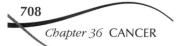

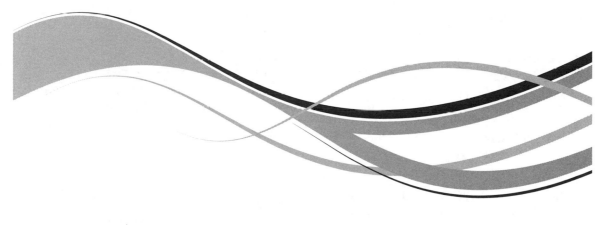

INDEX

ABC inventory
224

Absorption
24, 280, 287, 289-291, 296, 297, 316-319, 322, 323, 339, 342, 343, 441, 475, 488, 489, 490, 494, 501, 502, 514, 555, 569, 572, 577, 612, 613, 624, 635, 636, 640, 657, 670, 673, 676, 681, 697

Accredited
2, 98, 161, 164, 165, 168, 171, 172, 193

Acetylcholine
356, 357, 362, 396, 401, 527, 528

Acquired immune deficiency syndrome
541, 638, 642-646

Acromegaly
414, 586, 594, 595, 597, 601

Activated charcoal
280, 281, 284

Acute coronary syndrome
389, 413, 417, 438, 442, 444, 509, 510, 572, 573, 615, 619, 621-623

Acute myocardial infarction
442, 615

Acute organ rejection
638

Acute pain
402, 403

Acute renal failure
567, 568, 570, 578, 579

Adaptive immunity
631, 632, 648

Addison's disease
587, 599

Additive effect
294, 297, 342, 343

Adenosine triphosphate
358, 507, 610

Adequate intake
315, 316, 320, 322, 324

Adjuvant analgesics
404, 405

Adjuvant therapy
693, 707

Admixture
119, 137, 144, 145, 155, 186, 698, 701

Adrenal cortex
586, 587, 599

Adrenal glands
584-587, 599, 601

Adrenal medulla
586

Adulterated
207, 338, 345

Adverse drug reaction
99, 187, 204, 425, 430, 441, 443

Adverse events
4, 168, 270, 293, 327, 338, 408, 572

Aerosols
24

Affective disorder
366, 369, 390, 395

Agonist
355, 379, 382, 386, 388, 391, 401, 406,
409, 410, 414, 421, 422, 470, 471, 473-
476, 480, 481, 491, 499, 539, 540, 542,
550, 557, 580, 586, 595, 656, 661, 696

Albumin
291, 415, 507, 511, 512, 622, 694, 703

Aldosterone
507, 511, 512, 574, 579, 586, 587

Alkylating agents
690, 693, 694

Allergen
86, 452-455, 466, 469, 476, 477, 676, 679,
686

Allergic rhinitis
451, 452, 454-456, 459, 460, 463, 482

Alopecia
326, 699

Alveoli
466, 467, 473

Ambulatory pharmacy service
27

Amenorrhea
539

Ampule
24, 111, 120, 124, 125, 137, 140, 141, 144,
147

Amygdala
351, 352, 361

Amylase
489

Anaphylactic reactions
281, 511, 613

Anaphylaxis
261, 270, 274, 341, 477, 481, 616, 639

Androgens
671

Anemia
18, 308, 319, 322, 323, 547, 571, 572, 580,
594, 605, 606, 612-614, 619, 625-628,
634, 637, 638, 693, 700, 702

Angina
100, 212, 342, 389, 413, 442, 443, 509,
615

Angiotensin converting enzyme (ACE)
inhibitors
430, 549, 571-573

Angiotensin receptor blockers
430, 573, 574

Angular stomatitis
319

Anniversary filling
153

Anovulation
539

Antacids
52, 293, 489, 492-495, 500, 576, 612, 613,
616, 626, 635

Antagonize
379, 430, 637

Ante area
101, 119

Anterior Cingulate Gyros
351

Anterior lobe
585

Anticholinergic medications
475

Anticoagulant medications
616

Antidote
103, 244, 246, 277, 281, 283, 285, 328

Antiemetics
405, 491, 492

Antigen
260-262, 266, 274, 555, 696

Anti-inflammatory agents
470, 473, 475

Antimetabolites
694

Antimicrotubules
694

Antiplatelet medications
615

Antipyretics
451

Antithrombin III
611, 616, 619, 628

Anxiety
21, 282, 303, 304, 306, 307, 318, 338, 339,
342, 343, 351, 354, 356, 366, 371-377,
382-389, 392, 394, 397, 412, 413, 457,
495, 509, 533, 537, 585, 659, 660, 684,
691, 699

Aorta
427

Aortic valve
427

Arteries
17, 427-429, 440, 442, 443, 510, 615

Arthritis
307, 308, 311, 318, 327, 341, 415-417,
482, 498, 532-534, 556, 576, 641, 646,
651, 655, 657-662, 664, 674, 683, 685,
702, 703, 705

Ascites
510-513, 520, 522

Aseptic processing
112, 119, 131

Assisted reproductive technology
540

Asthma
7, 66, 251, 336, 341, 342, 355, 391, 431,
455, 458-460, 465, 466, 469-477, 479-485,
492, 498, 616, 646, 676, 678

Astrocytes
358, 362, 514

Ataxia
410

Atherosclerosis
442

Atherosclerotic
615

Atopic dermatitis
676, 679, 685

Atria
426, 443, 615, 617, 619, 628

Atrioventricular (AV) node
428

Attention deficit hyperactivity disorder
356, 380, 387, 388, 391-393, 560

Audit
4, 47, 49-51, 62, 68, 163, 165, 169, 170,
208

Automated dispensing cabinet
98-101, 108, 289

Autonomic nervous system
400, 401, 419-421, 428

Auxiliary labels
27, 53, 289

Average wholesale price
28, 63, 81

Axon
353, 358, 361, 407

Bacterial endotoxin test
119

Balance measures
187

Band leukocytes
608

Bank Identification Number
63

Basophils
453, 454, 607-609, 627, 632, 648

B-cell
607-609, 632, 638

Beaker
88, 94

Benign prostatic hyperplasia
303, 342, 553-555, 562

Benzoyl peroxide
308, 672-674, 686

Bergmann cells
358

Beta agonists
470, 474-476, 580

Beta blocker
188, 373, 389, 413, 421, 430, 431, 433,
434, 439, 443, 481, 508-510, 527, 580

Beta receptor antagonists
430

Beyond-use date
119

Bicuspid valve
427

Bile
292, 434, 441, 489, 506-508, 522, 620,
621

Bile acid sequestrants
441

Bile canaliculi
507, 522

Bile salts
489, 507

Biliary system
292

Bilirubin
507, 508, 522, 636

Bioavailability
290, 291, 295, 296, 635

Biofeedback
556

Biological response modifiers
658, 692, 693, 696

Biological safety cabinet
119, 131, 147

Bioterrorism
244, 246, 253, 266, 337

Biotin
316, 319, 321

Bipolar disorder
354, 355, 366, 369-371, 379, 380, 383-
386, 390, 391, 394, 396, 411, 412

Bladder
18, 114, 305, 342, 407-409, 488, 526, 527,
530, 542, 554-558, 560-562, 564, 569,
656, 691, 702

Blood Brain Barrier
358

Blood-Cerebrospinal Fluid Barrier
358

Blood pressure
8, 17, 21, 40, 57, 103, 156, 270, 279, 281,
301, 303-308, 311, 322, 323, 326, 336,
339, 340, 342, 346, 356, 367, 373, 380,
388, 389, 413, 428-431, 444, 445, 453,
492, 509, 510, 512, 528, 533, 536, 555,
560, 568, 569, 571-575, 579, 586, 591,
593, 614, 615, 658, 695

Blood urea nitrogen
570

Bone metabolism
652

Bone remodeling
652

Bone resorption
652, 656

Brachytherapy
692

Bradycardia
17, 428, 430, 431

Bradykinesia
409

Brain
23, 114, 279, 280, 292, 317-319, 322, 349-
354, 356-362, 368, 369, 372, 376, 377,
381, 400-403, 405, 406, 409, 410, 419,
429, 467, 490-492, 510, 514, 520, 528,
530, 585, 587, 615, 690, 702

Brand or trade name
300

Breakthrough bleeding
539

Bronchi
466, 473

Bronchioles
466

Buccal
23, 91, 290, 418

Buffer area
119, 123, 132, 133, 136, 137

Bullae
671, 679, 680

Calcium
26, 33, 300, 302, 307, 314, 316, 317, 322-324, 327, 331, 334, 358, 406, 410, 430, 431, 438, 446, 493-495, 503, 549, 556, 569, 570, 574, 576, 577, 579, 595, 610, 612, 624, 652, 655-657, 663, 665, 666, 677, 699

Calcium channel blocker
406, 430, 431, 438, 446, 549, 556

Cancer
5, 18, 101, 131, 229, 263, 308, 316, 326, 336, 338, 341, 342, 344, 402, 411, 473, 478, 515, 528, 532, 536-538, 541, 542, 545, 548, 549, 555, 572, 589, 594, 599, 602, 608, 609, 614, 619, 632, 640, 656, 679, 683, 689-696, 698-708

Caplet
24

Capsule (Cap)
3, 6, 7, 24, 34, 44-46, 48, 57, 84, 90, 91, 101, 153, 230, 232, 240, 261, 290, 296, 306, 346, 354, 355, 383-393, 411-419, 432-437, 456-459, 479-481, 495-499, 509, 510, 515, 518, 519, 532-534, 543, 546, 555, 559-561, 568, 575-577, 595, 616-621, 624, 634-636, 640-646, 657, 660-675, 683, 684, 702-705

Capsule filling machine
90

Carbohydrate metabolism
323, 507, 522

Carbohydrates
315, 317-319, 322, 323, 330, 410, 489, 490, 492, 507, 522, 592, 593, 613

Carcinogen
690

Cardiac cycle
426-428

Cardiac muscle
401, 654

Cardiac output
428, 430, 445

Cardiac toxicity
694

Cardiovascular system
425, 426, 444

Cartilage
653, 657

Cartilaginous joints
653

Catharsis
280

CBRNE
245, 250, 255

CCR5 receptor antagonists
637

Centers for Medicare and Medicaid Services
8, 62, 65, 79, 98, 165, 170

Central-fill pharmacy
4

Central nervous system
265, 281, 282, 292, 293, 340, 343, 344, 349, 359, 368, 400, 401, 404, 410, 419, 421, 431, 454, 455, 513, 584, 636

Cerebellum
351, 352, 358

Cerebrospinal fluid
358, 585

Cervix
529, 530, 549, 585

Chemical name
27, 288, 300, 310

Chemoprevention
691

Chemotherapy
4, 74, 101, 112, 162, 229, 288, 438, 491, 492, 503, 614, 619, 689, 690, 692-701, 706-708

CHEMPACK
244, 250

Chewable
24, 158, 354, 355, 384, 388, 393, 411, 412, 416, 417, 419, 437, 454, 457-459, 476, 482, 493, 495, 496, 482, 493, 495, 496, 498, 499, 532, 534, 544, 559, 576, 623, 660, 662, 663

Chicken pox
262

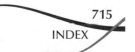

Child-resistant packaging
198, 210

Chlamydia
542, 550

Chloride (chlorine)
26, 136, 246, 305, 306, 322, 325, 331, 368, 491, 498, 576

Chromium
26, 322, 324

Chronic bronchitis
473

Chronic kidney disease
567, 568, 570-572, 574, 576, 578, 580, 613

Chronic liver disease
508, 517

Chronic obstructive pulmonary disease
473, 474, 478, 483

Chronic organ rejection
638

Chronic pain
354, 358, 367, 384, 387, 390, 399, 402, 403, 408, 412, 421

Cilia
358, 450, 456, 462, 466, 474, 638

Cirrhosis
263, 322, 505, 508, 509, 511, 512, 519, 520, 522, 523

Class I drug recall
205, 228

Class II drug recall
205, 229

Class III drug recall
205, 229

Class 100 area
121

Class 1,000 area
121

Class 10,000 area
121

Class 100,000 area
121

Clean room
108, 119, 122, 128, 129, 131-133, 136, 145, 147

Clitoris
529, 530, 549

Closed comedone
671

Closed system
117, 118, 142, 146

Coagulation
515, 521, 610, 611, 615, 620, 624-626

Cockcroft-Gault equation
292, 569

Code of ethics
213-216, 219

Cold chain
271, 273

Cold sterilization
118

Collaborative practice agreement
39, 40, 156

Collagen
319, 654, 665

Colonization
671, 672

Common bile duct
507

Complementary and alternative medicine
334, 335, 340, 342-347, 409

Complicated UTI
558

Compounded sterile products
91, 111, 112, 124, 145

Compounding
3, 6, 10-12, 38, 46, 83-87, 89, 91-94, 102, 108, 111-113, 119, 120, 122-133, 136, 137, 140, 143-145, 147, 162, 230, 246

Compounding aseptic containment isolator
119, 131, 147

Compounding aseptic isolator
120, 131, 147

Compulsions
375, 376

Computed tomography (CT) scan
350

Conjugation
292, 297

Conjunctivitis
452, 455, 459

Constipation
281, 293, 306, 317, 319, 322, 323, 336,
357, 367, 373, 378, 382, 391, 401, 403,
404, 421, 441, 490-493, 495, 497-499,
501, 514, 515, 531, 557, 591, 612, 699

Consultant pharmacist
3, 4, 151

Contamination
86, 88, 103, 112, 118, 120, 124, 131, 132,
136, 137, 147, 231, 232, 247, 248, 375,
585

Contraception
39, 525, 534-537, 541, 543, 544-546, 548

Controlled substance
39-44, 47, 52, 53, 56, 58, 71, 98, 101, 103,
107, 152, 159, 197, 205, 207-209, 211,
216, 226, 230, 338, 371, 373, 383, 404,
455, 490, 528

Controlled Substances Act
98, 200, 207, 219, 237

Cooperative buying group
225, 239

Copay
49, 50, 63, 64, 71, 76, 165, 223, 275

Copper
26, 322, 324, 326, 331, 508

Coronary arteries
442, 443

Coronary artery disease
417, 431, 438, 442, 454, 510, 536

Corpus cavernosum
526, 528

Cortex/cerebrum
351

Corticosteroids
342, 405, 408, 449, 452, 453, 456, 470,
471, 473-477, 480, 491-493, 639, 640,
658, 659, 666, 671, 677-679, 682, 685

Cosmetic
49, 200, 202, 207, 279, 344, 588, 671, 681

Cough
39, 77, 132, 207, 208, 260-262, 265, 274,
281, 308, 322, 430, 439, 445, 451-456,
459, 460-462, 469, 473, 476, 477, 479,
480, 482, 496, 556, 691

Covered entities
200

Creams
7, 24, 50, 68, 87, 89, 90, 232, 538, 541,
672, 680, 682, 695

Creatinine
292, 569, 570, 579, 638

Creatinine clearance (CrCl)
292, 569

Cretinism
323

Crew resource management
186

Critical area
120

Critical site
111, 120, 122, 124, 128, 130, 131, 133,
134, 137, 141, 143, 147

Current Procedural Terminology (CPT) codes
66

Cushing's syndrome
587, 599, 601

Cycle filling
153

Cystitis
557, 558

Cytomegalovirus
640, 642

DAW
21, 40, 42, 50, 57, 63, 64

DEA-222
226

DEA number
41, 98, 209

Decontamination
277, 279, 280, 284

Deep vein thrombosis
304, 615, 619, 620, 622, 656, 696

Dendrites
353

Deoxyribonucleic acid
28, 633, 693

Department of Health and Human Services
9, 65, 165, 200, 217, 252, 253, 314, 344,
548, 647

Depression
202, 246, 281, 282, 303-306, 317-319,
326, 339, 343, 356, 357, 366-373, 376,
379, 380, 382, 383, 385-388, 391, 393,
394, 396, 402, 403, 421, 431, 445, 454,
455, 533, 560, 660, 699

Dermis
670, 671

Desiccant
635

Desquamated
671

Diabetes mellitus
478, 531, 589, 600

Dialysis
65, 280, 284, 317, 516, 570-572, 580

Diaphragm
114, 115, 467, 506, 534, 541, 585

Diaphragm sellae
585

Diarrhea
264, 274, 280, 282, 318, 319, 322, 323,
326, 341, 367, 402, 441, 479, 487, 490,
492-495, 498, 501, 502, 510, 514, 515,
539, 591, 594, 612, 635, 638, 693, 695,
699

Diastole
427, 428

Diastolic
428, 429

Dietary Reference Intakes
315, 320, 324

Dietary supplement
39, 85, 202, 206, 207, 210, 314, 328, 329,
333, 336-338, 340, 344-347, 613, 635

Digital balance
88, 94

Diphtheria
261, 265, 266, 273, 275, 518

Direct Compounding Area
120

Dispensing process
7, 37, 44, 46, 162, 164, 165, 247, 250

Distribution
4, 86, 98, 101, 130, 150, 185, 207, 212,
214, 216, 221, 224, 230, 239, 245, 287,
289-291, 296, 297, 356, 635, 698

Diuretics
317, 326, 327, 370, 430, 431, 435-439,
511, 549, 556, 570

DMEPOS
161-165, 167-172, 234-236

Dominant follicle
531, 534

Dopamine
189, 355-357, 362, 366, 368, 369, 376-
379, 381, 385, 391, 396, 401, 409, 410,
414, 422, 492, 586, 595

Drug
2-10, 17, 19, 23-25, 27, 28, 30, 37-42, 44-54, 56-58, 62-69, 71, 73, 74, 76, 78-81, 84-86, 98-105, 107, 108, 112-114, 119, 120, 125, 128, 129, 137, 144, 145, 150-156, 159, 161, 162, 170, 176, 177, 185-190, 194, 197-200, 202-212, 217, 219, 222-232, 234-236, 238-240, 261, 263, 269-271, 278, 279, 281, 282, 287-297, 299-311, 317, 327-329, 336, 337-344, 346, 350, 354, 356-360, 366-379, 381-395, 397, 399, 402-405, 409-419, 425, 430-443, 446, 451, 453-461, 463, 465, 466, 468, 470, 474-477, 479-483, 487-503, 505, 507-510, 512-521, 525, 527, 528, 531-534, 536-540, 542-550, 553, 555-562, 564, 568-578, 585, 587, 589, 592-599, 602, 610, 612-626, 628, 631-647, 649, 656 666, 670, 672-678, 682-685, 690-698, 700-708

Drug Enforcement Administration (DEA)
8, 28, 39, 78, 98, 207, 238, 528

Drug utilization evaluations
187

Drug utilization review
28, 49, 67, 205

Dry powder inhaler
24, 468, 484

Duodenum
489

Durable medical equipment (DME), prosthetics, orthotics and supplies
161-165, 167-172, 234-236

Dysarthria
409

Dyslipidemia
439, 441, 442

Dysmenorrhea
388, 539, 550

Dyspareunia
539

Dysphagia
409

Dyspnea
473

Dysrhythmias
389, 413, 428, 432, 433, 439, 443, 509

Ectopic pregnancy
18, 531, 542

Eczema
338, 669, 670, 677, 679, 680, 686

Edema
19, 438, 482, 496, 511, 512, 529, 574, 575, 638, 639

Effervescent
24, 91, 210, 417, 437, 499, 576

Effervescent packet
91

Ejection fraction
428

Electrocardiogram
428

Electronic Mortar and Pestle
89

Elixir
24, 90, 388, 389, 392, 418, 456, 458, 459, 480, 496, 576, 577, 623, 624, 684

Embolus
615

Emergency Medical Technician
103

Emergency Prescription Assistance Program
252

Emesis
280, 284, 401, 419, 491

Emetogenic potential
699

Emphysema
431, 473

Emulsions
24, 25, 88, 90

Endocarditis
18, 608

Endocrine therapies
689, 693

Endocrinologists
584

Endocrinology
584, 585, 599

Endometriosis
525, 534, 539, 543-548, 550, 705

Endometrium
539

Endothelial cells
507, 522

Endothelium
610, 615

End-stage renal disease
65, 570, 571

Enemas
24, 514

Enteric-coated
21, 24, 616, 634

Enteric glial cells
358

Enuresis
388, 553, 554, 557, 561, 562, 564

Enzyme inhibitors
549, 694, 695

Eosinophils
454, 607-609, 627, 632, 648

Ependymocytes
358, 362

Epidermis
670, 671

Epididymis
526

Epilepsy
410, 411, 419, 420

Epistaxis
456, 656

Equianalgesic
404

Equipotent
402, 404

Erectile dysfunction
342, 525, 527, 528, 548, 550

Erythrocytes
605-607, 625, 627

Erythropoiesis
606, 700

Erythropoietin
569, 571, 572, 579, 606, 614

Esophagus
488, 489, 492-494, 509, 588, 656, 693,
699

Estrogen
210, 342, 507, 525, 529-531, 533-540,
542, 543, 546, 547, 557, 562, 564, 586,
594, 615, 656, 661, 662, 676, 690, 691,
695, 705

Exposure
10, 120, 122, 124, 145, 146, 185, 229, 231,
245-248, 250, 263, 278-281, 283, 302,
320, 353, 359, 372, 452, 455, 476, 491,
508, 520, 541, 550, 637, 647, 672, 676,
679, 680, 690, 691, 697

Extended-release
24, 280, 281, 354, 355, 373, 379, 384-389,
391, 392, 412-418, 432-437, 441, 456-459,
481, 482, 497, 498, 500, 509, 510, 515,
532, 557, 559, 560, 574-577, 621, 623,
624, 674

Extrapyramidal side effects
378

Eye insert
24

Failure mode and effect analysis
183, 193

Fallopian tubes
529, 531, 539, 549

Fasting blood glucose
590

Fats and oils
24, 315

Fat-soluble vitamins
316, 508

Federal Hazardous Substance Act
211

Federal Trade Commission
202

Fibrates
435, 436, 441

Fibrinogen
507, 611

Fibromyalgia
367, 384, 387, 402, 412, 588, 651, 655,
659, 660, 664, 666

Fibrous joints
653

Filtration
118, 131, 146, 280, 292, 568, 569, 579, 585

First air
120

First-pass effect
290, 296

Flaccid
527

Flash pulmonary edema
639

Flask
87, 94

Flat bones
652

Flatulence
441, 487, 489, 496, 514

Fluoride
322-324, 331, 588

Folic Acid (Folate)
318

Follicular phase
531

Follicular stimulating hormone
530

Food
9, 20, 38, 39, 52, 86, 100, 112, 124, 144, 151, 183, 190, 193, 197, 200, 202, 207, 226, 261, 263, 271, 288, 300, 314-316, 318-324, 326, 336, 340, 344, 345, 356, 367, 368, 375, 397, 405, 406, 451, 454, 476, 479, 487-490, 492-494, 501-503, 507, 516, 520, 538, 557, 572, 586, 591, 592, 612, 616, 617, 634-636, 640, 654, 656, 659, 664, 673, 685, 693

Food and Drug Administration
9, 86, 190, 197, 202, 226, 261, 288, 300, 336, 367, 451, 494, 501, 520, 528, 557, 617, 626, 634, 656, 659, 664, 673, 685, 693

Food, Drug, and Cosmetic Act
200, 202, 207

Forebrain
351, 356-358, 361, 372, 376, 377, 381

Formulary
64, 68, 85, 99, 156, 159, 221-223, 239, 548, 562

Formulary system
64, 221, 222

Free radicals
317, 319, 326

Frontal lobe
351

Functional incontinence
556

Functional pain
402

Gall bladder
18, 488, 656

Gamma-aminobutyric acid
356, 513

Gastric lavage
280, 284

Gastroesophageal reflux disease
492, 501

Gels
24, 89, 91, 538, 676, 682

Generalized anxiety disorder
372, 383-387, 394

Generalized seizures
410

Generic name
27, 41, 288, 299, 300, 302-310, 383-393, 407, 411-419, 446, 456-459, 480-482, 509, 510, 513, 519, 559, 561, 573, 575, 577, 619, 621, 623, 641, 643, 645, 673, 675, 677, 683, 703, 705

Geriatrics
84, 151, 562

Gestational diabetes
531, 590, 600, 602

Gigantism
586, 601

Gingival hyperplasia
639

Glands
263, 336, 371, 401, 452, 466, 488, 489, 511, 526, 529, 583-587, 599, 601, 671

Glans penis
526, 527

Glial cells
349, 353, 358, 362

Glomerular filtration rate
292, 569

Glomerulus
568

Glossitis
318, 319

Glucocorticoids
586, 587

Glucose
3, 151, 170, 180, 201, 218, 279, 322, 323, 342, 366, 507, 508, 522, 570, 586, 589-593, 602, 640

Glutamate
356, 359, 362, 377, 406, 410

Glycogen
507

Glycoprotein
345, 435, 436, 443, 613, 615, 622

Gonadotropin-releasing hormone
530, 539, 550

Gonorrhea
541, 550

Good faith effort
201, 202

Gout
307, 308, 311, 326, 336, 416, 417, 430, 441, 482, 498, 534, 576, 646, 651, 655, 659-662, 664, 666

Graduated cylinders
87

Granulocytes
607, 608, 626, 627

Group purchasing organization
207, 225

Growth hormones
586

Gynecomastia
511

Hazardous drugs
86, 119, 120, 706

Hazardous substance
211, 219, 697

Headache phase
405, 406

Health Insurance Portability and Accountability Act
61, 62, 75, 197, 200

Heart
17, 18, 19, 23, 66, 103, 114, 212, 246, 262, 282, 308, 315, 317-319, 322, 323, 326, 336, 338, 341-343, 352, 371, 373, 374, 379, 389, 401, 402, 413, 417, 425-446, 453, 454, 466, 473, 474, 477, 479, 483, 491-493, 495, 498, 499, 507-509, 512, 528, 530, 533, 537, 538, 569, 570, 572-575, 591-593, 608, 610, 615, 617, 618, 622, 623, 626, 638, 648, 654, 658, 690, 694, 697

Heart failure
66, 282, 308, 317, 319, 323, 336, 342, 413, 429-439, 443, 444, 509, 512, 533, 570, 572-575

Heat sterilization
118

Hematopoiesis
606

Hematopoietins
606

Hemodialysis
280, 284, 516, 571

Hemoglobin
590, 606, 607, 612, 614, 696, 700

Hemoglobin A1c (HbA1c)
590

Hemophilia
605, 606, 614, 620, 625, 628, 635

Hepatic encephalopathy
513, 515, 520, 521, 523

Hepatic sinusoids
506, 507

Hepatic veins
506, 507

Hepatitis
17, 263, 266, 267, 270, 273, 275, 342, 505,
508, 515-519, 521, 523, 614, 638, 642,
644, 646, 690

Hepatitis A
263, 266, 273, 342, 515-518, 523

Hepatitis B
263, 266, 267, 270, 275, 515-519, 521,
523, 642, 644, 646, 690

Hepatocytes
506, 507, 522

Herbal supplement
105, 333-338, 340, 344, 347, 563

Herpes Simplex Virus
541

High density lipoprotein
439

High-Efficiency Particulate Air
120

Highly active antiretroviral therapy
637

High-risk level CSP
125, 127

Hindbrain
351, 352, 356, 358, 361

Hippocampus
351, 352, 361

Hirsutism
529, 539, 676

Histamine
17, 356, 357, 362, 368, 402, 452-455, 461,
476, 477, 608, 679

Histamine-2 receptor antagonists
493

Histological
638

HMG-CoA reductase inhibitors
300, 440

Homeostasis
585

Homogenizer
89

Horizontal Laminar Flow Workstation
120, 121, 130

Hormone replacement therapy
525, 528, 538, 690

Hormones
91, 316, 322, 319, 323, 326, 342, 356, 357,
368, 379, 391, 499, 507, 508, 510, 525,
526, 528-531, 533-539, 542-548, 550, 555,
560, 562, 572, 583-589, 596, 598, 599,
601, 606, 646, 648, 652, 656, 661-663,
676, 690, 693, 695, 696, 705, 707

Human chorionic gonadotropin
531

Human factors engineering
180, 192, 193

Human immunodeficiency virus
519, 541, 632-646

Human papillomavirus
263, 273, 275, 541, 690

Hydrolysis
292

Hyperacute organ rejection
638

Hyperalimentation
23

Hypercholesterolemia
100, 323

Hyperinsulinemia
592

Hyperkalemia
327, 430

Hyperlipidemia
66, 316, 434-436, 439-442, 444, 621, 635

Hypersomnia
382, 383

Hypertension
21, 66, 100, 246, 281, 303, 316, 323, 327,
338, 356, 373, 381, 413, 429-440, 442-
444, 446, 454, 508-510, 520, 522, 523,
546, 555, 570-572, 591, 614, 639

Hypertensive emergency
429

Hyperthyroidism
589, 595

Hypodermis
670

Hypogonadism
525, 527, 528, 548

Hypomania
369

Hypophysis
351, 585

Hypotension
17, 281, 293, 319, 410, 430, 492, 555, 563

Hypothalamic-pituitary axis
585

Hypothalamic-pituitary-ovarian (HPO) axis
530

Hypothalamus
351, 357, 530, 531, 539, 540, 584-587, 599, 601

Hypothyroid goiter
323

Hypothyroidism
323, 391, 589, 598, 646

Hypoxia
606

Hysterectomy
538

ID-me
248, 249

Immediate-use CSP
125, 127

Immune globulin (antibodies)
632, 648

Immunoglobulins
607, 609

Immunomodulator
415, 477, 482, 519, 534, 704

Immunosuppressant
341, 638-640, 649, 682

Implantable pellets
90

Incontinence
408, 553-557, 561-564, 596

Indication
18, 64, 105, 202, 203, 206, 210, 293, 302, 303-308, 336, 354, 355, 359, 369, 377, 382-393, 411-419, 425, 432-438, 451, 456-459, 465, 480-482, 495-500, 509, 510, 512, 513, 515, 518-521, 532-534, 542-547, 559-561, 572-577, 594-598, 613, 619-625, 641-646, 660-663, 673-675, 677, 678, 680, 683, 684, 693, 697, 702-705

Infarction
18, 428, 442, 615

Infection Control Committee
99, 107

Infectious prostatitis
558

Infectious pyelonephritis
557, 558

Infectious urethritis
557

Inferior vena cava
427, 506-509

Infertility
341, 525, 528, 539, 540, 542, 547, 548, 550, 694, 699

Influenza
245, 250, 251, 260-267, 269, 270, 273, 274, 452, 465, 466, 474, 478, 479, 485, 518, 643

Infusion
4, 23, 92, 113, 155, 281, 282, 484, 510, 511, 614, 616, 639, 660, 682, 695, 696

Inhalation
23, 24, 278, 290, 450, 451, 458, 467, 475, 480-482, 518, 642, 643, 678, 697

Inhalers
24, 44

Innate immunity
632

Insomnia
281, 305, 307, 318, 338, 342, 340, 356, 367, 368, 371, 381-383, 386-388, 391, 392, 454, 457, 458, 476, 495, 496, 537, 539, 640, 684

Institute for Safe Medication Practices
20, 185, 190, 192, 193, 288, 295

Institutional Review Board
99, 107, 203

Insulin
113, 144, 189, 210, 317, 322, 342, 489,
530, 570, 586, 589, 590-593, 596, 597,
599, 602, 636

Intake process
165

Interactive voice-response (IVR) system
45, 46

Internal Revenue Service
9

Internet pharmacy
5

Intra-arterial
113, 114

Intra-articular
114

Intracardiac
23, 114

Intradermal
23, 113, 145, 146

Intramuscular
21, 23, 33, 101, 113, 145, 146, 261, 262,
268, 274, 290, 319, 379, 390, 404, 452,
538, 541, 593, 613

Intranasal
23, 261, 262, 406, 453, 454, 456, 463, 557,
564, 656, 661

Intraoseous
23, 34

Intraperitoneal
114

Intrapleural
114

Intrathecal
23, 34, 114

Intravenous
3, 21, 23, 31, 33, 34, 91, 101, 103, 113,
114, 144-146, 149, 180, 186, 278, 290,
404, 439, 443, 470, 476, 478, 483, 484,
510-514, 540, 541, 572, 593, 614, 616,
634, 682, 695, 698, 699

Intraventricular
114

Intravesicular
114

Intravitrial
114

Intrinsic renal failure
570

Investigational New Drugs
203

In vitro fertilization
540

Iodine
26, 322-324, 331, 587-589

iPLEDGE program
675

Iron
26, 33, 52, 280, 282, 284, 285, 319, 322-
324, 328, 331, 339, 340, 508, 544, 572,
576, 577, 580, 606, 612, 613, 623-627

Irregular bones
652

Ischemia
442

ISO Class 5 Area
121, 123

ISO Class 6 Area
121

ISO Class 7 Area
121

ISO Class 8 Area
121

Isthmus
587

Jaundice
263, 508, 517

The Joint Commission (TJC)
30, 98, 106, 175, 176, 187, 200, 233, 295

Joints
17, 326, 334, 614, 651-654, 657-659, 663,
665

Junction
353, 358, 361, 526, 529, 540

Just-in-time
224

Kegel exercises
556

Keratinization
671, 673

Keratolytic
673

Ketoacidosis
593, 600, 602

Ketones
593

Kidneys
280, 282, 292, 297, 316, 318, 319, 322,
323, 326, 403, 429, 430, 438, 510, 511,
554, 557, 558, 564, 568-571, 578, 579,
585, 591, 592, 593, 682

Kinase inhibitors
695

Kupffer cells
507, 522

Labia majora
529, 530

Labia minora
529, 530

Lactic acidosis
317, 319, 634

Lactulose
491, 499, 514, 515

Laminar flow
119-123, 128, 130-132, 137, 139, 142,
143, 145, 697, 708

Large intestine
488-490

Larynx
450, 462

Leukemia
411 , 609, 610, 693, 694, 696, 702-705

Leukocytes
605-609, 625-627

Leukopenia
634, 639, 640

Leukotrienes
402, 454, 465, 476

Ligaments
652, 654, 663, 665

Liniments
25

Lipase
671

Lipid metabolism
507, 522

Lipid panel
439

Lipodystrophy
596, 634, 635, 649

Liver
17, 263, 281, 282, 290-293, 297, 316-319,
322, 323, 326, 338, 339, 341, 368, 370,
403, 440, 441, 477, 478, 488, 489, 492,
502, 505-509, 511, 513-515, 517, 519-523,
570, 580, 585, 586, 592, 593, 608, 613,
634-636, 638, 639, 649, 656-658, 676,
682, 686, 687, 690, 696, 700, 704

Lollipops
90

Long bones
652

"Look-Alike, Sound-Alike" drugs
288

Lotions
25, 89, 672, 682

Low density lipoprotein
439

Low-risk level CSP
123, 124, 126, 133

Low-risk level CSP with 12-hour or less BUD
124

Lozenges
25, 452

Luteinizing hormone
530, 696

Lymphocele
640

Lymphocytes
607-609, 627, 632, 648

Lymphoma
18, 609, 690, 693, 696, 702, 703, 705

M.A.S.S.
248, 249

Macrocytic anemia
18, 605, 612, 613, 625, 627

Macro minerals
322

Magnesium
26, 30, 33, 280, 282, 322-324, 327, 331,
409, 417, 430, 491, 493, 495, 499, 586

Magnetic Resonance Image
350

Mail-order pharmacy
10, 67, 75

Malaise
318, 451, 638

Malpractice
188, 198, 199, 211, 212

Mammary glands
511, 529

Manganese
26, 33, 322-325, 513, 523

Mast cell stabilizers
449, 455, 465, 470, 476

Matrix
25, 652

Measles
260, 263, 267, 273, 275

Media fill test
122

Medicaid
7, 9, 12, 43, 49, 50, 61, 62, 65, 71, 78-81,
98, 151, 161-165, 169-171, 198, 205, 206,
219

Medical Executive Committee
99, 107

Medical team training
186, 193

Medicare
7, 9, 12, 50, 61, 62, 65, 66, 71, 76, 78-80,
98, 151, 153, 161-165, 167-172, 198, 235,
270, 275

Medicare Administrative Contractor
163, 165

Medicare Detailed Written Order
163

Medicare Part D
50, 65, 66, 71, 78, 80, 270

Medicare Prescription Drug, Improvement and
Modernization Act (MMA) of 2003
65

Medication administration record
100

Medication event reporting system
177

Medication order
4, 6-8, 23, 30, 97, 99, 149, 151, 153, 155,
158, 185

Medication profile
27, 100, 102

Medication reconciliation
105, 278

Medication therapy management services
65, 81

Medium-risk level CSP
124, 126

Medulla oblongata
352, 361

Megakaryocytes
610

Megaloblastic anemia
612, 625

Melanin
670

Meningitis
264, 265, 381

Meningococcal disease
265

Meniscus
87

Menopause
19, 334, 342, 406, 525, 537, 538, 655

Metabolism
281, 287, 289, 290, 292-297, 317-319,
322, 323, 326, 339, 507, 520, 522, 584,
586, 587, 589, 635, 636, 652

Metabolites
281, 292, 568, 635

Metastasize
690

Metered-dose inhaler
24, 465, 468, 469, 484

Microcomedone
671

Micrographia
409

Midbrain
351, 352, 358, 361

Migraines
304, 307, 308, 311, 355, 389, 405, 406,
413, 414

Migraine triggers
406

Misbranded
207

Mitosis
613

Mixed incontinence
556

Modification of Diet in Renal Disease
569

Molybdenum
322-326, 331

Monoamine oxidase inhibitors
368

Monoclonal antibodies
639, 695

Monocyte macrophages
607-609

Monocytes
609, 632

Mons pubis
529

Mortar
7, 45, 87, 89

Motility
488-491

Motor (efferent or outgoing) neurons
421

Mucositis
693-695, 699

Mucus
246, 247, 255, 263, 373, 450-453, 455,
456, 466, 470, 473, 474, 476, 489

Muller cells
358

Multiple sclerosis
341, 399, 407-409, 411, 415, 419, 420,
422, 556

Mumps
263, 267, 275

Musculoskeletal system
651, 652, 654, 655, 663

Mycobacterium avium complex infection
638

Myelin
353, 358, 362, 407

Myelosuppression
693-695

Narcolepsy
382, 383, 392, 393

Nasogastric
23

National Association of Boards of Pharmacy
66, 79, 86, 92, 213

National Coordinating Committee for
Medication Error Reporting and Prevention
178, 190, 192

National Drug Code
46, 53, 66, 226, 299, 301

National Patient Safety Goals
105, 187

National Provider Identifier
41

Nebulizers
3

Necrosis
508, 515, 682

Negative feedback loop
585

Nephrons
568, 579

Nephrotoxic agent
570

Nerves
318, 322, 351-353, 358, 361, 400, 402,
405, 526, 529, 556, 593

Nerve tracts
351, 353, 356

Nervous system
265, 281, 282, 292, 293, 317, 318, 326,
343, 344, 349, 350, 358-360, 368, 399-
402, 404, 410-416, 419-421, 428, 430,
431, 454, 455, 491, 513, 528, 542, 554,
556, 557, 584, 636, 654, 659

Neoadjuvant therapy
693, 707

Neuraminidase inhibitors
479

Neuroglia
358

Neurons
352, 353, 356-358, 362, 368, 372-374,
400, 401, 409, 410, 419, 421

Neuropathic pain
355, 373, 384, 402-404, 412

Neurotransmitters
318, 350, 354, 356-359, 366, 368, 372,
377, 385, 396, 401, 410, 419, 527

Neutropenia
609, 616, 638, 693, 700, 708

Neutrophils
607-609, 627, 632, 648

Niacin
318, 321, 327, 330, 341, 441, 445

Nociceptive pain
402

Nociceptors
402

Nodes
18, 247, 255, 353, 452, 608, 658, 692

Noninflammatory acne
671

Nonnucleoside reverse transcriptase inhibitors
636

Nonprescription
27, 28, 38, 104, 105, 108, 197, 203, 206,
210, 236, 288, 327, 329, 338, 460, 528,
531, 557, 685

Norepinephrine
356, 359, 362, 366-369, 372-374, 376,
381, 385-387, 391, 396, 401, 404, 405,
586

Nuclear pharmacy
5

Nucleoside reverse transcriptase inhibitors
631, 633, 634

Nutrient
23, 279, 313-315, 317, 322, 323, 329, 330,
358, 426, 438, 489, 502, 506, 507, 539,
568, 606, 626

Obsessions
375

Obsessive-compulsive disorder
372, 375, 394, 395

Ointment mill
89, 94

Ointments
4, 25, 50, 89, 90, 94, 154, 232, 269, 433,
458, 481, 482, 660, 674, 676-678, 680,
682, 684, 686, 695

Oligodendrocytes
358, 362

Omega-3 fatty acids
314, 337, 345

Omnibus Budget Reconciliation Act of 1990
198, 201, 205

Oncology
689, 692, 695, 698, 699, 706

On-demand filling
153

Open system
114, 115, 140

Ophthalmic
23, 25, 91, 411, 413, 414, 416, 421, 455,
458, 459, 495, 513, 559, 641, 677, 683

Opioid analgesics
399, 402-405, 658

Oral glucose tolerance test
590

Orange Book
204, 226

Orthography
188

Osteoarthritis
341, 402, 415-417, 419, 459, 482, 498,
549, 576, 646, 651, 655, 657-662, 664,
666, 684

Osteoblasts
652, 655

Osteoclasts
652, 655, 656

Osteocytes
652

Osteomalacia
317, 495, 577, 624, 634, 651, 655-657,
663, 666

Osteoporosis
18, 317, 322, 323, 346, 476, 494, 495, 533,
537, 538, 542, 543, 544, 577, 594-596,
624, 640, 651, 655-657, 659-665

Otic
23, 91, 513, 559, 677

Outcome measures
182, 186, 187

Ovaries
529-531, 534, 537, 539, 540, 584, 676

Overflow incontinence
556

Ovulation
531, 534, 537, 539, 540, 542, 543, 545,
546, 705

Ovum
526, 529, 531, 537

Oxidation
292

Oxytocin
585

Pain
12, 17, 21, 39, 42, 56, 73, 100, 155, 212,
261, 262, 274, 281, 282, 292, 303-308,
316, 318, 322, 326, 336, 341-343, 351,
354, 355, 358, 361, 366, 367, 373, 383,
384, 385, 387, 388, 390, 391, 399, 400,
402-406, 408, 410, 412, 415-421, 440-443,
445, 452, 453, 477, 479, 480, 489, 491,
492, 496, 508, 510-512, 514, 517, 528,
537, 539, 541, 542, 550, 558-560, 591-
594, 612, 614, 621 635, 637, 638, 646,
655, 657-659, 680, 687, 691, 692, 694,
696, 699

Palliation
692

Palliative therapies
693

Pancreas
323, 488, 489, 584, 589, 591, 592, 601,
638, 656

Pandemic
245, 250, 251, 253, 256, 262

Panic attacks
374

Panic disorder
372, 374, 375, 383, 385-387, 392, 394,
533, 560

Papule
671, 672

Paracentesis
511

Paralytic poliomyelitis
264

Parasomnias
382

Parasympathetic nervous system
421, 428, 554, 557

Parenteral solutions
144, 290

Paresthesia
317, 408, 635

Pareto's Law (80/20 analysis)
224, 239

Parkinson's disease
304, 306, 307, 355, 356, 362, 389, 399,
409-412, 414, 415, 419, 420, 422, 549,
556, 595

Partial seizures
410

Partial thromboplastin time
616

Pathogens
131, 607, 632, 648

Patient medication profile
27

Peak flow monitoring
472

Pellagra
318

Pellets
25, 90, 538

Penis
526-528

Peptic ulcer
487, 493, 503

Perennial
452, 463

Perfusion
280, 291

Peripheral nervous system
358, 399-422

Peripheral neuropathy
322, 326, 384, 387, 412, 634, 694, 699

Peristalsis
401, 490, 491, 502

Peritoneal dialysis
571, 580

Pertussis
260, 265, 266, 273, 275, 518, 523

Pestle
7, 45, 87, 89, 94

pH
280, 291, 492

Phagocytes
607, 608, 632

Phagocytize
608

Pharmacodynamics
287-289, 293, 295, 296

Pharmacokinetics
287-290, 295, 296

Pharmacy and Therapeutics (P&T) or Formulary
Committee
99

Pharmacy benefit manager
44, 63, 67, 81, 222

Pharmacy Compounding Accreditation Board
83, 91, 92

Pharyngitis
449, 451, 452, 460, 475

Pharynx
450, 452, 488, 489

Phase I investigational drug
203

Phase II investigational drug
203

Phase III investigational drug
203

Phase IV investigational drug
203

Phonology
188

Phosphorus
322, 335, 326, 331, 576, 652, 699

Phytoestrogens
538

Pipette
87, 94

Pituitary gland
528, 530, 539, 540, 583-588, 599, 601

Plaque
442, 615, 671, 682

Platelets
402, 507, 605, 606, 610, 615, 616, 625,
627, 696, 700, 708

Pledgets
25

Plenum
121, 122, 130, 132

Pneumococcal disease
264, 273

Pneumonia
261, 262, 264, 265, 280, 465, 466, 477-479, 483, 485, 512, 513, 559, 631, 632, 637

Poison
19, 27, 103, 200, 210, 277, 278, 281, 283, 284, 285, 381, 431, 492, 612

Poison Prevention Packaging Act
200, 210

Polymorphonuclear leukocytes
608

Pons
352

Portal hypertension
413, 508, 510, 520, 522, 523

Portal triad
507

Posterior lobe
585

Postexposure prophylaxis
637, 647

Post-renal obstruction
570

Post-synaptic neuron
354, 368

Postural hypotension
319, 555, 563

Potassium
26, 33, 210, 280, 282, 303-306, 314, 322-325, 327, 430, 437, 439, 511, 512, 559, 570, 574-577, 586, 623, 676, 699

Powders
24, 25, 87, 94, 142

Prefix
16, 17

Premonitory symptoms
405

Pre-renal failure
570, 580

Prescribe
3, 6-8, 37, 39-41, 56, 99, 206, 209, 275, 370, 442, 592, 675

Prescription
4, 6-8, 16, 20, 27, 37-58, 61-76, 78-81, 85, 86, 88, 100, 104, 105, 108, 112, 132, 150, 152, 156, 159, 162-164, 181, 188, 197-203, 205-212, 218, 219, 222, 223, 226, 231, 232, 235, 236, 251, 252, 269, 272, 275, 278, 281, 288, 299, 301, 302, 309, 313, 334-337, 339, 341, 342, 344, 345, 370, 372, 403, 406, 441, 452, 455, 460, 468, 487, 488, 491-494, 503, 531, 537, 538, 541, 542, 558, 613, 656, 672, 673, 679, 700

Pre-synaptic neuron
354

Primary Engineering Control
111, 119, 120, 122, 146

Primary hemostasis
610

Primary hypogonadism
528

Primary-progressive multiple sclerosis
408

Prime vendor agreement
225, 239

Prior authorization
5, 48, 68, 69, 74, 79, 155, 156, 223

Prior authorization request
69

Privacy Rule
197, 200-202, 217, 218

PRN
21, 42, 57, 101, 373, 396

Process measures
186, 187

Processor Control Number
63

Productive
178, 369, 455, 456, 469, 477, 547

Progesterone
525, 529-531, 534, 535, 537, 540, 546, 547, 586, 662

Progressive-relapsing multiple sclerosis
407

Prostaglandin
402, 657, 680

Prostate
305, 316, 334, 411, 526, 527, 542, 545,
554-556, 558, 559, 561, 690, 691, 693,
695, 696, 703-705

Protease inhibitors
631, 633, 635

Protected health information
76, 197, 200

Protein metabolism
322, 323, 507, 522

Proteins
291, 315, 318, 319, 441, 478, 506, 507,
514, 526, 606-608, 615, 633, 694

Prothrombin
23, 507, 515, 616

Proton pump inhibitors
494, 501, 636

Psoriasis
327, 341, 347, 532, 594, 641, 669, 670,
682, 683, 685, 687, 703

Pulmonary embolism
532, 615, 619, 620, 622, 623

Pulmonary valve
427

Pustules
671, 672

Pyrogen
118, 134

Radial glial cells
358, 362

Radiation therapy
586, 692, 693, 707

Radioactive contrast dyes
6

Rebound congestion
452, 454

Recommended Dietary Allowance
315

Rectal
23, 24, 263, 290, 383, 404, 405, 495, 514,
555, 678

Reduction
63, 89, 178, 192, 279, 292, 293, 318, 366,
376, 379, 402, 409, 430, 431, 440, 493,
515, 538, 612, 658, 659, 672, 691, 697

Relapsing-remitting multiple sclerosis
408

Renal artery
568, 579

Renal capsule
568

Renal tubule
568, 579

Renal vein
569, 579

Renin
430, 569, 574, 579, 586

Renin-angiotensin-aldosterone system
586

Resolution phase
405

Reticulocytes
606

Reticuloendothelial system
606

Reverse distributor
54, 103, 227

Reverse transcriptase
519, 631, 633, 634, 636, 642

Rhabdomyolysis
327, 441

Rheumatoid arthritis
307, 308, 311, 327, 341, 415-417, 482,
576, 641, 646, 651, 655, 657-659, 664,
674, 683, 702, 703, 705

Rhinitis
449, 451-456, 459, 460, 463, 482, 656

Rhinorrhea
19, 451

Rhinosinusitis
453

Ribonucleic acid
633

Root cause analysis
175, 181, 192, 193

Rotating the stock
226

Rubella
263, 267, 275

Rx Response
252

Saliva
401, 411, 473, 489

Salivary glands
263, 488, 498

Salvage therapy
693, 707

Satellite cells
358

Saturated fats
314, 315, 440

Schizophrenia
354, 356, 359, 362, 371, 377-382, 384,
389-391, 394-397, 411, 497, 522

Schwann cells
353, 358

Scrotum
526, 527

Scurvy
319

Sebum
671, 672, 676

Secondary Engineering Control
123, 132

Secondary hemostasis
610

Secondary hypogonadism
528

Secondary progressive Multiple Sclerosis
408

Segregated Compounding Area
123, 124, 126, 133

Selective estrogen receptor modulators
538, 691

Selective serotonin reuptake inhibitors
366, 405, 406

Selenium
322, 325, 326, 331

Sella turcica
58

Semen
526, 529

Semi-closed system
116

Seminal vesicle
526, 527

Sensory (afferent or incoming) neurons
401, 421

Sentinel event
187, 193

Sepsis
264, 265, 510, 512, 558

Serotonin
343, 354, 356, 357, 366-368, 372, 373,
374, 376, 378, 385-387, 395, 396, 402,
404-406, 491, 492, 496, 497, 499, 533,
699

Serotonin/norepinephrine reuptake inhibitors
367

Sexually transmitted diseases
540, 547, 548

Short bones
652

Sickle cell anemia
605, 612, 614, 625, 628, 702

Side effect
293, 297, 339, 366-368, 370, 378, 379,
403, 405, 430, 441, 445, 475, 476, 492,
494, 539, 555, 563, 591, 614, 616, 634,
640, 682, 686, 693-695, 699, 700, 708

Sinoatrial (SA) node
428

Sinuses
450, 453, 462

Sinusitis
449-451, 453, 460, 463

Six Sigma method
188

Skeletal muscle
247, 255, 352, 401, 441, 654, 655

Sleep apnea
382, 392, 429, 591

Small intestine
290, 292, 297, 317, 488, 489, 507, 508, 613, 616

Smooth muscle
403, 453, 466, 470, 474-476, 555, 556, 654

SNS Pushpack
249

Sodium
24, 26, 136, 280, 304, 306, 307, 314, 322, 325, 326, 354, 384, 406, 410, 411, 438, 491, 499, 500, 503, 510, 511, 576, 577, 586, 595, 598, 623, 624, 658, 661, 673

Soluble mediators
632

Solutions
25, 31, 67, 68, 79, 84, 91, 92, 101, 112, 114, 118, 142, 144, 280, 290, 474, 694

Somatic
375, 400-402, 419, 421

Somatic nervous system
400, 401, 419, 421

Somatotropes
586

Spacer
468, 469

Spasticity
407-409

Sperm
526, 528, 529, 531, 534, 540

Sphincter muscle
554, 556

Spinal cord
23, 114, 319, 351, 352, 401-403, 419

Spirometry
472

Spontaneous bacterial peritonitis
512, 513, 520, 522, 523

Sprays
25, 42, 44, 154, 405, 407, 454, 682

Stable angina
442, 443

Stat
22, 98, 100, 101, 107, 150, 155, 159, 307, 355, 389, 414, 698

Statin
300, 440, 621

Step therapy
74, 79, 155, 156

Sterile
24, 85, 86, 89, 91, 93, 101, 108, 111-113, 118-121, 123-127, 130, 133, 134, 137, 139, 140-145, 155

Sterile products
91, 111, 112, 119, 123-127, 134, 137, 145

Sterilize
27, 118

Steven-Johnson's syndrome
675

Stomach
18, 23, 24, 52, 100, 261, 263, 279, 280, 290, 293, 321, 322, 326, 341-343, 354, 402, 441, 455, 476, 488, 489, 492, 493, 506, 509, 539, 572, 615-617, 634, 636, 640, 658, 666, 704

Strategic National Stockpile
249

Stress incontinence
556, 557, 564

Striated
654

Stroke volume
428

Structural name
288, 300, 310

Subcutaneous
22, 23, 25, 113, 145, 146, 268, 290, 404, 477, 510, 613, 614, 616, 656

Sublingual
19, 22, 25, 31, 34, 100, 210, 290, 380, 390, 413, 436, 443, 500, 624

Suffix
17

Superior vena cava
427

Supplemental New Drug
203

Suppositories
3, 7, 11, 25, 91, 232, 405, 490, 541

Suspensions
3, 6, 24, 25, 87-90, 232, 493

Swiss Cheese Model of System Accidents
179

Sympathetic nervous system
401, 419, 421, 428, 430, 431

Sympathomimetics
454

Synapse
353, 354, 357, 361, 366, 372, 419

Synaptic cleft
368

Synergistic effect
294

Synergistic response
27

Synovial joint
653, 657, 665

Syphilis
541, 550

Syrup
25, 39, 280, 284, 354, 384, 388, 392, 411,
455-549, 480-482, 496, 498, 542, 560,
576, 623, 646, 684

Systemic autoimmune disorder
658

Systemic disease
658

Systems approach
177

Systole
427, 428

Systolic
428, 429

Tablets
3, 6, 7, 21, 24, 25, 40, 42, 44, 45, 46, 48,
50, 52, 53, 57, 75, 84, 87, 100, 101, 152,
153, 155, 210, 225, 228, 230, 231, 232,
240, 280, 282, 290, 301, 304, 306, 354,
355, 379, 380, 383-393, 403, 406, 407,
411-419, 421, 432-438, 442, 443, 454,
456-459, 474, 476, 477, 480-482, 493,
495-500, 509, 510, 512, 513, 515, 518,
519, 532-537, 542-547, 555, 559, 560,
572-576, 587, 594-598, 612, 613, 620-625,
640-646, 660-663, 674, 675, 683, 684,
702-705

Tachycardia
19, 319, 338, 356, 357, 367, 373, 382, 428,
431, 443, 445, 474, 477, 492

Tamper-resistant packaging
197, 210

Tardive dyskinesia
378, 395

T-cell
607-609, 632, 638-640, 682, 683

Tendon
319, 513, 654, 663, 665

Testes
526, 528, 584

Testosterone
308, 406, 525, 527-530, 534, 546, 547,
550, 586, 594

Tetanus
261, 265, 266, 275, 518

Thalamus
351, 357

Theophylline
294, 343, 355, 391, 470, 471, 473, 476,
477, 484, 494, 537

Therapeutic substitution
156, 159, 222

Therapeutic window
294

Thrombocythemia
610

Thrombocytopenia
610, 616, 619, 620, 634, 639, 693, 700

Thrombolytics
437, 443, 615, 616, 618, 625

Thrombopoietin
610

Thrombosis
304, 532, 614, 615, 619, 620, 622, 656, 696

Thrombotic thrombocytopenic purpura
610, 616

Thrush
475

Thyroidectomy
588, 589

Thyroid gland
323, 584, 587-589, 599, 601

Thyroid goiter
323, 588

Thyroid hormone
323, 326, 368, 507, 587-589, 598, 652

Tincture
25, 490

Tolerable Upper Intake Level
315

Topical
3, 23-25, 50, 51, 102, 112, 152, 308, 387, 411, 415, 452, 454-456, 541, 542, 560, 646, 657, 658, 672-680, 682, 685, 686, 695, 702

Topical antibiotic
672, 673, 679, 680, 686

Topical retinoid
672, 673, 682

Torsion balance
46, 87, 88

Toxicities
284, 293, 294, 317-319, 431, 476, 493, 514, 639

Toxicity
27, 261, 281, 282, 284, 285, 293, 294, 316-319, 322, 323, 326, 237, 341, 370, 381, 439, 441, 461, 477, 493, 514, 639

Toxin
27, 91, 103, 247, 255, 265, 280, 281, 318, 409, 490, 508, 571

Trace mineral
322

Trachea
466, 587, 588

Transdermal
23, 25, 91, 290, 303, 403, 404, 421, 443, 538, 555, 557

Transient ischemic attack
615

Transurethral microwave thermotherapy
555

Transurethral needle ablation
555

Transurethral resection of the prostate
555

Trichomoniasis
542, 550

Tricyclic antidepressants
293, 367, 405, 406, 408, 409

Trigeminal nerve
405

Troche
25, 91

Tumor
18, 490, 586, 587, 682, 690, 692-694, 696, 699

Turbinates
450, 462

Type 1 diabetes
589, 592, 593, 602

Type 2 diabetes
589, 590, 592, 600, 602

Uncomplicated UTI
558

Unit-dose
77, 101, 153, 154, 210, 231-233

United States Pharmacopeia
28, 83, 85, 92, 93, 112, 145, 178, 190

Unit-of-use
101, 231-233, 240

Unstable angina
442, 615

Upper parietal lobe
351

Ureters
554

Urethra
25, 526-528, 530, 541, 549, 554-557, 561

Urge incontinence
556

Urinary tract infection (UTI)
339, 407, 531, 553, 554-557, 562

Usual and customary price
69

Uterus
18, 529-531, 534, 537, 538, 540, 549

Vaccine Information Statement (VIS)
269

Vagina
22-25, 529, 530, 549, 557, 585

Vaginal
23, 25, 533-535, 537-539, 541-544, 546, 556, 661, 675

Vaginal candidiasis
541

Validation
123, 137, 165

Varice
508-510, 513, 520-522, 594

Varicella
261, 262, 268, 275, 641

Vasculature
427, 454

Vas deferens
526, 527, 549

Vasodilator
431, 437-439, 547

Vasomotor symptom
537

Vasopressin
510, 585, 586, 598

Vein
19, 21, 23, 144, 176, 279, 290, 304, 427, 506-508, 532, 569, 579, 615, 619, 620, 622, 656, 696, 699

Velometer
132

Ventricles
358, 426

Vertical Laminar Flow Workbench
119, 122, 123, 130

Viron
633

Visceral
402, 491, 506

Vital signs
3, 249, 279

Vitamin
21, 72, 105, 144, 202, 279, 313-331, 334, 336, 343, 345, 409, 441, 451, 494, 500, 508, 515, 532, 547, 569, 577, 606, 611-613, 617, 620, 624, 625, 627, 652, 655-657, 663, 665, 666, 670, 682, 691, 708

Vitamin A
316, 320, 327, 330, 331, 336, 409

Vitamin B_1
279, 317

Vitamin B_2
317, 318

Vitamin B_3
318, 441

Vitamin B_5
318

Vitamin B_6
318, 327, 627

Vitamin B_{12}
319, 500, 508, 606, 612, 613, 624, 625, 627, 708

Vitamin C
316, 319, 330, 334, 345, 451, 612, 627, 666

Vitamin D
314, 316, 317, 320, 329-331, 334, 409, 494, 508, 569, 577, 624, 656, 657, 663, 665, 666, 682

Vitamin E
317, 327, 331

Vitamin K_1
317, 327

Vulva

529, 549

Warfarin

153, 155, 194, 285, 304, 317, 328, 330, 341-343, 403, 490, 494, 532, 611, 617, 620, 624, 625, 628

Water soluble

290, 292, 297, 316, 317, 409, 500, 547, 624, 625

Water-soluble vitamins

316, 317, 409

Wholesale acquisition cost

69

Wholesaler

3, 6, 46, 63, 69, 81, 86, 223-226, 228, 239, 240, 249

Wilson's disease

322

Word root

17

Zinc

26, 322, 325, 326, 334, 451, 513, 514, 523, 681

Zona fasiculta

586

Zona glomerulosa

586

Zona reticularis

586